JOHN CAMPBELL
DAVID FOSKETT
NEIL RIPPINGTON
PATRICIA PASKINS

PRACTICAL COOKERY

FOR THE LEVEL 2 VRQ DIPLOMA

With contributions from Olly Rouse, Chris Barker and Stephanie Conway

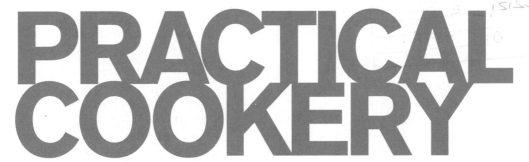
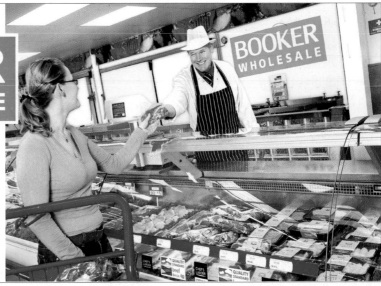
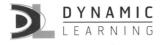
DYNAMIC LEARNING

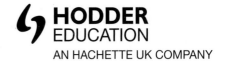
HODDER EDUCATION
AN HACHETTE UK COMPANY

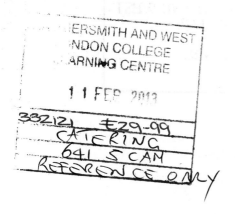
Orders: please contact Bookpoint Ltd, 130 Milton Park, Abingdon, Oxon OX14 4SB. Telephone: (44) 01235 827720. Fax: (44) 01235 400454. Lines are open from 9.00 to 5.00, Monday to Saturday, with a 24-hour message answering service. You can also order through our website www.hoddereducation.co.uk.

If you have any comments to make about this, or any of our other titles, please send them to educationenquiries@hodder.co.uk

British Library Cataloguing in Publication Data
A catalogue record for this title is available from the British Library

ISBN: 978 1444 17911 8

First edition published 2010 as Practical Cookery Level 2
This edition published 2012
Impression number   10 9 8 7 6 5 4 3 2 1
Year   2016, 2015, 2014, 2013, 2012

Copyright © 2010 John Campbell, David Foskett, Neil Rippington, Victor Ceserani

Hachette UK's policy is to use papers that are natural, renewable and recyclable products and made from wood grown in sustainable forests. The logging and manufacturing processes are expected to conform to the environmental regulations of the country of origin.

Typeset by Fakenham Prepress Solutions, Fakenham, Norfolk NR21 8NN
Printed in Italy for Hodder Education, an Hachette UK Company, 338 Euston Road, London NW1 3BH

Contents

Preface   vi
Introduction   vii
Acknowledgements   ix
Reasons to come to Booker   xii

Chapter 1 **Investigate the catering and hospitality industry**   **1**

The structure of the catering and hospitality industry   1
The UK hospitality industry   3
Product and service   6
Types of establishment   8
Food provision in the leisure industry   11
Travel   14
Public sector catering (secondary service sector)   16
Catering for business and industry   18
The contract food service sector   19
Franchising   20
Employment in the hospitality industry   21

Chapter 2 **Food safety**   **28**

The importance of food safety   28
Bacteria and contamination   30
Personal hygiene   32
Cross-contamination   33
The importance of temperature   36
Food deliveries and storage   37
Cleaning   40
Pests   43
Premises   44
Food safety management systems   45

Chapter 3 **Health and safety in catering and hospitality**   **51**

Working safely   51
Bullying and harassment   52
Injuries, accidents and disease   53
Control of substances hazardous to health   54
Identifying hazards and avoiding accidents   55
Safety in the workplace   57
Fire safety   63
Security in catering   65
Personal safety   67

Chapter 4 **Healthier foods and special diets**   **69**

Why healthy eating is important   69
A balanced diet   70
Carbohydrates   71
Protein   73
Fats   74
Vitamins   76
Minerals   78

Water		80
Healthy eating		80
Special diets		83
The chef's role – good practice		85
Chapter 5	**Catering operations, costs and menu planning**	**87**
The organisation of the kitchen		87
Staffing hierarchy and good working relationships		89
Planning a kitchen		91
Kitchen design		95
Planning and preparing menus for catering operations		99
Food purchasing		105
Portion control – controlling waste and costs		108
Cost control		110
Chapter 6	**Applying workplace skills**	**117**
Professional presentation		117
Workplace skills		118
Applying for a job		122
Personal development plans		124
Chapter 7	**Methods of cookery**	**128**
Cooking methods		128
Applying heat to food		128
The effect of cooking on food		129
Boiling, poaching and steaming		130
Stewing/casseroling and braising		134
Baking and roasting		137
Grilling and barbecuing		141
Shallow and deep frying		142
Other methods of cooking		147
Chapter 8	**Prepare and cook stocks, soups and sauces**	**153**
Health, safety and hygiene		154
Stocks		155
Soups		155
Sauces		156
Stock, soup and sauce recipes		158
Chapter 9	**Prepare and cook fruit and vegetables**	**203**
Fruit		204
Vegetables		205
Potatoes		208
Pulses		212
The vegetarian diet		215
Fruit and vegetable recipes		218
Chapter 10	**Prepare and cook meat and offal**	**267**
Meats		268
Lamb and mutton		274
Beef		279
Veal		283
Pork and bacon		287
Meat and offal recipes		291

Chapter 11 Prepare and cook poultry   340

Poultry   340
Turkey   344
Duck, duckling, goose, gosling   345
Poultry recipes   346

Chapter 12 Prepare and cook fish and shellfish   362

Fish   363
Shellfish   376
Fish and shellfish recipes   381

Chapter 13 Prepare and cook rice, pasta, grains and egg dishes 412

Rice   413
Pasta   414
Grains   417
Eggs   419
Rice, pasta, grain and egg recipes   421

Chapter 14 Produce hot and cold desserts and puddings 446

Ingredients used in the pastry kitchen   447
Healthy eating and puddings and desserts   454
Egg custard-based desserts   455
Ice creams and sorbets   458
Fruit-based recipes   461
Dessert and pudding recipes   462

Chapter 15 Produce paste products   498

Techniques   499
Paste product recipes   500

Chapter 16 Produce biscuits, cake and sponge products 521

Cake mixtures   521
Biscuit mixtures   526
Decorating and finishing for presentation   527
Biscuit, cake and sponge product recipes   529

Chapter 17 Produce fermented dough products   541

Dough products   541
Dough product recipes   545

Appendix: Savouries, hors d'oeuvre and canapés   560
Glossary   571
Index   575

Preface

When David Foskett and Victor Ceserani invited me to join their writing team several years ago I jumped at the opportunity. Education has shaped the person I am today – through college and higher education where my skills were developed and nurtured by some inspirational teachers, and through the day-to-day contact I have with my staff and professional peers who continually help me to develop and refine my knowledge and skills in the profession I love.

At the heart of *Practical Cookery* is a strong partnership with industry. This close connection ensures that the book reflects modern practice and will effectively help prepare you for your career. It will also continue to support you long after your career has started, so keep it close to hand!

This book has been the product of a huge amount of work both by the authors and the supporting team. I hope it makes the theoretical parts of the course understandable and the practical elements truly inspiring. To play a part in helping to shape the education of students using this book is a privilege. It provides me with an opportunity to give something back in return for the education I have been lucky enough to receive. My hope is that this book will help motivate you to succeed in your studies and go on to have a rewarding and fulfilling career. We think it represents the best we can give you.

Good luck!

John Campbell

Introduction

This book has been written to cover everything you need for the Level 2 Diploma in Professional Cookery course. It is also a great resource for catering students on other courses, and for anyone training in a hospitality and catering workplace. The purpose of the book is to give you a good foundation for a career in professional cookery.

The key outcomes of this course are:

- To behave in a professional way, with a good attitude, smart appearance and all the necessary skills
- To learn about food commodities, their costs and quality points, and how to use them
- To be able to use recipes to prepare, cook and serve dishes of good quality, with good presentation
- As you gain more experience, to start developing your own original recipe ideas
- To understand the principles of healthy eating and basic nutrition
- To carry out healthy, hygienic and safe procedures at all times when storing, preparing, cooking and serving food, and understand why this is essential.

In Chapters 8 to 17 you will find a large selection of recipes including basic dishes, many classical dishes that have their origins in the traditional French kitchen, international recipes, and 'eclectic' cuisine – dishes in which influences from around the world are mixed together.

Nutritional analysis

There is no such thing as unhealthy food, but eating in an unhealthy way may lead to obesity, ill health and even early death. Obesity is increasing in the UK, especially among young people.

Nutritional data is provided for some of the recipes in this book, to help you make informed choices about what to cook and eat.

The recipes were analysed by Jenny Arthur, nutrition consultant, Dr Jenny Poulter, Jane Cliff and Pat Bacon. Jenny Poulter and Jane Cliff provided the following information about the nutritional analysis.

The analysis was performed using the computer software CompEat Pro version 5.8.0 (2002). This holds the UK integrated databases of McCance and Widdowson's *The Composition of Foods, 6th Summary Edition* and associated supplements (RSC).

Weights and measures were used as given in the recipe; if the recipe gave a number of items (e.g. 1 egg), exact data was taken from *Food Portion Sizes, 3rd Edition* (Defra).

Sometimes the waste produced during preparation would have distorted the nutritional data, for example where a whole chicken was prepared but only the leg and wing quarters were used. In these cases, only the edible portion of the ingredient was included.

Except where stated:

- The oil used was vegetable oil
- Butter was used, instead of margarine
- The milk used was semi-skimmed.

How to use this book

To help make sure that you develop all the practical skills you need for your course, each recipe has icons showing which method(s) of cookery it uses. So if you want to practise shallow frying, look for that icon. The icons look like this:

 Boiling

 Stewing or casseroling

 Roasting

 Steaming

 Grilling

 Shallow frying

 Poaching

 Baking

 Deep frying

Some of the photos show garnishes and presentations that are not mentioned in the recipe. This is intended to be a source of inspiration and ideas.

There are free videos on the website. Look out for the QR codes throughout the book. They look like this.

Principles of poaching
http://bit.ly/wutwTE

To use the QR codes to view the videos you will need a QR code reader for your smartphone/tablet. There are many free readers available, depending on the smartphone/tablet you are using. We have supplied some suggestions below, but this is not an exhaustive list and you should only download software compatible with your device and operating system. We do not endorse any of the third-party products listed below and downloading them is at your own risk.

- for iPhone/iPad, Qrafter – http://itunes.apple.com/app/qrafter-qr-code-reader-generator/id416098700

- for Android, QR Droid – https://market.android.com/details?id=la.droid.qr&hl=en

- for Blackberry, QR Scanner Pro – http://appworld.blackberry.com/webstore/content/13962

- for Windows/Symbian, Upcode – http://www.upc.fi/en/upcode/download/

Once you have downloaded a QR code reader, simply open the reader app and use it to take a photo of the code. The video will then load on your smartphone/tablet.

If you cannot read the QR code or you are using a computer, the web link next to the code will take you directly to the same video.

The terms and conditions which govern these free online resources may be seen at http://bit.ly/yfVC0P

Even more digital resources are available to centres that purchase Practical Cookery Level 2 VRQ Dynamic Learning – see the inside front cover for more information.

About the diploma

If you are a student taking the VRQ Level 2 Diploma in Professional Cookery you will find that the book has been carefully structured around the requirements of the course. Each chapter covers one unit of your course.

The units on preparing, cooking and producing dishes are assessed by practical tests. In this book, recipes marked **Assessment** are suitable for use in City and Guilds practical tests (at the time of writing). Always check the requirements of the test carefully. Other awarding bodies have different requirements for practical tests; the wide variety of recipes in this book means that you can find suitable recipes for most tests here.

Please note that Chapter 7, Methods of cookery, is not a unit of the qualification. It is designed to help you understand the key methods of cooking and develop the practical skills that underpin this course.

Acknowledgements

We are most grateful to the following for their assistance in preparing this book:

Booker PLC, in particular Ron Hickey and Niall Brannigan, for their support in the development of the book, including the provision of all the food shown in the photographs in Chapters 14 to 17.

Jenny Arthur, nutrition consultant, Dr Jenny Poulter, Jane Cliff and Pat Bacon for their nutritional analysis of some of the recipes included in this book.

Iain Middleton, Steve Thorpe and Stephen Stackhouse for their advice and input.

The staff at Coworth Park, part of the Dorchester Collection, especially Peter Eaton.

Russums Catering Clothing and Equipment for supplying some of the photographs.

Compass Group UK for supplying some of the photographs.

Alexia Chan, Deborah Edwards Noble, Colin Goodlad, Neil Fozzard and Melissa Brunelli at Hodder Education, and Rick Jackman, Alison Walters, Jo Kemp and Lynn Brown.

Photography

Most of the photos in this book are by Andrew Callaghan of Callaghan Studios. The photography work could not have been done without the help of the authors and their colleagues and students at Thames Valley University (TVU, now the University of West London) and Colchester Institute. The publishers would particularly like to acknowledge the following people for their work.

John Campbell and Olly Rouse organised the photography at TVU. They were assisted in the kitchen by:

- James Breslin
- Kate Carrington
- Juan Sanchez Chavez
- Axel Herve
- Sergei Kuzmin
- Andrew Lewis
- Samantha Oliver Munt
- Tony Rose
- Jack Shaw
- Daniel Waldock

- Jamie Woodstock

and also by Professor David Foskett and the TVU staff.

Neil Rippington, Chris Barker and Stephanie Conway organised the photography at Colchester Institute. They were assisted in the kitchen by:

- Roddy Isbister
- Chariz de Leon

- Amy McCormick
- Richard Mitchell
- Daniel Pitts
- Thomas Smith.

The authors and publishers are grateful to everyone involved for their hard work, without which this book would be much poorer.

About the contributors

Olly Rouse is Head Chef of Restaurant John Campbell at The Dorchester Collection's Coworth Park, Surrey. Formerly sous chef at the two Michelin starred restaurant The Vineyard at Stockcross, Olly consults internationally on the modern use of cooking techniques including sous vide.

Stephanie Conway has worked in some of the finest country house hotels including Rhinefield House Hotel under Richard Bertinet. After a stint at the White Barn Inn in Maine USA, Stephanie worked at London's Royal Garden Hotel under Nick Hollands, later becoming Chef

Patissier at the London Marriott County Hall. Stephanie is currently employed as a chef lecturer at Colchester Institute, teaching patisserie.

Chris Barker completed his apprenticeship with Trust House Forte before working at The Intercontinental Hotel, London in the pastry section under Michael Nadell. He then moved to The Ritz Hotel as Chef Patissier. As well as teaching patisserie at Colchester Institute, Chris is currently Curriculum Manager with responsibility for part-time and Level 3 full-time chefs' programmes.

Picture credits

Every effort has been made to trace the copyright holders of material reproduced here. The authors and publishers would like to thank the following for permission to reproduce copyright illustrations:

p.4 © Stockbyte/Getty Images; p.8 © Bananastock/Photolibrary Group Ltd/Getty Images; p.10 © Ingram Publishing Limited; p.11 © Photodisc/Getty Images; p.12 © Clover/Amana Images/Photolibrary; p.13 © Andrew Ward/Life File/Photodisc/Getty Images; p.14 © Photodisc/ Getty Images; pp.17–19 Compass; p.26 Booker; p.29 (bottom) Oxford Designers and Illustrators; p.31 by Eric Erbe (digital colorization by Christopher Pooley/material produced by ARS is in the public domain); p.34 (right) Russums; p.35 Sam Bailey/Hodder Education; p.36 Russums;

p.38 Sam Bailey/Hodder Education; p.42 Booker; p.43 © Bananastock/Photolibrary Group Ltd/Getty Images; p.47 Booker; p.54 Barking Dog Art; p.56 © Royalty-Free/Corbis; p.57 © Bananastock/Photolibrary Group Ltd/Getty Images; p.60 © Thomas Perkins/iStockphoto. com; p.61 © Bananastock/Photolibrary Group Ltd/Getty Images; pp.62–3 Barking Dog Art; p.66 © xyno/istockphoto.com; p.71 © ranplett/ iStockphoto.com; p.72 © eyewave/Alamy; p.73 (top left, bottom) Barking Dog Art; p.74 © Photolibrary.com; p.75 (top) Barking Dog Art; p.77 (top) © Ingram Publishing Limited; pp.77 (bottom), 78 Barking Dog Art; pp.79–81 Sam Bailey/ Hodder Education; p.83 © Ingram Publishing Limited; p.85 Sam Bailey/Hodder Education; p.88 © Bananastock/Photolibrary Group Ltd/

Getty Images; pp.94–7 Sam Bailey/Hodder Education; p.101 © Bananastock/Photolibrary Group Ltd/Getty Images; p.104 © iStockphoto.com; pp.111–14 Sam Bailey/Hodder Education; p.115 Booker; p.117 Compass; p.118 Barking Dog Art; p.119 © Bananastock/Photolibrary Group Ltd/Getty Images; p.120 Sam Bailey/Hodder Education; pp.121–4 © Bananastock/Photolibrary Group Ltd/Getty Images; pp.132, 133 (left) Sarah Bailey/Hodder Education; p.133 (right) Sam Bailey/Hodder Education; p.139 © Ingram Publishing Limited; p.142 Sam Bailey/Hodder Education; pp.144, 148 (left) Sarah Bailey/Hodder Education; p.148 (right) Sam Bailey/Hodder Education; p.150 Compass; p.167 (bottom) Sam Bailey/Hodder Education; p.188 Sarah Bailey/Hodder Education; p.208 Sam Bailey/Hodder Education; p.210 Potato Council; pp.214, 219, 220 (top), 221, 227, 230 (top), 245 (bottom), 250 (bottom), 256 (bottom), 258–9, 266 Sam Bailey/Hodder Education; p.277 (left and top) Meat and Livestock Commission; pp.277 (bottom), 278 Sam Bailey/Hodder Education; pp.281, 284 (top), 288, 289 (top) Meat and Livestock Commission; p.297 (top) Sarah Bailey/Hodder Education; p.317 Sam Bailey/Hodder Education; pp.345, 347, 350 (bottom), 355, 358 (bottom) Sam Bailey/Hodder Education; p.369 Adrian Moss; p.370 (top) Sam Bailey/Hodder Education; p.371 Sam Bailey/Hodder Education; p.372 (top, bottom) Sam Bailey/Hodder Education, (middle) Adrian Moss; pp.381 (middle), 386 (top), 387 (bottom), 395, 402, 416, 427, 429, 432 (top), 443 (bottom), 452–7 Sam Bailey/Hodder Education; pp.494 (top), 511, 519, 539 (top), 540 (bottom) Sam Bailey/Hodder Education; p.543 (right) Booker; pp.548 (bottom), 561, 564 (left), 568 Sam Bailey/Hodder Education.

Except where stated above, photographs are by Andrew Callaghan, and illustrations by Richard Morris. Cookery icons designed by Art Construction. Crown copyright material is reproduced with the permission of the Controller of HMSO and the Queen's Printer for Scotland.

Figures in Table 1.1 produced by Horizons for *British Hospitality: Trends and Developments*, published by the British Hospitality Association. Table 4.2 reproduced from Fox and Cameron's *Food Science, Nutrition and Health*, 7th edition (Michael E. J. Lean, Hodder Arnold, 2006).

Metric and Imperial units

Weights and measures in this book are given in metric units. You can use the tables on the inside of the back cover to convert to Imperial units.

Reasons to come to Booker
the UK's biggest wholesaler
To find your nearest branch visit www.booker.co.uk

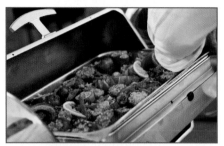

choice up

Huge range
The average branch carries over 10,000 lines in stock the whole time, with even more available to order.

New Lines
Our expert buyers are constantly sourcing great new lines for you. Look for the 'New Line shelf' cards in branch, every week.

prices down

Catering Price check
Our catering price check service allows you to enter your current Brakes or 3663 prices and, with one click, instantly see if you can buy cheaper from Booker. Why not compare our prices for yourself by visiting www.booker.co.uk today!

Essentials - every day low price
We have lock down prices on a range of products that are essential to your business. From bread, milk, eggs and potatoes through to sugar, tuna, chips and peas we will give you a low price, every day to help you plan your menu and your budget.

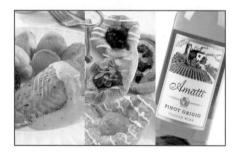

better service

Internet ordering
The easiest way to place your order with your branch is via our website. Simply log on to www.booker.co.uk, and register for online ordering. Its so simple - start today!

Free, 7 days a week, delivery service*
All your fresh produce, frozen, wet and dry goods delivered to your door on the one vehicle - 7 days a week.

*Terms and conditions apply - see in branch for details.

1 Investigate the catering and hospitality industry

In this chapter you will learn how to:

1. understand the hospitality and catering industry including:
- the features and operations of different establishments
- the structure, size, importance, influences on, and development of the industry

2. understand the national and international employment opportunities available in the hospitality and catering industry including:
- the main job roles and differences between them within the hospitality and catering industry
- the legal requirements to work within the law
- the functions of professional associations.

The structure of the catering and hospitality industry

The word 'hospitality' encompasses all aspects of the hotel and catering industry. It is a relatively modern word, meaning the friendly and generous treatment of guests and strangers. The word 'catering' refers to offering facilities to people, especially the provision of food.

Wherever there are groups of people there is likely to be some kind of hospitality provision, in other words, somewhere where people can get food, drink and accommodation.

The hospitality industry in Britain employs around 1.7 million people and is growing all the time. It provides excellent opportunities for training, employment and progression.

Hotels, restaurants, bars, pubs and clubs are all part of what is known as the **commercial sector**. Businesses in the commercial sector need to make a profit so that they can survive.

Catering provided in places like hospitals, schools, colleges, prisons and the armed services also provides thousands of meals each day. This sort of catering is part of what is known as the **public sector** (also known as the secondary service sector). Businesses in the public sector do not need to make a profit, but these days many catering services in the public sector are run by profit-making contract caterers (described later in this chapter).

The **service sector** usually refers to the contract catering market, now sometimes referred to as the **'primary service sector'**. This includes hospitality in banks, insurance companies, law firms and large corporate businesses.

Traditionally the public service sector was known as the 'non-profit making sector', as it was run by the public sector, catering for establishments like schools, college refectories, hospitals and prisons. As a large percentage of it is now run by commercial companies like Compass and Sodexo, for a profit, this sector now is referred to as 'cost sector catering' or the **'secondary service sector'**.

The three main types of business

The industry can be divided into three main types of business: SMEs, public limited companies and private companies.

Small to medium-sized business enterprises (SMEs)

These have up to 250 employees. In the UK as a whole, SMEs account for over half of all employment (58.7 per cent). These are usually private companies that may become public limited companies if they become very large.

Public limited companies and private companies

The key difference between public and private companies is that a public company can sell its shares to the public, while private companies cannot. A share is a certificate representing one unit of ownership in a company, so the more shares a person has the more of the company they own.

Before it can start in business or borrow money, a public company must prove to Companies House (the department where all companies in the UK must be registered) that at least £50,000 worth of shares have been issued and that each share has been paid up to at least a quarter of its nominal value (so 25 per cent of £50,000). It will then receive authorisation to start business and borrow money.

Other types of business

The types of business in the catering and hospitality industry can also be divided into sole traders, self-employed, partnership and limited liability companies. These are usually private companies.

Sole trader

A sole trader is the simplest form of setting up and running a business. It is suited to the smallest of businesses. The sole trader owns the business, takes all the risks, is liable for any losses and keeps any profits. The advantage of operating in business as a sole trader are that very little formality is needed. The only official records required are those for HM Revenue and Customs (HMRC), National Insurance and VAT. The accounts are not available to the public.

Self-employed

There is no precise definition of self-employment, although guidance is offered by HMRC.

In order to determine whether an individual is truly self-employed, the whole circumstances of his or her work need to be considered. This may include whether he or she:

- is in control of their own time, the amount of work they take on and the decision making
- has no guarantee of regular work
- receives no pay for periods of holiday or sickness
- is responsible for all the risks of the business
- attends the premises of the person giving him or her the work
- generally uses her or his own equipment and materials
- has the right to send someone else to do the work.

> **HM Revenue and Customs (HMRC):** The government department responsible for collecting tax.
>
> **Personal assets:** Possessions or belongings of value that an individual owns and which may not be related to the business (e.g. personal car, house, clothes, personal bank account, stocks and shares).

Partnership

A partnership consists of two or more people working together as the proprietors of a business. Unlike limited liability companies (see below), there are no legal requirements in setting up as a partnership. A partnership can be set up without the partners necessarily being fully aware that they have done so.

The partnership is similar to a sole trader in law, in that the partners own the business, take all the risks, stand any losses and keep any profits. Each partner individually is responsible for all the debts of the partnership. So, if the business fails, each partner's personal assets are fully at risk. It is possible, though not very common, to have partners with limited liability. In this case the partner with limited liability must not play any active part in the management or conduct of the business. In effect, he or she has merely invested a limited sum of money in the partnership.

The advantages of operating a business as a partnership can be very similar to those of the sole trader. Very little formality is needed, although everyone contemplating entering into a partnership should seriously consider taking legal advice and having a partnership agreement drawn up.

The main official records that are required are records for the Inland Revenue, National Insurance and VAT. The accounts are not available to the public. There may be important tax advantages, too, when compared with a limited company. For example, they might be able pay the tax they owe at a later date, or treat deductible expenses more generously.

Limited liability companies

These are companies that are incorporated under the Companies Acts. This means that the liability of their owners (the amount they will have to pay to cover the business's debts if it fails, or if it is sued) is limited to the value of the shares each shareholder (owner) owns.

Limited liability companies are much more complex than sole traders and partnerships. This is because the owners can limit their liability. As a consequence it is vital that people either investing in them or doing business with them need to know the financial standing of the company. Company documents are open to inspection by the public.

The UK hospitality industry

Hospitality and catering, like all leisure markets, benefits from improving economic conditions. For many people, real disposable income has grown over the last 20 years, and the forecasts are that it will continue to grow. In wealthy markets, the leisure and pleasure sectors outperform the economy in general. It is usually the case that, as people become wealthier, their extra income is not spent on upgrading the essentials but on pleasure and luxury items. However, whenever there is a downturn in the economy, the leisure sectors suffer more than others.

> **Real disposable income:** The amount of money available to spend after taxes have been deducted and any state benefits have been added.

The leisure sector has been described as the biggest, fastest-growing industry in the UK. Within the leisure sector, some areas have slowed down, while others are consolidating and concentrating on core businesses. One of the most useful ways of categorising the leisure sector is to separate it into popular leisure activities, for example: theatre, ten-pin bowling, cue sports, casinos, bingo, golf, health and fitness. The venues of all these leisure activities will offer some form of hospitality and catering, whether this is in the form of bars, snack bars, cafés or vending machines.

Traditionally, catering activity has been divided into either profit or cost sector markets. The profit sector includes such establishments as restaurants, fast-food outlets, cafés, takeaways, pubs, and leisure and travel catering outlets. The cost sector refers to catering outlets for business and industry, education and health care. Recent developments, such as the contracting out of catering services (see page 20) have blurred the division between profit- and cost-orientated establishments.

Despite its complexity, catering represents one of the largest sectors of the UK economy and is fifth in size behind retail food, cars, insurance and clothing. It is also an essential support to tourism, another major part of the economy, and one of the largest employers in the country.

The number of businesses

The leisure sector, including hospitality, travel and tourism, is large and employs about 2 million people. Around 7 per cent of all jobs in the UK are in the sector, that is, the sector accounts for about one in every 14 UK jobs, and it is predicted to grow even more.

There are approximately 142,000 hospitality, leisure, travel and tourism businesses in the UK that operate from 192,100 outlets. The restaurant industry is the largest within the sector (both in terms of the number of outlets and size of the

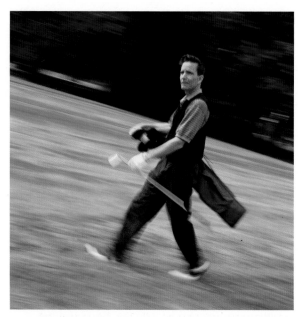

Golf courses usually have bars, serve food and offer a range of other hospitality services

workforce), followed by pubs, bars and nightclubs and the hotel industry.

The UK leisure industry (tourism and hospitality) is estimated by the Government to have been worth £85 billion in 2009. Including all business expenditure, the total market is worth much

Table 1.1 Number of businesses (enterprises) by industry

Industry	Number of businesses	%
Restaurants	63,600	45
Pubs, bars and nightclubs	49,150	35
Hotels	10,050	7
Travel and tourist services	6,750	5
Food and service management (contract catering)	6,350	4
Holiday centres and self-catering accommodation	3,650	3
Gambling	1,850	1
Visitor attractions	450	*
Youth and backpacker hostels	150	*
Hospitality, leisure, travel and tourism total	142,050	100

* Negligible

more than this. Expenditure on accommodation is difficult to pin down, but it is estimated that it contributes £10.3 billion (excluding categories such as camp sites and youth hostels) to the total leisure market.

Size

2.44 million people employed

£90 billion annual turnover, worth £46 billion to the UK economy

£7.5 billion on accommodation

The hospitality industry consists of all those business operations that provide for their customers any combination of the three core services of food, drink and accommodation. While there is a clear overlap with tourism, there are a number of sectors within the hospitality industry that can be regarded as separate from tourism, for example, industrial catering and those aspects of hospitality that attract only the local community.

Restaurants in the UK have approximately 40 per cent of the commercial hospitality market, and small establishments employing fewer than ten staff make up the majority of the industry. The south-east of England has the highest concentration of catering and hospitality outlets.

The hotel sector

The hotel sector is predominantly independently owned. The properties come in all shapes, sizes and locations. More than three-quarters of them have fewer than 20 rooms and are invariably family run.

The hotel sector, despite its disparate nature, can be divided into distinct categories, such as luxury, business, resort, town house and budget properties. Each category has its own characteristics. Business hotels, as the name suggests, are geared to the corporate traveller; the emphasis therefore tends to be on functionality. These hotels will usually have a dedicated business centre, up-to-date communication technology in the rooms, and ample conference and meeting facilities. Business hotels are more likely to be chain operated, often with a strong brand element. Town houses, meanwhile, are notable for their individuality, intimacy and emphasis on service. These hotels are invariably small and, as the name suggests, located in converted town houses with a domestic feel that is emphasised by their decor. The fastest-growing sector is budget hotels (e.g. Travel Lodge, Travel Inn).

Formal dining and buffet set-ups, traditional fare and theme restaurants, room service and public bars ... clearly the provision of food and beverage (F&B) varies greatly between establishments. Again, some general differences can be discerned between the various hotel categories. Upmarket hotels are likely to provide a full range of F&B services, usually with at least one *à la carte* restaurant, 24-hour room service and a well-stocked bar. Some smaller and budget establishments may have a very limited food provision or none at all.

Recently many hotels have been re-examining the place of F&B in their operations. While many town houses open with no restaurant at all, other hotels believe that F&B provision is an essential guest service. This has led them to consider alternative methods of running a restaurant, such as contracting out to a third party or introducing a franchise operation.

The economics of running a restaurant in a hotel show why hotels have been reluctant to take this on. While F&B receipts traditionally provide about 20–30 per cent of a hotel's total revenue, over three-quarters of this will be absorbed by departmental expenses, including payroll costs of approximately a third. A hotel's room department typically provides 50–60 per cent of revenue, but departmental costs account for only 25–30 per cent of this.

An international industry

Businesses today find themselves competing in a world economy for survival, growth and profitability. Managers working in the industry have to learn to adjust to change in line with market demands for quality and value for money, and increased organisational attention must be devoted to profitability and professionalism.

The globalisation of the hospitality and tourism industries has advanced under the pressures of increased technology, communication, transportation, deregulation, elimination of political barriers, socio-cultural changes and global economic development, together with growing competition in a global economy. An international hospitality company must perform successfully in the *world's* business environment.

Disparate: Made up of elements which are so different that they cannot be compared.

Deregulation: The removal of regulations or government controls, allowing businesses to operate with more freedom.

Travel, tourism and hospitality together make up the world's largest industry. According to the World Travel and Tourism Council (WTTC), the annual gross output of the industry is greater than the gross national product (GNP) of all countries except the United States and Japan. Worldwide, the industry employs over 112 million people. In many countries, especially in emerging tourist destinations, the hospitality and tourism industry plays a very important role in the national economy, being the major foreign currency earner.

Travel
Tourism
Hospitality
The world's largest industry.

As the world economy continues to become more interdependent, this will give rise to increasing amounts of business travel. With this in mind, it is clear that the global economic environment plays a significant role in the internationalisation opportunities available to hospitality and tourism companies, and that global economic policies and developments play a critical role in the hospitality and tourism industry.

Key influences affecting the hospitality industry	
Social trends/lifestyle	Cultural factors – people using hospitality to celebrate occasions: birthdays, weddings, etc.
Amount of disposable income people have to spend	Regulation – taxation, VAT, tourism
Inflation	Media – television, advertising, magazines, celebrity chefs
Available credit	

Product and service

The hospitality product consists of elements of food, drink and accommodation, together with the service, atmosphere and image that surround and contribute to the product

The hospitality industry contains many of the characteristics of service industries with the added complications of the production process. It is the production process that is the complicated element as it focuses on production and delivery, often within a set period of time.

ACTIVITY

What do you think of as good service? Give an example where you have experienced good service.

The need to provide the appropriate environment within which hospitality can be delivered, means that most hospitality businesses need to invest a substantial amount in plant and premises. This creates a high fixed cost/low variable cost structure. Fixed costs are those that remain the same or similar regardless of how much business is being carried out, such as rent and salaries. Variable costs, on the other hand, are those that change depending on the volume of business, such as food costs. The variable costs in servicing a room are minimal, although the hotel itself – particularly in the luxury hotel market – has a high fixed cost. In general, the financial break-even point for hospitality businesses is fairly high. The break-even point is the point when the total expenditure (the amount the business is spending

to operate) matches the income from the sales. Exceeding this level will result in profits, but when income is below the break-even point, the low volumes will result in losses.

Forecasting

Hospitality services suffer from fluctuations in demand: demand fluctuates over time and by type of customer. Therefore, because of the mixture of patterns and variables that can affect demand, forecasting business is often difficult, making planning, resourcing and scheduling difficult. Hospitality cannot be delivered without customers. Achieving a satisfactory balance between demand patterns, resource scheduling and operational capacity is a difficult task for managers in hospitality.

Scheduling of resources is also difficult. If too many staff are on duty to cover the forecast demand, then profitability suffers – too many people are being paid for too little work. Insufficient staffing creates problems with servicing and staff morale – there is too much work to do and too few people to do it. Forecasting is therefore a crucial function, which contributes to the successful operation of the hospitality business.

Interacting with the customer

The ability to deliver a consistent product to every customer is also an important consideration. Staff must be trained in teams to deliver a consistent standard of product and service. This means being

Definitions

Fluctuations in demand – when demand for a product or service varies from time to time. This could be day to day, month to month or at certain times of the year. For example, January is not usually a good time of the year for hotels and restaurants as many people do not have the money to spend straight after Christmas, so business may go down.

Variables – other changes that may affect business, e.g. changes in people's income, higher taxation so people have less money to spend, or changes in the weather which can affect whether people decide to go out or stay at home. Also, supermarkets producing restaurant-style food at a reasonable price may mean that more people eat at home rather than go out

Resourcing – providing the food, labour and equipment to do the job.

Demand patterns – patterns of customer behaviour, e.g. when the weather is bad people tend to stay at home; at the weekend more people go out to eat; at certain times of the year restaurants get very busy, for example during the Christmas period. National and international events also make a difference, such as the Olympics or royal events.

Resource scheduling – planning and making sure that all the resources are in place when they are needed, such as the food, staff and equipment.

Operational capacity – how much work (number of customers/orders/functions) the operation is able to cope with to deliver a product at the required standard to satisfy the customer.

able to cater not just for individual customers, but also to the needs of many different groups of customers, all with slightly different requirements. The success of any customer experience will be determined at the interaction point between the customer and the service provider.

The service staff have an additional part to play in serving the customer: they are important in the future selling process, in other words, if they provide the customer with a good experience the customer is more likely to return in the future. Staff should, therefore, be trained to use the opportunity to generate additional revenue.

There are four main characteristics of the hospitality industry that make it a unique operation.

1. Hospitality cannot be delivered without customers. The customer is directly involved in many aspects of the delivery of the hospitality service, and is the judge of the quality of the hospitality provided.

2. Achieving a satisfactory balance between demand patterns, resource scheduling and operations is a particularly difficult task in the hospitality industry.

3. All hospitality operations require a combination of manufacturing expertise and service skill, in many cases 24 hours a day. To deliver a consistent product to each individual customer requires teams of people well trained to deliver to a set standard every time.

4. No matter how well planned the operation, how good the design and the environment, if the interaction between customer and service provider is not right this will have a detrimental effect on the customer experience of the total product. It will be a missed opportunity to sell future products. Good interaction between customers and service providers can also increase present sales – for example, waiting staff can 'up sell' by suggesting, in a positive way, additions to the meal, perhaps items the customer may not even have considered but which they are delighted to have recommended.

Standard Operational Procedures (SOP) are put in place by an establishment to ensure standards remain consistent. Examples include the way guests are greeted or the way tables are laid.

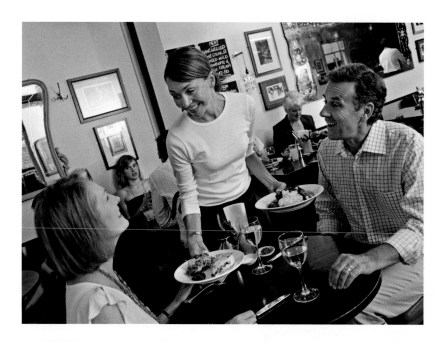

Types of establishment

Hotels

Hotels provide accommodation in private bedrooms. Many offer other services such as restaurants, bars and room service, reception, porters and housekeepers. What a hotel offers will depend on the type of hotel it is and its star rating.

Hotels are rated from five-star down to one-star. A luxury hotel will have five stars while a more basic hotel will have one star. There are many international hotel chains, such as the Radisson group, Mandarin Oriental, Intercontinental and Dorchester Collection in the five-star hotel market. There are also budget hotels, guesthouses and bed and breakfast accommodation (see below).

In the UK there are more hotel bedrooms in the mid-market three-star hotels than in any other category. Most hotels in this market are independent and privately owned, in other words they are not part of a chain of hotels.

Some hotels have speciality restaurants, run by a high-profile or 'celebrity' chef, for example, or specialising in steaks, sushi or seafood.

To attract as many guests as possible, many hotels now offer even more services. These may include office and IT services (e.g. internet access, fax machines, a quiet area to work in), gym and sports facilities, swimming pool, spa, therapy treatments, hair and beauty treatments and so on.

 ACTIVITY

Give an example of a five-star and a four-star hotel that you have heard of. What additional services do they offer?

Country house hotels

Country house hotels are mostly in attractive old buildings, such as stately homes or manor houses, in tourist and rural areas. They normally have a reputation for good food and wine and a high standard of service. They may also offer the additional services mentioned above.

 ACTIVITY

Give an example of a country house hotel. Where is it located?

Outsourcing: a growing trend

The contracting-out of food and beverage services to third parties will continue to be a major trend in the hotel catering sector over the next few years, although this will probably be much stronger in London than in the provinces. As many hotels continue to remain slow in response to evolving consumer demand for food and beverages, and intense competition from the high street, the attraction of outsourcing food and beverage services will become increasingly appealing.

Outsourcing is not always a straightforward option for hotels, however. To attract walk-in dining customers, a hotel ideally needs to be located where there is easy access to the restaurant, and the location of the hotel itself (city centre, countryside, etc.) needs to fit with the clientele that are being targeted – that is, the product must be attractive to the passing trade. Despite these constraints, the number of outsourced restaurants is expected to increase considerably, for example, Gordon Ramsey at Claridges and Gary Rhodes at the Cumberland in London.

In-house dining development

With increased consumer interest in food and eating out, hotels are becoming more focused on developing attractive food and beverage facilities in-house. The success of in-house dining development will depend on the willingness of hotels to deliver a product that will be attractive to the outside market, and to maintain this product so that it evolves with changing consumer tastes and trends. According to human resource specialists within the hotel sector, key factors holding back further development are that food and beverage managers in hotels tend to be hoteliers rather than restaurateurs; further difficulties are caused by the shortage of experienced culinary and service staff.

Consortium

A consortium is a group of independent hotels that make an agreement to buy products and services together. For example, they might all pay a specialist company to do their marketing (advertising and so on). This might mean, for example, that the members of the consortium could then use international reservation systems and compete against the larger hotel chains.

Budget hotels

Budget hotels like motels and Travel Lodges are built near motorways, railway stations and airports. They are aimed at business people and tourists who need somewhere inexpensive to stay overnight. The rooms are reasonably priced and have tea and coffee making facilities. No other food or drink is included in the price. Staff members are kept to a minimum and there is often no restaurant. However, there may be shops, cafés, restaurants or pubs close by, which are often run by the same company as the motel. The growth and success of the budget hotel sector has been one of the biggest changes in the hospitality industry in recent years.

 ACTIVITY

Why are budget hotels often built near motorways, railway stations and airports?

Guesthouses and bed and breakfasts

There are guesthouses and bed and breakfast establishments all over the UK. They are small, privately owned businesses. The owners usually live on the premises and let bedrooms to paying customers. Many have guests who return regularly, especially if they are in a popular tourist area. Some guesthouses offer lunch and an evening meal as well as breakfast.

Clubs and casinos

People pay to become members of private clubs. Private clubs are usually run by managers (sometimes known as club secretaries) who are appointed by club members. What most members want from a club in Britain, particularly in the fashionable areas of London, is good food and drink and informal service often in the old English style.

Most nightclubs and casinos are open to the public rather than to members only. As well as selling drinks to their customers, many now also provide food services, such as restaurants.

Restaurants

The restaurant sector has become the largest in the UK hospitality industry. It includes exclusive restaurants and fine-dining establishments, as well as a wide variety of mainstream restaurants, fast-food outlets, coffee shops and cafés.

Many restaurants specialise in regional or ethnic food styles, such as Asian and Oriental, Mexican and Caribbean, as well as a wide range of European-style restaurants. New restaurants and cooking styles are appearing and becoming more popular all the time.

Speciality restaurants

Moderately priced speciality restaurants continue to increase in popularity. In order for them to succeed, it is essential that they understand what customers want and plan a menu that will attract enough customers to make a good profit. A successful caterer is one who gives customers what they want; they will be aware of changing trends and adapt to them. The most successful catering establishments are those that maintain the required level of sales over long periods and throughout the year.

Fast food

Many customers now want the option of popular foods at a reasonable price, with little or no waiting time. Fast-food establishments offer a limited menu that can be consumed on the premises or taken away. Menu items are quick to cook and have often been partly or fully prepared beforehand at a central production point.

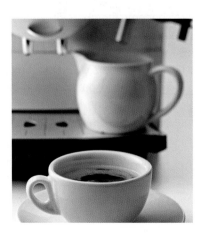

Drive-ins (or drive-throughs)

The concept of drive-ins came from America, and there are now many of them across the UK. The most well known are the 'drive-thrus' at McDonald's fast-food restaurants. Customers stay in their vehicles and drive up to a microphone where they place their order. As the car moves forward in a queue, the order is prepared and is ready for them to pick up at the service window when they get there.

Delicatessens and salad bars

These offer a wide selection of salads and sandwich fillings to go in a variety of bread and rolls at a 'made-to-order' sandwich counter. The choice of breads might include panini, focaccia, pitta, baguette and tortilla wraps. Fresh salads, homemade soups, chilled foods and a hot 'chef's dish of the day' may also be available, along with ever-popular baked jacket potatoes with a good variety of fillings.

With such a wide variety of choices these establishments can stay busy all day long, often serving breakfast as well.

Chain catering organisations

There are many branded restaurant chains, coffee shops, and shops with in-store restaurants. Many of these chains are spread widely throughout the UK and, in some cases, overseas. These are usually well-known companies that advertise widely. They often serve morning coffee, lunches and teas, or may be in the style of snack bars and cafeterias.

Coffee shops

The branded coffee shop has been a particularly fast-growing area, providing a wide variety of good quality coffee and other drinks, along with a limited selection of food items. They provide for both a fast 'takeaway' or a more leisurely café style consumption.

Licensed-house (pub) catering

Almost all of the tens of thousands of licensed public houses (pubs) in the UK offer food of some sort or another. The type of food they serve is ideal for many people. It is usually quite simple, inexpensive and quickly served in a comfortable atmosphere. In recent years there have been a number of pub closures due to the availability of alcohol in supermarkets, and the smoking ban, which has had a major effect on business. For this reason, many pubs have moved into selling food, revisiting their product offer (what they have to offer the customer) and the total pub experience for their customers in order to stay in business, for example adding restaurants, offering more bar food and putting on live entertainment.

There is a great variety of food available in pubs, from those that serve simple sandwiches and rolls to those that have exclusive *à la carte* restaurants. Pub catering can be divided into five categories:

1. luxury-type restaurants
2. gastro pubs that have well-qualified chefs who develop the menu according to their own specialities, making good use of local produce
3. speciality restaurants like steak bars, fish restaurants, carveries and theme restaurants
4. bar-food pubs where dishes are served from the bar counter and the food is eaten in the normal drinking areas rather than in a separate restaurant
5. bar-food pubs that just serve simple items such as rolls and sandwiches.

(Note: data in this section comes from the BHA and Hospitality.net.)

 ACTIVITY

Choose a local restaurant which you are familiar with. List the types of food it has on offer and what special features the restaurant has.

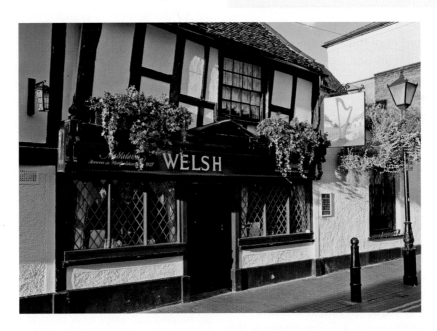

Food provision in the leisure industry

Timeshare villas and apartments

A timeshare owner buys a particular amount of time (usually a few weeks) per year in a particular self-catering apartment, room or suite in a hotel or a leisure club. The arrangement may be for a period of years or indefinite. There will usually be a number of restaurants, bars and other leisure facilities within the same complex for timeshare owners to use.

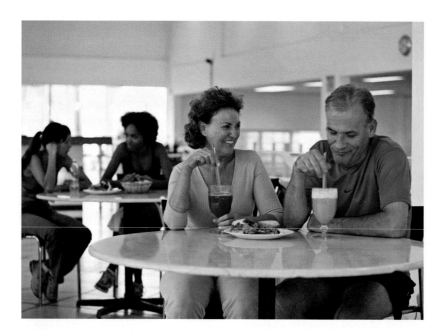

Health clubs and spas

These may be establishments in their own right, or provided within other luxury establishments or hotels, and offer a variety of treatments and therapies. The number of these has increased rapidly over recent years and they have become very popular. They usually offer healthy food, therapies and activities that fit in with people's modern-day lifestyles and their interest in health, fitness and well-being.

Museums

In order to diversify and to extend their everyday activities, some museums now provide hospitality services. For example, many museums have one or more cafés and restaurants for visitors. Some run events such as lunch lectures, family events and children's discovery days where food is provided as part of the event. Museums can even be used as an interesting venue for private events and banqueting during the hours they are closed to the general public. Sometimes outside caterers are employed for the occasion, but many museums employ their own catering team to provide a wide range of food.

Theme parks

Theme parks are now extremely popular venues for a family day out or even a full holiday. The larger theme parks include several different eating options ranging from fast food to fine dining. Some include branded restaurants (such as McDonald's and Burger King), which the visitor will already know. Theme parks are also used for corporate hospitality, in other words, they are used by companies for conferences or other events. Several have conference and banqueting suites for this purpose, and larger theme parks may even have their own hotels.

Holiday centres

Holiday centres around the UK provide leisure and hospitality facilities all together in the same place, on a single site. They cater for families, single people and groups of people. Many holiday centres have invested large amounts of money to improve the quality of the holiday experience. Centre Parcs, for example, have developed sub-tropical pools and other sporting and leisure activities that can be used even if the weather is bad. The holiday centres (sometimes called complexes) include a range of different restaurants and food courts, bars and coffee shops. These are examples of year-round holiday centres that encourage people to take holidays and weekend breaks from home.

Historical buildings

Numerous historical buildings and places of interest have food outlets such as cafés and restaurants. Many in the UK specialise in light lunches and afternoon tea for the general public. Some are also used as venues to host large private or corporate events.

Visitor attractions

Places like Hampton Court, Kew Gardens and Poole Pottery can be categorised as visitor attractions. They will usually have refreshments outlets serving a variety of food and drinks. Some, like Kew Gardens, are also used to stage large theatrical events or concerts in the summer.

Event management

Event management is when a person or company plans and organises events, such as parties, dinners and conferences, for other people or companies. This will include such tasks as hiring the venue, organising the staff, the food and drink, music, entertainment and any other requests the host may have.

Farms

The tourism industry in the countryside is very important in the UK. Farmers understand this and have formed a national organisation called the Farm Holiday Bureau. The farms in the organisation usually offer bed and breakfast and holiday cottages. Most members of the organisation have invested money to improve their bedrooms to meet the standards required by the National Tourist Board. The Tourist Board inspects every member property to ensure that it is good value and that the accommodation is good quality. The accommodation is usually on or near a working farm.

Youth hostels

The Youth Hostels Association runs hostels in various locations in England and Wales. These establishments cater for single people, families and groups travelling on a limited budget. They mainly provide dormitory accommodation, but some also have a few private rooms. In some locations they include a number of sports and leisure facilities. Basic, wholesome meals are provided at a low cost in some hostels, and they all have a kitchen that can be used by visitors to store and prepare their own food.

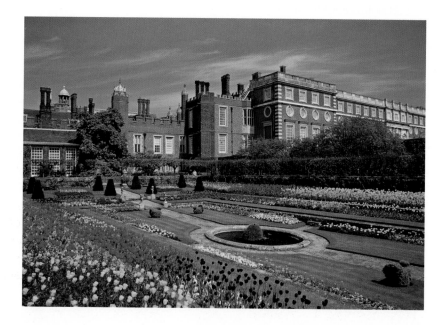

Travel

Catering at sea

There is a variety of types of sea-going vessels on which catering is required for both passengers and crew. Catering for passengers on ferries and cruise liners is becoming increasingly important in today's competitive markets.

Sea ferries

There are several ferry ports in the UK. Ferries leave from these every day, making a variety of sea crossings to Ireland and mainland Europe. As well as carrying passengers, many ferries also carry the passengers' cars and freight lorries. In addition to competing against each other, ferry companies also compete against airlines and, in the case of English Channel crossings, Eurostar and Le Shuttle. In order to win customers they have invested in (spent money on) improving their passenger services, with most ferries having several shops, bars, cafés and lounges on board. Some also have very good restaurant and leisure facilities, fast food restaurants and branded food outlets. These are often run by contract caterers (sometimes known as 'contract food service providers' – see page 20) on behalf of the ferry operator. More recently, well-known chefs have become involved in providing top-quality restaurants on popular ferry routes.

Cruise liners

Cruise ships are floating luxury hotels, and more and more people are becoming interested in cruising as a lifestyle. The food provision on a large cruise liner is of a similar standard to the food provided in a five-star hotel and can be described as excellent quality, banquet-style cuisine. Many shipping companies are known for the excellence of their cuisine.

As cruising becomes more popular, cruise companies are getting more and bigger cruise liners. This means that there are excellent hospitality career opportunities. Many companies provide good training and promotion prospects, and the opportunity to travel all over the world. The caterers produce food and serve customers to a very high standard in extremely hygienic conditions. All of these things mean that working on cruise liners can be an interesting and rewarding career. As an example of working conditions, staff may work for three months and then have, say, two months off. On-board hours of work can be long, perhaps 10 hours a day for 7 days a week, but this appeals to many people who want to produce good food in excellent conditions.

On cruises where the quality of the food is of paramount importance, other factors such as the

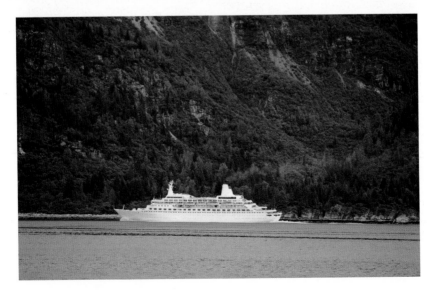

dining room's ambience of refinement and elegance are also of great significance. Ship designers generally want to avoid Las Vegas-type glittery dining rooms, but also those that are too austere. Ships must also be designed with easy access to the galley (ship's kitchen) so waiters are able to get food quickly and with as little traffic as possible.

> **Austere:** Stern or severe; without comforts or luxuries.

A distinction can be made between dining and eating on cruises, as shown in table 1.2.

Table 1.2 The differences between dining and eating on cruises

Dining	Eating
Dining room	Buffet style
Set times	Any time
Assigned tables	Choice of seating
Elegance	Cafeteria-like ambience
Elaborate table settings	Informal tables
Carefully planned menus	Choice from selection
Waiters	Self-serve
Sociability	Separation − informal

This set of polarities doesn't apply as much to the new giant ships that have many different dining rooms. On such ships passengers can eat in the dining room of their choice, more or less whenever they want, at tables of various sizes. This gives passengers maximum freedom.

Dining is one of the most important − and selling − points for cruise lines. People who take cruises want to dine well and generally they do, though cooking dinner for 800 people per sitting and giving people what they want takes skill and good management.

Other vessels

As well as luxury liners, catering at sea includes smaller cargo and passenger ships, and the giant cargo tankers. The food provision for crew and passengers on these ships will vary from good restaurants and cafeterias to more industrial-style

catering on the tankers. On all types of ship, extra precautions have to be taken in the kitchen in rough weather.

 ACTIVITY

Name two companies that operate cruises.

Air travel

With increased air travel, the opportunities and need for food services catering to the industry have also increased. The food provision varies greatly both from airport to airport and airline to airline.

Airline services

Airline catering is a specialist service. The catering companies are usually located at or near airports in this country and around the world. The meals provided vary from snacks and basic meals to luxury meals for first-class passengers. Menus are chosen carefully to make sure that the food can safely be chilled and then reheated on board the aircraft.

The price of some airline tickets includes a meal served at your seat. The budget airlines usually have an at-seat trolley service from which passengers can buy snacks and drinks.

At the airport

Airports offer a range of hospitality services catering for millions of people every year. They operate 24 hours a day, 365 days a year. Services include a wide variety of shops along with bars, themed restaurants, speciality restaurants, coffee bars and food courts.

All of these outlets need to have the ability to respond rapidly to fluctuations in demand caused by delayed and cancelled flights and high-volume periods such as bank holidays.

Roadside services

Roadside motoring services (often referred to as 'service stations') provide a variety of services for motorists. These include fuel, car washing and maintenance facilities and a variety of shops. Many are becoming more sophisticated, with baby changing, infant and pet feeding facilities, bathrooms and showers, a variety of branded food and drinks outlets (such as Burger King, Costa Coffee and M&S Simply Food) and often accommodation. The catering usually consists of food courts offering travellers a wide range of meals 24-hour, 7 days a week. MOTO is an example of a company that provides these sorts of services nationwide.

Rail travel

Snacks can be bought in the buffet car on a train, and some train operators also offer a trolley service so passengers can buy snacks without leaving their seats. Main meals are often served in a restaurant car. However, there is not much space in a restaurant car kitchen, and with a lot of movement of the train, it can be quite difficult to provide anything other than simple meals.

Two train services run by separate companies run through the Channel Tunnel. One is Euro Tunnel's Le Shuttle train, which transports drivers and their vehicles between Folkestone and Calais in 35 minutes. Passengers have to buy any food and drink for their journey before they board the train.

The other company, Eurostar, operates between London St Pancras and Paris or Brussels. This carries passengers only. Eurostar is in direct competition with the airlines, so it provides catering to airline standards for first and premier class passengers. Meals are served by uniformed stewards and stewardesses in a similar service to an airline's club class. This food is included in the ticket price. Economy travellers usually buy their food separately from buffet cars or trolley services.

This is another area where catering is often provided by contract food service providers.

Public sector catering (secondary service sector)

Public sector organisations that need catering services include hospitals, universities, colleges, schools, prisons, the armed forces, police and ambulance services, local authorities and many more.

The aim of catering in hotels, restaurants and other areas of the leisure and travel industry (known as the private sector) is to make a profit. The aim of public sector catering is to keep costs down by working efficiently. However, these days the business of catering for public sector organisations is tendered for. This means that different companies will compete to win a contract to provide the catering for these organisations. Many public sector catering tenders have been won by contract caterers (contract food service providers), which have introduced new ideas and more commercialism (promoting business for profit) into the public sector. Because much of the public sector is now operated by profit-making contractors, it is sometimes referred to as the secondary service sector.

For a variety of reasons, the types of menu in the public sector may be different from those in the private sector. For example, school children,

hospital patients and soldiers have particular nutritional needs (they may need more energy from their food, or more of certain vitamins and minerals), so their menus should match their needs. Menus may also reflect the need to keep costs down. However, the standards of cooking in the public sector should be just as good as they are in the private sector.

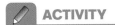 **ACTIVITY**

Find out the name of three major contract catering companies.

Prisons

Catering in prisons may be carried out by contract caterers or by the Prison Service itself. The food is usually prepared by prison officers and inmates. The kitchens are also used to train inmates in food production. They can gain a recognised qualification to encourage them to find work when they are released.

Prisons used to have something called Crown Immunity, which meant that they could not be prosecuted (taken to court) for poor hygiene and negligence in the kitchen. However, they no longer have this and they must operate to the same standards as other kitchens in the public sector.

In addition to catering facilities for the inmates, there are also staff catering facilities for all the personnel (staff) who work in a prison, such as administrative staff and prison officers.

The armed forces

Catering in the armed forces includes providing meals for staff in barracks, in the field and on ships. Catering for the armed forces is specialised, especially when they are in the field, and they have their own well-established cookery training programmes.

However, like every other part of the public sector, the forces need to keep costs down and increase efficiency. Consequently, they also have competitive tendering for their catering services. The Ministry of Defence contracts food service providers to cater for many of their service operations.

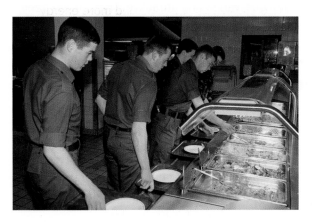

The National Health Service

The scale of catering services in the NHS is enormous. Over 300 million meals are served each year in approximately 1,200 hospitals. NHS Trusts must ensure that they get the best value for money within their catering budget.

Hospital caterers need to provide well-cooked, nutritious, appetising meals for hospital patients and must maintain strict hygiene standards.

As well as providing nutritious meals for patients in hospital (many of whom need special diets), provision must also be made for out-patients (people who come into hospital for treatment and leave again the same day), visitors and staff. This service may be provided by the hospital catering team, but is sometimes allocated to commercial food outlets, or there may be a combination of in-house hospital catering and commercial catering.

The education sector school meals service

School meals play an important part in the lives of many children, often providing them with the only hot meal of the day. In 1944 the Education Act stated that all schools should provide a meal to any children who wanted one. The meal had to meet strict nutritional and price guidelines. The school meals service continued to work in this way until the 1980 Education Act. This stated that schools no longer had to provide school meals for everyone, and also removed the minimum nutritional standards and the fixed charge.

In April 2001, for the first time in over 20 years, minimum nutritional standards were re-introduced by the government. These are designed to bring all schools up to a measurable standard set down in law. Since this date, Local Education Authorities have been responsible for seeing that the minimum nutritional standards for school lunches are met. Schools also have to provide a paid-for meal, where parents request one, except where children are under five years old and only go to school part-time. This does not affect the LEA's or the school's duty to provide a free meal to those children who qualify for one.

In 2006 the government announced new standards for school food. These were phased in by September 2009. Together they cover all food sold or served in schools: breakfast, lunch and after-school meals; tuck shops, vending machines, mid-morning break snacks and anything sold or served at after-school clubs.

The standards are based on both foods and nutrients.

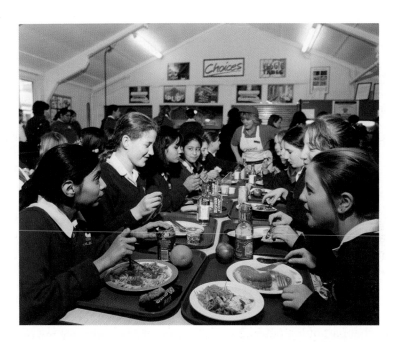

Residential establishments

Residential establishments include schools, colleges, university halls of residence, nursing homes, homes for the elderly, children's homes and hostels, where all the meals are provided. It is very important to consider the nutritional balance of food served in these establishments. It should satisfy all the residents' nutritional needs, as the people eating these meals will probably have no other food provision. Many of these establishments cater for children, who may lead energetic lives and will probably be growing fast so have large appetites, so the food should be well prepared from good ingredients and should be nutritious, varied and attractive. These often need to be provided within stringent financial controls.

Catering for business and industry

The provision of staff dining rooms and restaurants in industrial and business settings has provided employment for many catering workers outside traditional hotel and restaurant catering. Working conditions in these settings are often very good. Apart from the main task of providing meals, these services may also include retail shops, franchise outlets (see page 21) and vending machines. It will also include catering for meetings and conferences as well as for larger special functions.

In some cases a 24-hour, 7-days-a-week service is necessary, but usually the hours are more streamlined than in other areas of the hospitality industry. Food and drink is provided for all employees, often in high-quality restaurants and dining rooms. The catering departments in these organisations are keen to keep and develop their staff, so there is good potential for training and career development in this sector.

Many industries have realised that satisfied employees work more efficiently and produce better work, so have spent a great deal of money on providing first-class kitchens and dining-rooms. In some cases companies will subsidise (pay part of) the cost of the meals so that employees can buy the food at a price lower than it costs.

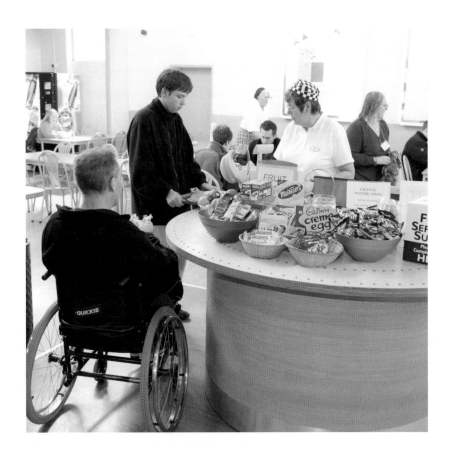

The contract food service sector

The contract food service sector, which has already been mentioned in relation to other sectors of the hospitality industry, consists of companies that provide catering services for other organisations. This sector has developed significantly over recent years.

Contract food service management provides food for a wide variety of people, such as those at work in business and industry, those in schools, colleges and universities, private and public healthcare establishments, public and local authorities, and other non-profit making outlets such as the armed forces, police or ambulance services.

It also includes more commercial areas, such as corporate hospitality events and the executive dining rooms of many corporations, special events, sporting fixtures and places of entertainment, and outlets such as leisure centres, galleries,

museums, department stores and specific retail stores, supermarket restaurants and cafés, airports and railway stations. Some contractors also provide other support services such as housekeeping and maintenance, reception, security, laundry, bars and retail shops.

Outside catering

When events are held at venues where there is no catering available, or where the level of catering required is more than the normal caterers can manage, then a catering company may take over the management of the event. This type of function will include garden parties, agricultural and horticultural shows, the opening of new buildings, banquets, parties in private houses, military pageants and tattoos, sporting fixtures such as horse racing, motor racing, football or rugby, and so on.

There is a wide variety in this sort of outside catering work, but the standards can be very high and people employed in this area need to be adaptable and creative. Sometimes specialist equipment will be required, especially for outdoor jobs, and employees need to be flexible as the work often involves travel to remote locations and outdoor venues.

Corporate hospitality

Corporate hospitality is hospitality provided by businesses, usually for its clients or potential clients. The purpose of corporate hospitality is to build business relationships and to raise awareness of the company. Corporate entertaining is also used as a way to thank or reward loyal customers.

Companies these days understand the importance of marketing through building relationships with clients and through the company's reputation. They are willing to spend large amounts of money to do this well.

Reasons for spending money on corporate hospitality include:

1. to build relationships with potential customers
2. to reward customers/thank them for loyalty
3. as a marketing tool/to raise company or product profile
4. to increase business/sales
5. to achieve closer informal contact in a relaxed environment
6. to raise and keep up the company's profile/ public relations
7. to encourage repeat business/to retain clients or customers
8. to keep the customers happy/to entertain them or act as a 'sweetener'
9. to talk about business/to network
10. to achieve better communication interaction/ improved understanding
11. to meet the expectations of customers or the industry
12. to reward/boost staff or team morale
13. for the social benefits/opportunity to relax.

Franchising

A franchise is an agreement where a person or group of people pay a fee and some set-up costs to use an established name or brand which is well known and is therefore likely to attract more customers than an unknown or start-up brand.

An example of this is where the contract caterer, Compass Group, buys a franchise in the Burger King brand from Burger King's owner. It pays a fee and a proportion of the turnover (the amount of money it makes). The franchisor (the branded company franchise provider) will normally lay down strict guidelines or 'brand standards' that the

franchise user has to meet. In this example these will affect things like which ingredients and raw materials are used and where they come from, as well as portion sizes and the general product packaging and service. The franchisor will check on the brand standards regularly to ensure that the brand reputation is not being put at risk. The franchisor will normally also provide advertising and marketing support, accounting services, help with staff training and development and designs for merchandising and display materials.

Employment in the hospitality industry

Staffing and organisation structure

Hospitality companies need to have a structure for their staff in order for the business to run efficiently and effectively. Different members of staff have different jobs and roles to perform as part of the team so that the business is successful.

In smaller organisations, some employees have to become multi-skilled so that they can carry out a variety of duties. Some managers may have to take on a supervisory role at certain times.

A hospitality team will consist of operational staff, supervisory staff, management staff and, in large organisations, senior management. These roles are explained below.

Operational staff

These are usually practical, hands-on staff. These will include the chefs de partie, (section chefs), commis chefs, waiters, apprentices, reception staff and accommodation staff.

Supervisory staff

Generally the supervisors work with the operational staff, supervising the work they do. In some establishments, the supervisors will be the managers for some of the operational staff.

A sous chef will have supervisory responsibilities, and a chef de partie will have both operational and supervisory responsibilities.

Management staff

- Managers have the responsibility of making sure that the operation runs smoothly and within the budget.
- They are accountable to the owners to make sure that the products and services on offer are what the customer expects and wants and provide value for money.
- Managers may also be responsible for planning future business.

- They will be required to make sure that all the health and safety policies are in place and that health and safety legislation is followed.
- In smaller establishments they may also act as the human resources manager employing new staff and dealing with staffing issues.

A hotel will normally have a manager, assistant managers, accommodation manager, restaurant manager and reception manager. So in each section of the hotel there could be a manager with departmental responsibilities. A head chef is a manager, managing kitchen operations, planning purchasing and managing the employees in his/her area.

The main job roles for operational staff, such as Chef de cuisine, Sous chef, Chef de partie Commis and Apprentice can be found in Chapter 5.

Employment rights and responsibilities

For those employed in the hospitality industry it is important to understand that there is a considerable amount of legislation that regulates both the industry itself and employment in the industry. Employers who contravene (break) the law or attempt to undermine the statutory (legal) rights of their workers – for example, paying less than the national minimum wage or denying them their right to paid annual holidays – are not only liable to prosecution and fines but could be ordered by tribunals and courts to pay substantial amounts of compensation.

People have rights in employment.

Employers must provide the employee with:

- a detailed job description
- a contract of employment with details of the job itself, working hours, the annual holiday the employee will have and the notice period.

An essential feature of a contract of employment is the 'mutuality of obligation'. This means that the

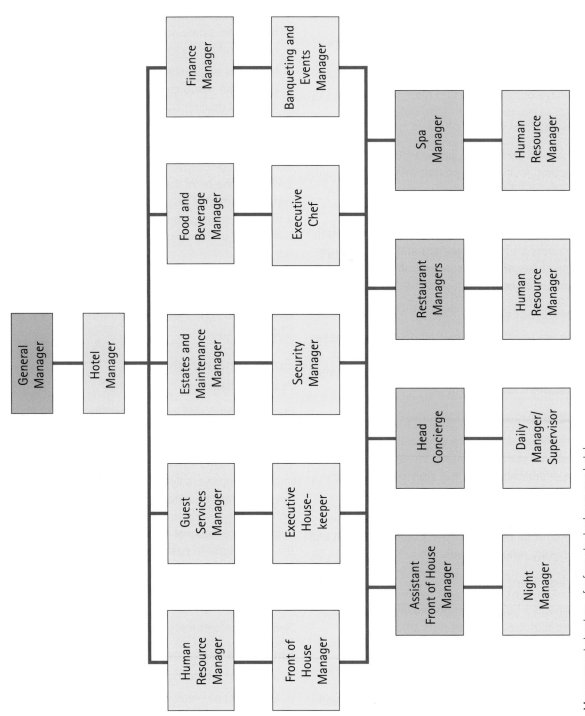

Management structure of a four-star bedroom spa hotel

employer will provide the employee with work on specified days of the week for specified hours and, if employed under a limited-term contract, for an agreed number of weeks or months. In return, the employee agrees to carry out the work for an agreed wage or salary.

Employers must follow the relevant laws, such as employment law, health and safety law, and food safety law.

Employees must work in the way that has been agreed to in the contract and job description and follow all the organisation's policies and practices.

Workers and employees

An employee is a person employed directly by a company under a contract of employment or service.

A worker or contractor is someone who works for another company (a sub-contractor) that has won a contract to carry out work or provide services, i.e. they are not actually an employee of the company itself.

Workers are still protected by:

- Health & Safety legislation
- Working Time Regulations 1998
- Equality Act 2010
- Public Interest Disclosure Act 1998
- National Minimum Wage Act 1998
- Part-time Workers (Prevention of Less Favourable Treatment) Regulations.

Recruitment and selection

When advertising for new staff it is important to be aware of the following legislation:

- Children and Young Persons Act 1933
- Licensing Act 1964
- Rehabilitation of Offenders Act 1974
- Data Protection Act 1988
- Asylum and Immigration Act 1996
- National Minimum Wage Act 1998
- Working Time Regulations 1998
- Equality Act 2010
- Human Rights Act 1998.

Job advertisements

It is unlawful to discriminate against job applicants on grounds of:

- sex, marital status or gender
- colour, race, nationality, or national or ethnic origins
- disability
- sexual orientation
- religion or beliefs
- trades union membership or non-membership.

The following words and phrases should be avoided in a job advertisement:

- young/youthful
- pleasing appearance
- strong personality
- energetic
- articulate
- dynamic
- no family commitments.

These could be construed (understood), or misconstrued, as indicating an intention to discriminate on grounds of sex, race or disability.

Use of job titles with a sexual connotation (e.g. 'waiter', 'barmaid', 'manageress') will also be taken to indicate an intention to discriminate on the grounds of a person's sex, unless the advertisement contains an indication or an illustration to the contrary.

Job applications

Job application forms must be designed with care. If 'sensitive personal information' is needed, such as a health record or disability disclosure, the reason for this should be explained, and the candidate reassured that the data will remain confidential and will be used and stored in keeping with the provisions of the Data Protection Act 1998.

Human Rights Act

Candidates must be informed at application stage, and at interview, if they have to wear uniforms or protective clothing on duty. Any surveillance

An example of a job description: Senior Sous Chef

Reporting to Head Chef

The Senior Sous Chef position reports to the Head Chef and is responsible for the day-to-day kitchen operation, overseeing the stores, preparation and production areas. The position involves supervising and managing the kitchen staff, with direct responsibility for rostering and scheduling production. In the absence of the Head Chef, the Senior Sous Chef will be required to take on the duties of the Head Chef and to attend Senior Management meetings in his/her absence.

Duties

- Monitor and check stores operation.
- Train new and existing staff in Health & Safety, HACCP (hazard analysis critical and control point), etc.
- Chair of the Kitchen Health and Safety Committee.
- Develop new menus and concepts together with Senior Management.
- Schedule and roster all kitchen staff.
- Maintain accurate records of staff absences.
- Maintain accurate kitchen records.
- Responsible for the overall cleanliness of the kitchen operation.
- Assist in the production of management reports.
- Establish an effective and efficient team.
- Assist with the overall establishment and monitoring of budgets.

Conditions

- Grade 3 management spine.
- Private health insurance.
- 5-day week.
- 20 days' holiday.
- Profit-share scheme after one year's service.

Personal specification: Senior Sous Chef

- Qualifications
  (i) Level 3 Diploma
  (ii) Level 4 Culinary Arts degree desirable
- Experience
  (i) Five years' experience in 4- and 5-star hotel kitchens; restaurant and banqueting experience
- Skills
  (i) Proficiency in culinary arts
  (ii) Microsoft Excel, Access, Word
  (iii) Operation of inventory control software
  (iv) Written and oral communication skills
  (v) Team-building skills
- Knowledge
  (i) Current legislation in Health & Safety
  (ii) Food hygiene
  (iii) HACCP
  (iv) Risk assessment
  (v) Production systems
  (vi) Current technology
- Other attributes
  (i) Honesty
  (ii) Reliability
  (iii) Attention to detail
  (iv) Initiative
  (v) Accuracy
- Essential
  (i) Basic computer skills
  (ii) High degree of culinary skills
  (iii) Good communication skills
  (iv) Supervisory and leadership skills
- Desirable
  (i) Knowledge of employment law
  (ii) Public relations profile

monitoring the company is likely to carry out must also be disclosed to applicants.

Asylum and Immigration Act

It is an offence under the Asylum and Immigration Act 1996 to employ a foreign national subject to immigration control (i.e. who needs a visa or work permit, for example) who does not have the right to enter or remain in the UK, or to take up employment while in the UK. Job application forms should caution future employees that they will be required, if shortlisted, to produce documents confirming their right to be in, and to take up employment in, the UK.

Job interviews

The purpose of the job interview is to assess the suitability of a particular applicant for the vacancy. The interviewer should ask questions designed to test the applicant's suitability for the job, covering qualifications, training and experience, and to find out about the individual's personal qualities, character, development, motivation, strengths and weaknesses.

If a job applicant resigned or was dismissed from previous employment, the interviewer may need to know why. Any health problems, injuries and disabilities the candidate has disclosed may also need to be discussed in order to determine the applicant's suitability for employment – for example, in a high-risk working environment.

Employers may lawfully ask an applicant if he or she has been convicted of any criminal offence, but must be aware of the right of applicants, under the Rehabilitation of Offenders Act 1974, not to disclose details of any criminal convictions that have since become 'spent' (i.e. were so long ago that they have been dealt with and no longer count).

The interviewer should not ask questions about sexuality or religion. However, questions on religion may be asked if, for example, aspects of the job may directly affect the beliefs of an individual – an example would be the handling of alcoholic drinks or meat, such as pork.

Job offers

An offer of employment should be made or confirmed in writing, and is often conditional on the receipt of satisfactory references from former employers. Withdrawing an offer of employment once it has been accepted could result in a civil action for damages by the prospective employee.

Statutory Sick Pay

Employers in Great Britain are liable to pay up to 28 weeks' Statutory Sick Pay to any qualified employee who is unable to work because of illness of injury.

Employers who operate their own occupational sick pay schemes may opt out of the Statutory Sick Pay scheme, as long as the payments available to their employees under such schemes are equal to or greater than payments they would be entitled to under Statutory Sick Pay, and so long as these employees are not required to contribute towards the cost of funding such a scheme. Payments made under Statutory Sick Pay may be offset against contractual sick pay, and vice versa.

Working Time Regulations

The Working Time Regulations apply not only to employees but also to every worker (part-time, temporary, seasonal or casual) who undertakes to do work or carry out a service for an employer.

The 1998 Regulations are policed and enforced by employment tribunals (in relation to a worker's statutory rights to rest breaks, rest periods and paid annual holidays) and by local authority Environmental Health Officers.

What about qualifications?

The hospitality industry provides many opportunities to learn because of its complexity and diversity. There are many different sectors, trends and themes, and there are new developments all the time.

Qualifications show that a person has studied a subject successfully, and a certificate is usually awarded as proof of the qualification. Successfully achieving a qualification usually involves some sort

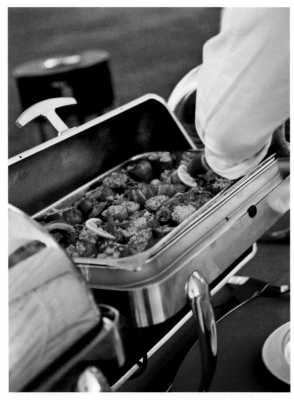

The Working Time Regulations apply to seasonal or part-time workers

of assessment, either in the form of examinations, coursework, observation by an assessor, or a combination of these things. The assessor decides whether the student had learned what they were supposed to and whether they have performed the skills to the required standard. Courses without assessment are not viewed very highly by potential employers.

Qualifications inform employers of what you should be able to do. They indicate to the employer whether you have the skills required to do the job. Qualifications differ all over the world and it is often difficult to make comparisons between qualifications in different countries. Even in the UK there are many different qualifications and that is why some employers ask job

applicants to do a practical test before they have an interview. Some employers ask chef applicants to do a trial day or more of work.

In spite of this, qualifications are important as they give you better career prospects and develop you personally. They help to boost your confidence and your self-esteem. There are a number of college-based courses that will help you to develop a range of practical skills and theoretical skills such as numeracy, language and information technology.

Apprenticeships are a way to learn skills within a workplace while also getting a qualification. Apprenticeship can be through a day-release course at college or may be completely work-based, where an assessor monitors the student's learning and development.

Whichever type of learning you choose, it is important to understand that learning is for life. In order to ensure that you have a job throughout your life you must continue to learn and develop your skills. You can improve your knowledge by reading hospitality journals, books and food magazines and by searching the internet for food sites. Find out how you learn best, and work at your own pace. Electronic learning (using CDs, DVDs and the internet) can help you to learn in the way that suits you best and to work at your own pace, testing yourself when you are ready to be tested. Assessment will help you to understand what you have achieved and what you must do to improve. It provides the building blocks for further learning and achievement.

 ACTIVITY

Give examples of statements in a job advertisement which could be deemed to be unlawful.

Test yourself • • • • • • • • • • • • • • •

1 How many people are employed in the UK hospitality industry?

2 Give three examples of hospitality outlets that would be included in the 'commercial sector.'

3 What is the maximum number of employees the business can have to be called a small- to medium-sized business enterprise?

4 Which type of businesses make up approximately 40 per cent of the commercial hospitality market?

5 Hospitality operations require a combination of two elements; what are they?

6 What type of hotel would have a five-star rating? Name two well-known five-star hotels.

7 What is meant by a hotel 'outsourcing'?

8 What are the main differences you would expect in food provision on a cruise liner and on a sea ferry?

9 Give four examples of public sector catering.

10 List six of the responsibilities of a Head chef in a four-star hotel.

• •

In this chapter you will learn how to:

1. understand how individuals can take personal responsibility for food safety including:

- food safety procedures, risk assessment, safe food handling
- reporting food safety hazards and legal responsibilities

2. understand the importance of keeping yourself clean and hygienic, including:

- the importance of personal hygiene in food safety, and effective personal hygiene practices

3. understand the importance of keeping the work areas clean and hygienic, including:

- safe use and storage of cleaning chemicals and materials, pest control and waste disposal
- how workflow, work surfaces and equipment can reduce contamination risks and aid cleaning

4. understand the importance of keeping food safe, including:

- the sources and risks to food safety from contamination and cross-contamination, and food spoilage
- safe food handling practices and procedures, temperature controls and stock control procedures.

The importance of food safety

Everyone consuming food prepared for them by others when they are away from home (e.g. in canteens, restaurants, etc.) has the right and expectation to be served safe food that will not cause illness or harm them in any way.

What is food safety?

Food safety means putting in place all of the measures needed to make sure that food and drinks are suitable, safe and wholesome through all of the processes of food provision, from selecting suppliers and delivery of food right through to serving the food to the customer.

Why is food safety important?

Eating 'contaminated' food can cause illness (food poisoning) and, in some cases, even death. The number of reported cases of food poisoning each year in England and Wales remains very high, between 70,000 and 94,000 reported cases each year. However, as a large number of food poisoning cases are not reported no one really knows the actual number.

Food poisoning is an illness of the digestive system that is the result of eating foods contaminated with pathogenic bacteria and/or their toxins. It can be an unpleasant illness for anyone, but it can be very serious or even fatal for some people. High-risk groups include:

- babies and very young children
- elderly people
- pregnant women
- those who are already unwell
- people with a repressed immune system.

It is therefore essential to take great care to prevent food poisoning, and The Food Standards Agency has committed to reducing the numbers of reported food poisoning cases significantly in the UK.

Food poisoning may also be caused by eating poisonous fish, plants or foods contaminated with chemicals, metal deposits or physical contaminants. Symptoms of food poisoning are often similar and may include:

- nausea
- vomiting
- diarrhoea
- fever
- dehydration.

Some people may also become ill after eating a food they are allergic to.

> **Digestive system:** The system in the body that processes food and turns it into energy. It is primarily the series of organs from the mouth to the anus including, for example, the stomach and intestines, through which food passes as it travels through the body before being excreted as waste. The liver and pancreas, which produce and store digestive chemicals, are also part of the digestive system.
>
> **Nausea:** A feeling of sickness with an urge to vomit.

 ACTIVITY

List the possible *disadvantages* a business may face if it *did not* have good food safety practices in place.

How is food contaminated?

There are four main ways that food can become contaminated:

- **Bacteria** are all around us in the environment – on raw food, on humans, animals, birds and insects. When bacteria multiply in food or use food to get into the human body they can make people ill.
- **Chemicals** can sometimes get into food accidentally and can make the consumer ill. The kinds of chemical that may get into food include cleaning fluids, disinfectants, machine oil, insecticides, pesticides etc.
- **Physical contamination** is caused when something gets into food that should not be there. This could be anything that a person should not eat, such as glass, pen tops, paperclips, blue plasters, hair, fingernails, etc.

- **Allergens** can cause allergic reactions. An allergy is when someone's immune system reacts to certain food (allergens). Allergic reactions can appear as swelling, itching, rashes, breathlessness and may even cause anaphylactic shock (a severe reaction often causing swelling of the throat and mouth that prevents breathing). **Food intolerance** is different and does not affect the immune system, but there may still be a reaction to some foods. Foods usually associated with allergies and food intolerances are nuts, dairy products, wheat-based products, eggs and shellfish.

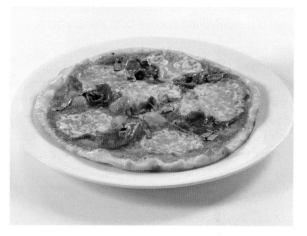

Some customers could be allergic to the cheese on this pizza, or intolerant of the gluten in the pizza base

All of these are potentially dangerous and great care must be taken to avoid contamination from any of them. However, the most dangerous of all is bacteria.

Poisoning from fish and vegetable items

Food poisoning can also be caused by poisons produced by some oily fish or shellfish, undercooked red or black kidney beans and items such as poisonous mushrooms, rhubarb leaves and daffodil bulbs.

Some moulds can produce dangerous toxins. Never risk using mouldy food. (Controlled mould such as in blue cheese is not dangerous.)

High-risk food

Some foods pose a greater risk to food safety than others; these are called high-risk foods. They are usually ready to eat, so do not need to be cooked to the high temperatures that would kill bacteria. They are moist, contain protein and need to be stored in the fridge or kept hot.

High-risk foods include:

- soups, stocks, sauces, gravies
- eggs and egg products
- milk and milk products
- cooked meat and fish, and meat and fish products
- any foods that need to be handled or reheated.

Bacteria and contamination

Not all bacteria are harmful. In fact, some are very useful and are used in foods and medicines. For example, the processes of making milk into yoghurt and making cheese both use bacteria.

The bacteria that are harmful are called 'pathogenic bacteria' (or 'pathogens') and can cause food poisoning. Bacteria are so small that you would need to use a microscope to see them – you cannot taste them or smell them on food. This is why pathogenic bacteria are so dangerous – you cannot tell when they are in food. If they have the right conditions (i.e. food, warmth, moisture and time) they can multiply approximately every 10–20 minutes by dividing in half. This is called binary fission.

Pathogenic bacteria can act in different ways to cause food poisoning. Bacteria may multiply in food until it is heated to very high temperatures, and will then cause infection when the food is eaten. Other pathogens use food to get into the body, where they then multiply. Some can produce toxins, while other can produce spores.

- As they multiply some pathogens produce **toxins** (poisons) that can survive boiling temperatures for half an hour or more. Because they are so heat resistant, the toxins are not killed by the normal cooking processes that kill bacteria, so remain in the food and can cause illness.
- Some bacteria produce toxins as they die, usually in the intestines of the person who has eaten the food.
- Others can produce **spores** to protect themselves. Bacteria form spores when

conditions surrounding them become hostile, for example, as temperatures rise, or in the presence of chemicals such as disinfectant. A spore forms a protective 'shell' inside the bacteria, protecting the essential parts from the high temperatures of normal cooking, disinfection, dehydration, etc. Once spores are formed the cells cannot divide and multiply as before but simply survive until conditions improve, for example the high temperatures drop to a level where multiplication can start again. Normal cooking temperatures will not kill spores.

- *Time* is crucial in preventing the formation of spores. If food is brought to cooking temperature slowly it allows time for spores to form. To avoid this, bring food to cooking temperature quickly and cool food quickly.

Some common food-poisoning bacteria

Salmonella

This used to be the most common cause of food poisoning in the UK, but since measures were put in place to reduce salmonella in chickens and eggs, food poisoning from this source has reduced. The main source of salmonella is the human and animal gut and excreta, but it is also carried by pests such as rodents, insects and birds, and in raw meat and poultry, eggs and shellfish. Salmonella poisoning can also be passed on through human carriers (someone carrying salmonella but not showing any signs of illness).

Staphylococcus aureus

The main source of this bacterium is the human body: on the skin, hair and scalp, nose and throat. Cuts, spots, burns and boils can also be a source of this organism. When it multiplies in food a toxin is produced which is very difficult to kill, even with boiling temperatures. To avoid food poisoning from this organism, food handlers need to maintain very high standards of personal hygiene. They should also tell their supervisor if they are ill, and not handle any food until the supervisor gives permission.

Clostridium perfringens

This is often present in raw meat, poultry and vegetables (also insects, soil, dust and sewage). It can also be passed on by humans, for example if they do not wash their hands properly after going to the toilet (it is present in human and animal faeces).

A number of incidents of *Clostridium perfringens* food poisoning have occurred when large amounts of meat have been heated slowly before cooking, then allowed to cool slowly before reheating it and using it later. *Clostridium perfringens* can produce spores during this heating and cooling process which are very resistant to further cooking and allow bacteria to survive in conditions that would usually kill them.

Bacillus cereus

This is another organism that can produce spores, and it can also produce toxins, so can be very dangerous. It is often associated with cooking rice in large quantities, cooling it too slowly and then reheating it. The temperatures the rice is reheated at are not high enough to destroy spores and toxins. It has also been linked with other cereal crops, spices, soil and vegetables.

Clostridium botulinum

Fortunately this type of bacterial infection is rare in this country. Symptoms can be very serious and even fatal. Sources tend to be soil, vegetables and the intestines of fish.

Other bacteria

Some bacteria cause food-borne illnesses but do not multiply in food. Instead, they use food to get into the human gut, where they then multiply and cause a range of illnesses, some of them serious, including severe abdominal pain, diarrhoea, vomiting, headaches, blurred vision, flu symptoms, septicaemia and miscarriage. These organisms may be transmitted from person to person, in water or through the air, as well as through food.

Food-borne pathogens include:

- *Campylobacter*, which now causes more food-related illness than any other organism. It is found in raw poultry and meat, sewage, animals, insects and birds.
- *E coli* 0157, which is present in the intestines and faeces of animals and humans. It is also found in raw meat and can be present on raw vegetables.

Septicaemia: Blood poisoning. It occurs when an infection in the bloodstream causes the body's immune system to begin attacking the body itself.

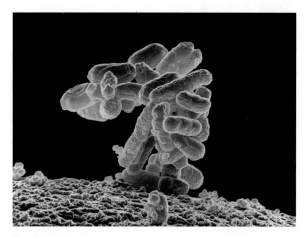

E coli bacteria

- Listeria, which is of particular concern because it can multiply slowly at fridge temperatures (i.e. below 5°C). It has been linked with such chilled products as unpasteurised cheeses, pâté and prepared salads as well as cook/chill meals (ready-prepared meals, which are cooked and then chilled ready for reheating).

- Norovirus which, like all viruses, will not multiply on food but may live for a short time on surfaces, utensils and food, and use these to get into the body. The most usual ways this is spread are through the air, from person to person, in water or sewage.

ACTIVITY

Answer 'true' or 'false' to the following questions about bacteria.

1 All bacteria produce spores.

2 Some bacteria are harmless and can be useful.

3 A pathogen is a bacterium that causes illness.

4 All toxins are killed by heating food to 70°C.

5 Salmonella could be found in the human gut.

6 Bacillus cereus has caused food poisoning through cooked rice.

7 Staphylococcus can be passed on to food by not covering a cut on your hand.

8 You can tell if a food has pathogens on it because it smells 'off'.

9 Under ideal conditions bacteria can multiply every 20 hours.

10 Bacteria need help to move from one area of the kitchen to another.

11 Bacteria will be killed by the low temperatures in freezers.

12 Bacteria need moisture to reproduce.

13 In the UK there are more reported cases of food poisoning from Campylobacter than any other pathogen.

14 The source of pathogenic bacteria is always raw meat.

15 It doesn't matter if you don't wash your hands before handling food because bacteria will be killed by heat when the food is cooked.

Personal hygiene

Because humans are a source of food poisoning bacteria it is very important for all food handlers to take care with personal hygiene and to adopt good practices when working with food.

- Arrive at work clean (bathe or shower daily) and with clean hair.
- Wear approved, clean kitchen clothing and only wear it in the kitchen. This must completely cover any personal clothing.
- Keep your hair neatly contained in a suitable hat/hairnet.
- Keep your nails short and clean and do not wear nail varnish or false nails.
- Do not wear jewellery or watches when handling food (a plain wedding band is permissible but could still trap bacteria).

- Avoid wearing cosmetics and strong perfumes.
- Smoking must not be allowed in food preparation areas (ash, smoke and bacteria from touching the mouth area could get into food).
- Do not eat food or sweets or chew gum when handling food as this may also transfer bacteria to food.
- Cover any cuts, burns or grazes with a blue waterproof dressing, then wash your hands.
- Report any illness to the supervisor as soon as possible. For example, you should report diarrhoea and/or vomiting (NB: you must not handle food until at least 48 hours after the last symptom), infected cuts, burns or spots, bad cold or flu symptoms or if you were ill while on holiday.

Hand washing

Hands are constantly in use in the kitchen and will be touching numerous materials, foods, surfaces and equipment. Contamination from hands can happen very easily and you must take care with hand washing to avoid this.

- A basin must be provided that is used only for hand washing. Make sure that you use this.
- Wet your hands under warm running water.
- Apply liquid soap.
- Rub your hands together, and rub one hand with the fingers and thumb of the other.
- Remember to include your fingertips, nails and wrists.
- Rinse off the soap under the warm running water.
- Dry your hands on a paper towel and use the paper towel to turn off the tap before throwing it away.

You should always wash your hands:

- when you enter the kitchen, before starting work and handling any food
- after a break (particularly if you have used the toilet)
- between different tasks, but especially between handling raw and cooked food
- if you touch hair, nose, mouth or use a tissue for a sneeze or cough
- after you apply or change a dressing on a cut or burn
- after cleaning preparation areas, equipment or contaminated surfaces
- after handling kitchen waste, external food packaging, money or flowers.

Cross-contamination

Cross-contamination is when bacteria are transferred from contaminated food (usually raw food), equipment or surfaces to ready-to-eat food. It is the cause of significant amounts of food poisoning and care must be taken to avoid it. Cross-contamination could be caused by:

- foods touching each other, e.g. raw and cooked meat
- raw meat or poultry dripping onto high-risk foods
- soil from dirty vegetables coming into contact with high-risk foods
- dirty cloths or dirty equipment
- equipment (e.g. chopping boards or knives) used with raw food and then used with cooked food
- hands touching raw food and then cooked food, without being washed between tasks
- pests spreading bacteria from their own bodies around the kitchen.

Controlling cross-contamination

Sources of bacteria (where they come from) include raw meat and poultry, pests, dirty vegetables and unwashed hands. Cross-contamination can be avoided by following hygienic working practices and storing, preparing and cooking food safely.

- Separate working areas and storage areas for raw and high-risk foods are strongly recommended. If this is not possible, keep them well away from each other and make sure that working areas are thoroughly cleaned and disinfected between tasks.
- Vegetables should be washed before preparation/peeling and again afterwards. Leafy vegetables may need to be washed in several changes of cold water to remove all of the soil clinging to them.
- Good personal hygiene practices by staff, especially frequent and effective hand washing, are very important in controlling cross-contamination and will avoid the significant amounts of contamination caused by faecal/

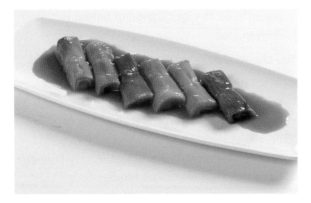

Vegetables like these leeks must be washed, several times if necessary, before they are prepared and cooked – this is to remove any soil and bacteria that are present on the raw leeks

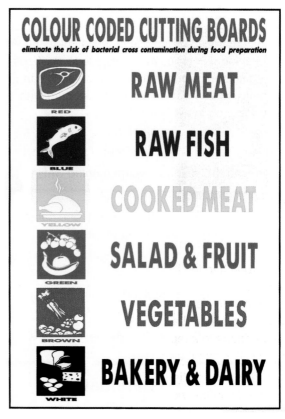

oral routes (when pathogens normally found in faeces are transferred to ready-to-eat foods, resulting in cross-contamination and illness). An obvious way that this may happen is when food handlers visit the toilet, do not wash their hands and then handle food.

- Avoid over-handling food, use spoons, slices, ladles and, where appropriate, disposable gloves (but change these frequently, especially between tasks).

Colour-coding equipment

Colour-coded chopping boards are a good way to keep different types of food separate. Worktops and chopping boards will come into contact with the food being prepared, so need special attention. Make sure that chopping boards are

in good condition – cracks and splits could trap bacteria which could be transferred to food.

As well as colour-coded chopping boards, some kitchens also provide colour coded-knives, cloths, cleaning equipment, storage trays, bowls and even staff uniforms to help prevent cross-contamination.

 ACTIVITY

Which colour-coded chopping board would you select to prepare each of these foods?

- Potatoes – peeling, cutting
- Cooked ham – slicing
- Bread – removing crusts
- Raw chicken – cutting, trimming
- Fresh herbs – chopping
- Raw haddock – skinning, trimming
- Sponge cake – cutting
- Fresh tomatoes – chopping

- Raw beef – cutting for stewing
- Cooked savoury flans – cutting
- Onions – chopping
- Choux pastries – cutting open
- Shredding lettuce
- Cooked smoked mackerel
- Fruit – preparing for fruit salad
- Cheese – cutting for sandwiches

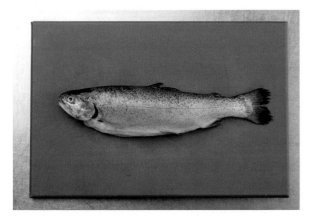

Cleaning and sanitising

As a food handler it is your responsibility, along with those working with you, to keep food areas clean and hygienic at all times. Clean and tidy as you go and do not allow waste to build up. It is very difficult to keep untidy areas clean. Clean up any spills straight away.

- Clean and sanitise worktops and chopping boards before working on them, and do this again after use, paying particular attention when they have been used for raw foods. Chopping boards can be disinfected after use by putting them through a dishwasher with a high rinse temperature of 82°C.

- Small equipment, such as knives, bowls, spoons, tongs, etc. can also cause cross-contamination. It is important to wash them thoroughly (once again a dishwasher does this well), especially when they are used for a variety of food and for raw foods.

- Take great care with kitchen cloths – they are a perfect growing area for bacteria. Different cloths for different areas will help to reduce cross-contamination and it is certainly good practice to use different cloths for raw food and cooked food preparation. Using disposable kitchen towel is the most hygienic way to clean food areas.

- Also take great care with tea towels, if they are used. Remember that they can easily spread bacteria, so do not use them as 'all-purpose' cloths and do not keep one on your shoulder (the cloth may touch your neck and hair and these can be sources of bacteria).

- In the same way as you can limit cross-contamination, you can help to control the spread and growth of bacteria by having good working practices. You need to protect food from bacteria and prevent bacterial growth by keeping it clean and covered.

- It is also important to clean fridges regularly and thoroughly (see page 39).

Cross-contamination and multiplication of bacteria

Here is an example of how quickly cross-contamination can spread bacteria.

Table 2.1

Time		Number of bacteria
10.00	A chicken has been cooked to 75°C and left in the kitchen, uncovered, to cool. No bacteria have survived.	0
10.20	Chef uses a dirty cloth to transfer chicken to a plate	6000
10.40	Bacteria start to multiply	12,000
10.40	and multiply	24,000
11am	and multiply	48,000
11.20	and multiply	96,000
11.40	and multiply	192,000
12 noon	and multiply	384,000
12.20	and multiply	768,000
12.40	and multiply	1.5 million
1pm	Probably enough to cause food poisoning	3 million

From one careless action with a dirty cloth, 6000 bacteria (pathogens) have multiplied to 3 million in 2 hours 40 minutes. One million pathogens per gram of food is enough to cause food poisoning.

The importance of temperature

Controlling bacteria

An important way of controlling bacteria is to ensure that food is kept in controlled temperatures as much as possible.

Temperatures between 5°C and 63°C are called the **danger zone** because it is possible for bacteria to multiply between these temperatures, with most rapid multiplication at around body temperature (37°C). Keep food held for service above 63°C, or cool it rapidly and keep it below 5°C.

Thorough cooking is one of the best methods available to control bacteria. Cooking to 75°C and holding that temperature for at least 2 minutes will kill most pathogens (but not spores and toxins).

Never put hot or warm food into a fridge or freezer as this will raise the temperature in the fridge or freezer and put food into the danger zone.

Temperature probes

Electronic temperature probes are very useful to measure the temperature in the centre of both hot and cold food. They are also good for recording the temperature of deliveries and checking food temperatures in fridges. Make sure the probe is clean and disinfected before use (disposable disinfectant wipes are useful for this). Place the probe into the centre of the food, making sure it is not touching bone or the cooking container. Check regularly that probes are working correctly

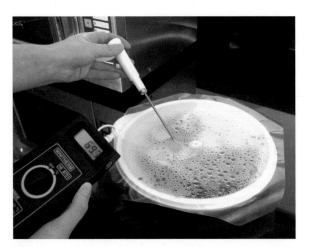

(calibration). This can be done electronically, but a simple and low-cost check is to place the probe in iced water – the reading should be between −1°C and +1°C. To check accuracy at high temperatures, place the probe in boiling water and the reading should be between 99°C and 100°C. If probes read outside of these temperatures they need to be repaired or replaced.

Using heat

The use of heat to make foods safe and to preserve it is one of the most useful procedures available to those involved in food production and manufacture. The following shows some commonly used temperatures.

Cooking
Cooked food generally keeps for longer than raw food. However, treat cooked items with care as, once cooked, foods move into the 'high-risk' category. Normal cooking (i.e. to 75°C for 2 minutes at the core of the food) will kill most pathogens, but not spores and toxins.
Pasteurisation
This involves heating food to a temperature similar to cooking temperatures but for a very short time (e.g. milk is heated to 72°C for 15 seconds), and then rapidly cooling it. These temperatures will kill most pathogens, bringing them to a 'safe level'. Toxins and spores will not be killed.
Sterilisation
The sterilisation of milk and other food items destroys all micro-organisms. Sterilisation involves heating to 100°C for 15–30 minutes by applying steam and pressure.
UHT
UHT or Ultra Heat Treatment gives milk a long shelf life without the need for refrigeration. The milk is heated under pressure to very high temperatures (135°C). UHT is also used for cream.
Canning
Canning processes use very high temperatures to make sure the food is safe from all micro-organisms, toxins and spores. The typical time/temperature used is 121°C for 3 minutes.

Cooking

Cooking food to a core temperature of 75°C for 2 minutes will kill most bacteria. These temperatures are especially important where large amounts are being cooked or the consumers are in the high-risk categories (see page 28). However, some popular dishes on hotel and restaurant menus are cooked to a lower temperature than this, according to individual dish and customer requirements.

Cooked food being held for service must be kept above 63°C (or below 5°C if chilled). If food is being cooled to serve cold or to reheat at a later time, it must be protected from contamination and cooled quickly to 8°C – within 90 minutes of being cooked. The best way to do this is in a blast chiller.

Any food that is to be chilled or frozen must be well wrapped or placed in a suitable container with a lid, or may be vacuum packed. Make sure that all food is labelled and dated before chilling or freezing.

Handling cold food

- Where possible, use plastic gloves when handling food.
- Keep all food (unprepared and prepared) refrigerated at a temperature no higher than 4–5°C. Refrigeration will not kill the bacteria that are present in the foods, but does help to prevent them from growing.
- Whenever possible, the food on display to the public should be kept under refrigeration and the temperature should be checked to ensure that it is being maintained at a safe level.

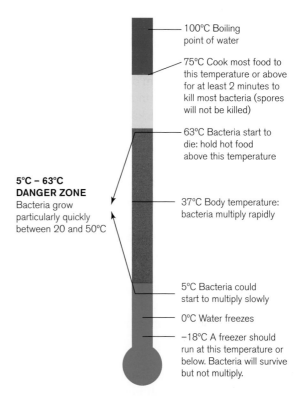

5°C – 63°C
DANGER ZONE
Bacteria grow particularly quickly between 20 and 50°C

100°C Boiling point of water

75°C Cook most food to this temperature or above for at least 2 minutes to kill most bacteria (spores will not be killed)

63°C Bacteria start to die: hold hot food above this temperature

37°C Body temperature: bacteria multiply rapidly

5°C Bacteria could start to multiply slowly

0°C Water freezes

−18°C A freezer should run at this temperature or below. Bacteria will survive but not multiply.

Important food safety temperatures

- Where customers can look at the food and are going to be close to it, ideally it should be displayed behind a sneeze screen.
- Dishes prepared in advance should be covered with film and refrigerated at 1–3°C to prevent them drying out.
- When working with cold foods, the highest standards of personal, food and equipment hygiene must be maintained.

Food deliveries and storage

For food to remain in the best condition and be safe to eat, it is essential that it is stored correctly. This should be planned and the procedures fully understood by kitchen staff. Only approved suppliers who can assure that food is delivered in the best condition should be used. Food must be delivered in suitable packaging, properly date coded and at the correct temperature.

- All deliveries should be checked and then moved to the appropriate storage area as soon

as possible. Chilled/frozen food should be put away in storage within 15 minutes of delivery.

- Use a food probe to check the temperature of food deliveries: chilled food should be below 5°C (reject it if it is above 8°C); frozen foods should be at or below −18°C (reject it if it is above −15°C). Record these temperatures.
- Many suppliers will now provide a printout of temperatures at which food is delivered.

- Dry goods should be in undamaged packaging, well within 'best before' dates, completely dry and in perfect condition on delivery.
- Remove food items from outer boxes before placing the products in fridge, freezer or dry store. Remove outer packaging carefully, looking out for any possible pests that may have found their way in.

Raw meat and poultry

Wherever possible, store in fridges that are used only for meat and poultry, running at temperatures between 0°C and 2°C. If not already packaged, place on trays, cover well with cling film and label. If it is necessary to store meat/poultry in a multiuse fridge, make sure it is covered, labelled and placed at the bottom of a fridge running below 5°C, well away from other items.

Fish

A specific fish fridge is preferable (running at 1°C to 2°C). Remove fresh fish from ice containers and place on trays, cover well with cling film and label. If it is necessary to store fish in a multiuse fridge, make sure it is well covered, labelled and placed at the bottom of the fridge well away from other items. Remember that odours from fish can get into other items such as milk and eggs.

Dairy products/eggs

Pasteurised milk and cream, eggs and cheese should be stored in their original containers at a temperature between 1–4°C. Sterilised or UHT milk can be kept in the dry store, following the storage instructions on the label. After delivery, eggs should be stored at a constant temperature and a fridge is the best place to store them. Prevent eggs touching other items in the fridge.

Frozen foods

Store in a freezer running at −18°C or below. Separate raw foods from ready-to-eat foods and never allow food to be re-frozen once it has thawed.

If you need to **defrost** frozen food, place it in a deep tray, cover with film and label it, including the date when defrosting was started. Place it at the bottom of the fridge where thawing liquid cannot drip onto anything else. Defrost food completely (there should be no ice crystals on any part), then cook thoroughly within 12 hours. Make sure that you allow enough time for this process – it may take longer than you think! (A 2 kg chicken will take about 24 hours to defrost at 3°C.)

Fruit, vegetables and salad items

Storage conditions will vary according to type, for example, sacks of potatoes, root vegetables and some fruit can be stored in a cool, well-ventilated storeroom but salad items, green vegetables, soft fruit and tropical fruit would be better in refrigerated storage. If possible, a specific fridge running at around 8°C would be ideal to avoid any chill damage.

Dry goods

Items such as rice, dried pasta, sugar, flour, grains, etc. should be kept in clean, covered containers on wheels, or in smaller sealed containers on shelves to stop pests getting into them. Storage should be in a cool, well-ventilated dry store area and well-managed stock rotation is essential. Retain packaging information as this may include essential allergy advice.

Canned products

Cans are usually stored in the dry store area, and once again rotation of stock is essential. Canned food will carry 'best before' dates and it is not advisable to use them after this date. 'Blown' (burst or swollen) cans must never be used, and do not use badly dented or rusty cans. Once opened, transfer any unused canned food to a clean bowl, cover and label it, and store in the fridge for up to 2 days.

Cooked foods

These include a wide range of foods, for example, pies, paté, cream cakes, desserts and savoury flans. They will usually be 'high-risk' foods, so correct storage is essential. For specific storage instructions see the labelling on the individual items, but generally, keep items below 5°C. Store carefully, wrapped and labelled and well away from and above raw foods, to avoid any cross-contamination.

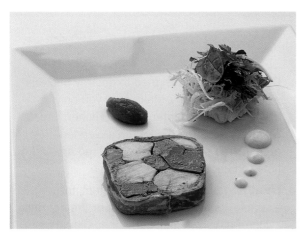

Cooked food, like this terrine, must be stored correctly

Storing food in a multiuse fridge

- Keep the fridge running at 1°C to 4°C.
- All food must be covered and labelled with name of the item and the date.
- Always store raw food at the bottom of the fridge, with other items above.
- Keep high-risk foods well away from raw foods.
- Never overload the fridge – to operate properly, cold air must be allowed to circulate between items.
- Wrap strong-smelling foods very well as the smell (and taste) can transfer to other foods such as milk.
- Record the temperature at which the fridge is operating. Do this at least once a day (this is an example of monitoring) and keep the fridge temperatures with other kitchen records.

Clean fridges regularly.

- Remove food to another fridge
- Clean according to cleaning schedule using a recommended sanitiser, (a solution of bicarbonate of soda and water is also good for cleaning fridges)
- Remember to empty and clean any drip trays, and clean door seals thoroughly
- Rinse then dry with kitchen paper
- Make sure the fridge front and handle is cleaned and disinfected to avoid cross contamination
- Make sure the fridge is down to temperature, 1°C-4°C, before replacing the food in the

 ACTIVITY

You have been asked to put away a chilled food delivery in a multiuse fridge. Show, in the grid below, where you would position the different foods.

The items in the delivery are: raw chicken, cooked ham, cream, salmon fillets, cooked vegetable quiche, eggs, cheese, sponge cakes filled with cream, pate, raw prawns, fresh pasta, rump steak, yoghurt, milk, sausages, butter, frozen chicken drumsticks that need to be defrosted for use tomorrow.

Four-shelf fridge:

Shelf 1
Shelf 2
Shelf 3
Shelf 4

proper positions (see above). Check dates and condition of all food before replacing.

'First in – first out'

This term is used to describe stock rotation, and is applied to all categories of food. It simply means that foods already in storage are used before new deliveries (providing stock is still within recommended dates and in sound condition). Food deliveries should be labelled with delivery date and preferably the date by which they should be used. Use this information along with food labelling codes (see below). Written stock records should form a part of a 'food safety management system'.

Food labelling codes

Use by dates appear on perishable foods with a short life. Legally, the food must be used by this date and not stored or used after it.

Best before dates apply to foods that are expected to have a longer life, for example, dry products or canned food. A 'best before' date advises that food is at its best before this date; using it after this date is legal but not advised.

Cleaning

Clean food areas play an essential part in the production of safe food and the team must plan, record and check all cleaning as part of a 'cleaning schedule'. Clean premises, work areas and equipment are important to:

- control the bacteria that cause food poisoning
- reduce the possibility of physical and chemical contamination
- make accidents (e.g. slips on a greasy floor) less likely
- create a positive image for customers, visitors and employees
- comply with the law
- avoid attracting pests to the kitchen.

The cleaning schedule needs to include the following information:

- **What** is to be cleaned.
- **Who** should do it (name if possible).
- **How** it is to be done and how long it should take.
- **When it is to be done**, i.e. time of day.
- **Materials** to be used, including chemicals and their dilution, cleaning equipment and protective clothing to be worn.
- **Safety** precautions that must be taken.
- **Signatures** of the cleaner and the supervisor checking the work, along with the date and time.

Cleaning products

There are different cleaning products for different tasks.

- **Detergent** is designed to remove grease and dirt. It may be in the form of liquid, powder, gel or foam and usually needs to be added to water. It will not kill pathogens (bacteria), although the hot water. It is mixed with may help to do this. Detergent will clean and degrease surfaces so that disinfectant can work properly. Detergents usually work best with hot water.

- **Disinfectant** is designed to destroy bacteria when used properly. Make sure you only use a disinfectant intended for kitchen use. Disinfectants must be left on a cleaned grease-free surface for the required amount of time (contact time) to be effective.
- **Heat** may also be used to disinfect, for example, using steam cleaners or the hot rinse cycle of a dishwasher. Items that should be both cleaned and disinfected include all items in direct contact with food, all hand contact surfaces, hand wash basins and cleaning equipment.
- **Sanitiser** cleans and disinfects. It usually comes in spray form. Sanitiser is very useful for work surfaces and equipment, especially when cleaning them between tasks.

Cleaning kitchen surfaces

One of the following two methods is recommended for cleaning a kitchen surface.

Six-stage method

1. Remove debris and loose particles.
2. Carry out main clean using detergent to remove soiling grease.
3. Rinse using clean hot water and a cloth to remove detergent.
4. Apply disinfectant and leave for contact time recommended on container.
5. Rinse off the disinfectant if recommended.
6. Allow to air dry or use kitchen paper.

Four-stage method

1. Remove debris and loose particles.
2. Carry out main clean using hot water and sanitiser.
3. Rinse using clean hot water and a cloth, if recommended on instructions
4. Allow to air dry or use kitchen paper.

ACTIVITY

Draw up a grid like Table 2.2, with items or surfaces from a kitchen you are familiar with.

Table 2.2

Surface/ item	When cleaned	Equipment/ chemicals	PPE	Safety measures	Method of cleaning	Cleaned by: (name)	Date/ time	Cleaning checked by: (name)
Solid stove tops (3) in main kitchen area 15 minutes for each solid top = 45 minutes	Daily at 6.30 a.m. before stoves are switched on	*Commercial Clean Ltd* stove-top cleaner + stove-top finisher Hot water – bucket Thick blue cleaning cloths Scraper Kitchen paper	Long-sleeved jacket Full apron Industrial gauntlet gloves Mask	Do not clean until 90 minutes after the solid top is switched off	Scrape off debris with scraper Wipe over with hot water and thick blue cloth Wash out the cloth in clean water Apply cleaning solution and leave for 2 minutes. Remove excess with kitchen paper. Rinse with clean water and dry with kitchen paper. Apply stove-top finisher and allow to air dry			
Bench in delivery area	After main morning deliveries, 10 a.m. approx.	Hot water – bucket Cleaning cloths *H 100 Sanitiser* spray Kitchen paper	Kitchen porter uniform Apron Rubber gloves	Wet floor sign Make sure surrounding area is dry when finished If boxes are removed from surface do not place on the floor	Remove any delivery boxes, etc. from surface Remove any small particles Wipe surface with hot water and cloth Spray evenly with *H 100 Sanitiser* (including sides and legs) Leave sanitiser in place for 1 minute contact time Rinse off with clean hot water Dry with kitchen paper			

ACTIVITY

Tick the items in Table 2.3 that you think should be both cleaned *and* disinfected.

Table 2.3

Item	Clean only	Clean and disinfect	Item	Clean only	Clean and disinfect
Cutlery			Staff lockers		
Milk cartons for recycling			Red chopping boards		
Delivery area floor			Fridge door handle		
Grater			Inside of deep fryer		
Food containers from a hot counter			Dishcloths		
Nailbrushes			Door frames		

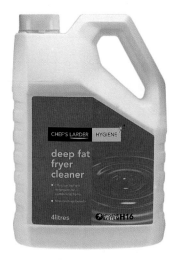

Dishwashing

Using a dishwashing machine

The most efficient and hygienic method of cleaning dishes and crockery is to use a dishwashing machine, as this will clean and disinfect items that will then air dry, removing the need for cloths. The dishwasher can also be used to clean/disinfect small equipment such as chopping boards. The stages in machine dishwashing are:

● Remove waste food.

● Pre-rinse or spray.

● Load onto the appropriate racks with a space between each item.

The wash cycle will run at 50°C to 60°C using a detergent. The rinse cycle will run at 82°C to 88°C and will disinfect items ready for air drying.

Dishwashing by hand

If items need to be washed by hand, the recommended way to do this is:

Scrape/rinse off residual food.

Wash items in a sink of hot water; the temperature should be 50°C to 60°C, which means rubber gloves will need to be worn. Use a dishwashing brush rather than a cloth – the brush will help to loosen food particles and is not such a good breeding ground for bacteria.

Rinse in very hot water – if rinsing can be done at 82°C for 30 seconds this will disinfect the dishes.

Allow to air dry; do not use tea towels.

Beware! Cleaning is essential to prevent health hazards, but if it is not managed properly it can become a hazard in itself. Do not store cleaning chemicals in food preparation and cooking areas, and take care with their use (avoid chemical contamination). Make sure that items such as cloths, paper towels and fibres from mops do not get into open food (avoid physical contamination). To avoid bacterial contamination, do not use the same cleaning cloths and equipment in raw food areas and high-risk food areas.

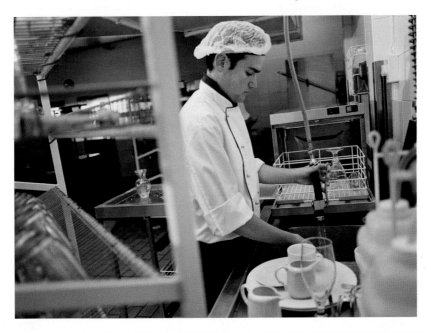

Pests

When there are reports of food premises being forcibly closed down, an infestation of pests is often the reason. As pests can be a serious source of contamination and disease, having them near food cannot be allowed and is against the law. Pests can carry food poisoning bacteria into food premises in their fur/feathers, feet/paws, saliva, urine and droppings. Other problems caused by pests include damage to food stocks and packaging, damage to buildings, equipment and wiring, blockages in equipment and piping.

Pests can be attracted to premises by food, warmth, shelter, water and possible nesting materials (e.g. cardboard boxes, packing materials). Everything must be done to keep them out. Any suspicion that pests may be present must be reported to the supervisor or manager immediately.

Common pests that may cause problems in food areas are rats, mice, cockroaches, wasps, flies, ants (pharaoh ants), birds and domestic pets. Measures to keep pests out of the building are important and need to be planned as part of food safety management. Pest control contractors can offer advice on keeping pests out and organise eradication systems for any pests that do get in.

Eradication: To remove or destroy completely.

Flying insects cause problems as they can find their way in through very small spaces, or from other parts of the building. They can then spread significant amounts of bacteria around the kitchen and onto open food. To eliminate flies, bluebottles, wasps etc an electronic fly killer is recommended (EFK). These use ultraviolet light to attract the insects that are then electrocuted on charged wires and fall into catch trays. Do not position EFK directly above food preparation areas and make sure the catch trays are emptied regularly.

Beware! Pest control measures can also introduce food safety hazards. The bodies of dead insects or even rodents may remain in the kitchen (causing physical and bacterial contamination). Pesticides, insecticides and baits could cause chemical contamination if not managed properly. Pest control is best managed by professionals.

Table 2.4 Signs of pest presence and how to keep them out

Pest	Signs that they are present	Ways to keep them out/ eliminate
Rats and mice	Sightings of rodent or droppings; gnawed wires; greasy marks on lower walls; damaged food stock; paw prints; unpleasant smell.	Block entry, e.g. no holes around pipe work. Fill all gaps and cavities where they could get in. Use sealed drain covers.
Flies and wasps	Sightings of flies and wasps; hearing them, sightings of dead insects; sightings of maggots.	Damage to the building or fixtures and fittings should be repaired quickly. Use window/door screening/netting.
Cockroaches	Sighting (dead or alive) usually at night. Unpleasant smell.	Check deliveries/packaging for pests.
Ants	Sightings, including in food. The tiny, pale coloured Pharaoh ants are difficult to spot but can still be the source of a variety of pathogens.	Use baits and traps. Use electronic Fly killer. Use sealed containers and ensure no open food is left out.
Weevils	Sightings of weevils in stored products, e.g. flour/cornflour. They are tiny black insects that are very difficult to see but can be spotted by their movement in flour, etc.	Do not allow build up of waste in kitchen. Do not keep outside waste too close to the kitchen.
Birds	Sighting; droppings in outside storage areas and around refuse.	**Arrange professional and organised pest management control, surveys and reports.**
Domestic pets	These must be kept out of food areas as they carry pathogens in fur, whiskers, saliva, urine, etc.	

Premises

Suitable buildings with well-planned fittings, layout and equipment allow for good food safety practices. Certain basics need to be available if a building is to be used for food production. There must be:

- electricity supplies and preferably gas supplies
- drinking water and good drainage
- suitable road access for deliveries and refuse collection
- no risk of contamination from surrounding areas and buildings, for example, chemicals, smoke, odours or dust.

Layout

- When planning food premises, a linear workflow should be in place, for example: **delivery → storage → preparation → cooking → hot holding → serving**. This means there will be no crossover of activities that could result in cross-contamination.

- There must be adequate storage areas – proper refrigerated storage is especially important.
- Staff hand washing/drying facilities suitable for the work being carried out must be provided.
- Clean and dirty (raw and cooked) processes should be kept apart.
- Cleaning and disinfection should be planned with separate storage for cleaning materials and chemicals.
- All areas should allow for good cleaning, disinfection and pest control.
- Personal hygiene facilities must be provided for staff, as well as changing facilities and storage for personal clothing and belongings.

Lighting and ventilation

Lighting (natural and artificial) must be sufficient and correctly placed for the tasks being carried out and for safe working. It must also allow for cleaning to be carried out efficiently.

Good ventilation is essential to prevent excessive heat, condensation, circulation of airborne contaminants, grease vapours and odours.

Drainage

Drainage must be adequate for the work to be carried out without causing flooding. If channels, grease traps and gullies are used they should allow for frequent and easy cleaning.

Floors

These need to be durable and in good condition; they must be impervious (not allow liquids to soak through them), non-slip and easy to clean. Suitable materials are non-slip quarry tiles, epoxy resins, industrial vinyl sheeting and granolithic flooring. Where the materials allow, edges between floor and walls should be coved (curved) to prevent debris collecting in corners.

Walls

Walls need to be non-porous, smooth, easy to clean and preferably light in colour. Suitable wall coverings are plastic cladding, stainless steel sheeting, ceramic tiles, epoxy resin or rubberised painted plaster or brickwork. Walls should be coved where they join the floor. Lagging and ducting around pipes should be sealed, and gaps sealed where pipes enter the building, to stop pests getting in.

Ceilings

Ceiling finishes must resist any build up of condensation which encourages mould. They should be of non-flaking material and washable. Non-porous ceiling panels and tiles are often used, and non-flaking paints are useful. Once again, edges should be coved where possible.

> **Non-porous:** With no pores or tiny holes, which means that air, water and other fluids cannot get through. Glass and steel are examples of non-porous materials.

Windows and doors

These provide possibilities for pests to enter the building, so should be fitted with suitable screening, strip-curtains, metal kick plates, etc. Doors and windows should fit well into their frames to prevent draughts and pests getting in.

Kitchen waste

This should be placed in waste bins with lids (preferably foot operated). Bins should be made of a strong material, be easy to clean and be pest proof. They should be emptied regularly to avoid waste build up, as this could cause problems with multiplication of bacteria and could attract pests. An overfull heavy bin is also much more difficult to handle than a regularly emptied bin.

Food safety management systems

It is good practice for all food businesses to have a food safety management system in place. In line with the Food Standards Agency's commitment to reduce food poisoning cases, it became a legal requirement from January 2006 for all foods businesses to operate such a system. When Environmental Health Officers/Practitioners inspect the premises of these businesses they will also check that food safety management systems are in place and are working well.

Hazard Analysis Critical Control Point (HACCP)

All systems must be based on the Hazard Analysis Critical Control Point (HACCP). This is an internationally recognised food safety management system that aims to identify the hazards that could occur at the critical points or stages in any process. The system must provide a documented record of the stages *all* food will go through right up to the time it is eaten and may include:

- purchase and delivery
- receipt of food

- storage
- preparation
- cooking
- cooling
- hot holding
- reheating
- chilled storage
- serving.

Once the hazards have been identified, measures are put in place to control the hazards and keep the food safe.

The HACCP system involves seven stages:

1. Identify hazards – what could go wrong.
2. Identify CCP (critical control points), i.e. the important points where things could go wrong.
3. Set critical limits for each CCP, e.g. the temperature that fresh chicken should be at when it is delivered.
4. Monitor CCPs and put checks in place to stop problems from occurring.
5. Identify corrective action – what will be done if something goes wrong.
6. Verification – check that the HACCP plan is working.
7. Documentation – record all of the above.

The system must be updated regularly, especially when the menu or systems change (e.g. a new piece of equipment is brought into the kitchen). Specific new controls must be put in place to include any changes. An example would be, when dealing with the roasting of pork loins, it is necessary to recognise the possible hazards at all of the identified stages.

Cooking fresh roast pork:

- Hazard – pathogens are likely to be present in raw meat.
- Control – the pork needs to be cooked thoroughly to 75°C+ to ensure pathogens are killed.
- Monitor – check the temperature right in the centre of the joint with a calibrated temperature probe; make sure the juices are running clear, not red or pink.
- Hot holding – before service the pork must be kept above 63°C; this can be checked with a temperature probe.
- Or chill and refrigerate – chill to below 8°C within 90 minutes. Cover, label and refrigerate below 5°C.
- Documentation – measure and record temperatures. Check hot holding equipment and record temperature. Record any corrective measures necessary.

For the cold storage/chilling of the cooked pork:

- Hazard – cross-contamination; multiplication of pathogens in the cooked meat.
- Control – protect from cross-contamination while cooling; store below 5°C.
- Monitor – check that the temperature of the pork is below 5°C and that the fridge is running below 5°C.
- Corrective action – if the pork has been above 8°C for two hours or more it should be thrown away.
- Documentation – record temperatures at least once a day and record any corrective action.

 ACTIVITY

You may like to complete this activity in pairs or as a group.

- A busy hotel/restaurant buys in 40 fresh chickens. The chicken breasts are removed and bread crumbed; these will be deep fried to order.
- The drumsticks are roasted and will be served cold on a buffet.

- The thighs are made into a chicken curry; this will be chilled, reheated the next day and then kept hot on a hot buffet counter.

Look at the possible hazards at each of the stages in table 2.5 and find suitable control measures to ensure that the chicken is safe for the consumers.

Table 2.5

	Possible hazards	**Controls**
Purchase, delivery, unloading		
Storage		
Preparation		
Cooking		
Hot holding		
Cooling		
Cold storage		
Reheating		
Serving		

'Safer food, better business' and 'CookSafe'

The HACCP system described above may seem complicated and difficult to set up for a small business. With this in mind, the Food Standards Agency launched its 'Safer food, better business' system for England and Wales. This is based on the principles of HACCP but is in a format that is easy to understand, with pre-printed pages and charts in which to enter the relevant information, such as temperatures for individual dishes. It is divided into two parts.

- The first part is about safe methods (e.g. avoiding cross-contamination, personal hygiene, cleaning, chilling and cooking).
- The second part covers opening and closing checks. These are checks that procedures are in place (e.g. safe methods, recording of safe methods, training records, supervision, stock control and the selection of suppliers and

contractors) to ensure that the operation is working to the standards required to produce safe food.

There is a diary entry page for every day that the business is open. Each day, the preset opening checks and closing checks are completed and

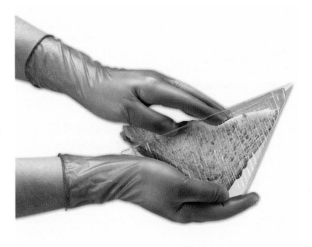

the diary page signed. Nothing else needs to be recorded unless something goes wrong, for example, a piece of equipment not working would be recorded along with the action that was taken.

A copy of 'Safer food, better business' is available from www.food.gov.uk.

A similar system called 'CookSafe' has been developed by the Food Standards Agency (Scotland) and details of this can also be found at www.food.gov.uk.

 ACTIVITY

For a kitchen you may be familiar with, suggest some opening checks and closing checks that could be completed each day to make sure the business is following good food safety procedures.

Table 2.6

Opening checks	Closing checks
E.g. Make sure all hand wash basins are clean/disinfected and that there is a good supply of liquid soap and paper towels.	E.g. Check that all waste bins are empty, cleaned and have new liners.

What the law says

The latest laws of importance to food businesses took effect from 1 January 2006. Almost all of the requirements in these regulations remain the same as the previous 1990/1995 regulations.

These set out the basic food safety requirements for all aspects of a food business, from premises to personal hygiene of staff, with specific attention to actual temperatures relating to food.

The main difference in the 2006 laws is that they provide a framework for EU legislation to be enforced in England and they require food establishments to have an approved Food Safety Management Procedure in place, with up-to-date records available.

Food safety legislation

Food safety standards and legislation are enforced by Environmental Health Officers (Environmental Health Practitioners). They may visit food premises as a matter of routine, after problems have occurred or after a complaint. The frequency of visits depends on the type of business, the food being handled, and whether there have been previous problems.

EHOs (EHPs) can enter a food business at any reasonable time, usually when the business is open. The main purpose of inspections is to identify any possible risks from the food business to the consumer, and to assess how well their food safety management systems are working.

Serving of notices

A **Hygiene Improvement Notice** will be served if the EHO (EHP) believes that a food business does not comply with regulations. The notice states the details of the business, what is wrong, why it is wrong, what needs to be put right and the time in which this must be completed (usually not less than 14 days). It is an offence if the work is not carried out in the specified time.

A **Hygiene Emergency Prohibition Notice** is served if the EHO (EHP) believes that the the business poses an imminent risk to people's health. These would include serious issues such as sewage contamination, lack of water supply, rodent infestation, etc. Serving this notice would mean immediate closure of the business for three days, during which time the EHO (EHP) must apply to magistrates for a **Hygiene Emergency Prohibition Order** to keep the premises closed. A Hygiene Prohibition Order prohibits a person (i.e. the owner/manager) from working in a food business.

Fines and penalties for non-compliance

Magistrates courts can impose fines of up to £5,000, a six-month prison sentence or both. For serious offences, magistrates could impose fines of up to £20,000. In a Crown Court, unlimited fines can be imposed and/or two years' imprisonment.

Due diligence

'Due diligence' can be an important defence under food safety legislation. This means that if there is proof that a business took all reasonable care and did everything it could to prevent food safety problems, legal action may be avoided. Proof would need to be provided in the form of accurate written documents such as pest control reports, staff training records, fridge temperature records, calibration of probes, staff sickness, lists of suppliers, etc.

Training

Food businesses must ensure that all staff who handle food are supervised and instructed and/or trained in food hygiene appropriate to the work they do. Basic food safety training should be given before starting to work with food, and more formal recorded training within four weeks of starting work. Training can take place in house or with a training provider. All records of staff training must be kept for possible inspection.

Food Standards Agency

The Food Standards Agency was set up in 2000 'to protect public health and to protect the interest of customers in relation to food'. The agency is committed to putting customers first, being open and accessible and being an independent voice on food-related matters.

'Scores on the Doors' is a strategy that has been introduced by the Food Standards Agency to raise food safety standards and reduce the incidence of food poisoning. Various schemes were piloted and tested, and in 2008 a star-rating scheme was selected for England and Wales. On inspection, food premises can be awarded up to 5 stars (0 stars = very poor food safety; 5 stars = excellent food safety). The intention is that the given star-rating certificate will be placed in a prominent position on the door or window of premises, but as yet it is not mandatory to do so.

It is expected that the 'Scores on the Doors' scheme will have a positive impact on food safety standards. No matter how good the food in a particular establishment, few people will want to eat there if the food safety score is low!

Test yourself ● ● ● ● ● ● ● ● ● ● ● ● ● ● ●

1 List the groups of people who are considered 'high risk' if they contract food poisoning.

2 Give three examples of foods that could cause an allergic reaction in some people.

3 Describe what happens when some bacteria produce spores.

4 There are certain illnesses/infections that you would need to report to a supervisor before being involved with food. What are they?

5 Give three examples of how cross-contamination could occur in a kitchen.

6 Why is essential to keep food above 63°C or below 5°C when holding food for service?

7 What temperature would you recommend storing: dairy foods, frozen fish, meat in a meat fridge, soft fruit?

8 When cleaning, what do each of the following do: detergent, disinfectant, sanitiser?

9 What are the main reasons why it is essential to keep pests out of food premises? Suggest three ways you could keep pests out.

10 What do the letters HACCP stand for? How is this applied in a kitchen situation?

● ●

In this chapter you will learn how to:

1. understand the importance of health and safety in the catering and hospitality industry including:

- the legal responsibilities of employers and employees and the power of enforcement officers
- common causes of ill health and accidents and the benefits of good health and safety practice

2. identify hazards in the catering and hospitality workplace including:

- the causes of and steps to minimise trips and falls, and injuries from manual handling, machinery/equipment, hazardous substances, fire and electrical dangers

3. control hazards in the workplace, including:

- the risk assessment process
- the control measures to reduce risk
- accident reporting, PPE and safety signs

4. maintain a healthy and safe workplace, including:

- the sources of information available, features in food preparation, welfare facilities, incident reporting, and emergency procedures.

Every day people are injured at work. Some may be permanently disabled and some may even die.

Be safe and do not let this happen to you or your work colleagues.

Working safely

Kitchens can be dangerous places. For this reason, it is important to work in a safe and systematic way in order to avoid accidents or injury to yourself or anyone else.

Absence due to sickness costs the UK economy approximately £400–£500 per employee each year. Over 200 people die in accidents at work each year; accidents can happen in any workplace.

If an employee works on a computer, they may be at risk of:

- problems with their eyes and eyesight
- epilepsy
- pain and discomfort in their arms, wrists and hands
- fatigue and stress.

Stress and accidents are currently the two biggest causes of absence from work.

You can report an accident at work by:

- email
- telephone
- fax
- letter.

The average number of days taken as sick leave each year in the UK is approximately 30 million.

Legal responsibilities

All chefs and kitchen workers need to know the laws on health and safety. The Health and Safety at Work Act gives employees and employers certain responsibilities while working.

- All employees and employers must take reasonable care of their own safety and the safety of others.
- Employees must inform their line manager if they see anything they think is unsafe and could cause an accident.
- Employers must make sure they do not put staff in dangerous situations where they could hurt themselves or others.

Who is responsible for health and safety?

Employers/employees
People in control of work premises
Self-employed people
Designers
Manufacturers
Suppliers
Local Authorities
Health & Safety Executive
Enforcement Officers
Environmental Health Officers
Health & Safety Inspectors

Under the Health and Safety at Work Act, an employer must make sure all staff are safe while at work. This means that they must:

- provide safe equipment and utensils
- train staff in safe practices
- provide first aid equipment
- keep an accident book/record
- produce a policy document telling everyone how to work safely.

 ACTIVITY

Write down potential dangers you have noticed in the kitchen where you have been working.

Bullying and harassment

Bullying and harassment can be when someone constantly finds fault with and criticises someone else. It can seem quite trivial, but it can feel very unpleasant. For example, people may:

- refuse to acknowledge you and your achievements
- undermine you, your position and your potential
- ignore you and make you and feel isolated and separated from your colleagues
- deliberately exclude you from what is going on at work
- humiliate, shout at and threaten you, often in front of others
- set you unrealistic tasks, which they keep changing
- attack you physically.

Employers should provide good welfare facilities for staff, rest facilities, drinking water, toilets, washing facilities, changing rooms and lockers

Who is bullied?

Bullying may occur at home, school/college and at work by peer groups, neighbours and work colleagues working at the same level as you or at different levels to you.

People who are being bullied can feel scared, vulnerable and isolated. If you are aware of any bullying, of you or of someone else, you must report it immediately so that it can be stopped. Nobody deserves to be bullied.

What is the difference between bullying and harassment?

Bullying tends to consist of many small incidents over a long period of time, whereas harassment may consist of one or more serious incidents. Harassment is the sort of unpleasant behaviour that creates an intimidating, hostile or offensive environment. This can take many forms and happen for many reasons. For example, it may be related to age, sex, race, disability, religion, sexuality or any personal characteristic of an individual.

Intimidating: From **intimidate** (to make someone feel timid or fearful, especially to control their behaviour). An 'intimidating environment' would be one in which people were made to feel fearful, and their actions were motivated by fear.

Injuries, accidents and disease

Common causes of accidents in kitchens

The following are some common causes of accidents in the kitchen:

- slipping on a wet or greasy floor
- walking into, tripping or falling over objects
- lifting objects
- being exposed to hazards such as hot or dangerous substances, e.g. steam, oven cleaner
- being hit or hurt by moving objects, such as being cut by a knife when chopping
- machines such as vegetable cutting machines, liquidisers, mincing machines
- fires and explosions
- electric shocks
- not wearing protective clothing
- poor lighting
- ignoring the rules.

RIDDOR (Reporting Injuries, Diseases and Dangerous Occurrences) Act 1996

The law says that all work-related accidents, diseases and dangerous occurrences must be recorded and reported. Employers must inform the Incident Contact Centre, Caerphilly Business Park, Caerphilly, CF83 3GG.

The following injuries must be reported:

- fractures (except fingers, thumbs or toes)
- amputation (cutting off) of limbs
- dislocation of a hip, knee or spine
- temporary or permanent loss of sight (blindness)
- eye injuries from chemicals getting into the eye,

a hot metal burn to the eye or any penetration of the eye

- any injury from electric shock or burning that leads to unconsciousness or the need to resuscitate the person or send them to hospital for more than 24 hours
- any injury resulting in hypothermia (when someone gets too cold), or illness due to heat, that leads to unconsciousness or the need to resuscitate the person or send them to hospital for more than 24 hours (e.g. an electric shock, or a gas flame blown back and causing burns)
- unconsciousness caused by exposure to a harmful substance or biological agents (e.g. cleaning products and solvents)
- unconsciousness or illness requiring medical treatment caused by inhaling a harmful substance or absorbing it through the skin (e.g. breathing in poisonous carbon monoxide leaking from a gas appliance)
- illness requiring medical treatment caused by a biological agent or its toxins or infected material (e.g. harmful bacteria used in laboratories).

Things that help to minimise risk

Health and safety training (COSHH, manual handling)

Good health and safety design

Wearing protective clothing

Strict enforcement of rules

Good housekeeping

Good lighting

Examples of reportable diseases:

- dermatitis
- skin cancer
- asthma
- hepatitis
- tuberculosis
- tetanus
- anthrax.

Solvent: A liquid that is able to dissolve other substances.

Dermatitis: A skin condition caused by contact with something that irritates the skin. Symptoms may include redness, scaling, blistering, weeping, cracking and swelling.

 ASSESS RISKS

Follow legal requirements

Report all accidents to management

Control of substances hazardous to health

The Control of Substances Hazardous to Health (COSHH) regulations state that an employer must not carry on any work that might expose employees to any substances that are hazardous to health, unless the employer has assessed the risks of this work to employees and has put the relevant controls in place.

Hazardous substances in catering

In catering establishments there are many chemicals and substances used for cleaning that can be harmful if not used correctly (see table 3.1).

Substances that are dangerous to health are labelled as very toxic, toxic, harmful, irritant or corrosive.

People using these chemical substances must be trained to use them. They must also wear protective clothing such as goggles, gloves and facemasks. Hazardous substances can enter the body through the skin, the eyes, the nose (by inhaling) and the mouth (by swallowing).

Ways to prevent an accident

COSHH says that the employer has to assess the risk from chemicals and decide what precautions are needed. The employer should make sure that measures are in place to control the use of chemical substances and monitor their use. If chemical substances are used you should:

- inform, instruct and train all staff in their use and safety
- always follow the manufacturer's instructions
- always store them in their original containers, away from heat

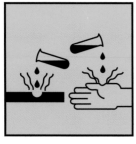
Corrosive

Flammable

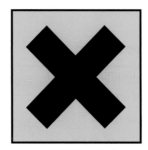
Harmful

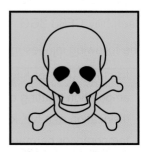
Toxic

Symbols to show hazardous substances

- keep the lids tightly closed
- not expose them to heat or to naked flames
- read all the labels carefully
- never mix chemicals
- know the first aid procedure
- get rid of empty containers immediately
- get rid of waste chemical solutions safely
- wear safety equipment and clothing.

Hazardous substance monitoring

In order to comply with legal obligations under the COSHH Regulations, all areas should be surveyed to ascertain which chemicals and substances are used. The table below lists the different work areas and the chemicals and substances likely to be found in them.

A COSHH register should be kept, by the manager, of all substances used in the establishment. Technical data sheets should be attached to the completed COSHH assessment sheet.

Table 3.1 Work areas and the chemicals and substances likely to be found in them

Area	Chemicals and substances
Kitchen	Cleaning chemicals including alkalis and acids, detergents, sanitisers, descalers Chemicals associated with burnishing; possibly some oils associated with machines Pest control chemicals, insecticides and rodenticides
Restaurant	Cleaning chemicals, polishes, fuel for flame lamps including methylated spirits, LPG
Bar	Beer-line cleaner, glass-washing detergent and sanitisers
Housekeeping	Cleaning chemicals including detergents, sanitisers, descalants, polishes, carpet-cleaning products, floor-care products
Maintenance	Cleaning chemicals, adhesives, solvents, paint, LPG, salts for water softening etc., paint stripper, varnishes etc.
Offices	Correction fluid, thinners, solvents, methylated spirits, toner for photocopier, duplicating fluids and chemicals, polishes

Identifying hazards and avoiding accidents

The Health & Safety at Work Act covers all full-time and part-time workers and unpaid workers. The Health & Safety Executive (HSE) is responsible for enforcing health and safety in the workplace.

- The HSE has the power to investigate premises, check, dismantle and remove equipment, inspect the records, ask questions, seize and destroy articles.
- It can give verbal or written advice, order improvement and prohibition notices and will, if necessary, prosecute, which can result in unlimited fines or even imprisonment.

What is a hazard?

When we assess health and safety we talk about hazards. A hazard is anything that can cause harm, such as:

- extremes of cold and heat
- uneven floors
- excessive noise
- chemicals
- electricity
- working using ladders
- moving parts and machinery
- dust and fumes.

The following aspects of the kitchen environment have the potential to give rise to hazards:

- equipment – knives, liquidisers, food processors, mixers, mincers, etc.
- substances – cleaning chemicals, detergents, sanitisers
- work methods – carrying knives and equipment incorrectly and not following a logical sequence
- work areas – spillages not cleaned up, overcrowded work areas, insufficient work space, uncomfortable work conditions due to extreme heat or cold.

Common causes of accidents

The majority of accidents in catering premises are due to people falling, slipping or tripping. Therefore, floor surfaces must be of a suitable construction to reduce this risk. A major reason for the high incidence of this kind of accident is that water and grease are likely to be spilt, and the combination of these substances is treacherous and makes the floor surface slippery. For this reason, any spillage must be cleaned immediately and warning notices put in place, where appropriate, highlighting the danger of the slippery surface. Ideally, a member of staff should stand guard until the hazard is cleared.

Another cause of falls is placing articles on the floor in corridors, passageways or between stoves and tables. People carrying trays and containers may have an obstructed view of where they are going, and may not see items on the floor and so may trip over them. They may fall onto a hot stove, or the item they are carrying may be hot. These falls can have severe consequences. The solution is to ensure that nothing is left on the floor that may cause an obstruction and be a hazard. If it is necessary to have articles temporarily on the floor, then they should be guarded so as to prevent accidents.

Kitchen equipment can also cause accidents or injury if misused. All staff must be trained in the correct use of equipment and machinery, especially young or inexperienced staff. Worn or faulty equipment must not be used and electrical equipment must be regularly maintained and checked.

Kitchen personnel should be trained to think and act in a safe manner so as to avoid this kind of accident.

Avoiding accidents

 ACTIVITY

List the common causes of accidents in the kitchen.

There are lots of precautions that can be taken to avoid accidents happening in catering premises.

- The main type of accident is people falling or tripping. Floors should be even, with no unexpected steps, and they should be kept dry. Clean up spillages immediately and use warning notices if a floor is slippery.

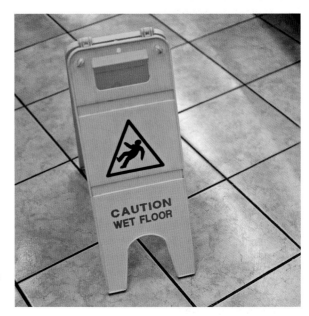

Wet floor warning

- Keep corridors and walkways clear so that people do not trip over objects that are in the way.
- There should be adequate lighting so that people can see clearly where they are going.
- There should be adequate ventilation so that any excess heat and fumes can escape.
- Kitchens should not be overcrowded. There should be enough space for people to move

around without bumping and pushing into one another.

- Follow the rules and working practices:
    - Always work in an organised way.
    - Clean up as you go.
- Follow the flow of traffic in the kitchen:
    - People should flow through the preparation area to the service area without backtracking or crossing over, so that they do not bump into each other.

- Food should flow through the preparation area to the service area. Ideally, raw food should never go into the area where there is cooked food. If this is unavoidable, make sure the raw food is safely wrapped/covered.
- Equipment should flow through the preparation area to the service area. Dirty equipment should not come into contact with or get mixed up with clean equipment.

Safety in the workplace

Managing health and safety

Employers must have appropriate arrangements in place (which must be recorded if there are five or more employees) for maintaining a safe workplace. These should cover the usual management functions of:

- planning
- organisation
- control.

Risk

Risk is the chance of somebody being harmed by the hazard. There may be a high risk or a low risk of harm.

> **Example**
>
> Using a liquidiser is a hazard. What is the likelihood of it causing harm?
>
> If it is overfilled, the contents can force the lid off. If the contents are hot, they may burst into the air and hit the chef, which may cause a burn.
>
> This risk is medium.

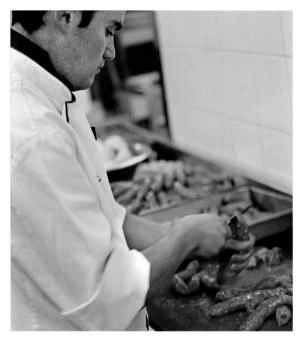

Knives are a hazard

Here are five steps to assessing risk:

1. Look for hazards, i.e. the things that can cause harm.
2. Identify who could be harmed and how.

Table 3.2

Common risks and hazards	Ways to minimise risks
Poor design and structure of building, poor signage, poor housekeeping standards, poor lighting and ventilation, dangerous working practices, distraction and lack of attention, working too quickly, ignoring the rules, not wearing protective clothing.	Improved and safe design of the building, correct and clear/visible signage, good housekeeping, well-lit and ventilated areas, well-trained staff, strict enforcement of rules, wearing correct protective clothing, concentrating on the work.

3. Work out the risks and decide if the existing precautions are good enough or whether more should be done to prevent any harm being caused.

4. Write down what the hazard is and what the risk is and keep this as a record.

5. Re-check the hazard and the risk at regular intervals and go back and change the risk assessment (the written record) if necessary.

Employers must examine the risks in the workplace, and write down what they are and what should be done about them. Risk in the workplace means anything that could cause harm to employees or other people (including customers, visitors and members of the public). After examining a risk carefully, you can estimate the size of the risk; then you can decide whether it is acceptable, or whether you need to take more precautions to prevent harm.

When the risk assessment has been done, employers are required to make any improvements that are identified as necessary. The aim is to make sure that no one gets hurt or becomes ill.

However, it is important to remember that employers only need to consider risks and hazards which are created by work activities. They do not need to consider every minor hazard or risk that we accept as part of our lives.

Table 3.3 Common risks and hazards in a hospitality operation, and ways to minimise them

Hazard	Risk level before control	Current control measures	Risk level with controls	Additional control required (action, person responsible and date)	Student initial understanding
Electricity		Maintain electrical equipment according to manufacturer instructions. Switch off from supply when not in use. Do not operate electrical switches with wet hands. Report electrical faults immediately.			
Hot liquids, e.g. water, oil		Everyone must be aware of the dangers of hot vessels. Do not overfill pans with water. When lifting the lid, always use the handle and stand to the side to allow steam to escape. Avoid drips, especially of oil. Drain condensation back into pan, not onto floor or feet.			
Hot surfaces		If the surface of the boiler becomes hot during use, then precautions must be taken to prevent burns. Place pans in a position that minimises the risk of contact. Do not over-reach.			
Knives		Ensure that knives are kept sharp, and have secure handles. Ensure that the correct size and type of knife is used. Do not leave knives lying on work surfaces or tables. When carrying knives, always do so with the point downwards.			

		Always use the correct chopping board or block, and ensure that it is placed securely on a firm work surface. Cutting movements must always be away from the body and downwards onto the chopping board.			

All staff need to receive training in the use of the equipment they use. This should be recorded and updated regularly.

Table 3.4 Learners must receive training in the use of each item of equipment: keep a log like this

Equipment name	Areas of safety covered in training	Authorised person/ trainer	Staff signature

Full name of injured person:			
Occupation:		Supervisor:	
Time of accident:	Date of accident:	Time of report:	Date of report:
Name of injury or condition:			
Details of hospitalisation:			
Extent of injury (after medical attention):			
Place of accident or dangerous occurrence:			
Injured person's evidence of what happened (include equipment/items and/or other persons):			
Witness evidence (1):		Witness evidence (2):	
Supervisor's recommendations:			
Date:		Supervisor's signature:	

An incident report form – this may be stored electronically

Incident/accident reporting

Health and safety has to be monitored regularly in the workplace, ideally by a designated Health & Safety Officer. Any incidents or near misses must be recorded, even if no one is injured.

All accidents should be reported to your line manager, chef or a supervisor. Each accident is recorded in an accident file or electronic system, which must be provided in every business. Below is an example of an incident report form showing all the details required.

Emergencies in the workplace

Emergencies that might happen in the workplace include:

- serious accidents
- outbreak of fire
- bomb scare
- failure of major system, e.g. water or electricity.

An organisation will have systems in place to deal with emergencies. Key staff are usually trained to tackle emergencies. There will be fire marshals and first aiders. These people will attend regular update meetings. Evacuation procedures will also be in place, which employees can practise (e.g. fire drill), and fire alarms will be tested regularly.

Ensure that you know the evacuation procedures in your establishment. If you have to leave the premises, ensure that the following procedures are adhered to.

- Turn off the power supplies, gas and electricity. Usually this means hitting the red button in the kitchen or turning off all appliances individually.
- Close all windows and doors.
- Leave the building by the nearest emergency exit. DO NOT USE THE LIFTS.
- Assemble in the designated area, away from the building.
- Check the roll-call of names to establish whether all personnel have left the building safely.

 ACTIVITY

List the health and safety points you would need to explain to new members of staff.

First aid

When people at work suffer injuries or fall ill, it is important that they receive immediate attention and that, in serious cases, an ambulance is called.

The arrangements for providing first aid in the workplace are set out in the Health and Safety (First Aid) Regulations 1981. First aiders and facilities should be available to give immediate assistance to casualties with common injuries or illness.

As the term implies, first aid is the immediate treatment given on the spot to a person who has been injured or is ill. Since 1982 it has been a legal requirement that adequate first aid equipment, facilities and personnel are provided at work. If the injury is serious, the injured person should be treated by a doctor or nurse as soon as possible.

 ACTIVITY

List items you would expect to find in a first aid box.

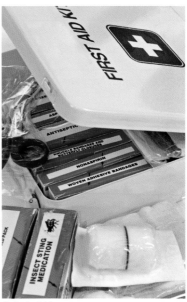

A first aid box

Potential costs of accidents in the workplace
Employees off work, illness, stress
Compensation/compensation claims
Prosecution
Fines
Legal costs
Damage to the business's reputation
High staff turnover

Potential benefits of good health and safety practices
Reduction in accidents and ill health
Motivated workers
Enhanced reputation
Increased productivity
Improved profitability

Clothing

It is most important that people working in the kitchen should wear suitable clothing and footwear. Suitable clothing must be:

- protective
- washable
- lightweight and comfortable
- strong
- absorbent.

Clothes worn in the kitchen must protect the body from excessive heat. For this reason chefs' jackets are double-breasted and have long sleeves; these protect the chest and arms from the heat of the stove and prevent hot foods or liquids burning or scalding the body.

- **Aprons** are designed to protect the body from being scalded or burned and particularly to protect the legs from any liquids that may be spilled; for this reason the apron should be of sufficient length to protect the legs.
- **Chefs' hats** are designed to enable air to circulate on top of the head and thus keep the head cooler. The main purpose of the hat is to prevent loose hairs from dropping into food and to absorb perspiration on the forehead. The use of lightweight disposable hats is both acceptable and suitable.

Personal protective equipment

According to the Personal Protective Equipment (PPE) at Work Regulations, 1992, employees must wear personal protective clothing and

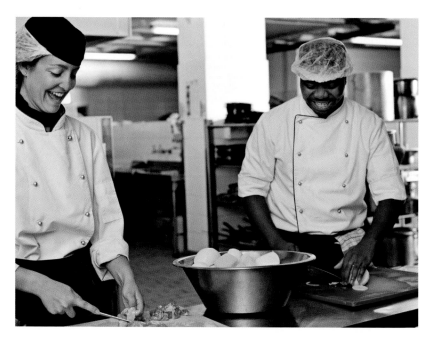

It is important to keep your hair covered while you work

equipment (e.g. safety shoes, eye protection such as goggles) for certain things. For example, chefs must wear chef's whites.

Manual handling

Picking up and carrying heavy or difficult loads can lead to accidents if it is not done properly. Handling loads wrongly is the main cause of back problems in the workplace. The safest way to lift objects is to bend your knees rather than your back. It is also better if two people lift the object together, rather than one person trying to do it on their own. This will help to prevent straining and damaging your back.

Handling checklist

- When you move goods on trolleys, trucks or other wheeled vehicles:
    - load them carefully
    - do not overload them
    - load them in a way that allows you to see where you are going.
- In stores, stack heavy items at the bottom.
- If steps are needed to reach higher items, use them with care.
- Take particular care when moving large pots of liquid, especially if the liquid is hot. Do not fill them to the brim.
- Use a warning sign to let people know if equipment handles, lids and so on might be hot.

This is traditionally done by sprinkling a small amount of flour, or something similar, onto the part of the equipment that might be hot or by wrapping a thick oven cloth around the handle.

- Take extra care when removing a tray from the oven or salamander. You do not want the tray to burn you or someone else.

Safety signs

We use safety signs to control a hazard. They should not replace other methods of controlling risks.

Yellow signs – warning signs

These are warning signs to alert people to various dangers, such as slippery floors, hot oil or hot water. They also warn people about hazards such as corrosive material.

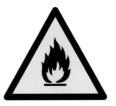

Corrosive: Something which can eat away or destroy solid materials.

Blue signs – mandatory signs

These signs inform people about precautions they must take. They tell people how to progress

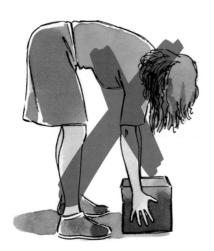
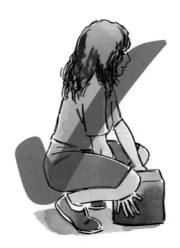

How to lift correctly

safely through a certain area. They must be used whenever special precautions need to be taken, such as wearing protective clothing.

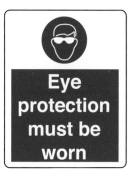 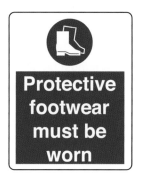

Red signs – prohibition signs – fire fighting signs

Red signs tell people that they should not enter. They are used to stop people from doing certain tasks in a hazardous area. Red signs are also used for fire fighting equipment.

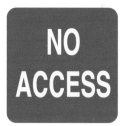 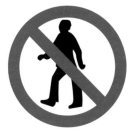

Green signs – safe signs

These are route signs designed to show people where fire exits and emergency exits are. Green is also used for first aid equipment.

Electricity and gas

Great care must be taken when dealing with electricity. If a person comes into direct contact

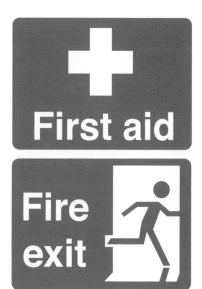

with electricity the consequences can be very serious and sometimes fatal. If a person has an electric shock, switch off the current. If this is not possible, free the person using something that is dry and will insulate you from the electricity, such as a cloth, or something made of wood or rubber. You must take care not to use your bare hands otherwise the electric shock may be transmitted to you. If the person has stopped breathing, send for a doctor. If you have been trained how to, you can give artificial respiration.

In an emergency:

- switch off the current
- raise the alarm
- call for a doctor/first aid help.

Gas is also potentially hazardous. On leaving the kitchen, turn off all the gas. It is important to report any gas leaks or smell.

Fire safety

Every employer has an explicit duty for the safety of his or her employees in the event of a fire. The Regulatory Fire Safety Order 2005 emphasises that fires should be prevented. It says that fire safety is the responsibility of the occupant of premises and the people who might be affected by fire, so in catering this will usually be the

employer (the occupant) and the employees (who will be affected by fire).

The responsible person must:

- make sure that the fire precautions, where reasonably practicable, ensure the safety of all employees and others in the building

- make an assessment of the risk of and from fire in the establishment; special consideration must be given to dangerous chemicals or substances, and the risks that these pose if a fire occurs
- review the preventative and protective measures.

Fire safety requires constant vigilance to reduce the risk of a fire, using the provision of detection and alarm systems, and well-practised emergency and evacuation procedures in the event of a fire.

For a fire to start, three things are needed:

1. a source of heat (ignition)
2. fuel
3. oxygen.

If any one of these three things is missing a fire cannot start. So, taking precautions to avoid the three coming together will reduce the chances of a fire starting.

Methods of extinguishing fires concentrate on cooling (as in a water extinguisher or fire hose) or depriving the fire of oxygen (as in an extinguisher that uses foam or powder to smother it).

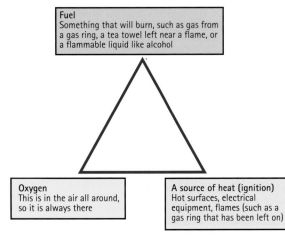

The fire triangle

Fire precautions

Below are some guidelines for good practice.

- Remove all hazards or reduce them as much as possible.
- Make sure that everyone is protected from the risk of fire and the likelihood of a fire spreading.

- Make sure that all escape routes are safe and used effectively, in other words they are signposted, easy to access and people know where they are.
- Some way of fighting fires (e.g. a fire extinguisher or fire blanket) must be available on the premises.
- There must be some way of detecting a fire on the premises (e.g. smoke alarms) and instructions as to what to do in case of fire.
- There must be arrangements in place for what to do if a fire breaks out on the premises. Employees must be trained in what to do in the event of a fire.
- All precautions provided must be installed and maintained by a competent person.

Competent: With enough relevant skills or knowledge.

Fire risk assessments

A fire risk assessment will:

- help to find out how likely it is that a fire might happen
- help to highlight the dangers from fire in the workplace.

Report:

dangerous electrical equipment

gas leaks

faulty equipment.

Always use qualified professionals for problems with gas, electricity and water.

There are five steps to complete for a fire risk assessment:

1. Identify the potential fire hazards in the workplace.
2. Decide who will be in danger in the event of a fire, e.g. employees, visitors.
3. Identify the risks caused by the hazards. Decide whether the existing fire precautions are adequate or whether more needs to be done, for example to remove a hazard to control the risk.
4. The things that are found out and changes that are made in numbers 1 to 3 should be written

down and kept on record, and all staff should be informed of them.

5. The risk assessment should be reviewed regularly to check that it is up to date. If things change it should be revised when necessary.

Fire detection and fire warning

There needs to be an effective way of detecting fire and warning people about it quickly enough to allow them to escape before it spreads too far.

In small workplaces, such as small restaurants, a fire will be detected easily and quickly and is unlikely to cut off the escape routes. In this case, if people can see the exits clearly, shouting 'FIRE!' may be all that is necessary.

In larger establishments fire warning systems are needed. Manually operated call points are likely to be the least that is needed. These are the type of fire alarm where you break glass to set off the alarm (as seen on the wall in schools, etc.).

Fire-fighting equipment

Portable fire extinguishers enable people to tackle fire in its early stages. People should be trained to use extinguishers and only use them if they can do so without putting themselves in danger.

Fires are classified in accordance with British Standard EN2 as follows:

- Class A – fires involving solid materials where combustion (burning) normally forms glowing embers, e.g. wood.
- Class B – fires involving liquids (e.g. methylated spirits) or liquefiable solids (e.g. any a kind of flammable gel used under a burner).
- Class C – fires involving gases.
- Class D – fires involving metals.
- Class F – fires involving cooking oils or fats.

There are different types of fire extinguishers that are suitable for different types of fire. Portable extinguishers all contain a substance that will put out a fire. The substance will vary, but whatever it is it will be forced out of the extinguisher under pressure. Generally, portable fire extinguishers contain one of the following five substances (extinguishing mediums):

- water
- foam
- powder
- carbon dioxide
- vaporising liquids.

The most useful form of general-purpose fire-fighting equipment is the water-type extinguisher or hose reel. Areas of special risk, such as kitchens where oil, fats and electrical equipment are used, may need other types of extinguisher such as carbon dioxide, dry powder or wet chemical. Your local fire authority will be able to advise you on everything to do with fire safety.

Where hose reels are provided, they should be located where they are conspicuous and always accessible, such as in corridors.

Conspicuous: Easy to notice; clearly visible.

In smaller workplaces, portable fire extinguishers will probably be sufficient to tackle small fires. However, in more complex buildings, or where it is necessary to protect the means of escape and/or the property or contents of the building, it may be necessary to consider a sprinkler system. Sprinkler systems are traditionally acknowledged as an efficient means of protecting buildings against extensive damage from fire. They are also now acknowledged as an effective means of reducing the risk to life from fire.

Security in catering

Security in catering premises is a major concern these days. The main security risks in the hotel and catering industry are:

- theft: where customers' property, employers' property (particularly food, drink and equipment) or employees' property is stolen

- burglary: where the burglar comes onto the premises (trespasses) and steals customers' property, employers' property or employees' property
- robbery: theft with assault, for example when staff are banking or collecting cash
- fraud: false insurance claims; counterfeit money; stolen credit cards
- assault: fights between customers; assaults on staff by customers (e.g. if a customer is not happy with the service, and may also be drunk, they may become violent towards staff); attacks on staff while they are taking cash to or collecting cash from the bank
- vandalism: damage to property caused by customers, intruders or employees
- arson: setting fire to the property
- undesirables: having people such as drug traffickers and prostitutes on the premises
- terrorism: bombs, telephone bomb threats.

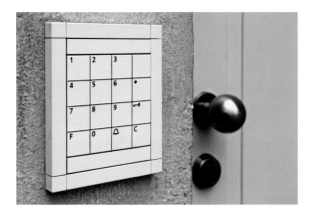

A security keypad

The Health & Safety at Work Regulations now require employers to conduct a risk assessment regarding the safety of staff in the catering business. Preventing crime is better than having to deal with it once it has happened. Here are some ideas for helping to prevent crime.

- The best way to prevent theft is to stop the thief entering the premises in the first place. Reception staff should be trained to spot suspicious individuals. Everyone who comes in should be asked to sign in at reception and, if they are a legitimate visitor, be given a security

badge. It is also essential to make sure that any suspicious person does not re-enter the building.

- All contract workers should be registered and given security badges, and they may be restricted to working in certain areas.
- There should also be a good security system at the back door, where everyone delivering goods has to report to the security officer.
- All establishments should try to reduce temptation for criminals, for example by reducing the amount of cash that is handled. The use of credit and debit cards does cost the establishment a small amount of money (they have to pay a fee to the credit card companies), but it reduces the amount of cash that is used, so it reduces the risk of cash being stolen. However, there is also more and more crime due to fraud (e.g. using stolen credit cards).
- Staff who handle money should be trained in simple anti-fraud measures such as checking bank notes, signatures on plastic cards, etc.
- It is impossible to remove all temptation, so equipment (e.g. computers, fax machines, photocopiers) should be marked with some sort of security tag or identification.
- There are many simple and obvious security measures that can also be taken, such as locking doors and windows.
- Good lighting is also important for security reasons – criminals are less likely to come onto the premises at night if people can see them easily. Supervisors and managers should regularly check the lighting in all areas. Leaving lights on in some areas that can be seen by passers-by can also help.
- Closed-circuit television (CCTV) camera recordings are also used as a deterrent against crime.
- With regard to staff, the first step is to appoint honest staff by checking their references from previous employers.
- Some companies write into employee contracts the 'right to search'. This means that from time to time the employer can carry out searches of the employees' lockers, bags and so on. This

discourages employees from stealing. It is not legal to force a person to be searched even if they have signed a contract about it, but if they refuse they may be breaking their employment contract.

Personal safety

Below is a personal safety checklist to help you stay safe.

- Wear protective clothing.
- Do not work under the influence of alcohol or drugs.
- Keep hair short, or tied back if long.
- Do not wear jewellery as this, like long hair, can be caught in machinery.
- Walk – do not run.
- Use the walkways provided and never take short cuts.
- Look out for and obey all warning notices and safety signs.
- Back problems can cause a lot of pain and may last a lifetime. Always use trolleys or other appropriate lifting equipment if available.
- You must be shown how to lift and carry items correctly. Take care that you:

   (a) lift or carry only what you can manage

   (b) can see clearly where you are going

   (c) get help with anything that you think might be too heavy or awkward to manage on your own

- If in doubt, don't do it – ask for help!

Sources of information

Acts of Parliament

European Union Directives

Health and Safety Executive

Local Authorities

Environmental Health Officers

Health and Safety Inspectors

 ACTIVITY

Assess a risk and the hazard when using each of the following pieces of equipment:

- a liquidiser
- a mandolin
- a thermostatically controlled deep fat fryer.

 ACTIVITY

Do you know:

- what to do if there is a fire?
- how to raise the alarm?
- what the alarm sounds like?
- where the fire exits are?
- where the assembly point is?

You should know all of the above. If you do not then you must find out.

ACTIVITY

State why risk assessment is important.

Draw up a risk assessment for a working area or piece of equipment in the establishment where you work.

Test yourself • • • • • • • • • • • • • • •

1 Under the Health and Safety at Work Act what must an employer do to ensure that staff are safe at work?

2 List four common causes of accidents in a kitchen.

3 What do the letters COSHH stand for? What are COSHH regulations in place to protect?

4 In relation to health and safety at work, who has the power to enter premises, check or dismantle equipment, inspect records, ask questions and seize/destroy dangerous articles?

5 Employers must now complete a risk assessment to identify risk. What are the five steps in a risk assessment?

6 What is meant by PPE? Give an example of PPE in a kitchen.

7 Health and safety signs are grouped into different colours. What are **red** signs used for? Give two examples of red signs.

8 For a fire to start there are three requirements – what are they?
   Name two different types of fire extinguisher and state the kind of fire each should be used for.

9 If you have been asked to move a heavy or awkward load what are the rules you should follow?

10 Name four areas in a large hotel that need to be kept secure. What security method/methods would you suggest for each?

• •

4 Healthier foods and special diets

In this chapter you will learn how to:

1. understand balanced diets, including:
- the sources of essential nutrients
- the impact of diet on health
- how to help maintain the nutritional value of food

2. plan and provide special diets:
- know the main features of special diets and their impact on health
- be able to plan and provide meals for those on special diets.

Why healthy eating is important

With more and more people eating outside the home, caterers are in a strong position to influence customers in the food choices they make.

The need for healthier menu options

Nearly 24 million adults in the UK today are overweight or obese. Levels of obesity have trebled in the UK over the past 20 years and are still increasing. However, healthy eating is not just about reducing obesity. Medical research suggests that a third of all cancers are caused by poor diet. Diet can be linked to bowel cancer, stomach and lung cancer, high blood pressure, diabetes, osteoporosis and tooth decay. Eating a balanced nutritional diet can help to protect us from these illnesses. Caterers should therefore know about healthy eating, and chefs should provide a range of healthy menu options.

> **Diabetes:** An illness in which the body is unable to cope with sugar, causing thirst, frequent urination, tiredness and other symptoms. There are different kinds of diabetes, not all of which need to be treated with insulin. Type 2 diabetes is more common in overweight and older people and can sometimes be controlled by diet alone.
>
> **Osteoporosis:** A disease in which the density or thickness of the bones breaks down, putting them at greater risk of fracture. Exercise and good nutrition can reduce the risk of developing osteoporosis.

What is healthy eating?

Food, nutrition and exercise are crucial to our health and wellbeing. There is no doubt that making the right choices of food and drink, combined with taking regular exercise, can protect us against many diseases like coronary heart disease and cancer. There are also lots of immediate health and lifestyle benefits to be gained from healthy eating.

Although scientists all agree on what makes a healthy style of eating, the information presented in the media may seem confusing, and there are still many myths about healthy eating. Contrary to popular opinion, it is not just a case of taking chips off the menu or sticking to salad. We do need to eat lots of fruit and vegetables and less of the high-fat sugary foods, but if we eat more bulky, filling foods, we can still feel satisfied. Some of the greatest dishes and most exciting cuisines in the world are based on these principles (e.g. paella, biryani, Chinese vegetables stir-fried with noodles, sushi and rice, couscous, and cannelloni stuffed with ricotta and spinach). See also the 'Healthy eating' section later in this chapter.

Table 4.1 Summing up healthy eating

What it is about	What it is not about	Immediate benefits
Eating more fruit and vegetables	Cutting down on food	Better weight control
Filling up on bread, pasta, rice and potatoes	Going hungry	Improved self-esteem
Eating a little less of some food items	Depriving yourself of treats	Looking and feeling better
Enjoying good food	Spending more money on food	Feeling fitter, with more energy
Making small, gradual changes	Not enjoying food	Enjoying a wide variety of foods
Knowing more about food	'Brown and boring food'	Not buying expensive 'diet' products
Altering food shopping patterns	Just salads	Knowing that changes made today will have long-term benefits
Feeling satisfied and good about food	Making major changes	
	Going on a 'special diet'	

Use the eatwell plate to get the balance right. It shows how much of what you eat should come from each food group.

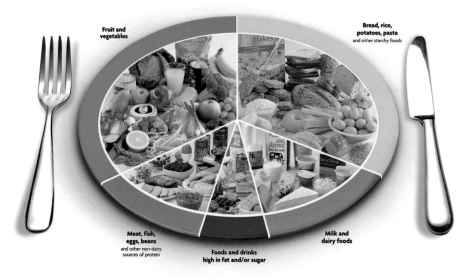

The eatwell plate

A balanced diet

Foods are not 'good' or 'bad'; it is the overall balance of the diet that matters.

There is no perfect food that gives you everything you need. No single food provides all the nutrients essential to keep us healthy. Different foods have different nutritional contents (in other words, they are good for us in different ways). So we need to eat a variety of foods to give us all the nutrients we need for a healthy diet. A balanced diet also makes our meal times more interesting.

Nutrients in foods help our bodies to do essential everyday activities. They also help our bodies to heal themselves if they are injured, and a balanced diet can help to prevent illness and disease. In ancient times, many foods (e.g. olive oil, pomegranates, spices such as ginger) were used for their healing properties.

The main nutrients are:

- carbohydrates
- proteins
- fats
- vitamins
- minerals
- water.

We will now look at each of these in more detail to find out what they do and which foods they are in.

> **Nutritionally balanced diet:** A diet which includes all the nutrients necessary for good health (from all the food groups) without too much or too little of any of the nutrients an individual needs. The Eatwell plate is a guide to the proportion of food which should be eaten from each food group. Different people have different nutritional requirements, depending on their age and occupation.

Carbohydrates

We need carbohydrates for energy. They are made by plants and then either used by the plants as energy or eaten by animals and humans for energy or as dietary fibre.

There are three main types of carbohydrate:

- sugar
- starch
- fibre.

Sugars

Sugars are the simplest form of carbohydrates. When carbohydrates are digested they turn into sugars.

There are several types of sugar:

- glucose – found in the blood of animals and in fruit and honey
- fructose – found in fruit, honey and cane sugar
- sucrose – found in beet and cane sugar
- lactose – found in milk
- maltose – found in cereal grains and is used in beer-making.

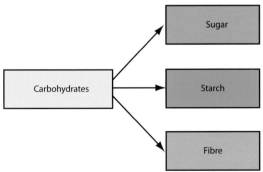

Types of carbohydrate

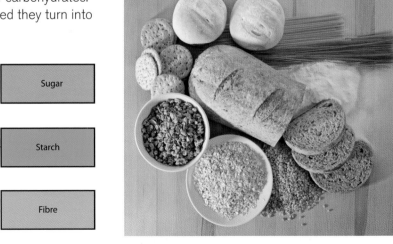

These foods are high in carbohydrates

Starches

Starches break down into sugars. Starches are present in many foods, such as:

- pasta, e.g. macaroni, spaghetti, vermicelli
- cereals, e.g. cornflakes, shredded wheat
- cakes, biscuits, bread (cooked starch)
- whole grains, e.g. rice, barley, tapioca
- powdered grains, e.g. flour, cornflour, ground rice, arrowroot
- vegetables, e.g. potatoes, parsnips, peas, beans
- unripe fruit, e.g. bananas, apples, cooking pears.

	Per 100 g
Energy	1760 kJ/417 kcal
Fat of which saturated fat	9.3 g 4.1 g
Carbohydrate of which sugars	79.5 g 57.9 g
Protein	3.9 g
Sodium	trace
Contains gluten and soya. May contain traces of nuts.	

Example of nutritional values on a food label

Where to find the nutritional values of different foods
Manual of nutrition
Internet
Food labels (like the example below)
Promotional leaflets
British Nutrition Foundation
Department of Health
Food Standards Agency

Fibre

Dietary fibre is a very important form of starch. Unlike other carbohydrates, dietary fibre cannot be digested and does not provide energy to the body.

However, dietary fibre is essential for a balanced diet because it:

- helps to remove waste and toxins from the body and maintain bowel action
- helps to control the digestion and processing of nutrients
- adds bulk to the diet, helping us to stop feeling hungry; it is used in many weight reduction foods.

Fibre is found in:

- fruits and vegetables
- wholemeal and granary bread
- wholegrain cereals
- wholemeal pasta
- wholegrain rice
- pulses (peas and beans) and lentils.

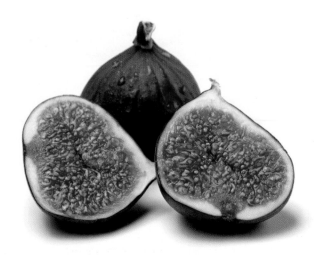

Fruit is a source of fibre

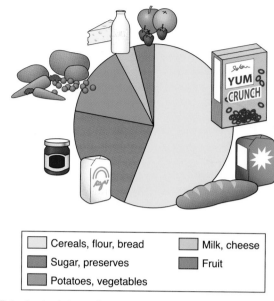

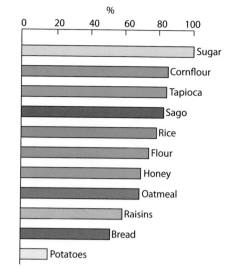

This graph shows what percentage of each food is made up of carbohydrates

This pie chart shows the sources of carbohydrates in the average diet: more than half come from cereal products

Protein

Protein is an essential part of all living things. Every day our bodies carry out millions of tasks (bodily functions) to stay alive. We need protein so that our bodies can grow and repair themselves.

There are two kinds of protein:

- animal protein
- vegetable protein.

The lifespan of the cells in our bodies varies from a week to a few months. As the cells die they need to be replaced. We need protein for our cells to repair and for new ones to grow.

We also use protein for energy. Any protein that is not used up in repairing and growing cells is converted into carbohydrate or fat.

What is protein?

Protein is made up of chemicals known as amino acids. The protein in cheese is different from the protein in meat because the amino acids are different. Some amino acids are essential to the body, so they must be included in a balanced diet. Ideally our bodies need both animal and vegetable protein so that we get all the amino acids we need.

- Animal protein is found in meat, game, poultry, fish, eggs, milk, cheese.
- Vegetable protein is found in vegetable seeds, pulses, peas, beans, nuts, wheat.

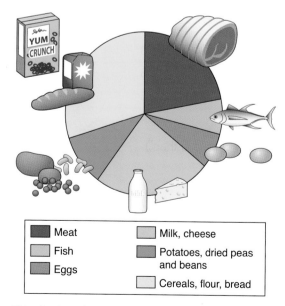

This pie chart shows the sources of protein in the average diet: the biggest sources are meat, cereals and dairy products

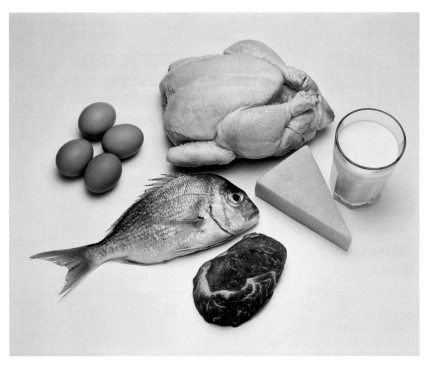

These foods are high in protein

Table 4.2 The proportion of protein in some common foods

Animal foods	Protein (%)	Plant foods	Protein (%)
Cheddar cheese	25	Soya flour, low fat	45
Bacon, lean	20	Soya flour, full fat	37
Beef, lean	20	Peanuts	24
Cod	17	Bread, wholemeal	9
Herring	17	Bread, white	8
Eggs	12	Rice	7
Beef, fat	8	Peas, fresh	6
Milk	3	Potatoes, old	2
Cream cheese	3	Bananas	1
Butter	< 1	Apples	< 1

(Note: < means 'less than'.)

Fats

Fats are naturally present in many foods and are an essential part of our diet. The main functions of fat are to protect the body, keep it warm and provide energy. Fats form an insulating layer under the skin and this helps to protect the vital organs and to keep the body warm. Fat is also needed to build cell membranes in the body.

Some fats are solid at room temperature and others are liquid at room temperature. Hard fats are mainly animal fats.

- Animal fats are butter, dripping (beef), suet, lard (pork), cheese, cream, bacon, meat fat, oily fish.
- Vegetable fats are margarine, cooking oils, nut oils, soya bean oils.

Too much fat is bad for us. It can lead to:

- being overweight (obesity)
- high levels of cholesterol, which can clog the heart's blood vessels (arteries)
- heart disease
- bad breath (halitosis)
- type 2 diabetes (the other type of diabetes, type 1, is something people are born with and is not from eating too much fat).

There are two types of fats:

- saturated fats
- unsaturated fats.

A diet high in saturated fat is thought to increase the risk of heart disease.

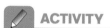 **ACTIVITY**

Produce a leaflet for a local catering establishment on the importance of maintaining a healthy diet.

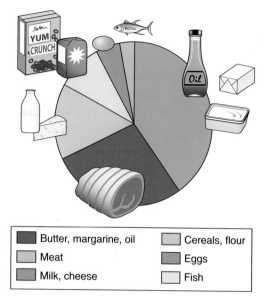

Butter, margarine, oil | Cereals, flour
Meat | Eggs
Milk, cheese | Fish

This pie chart shows the sources of fat in the average diet: butter and oil are the biggest source because they are used to make lots of fatty foods such as cake

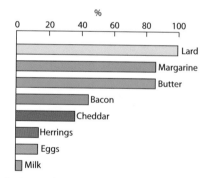

This graph shows what percentage of each food is made of fat

Table 4.3 The percentage of saturated fat in an average diet

Type of food	% saturated fat
Milk, cheese, cream	16.0
Meat and meat products *This splits down into:*	25.2
Beef	4.1
Lamb	3.5
Pork, bacon and ham	5.8
Sausage	2.7
Other meat products (e.g. burgers, faggots, paté)	9.1
Other oils and fats (e.g. olive oil, margarine, sunflower oil)	30.0
Other sources, including eggs, fish, poultry	7.4
Biscuits and cakes	11.4

Vitamins

Vitamins are chemicals which are vital for life. They are found in small amounts in many foods. If your diet is deficient in any vitamins, you can become ill or unhealthy.

Vitamins help with many of our bodily functions, such as growth and protection from disease.

> **Deficient:** Not having enough of; lacking.
> **Nervous system:** The system which controls the body's responses to internal and external stimuli, coordinating actions and transmitting signals between different parts of the body. It includes the brain, spinal cord and nerves.

Vitamin A

Vitamin A:

- helps children to grow
- helps the body to resist infection
- helps to prevent night blindness.

Vitamin A is found in fatty foods. Dark green vegetables are a good source of vitamin A.

Other sources of vitamin A are:

- halibut and cod liver oil
- milk, eggs and cheese
- butter and margarine
- watercress
- herrings
- carrots
- liver and kidneys
- spinach
- tomatoes
- apricots.

Fish liver oils are the best source of vitamin A.

Vitamin D

Vitamin D:

- controls the way our bodies use calcium (a mineral that you will read about later)

- is necessary for healthy bones and teeth.

An important source of vitamin D is sunlight. Other sources are fish liver oils, oily fish, egg yolk, margarine and dairy produce.

Vitamin B

There are two main types of vitamin B:

- Thiamin, also known as B1 – this helps our bodies to produce energy and is necessary for our brain, heart and nervous system to function properly
- Riboflavin, also known as B2 – this helps with growth, and helps us to have healthy skin, nails and hair, among other things.

As well as these two main types of vitamin B there is a third, Niacin or Nicotinic acid. This is vital for normal brain function and it improves the health of the skin, the circulation and the digestive system.

Vitamin B:

- helps to keep the nervous system in good condition
- enables the body to get energy from carbohydrates
- encourages the body to grow.

When you cook food the vitamin B in it can be lost. It is important to learn how to preserve vitamin B when you cook foods. You will learn about this as you study cookery in more depth.

Vitamin C (also called Ascorbic Acid)

Vitamin C:

- is needed for children to grow
- helps cuts and broken bones to heal
- prevents gums and mouth infections.

When you cook food the vitamin C in it can be lost. It is important to learn how to preserve vitamin C when you cook foods – one of the most important sources of vitamin C in our diet is potatoes. You will find more references to vitamin C and how to preserve it in other sections in this book.

Table 4.4 sources of vitamin B

Thiamin (B1)	Riboflavin (B2)	Nicotinic acid
Yeast	Yeast	Meat extract
Bacon	Liver	Brewers' yeast
Oatmeal	Meat extract	Liver
Peas	Cheese	Kidney
Wholemeal bread	Egg	Beef

Sources of vitamin C are:

- blackcurrants
- green vegetables
- lemons
- grapefruit
- bananas
- potatoes
- strawberries
- oranges
- tomatoes
- fruit juices.

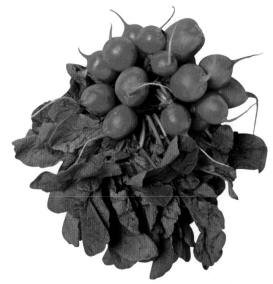

Lots of vegetables are high in vitamin C, including radishes

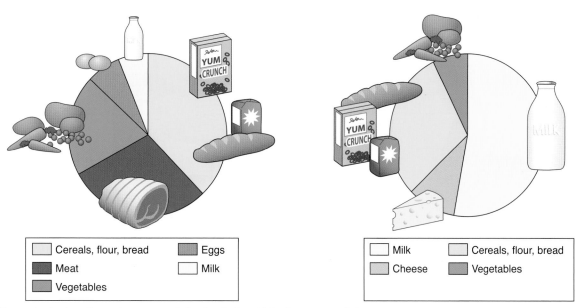

These charts show the main sources of vitamins A, C and D in the average diet

Minerals

There are 19 minerals in total, most of which our bodies need, in very small quantities, to function properly.

- We need minerals to build our bones and teeth.
- Minerals help us to carry out bodily functions.
- Minerals help to control the levels of fluids in our bodies.

We will now look at a few of the most important minerals for our bodies.

Calcium

We need calcium to:

- build bones and teeth
- help our blood to clot
- help our muscles to work.

In order for our bodies to use calcium effectively they also need vitamin D.

Sources of calcium are:

- milk and milk products
- green vegetables

- the bones of tinned oily fish (e.g. sardines)
- drinking water
- wholemeal bread and white bread if calcium has been added.

Iron

We need iron to build haemoglobin, which is a substance in our blood that transports oxygen and carbon dioxide around the body.

Sources of iron include:

- lean meat
- wholemeal flour
- offal (animals' internal organs, such as the heart, liver and kidneys)
- green vegetables
- egg yolk
- fish.

Our bodies absorb iron more easily from meat and offal. Iron is also absorbed better if vitamin C is present.

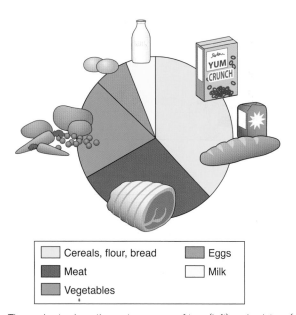

Cereals, flour, bread	Eggs
Meat	Milk
Vegetables	

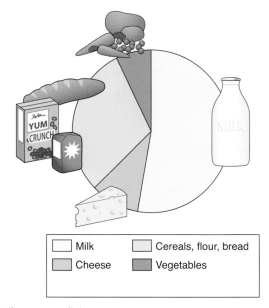

| Milk | Cereals, flour, bread |
| Cheese | Vegetables |

These charts show the main sources of iron (left) and calcium (right) in the average diet

Phosphorus

We need phosphorus to:

- build bones and teeth (together with calcium and vitamin D)
- control the structure of our brain cells.

Sources of phosphorous include:

- liver
- bread
- cheese
- eggs
- kidney
- fish.

Sodium

We need to have sodium in all our body fluids. It regulates the amount of water we have in our bodies. It also helps with the functioning of our muscles and nerves.

If we eat too much salt our bodies can excrete some of it in our urine. Our kidneys control how much salt we get rid of through our urine. We also lose sodium when we sweat, but our bodies cannot control how much salt we lose in this way.

Sodium is found in salt (sodium chloride).

Many foods:

- are cooked with salt
- or have salt added to them (e.g. bacon and cheese)
- or already contain salt (e.g. meat, eggs, fish).

Too much sodium can cause hypertension (high blood pressure) and can increase the risk of a stroke. It is recommended that we do not eat more than 6g of salt per day. Our bodies only need 4.1g.

Iodine

We need iodine so that our thyroid gland can function properly. The thyroid gland produces hormones that control our growth. If it is not working properly it can make us underweight or overweight.

Sources of iodine include:

- seafood
- iodised salt
- drinking water obtained near the sea
- vegetables grown near the sea.

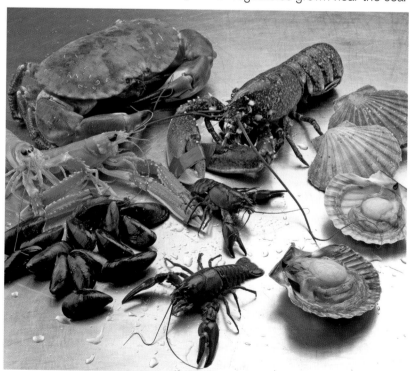

Water

Water is vital to life. Without it we cannot survive for very long. We lose water from our bodies through urine and sweat, and we need to replace it regularly to prevent dehydration. It is recommended that we drink eight glasses of water a day.

Our organs require water to function properly.

- Water regulates our body temperature – when we sweat the water evaporates from our skin and cools us down.
- Water helps to remove waste products from our bodies. If these waste products are not removed they can release poisons, which can damage our organs or make us ill.
- We need water to help our bodies absorb nutrients, vitamins and minerals and to help our digestive system.
- Water acts as a lubricant, helping our eyes and joints to work and stay healthy.

Sources of water:

- drinks of all kinds
- foods such as fruits, vegetables, meat, eggs
- fibre.

As you have already read, fibre cannot be digested, but we need it to remove waste from our bodies.

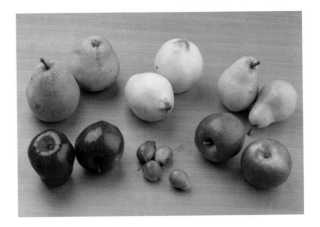

Healthy eating

If you eat a healthy diet you will reduce the risk of a number of diseases including stroke, heart disease, diabetes and some cancers.

The best way to stay fit and healthy is to eat a diet high in fruit, vegetables, whole grains and plant-based foods like beans and lentils, but low in fat, sugar and salt.

Fruit and vegetables

Fruit and vegetables contain valuable vitamins, minerals, fibre and folate acid, which help to protect us from illness. They also contain substances called phytochemicals, which are antioxidants. Antioxidants help to protect the body's cells from damage.

- There are some vegetables and fruits that protect us particularly well against strokes because they have such high levels of antioxidants. The vegetables include cauliflower,

cabbage, broccoli and Brussels sprouts. The fruits include blackcurrants, oranges, kiwis, and red and yellow peppers.

- The fibre found in fruit and vegetables plays an important role in preventing a stroke too. It also helps to lower cholesterol and maintain a healthy digestive system.

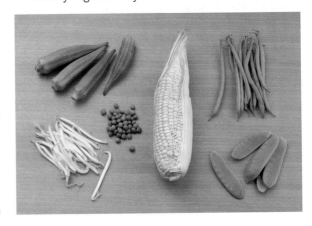

- Folate or folic acid is found in dark green vegetables like broccoli and spinach. This also helps to protect us against strokes.
- Potassium is another essential mineral, like sodium, that we need to balance the fluids in our bodies. It is also important in keeping our heart rate normal and helps our nerves and muscles to function. It is found in bananas, avocados, citrus fruits and green leafy vegetables.

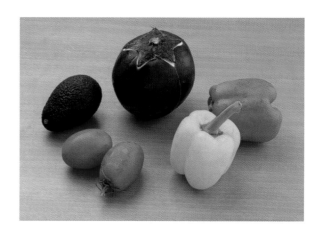

Ideally you should aim to eat at least five portions of fruit and vegetables a day, e.g. 1 apple, 1 banana, 2 plums, a heaped tablespoon of dried fruit like raisins (15g) or three broccoli or cauliflower florets.

The nutrient content of different foods

Table 4.5 The different nutrients, what foods they are found in and their use in the body

Nutrient	Food in which it is found	Use in body
Protein	Meat, fish, poultry, game, milk, cheese, eggs, pulses, cereals	For building and repairing body tissues Provides some heat and energy
Fat	Butter, margarine, cooking fat, oils, cheese, fat meat, oily fish	Provides heat and energy
Carbohydrate	Flour, flour products and cereals, sugar, syrup, jam, honey, fruit, vegetables	Provides heat and energy
Vitamin A	Oily fish, fish liver oil, dairy foods, carrots, tomatoes, greens	Helps growth Provides resistance to disease
Vitamin B1 (thiamin)	Yeast, pulses, liver, whole grain, cereals, meat and yeast extracts	Helps growth Strengthens the nervous system
Vitamin B2 (riboflavin)	Yeast, liver, meat, meat extracts, wholegrain cereals	Helps growth Helps in the production of energy
Nicotinic acid (niacin)	Yeast, meat, liver, meat extracts, wholegrain cereals	Helps growth
Vitamin C (ascorbic acid)	Fruits such as strawberries, citrus fruits, green vegetables, root vegetables, salad	Helps growth Promotes health
Vitamin D (sunshine vitamin)	Fish liver oils, oily fish, dairy foods	Helps growth Builds bones and teeth
Iron	Lean meat, offal, egg yolk, wholemeal flour, green vegetables, fish	Builds up the blood
Calcium	Milk and milk products, bones of fish, wholemeal bread	Building bones and teeth Helps with blood clotting Helps the muscles to work

Phosphorus	Liver and kidney, eggs, cheese, bread	Builds bones and teeth
		Regulates body processes
Sodium (salt)	Meat, eggs, fish, bacon, cheese	All bodily fluids need it, to help regulate water content
		Prevents muscular cramp

Table 4.6 The main functions of different nutrients

Energy	Growth and repair	Regulation of body processes
Carbohydrates	Proteins	Vitamins
Fats	Minerals	Minerals
Proteins	Water	Water

The effects of too little or too much of some nutrients in the diet

Table 4.7 The effects of having too little or none of some nutrients in your diet

Nutrient	Effect of absence in diet
Carbohydrate	Lack of energy
	Weight loss
	Low immune system
Fat	Weight loss
	Lack of energy
	Low immune system
Protein	Water retention (when the body does not get rid of enough water)
	Muscle wastage (when muscles wither away)
	Hair loss
Dietary fibre	Bowel disorders
	Bowel cancer
	Constipation
Vitamin A	Sight problems
	Hydration problems
Vitamin B1	Nervous disorders
Vitamin B2	Growth disorders
	Skin disorders
Vitamin B6	Anaemia
	Blood disorders
Vitamin B12	Anaemia
	Blood disorders
	Possible mental problems
Vitamin C	Scurvy (a disease that can cause bleeding gums and other symptoms)
	Tiredness
	Blood loss if injured, as blood does not clot properly
	Bruising

Vitamin D	Rickets (a disease of the bones)
Niacin	Possible mental problems and depression
	Diarrhoea
Iron	Tiredness
	Lack of energy and strength
Calcium	Rickets
Potassium	High blood pressure
Magnesium	Slower recovery from injury or illness
Folic acid	Blood disorders

Table 4.8 The effects of having too much of some nutrients in your diet

Nutrient	Effect of excess in diet
Fat	Obesity
	Heart disease and heart attacks
	High blood pressure
Carbohydrate	Obesity
	Tooth decay
	Diabetes caused by too much sugar
Salt	High blood pressure and stroke

Special diets

There are various reasons why people may follow a particular type of diet.

Groups with special dietary requirements

There are certain groups of people who have special nutritional needs. You may have different needs at different points in your life, for example, if you change your lifestyle or occupation and when you grow older.

Pregnant and breastfeeding women

Pregnant and breastfeeding women should avoid soft mould-ripened cheese, paté, raw eggs, undercooked meat, poultry and fish, liver and alcohol.

Children and teenagers

As children grow their nutritional requirements change. Children need a varied and balanced diet rich in protein.

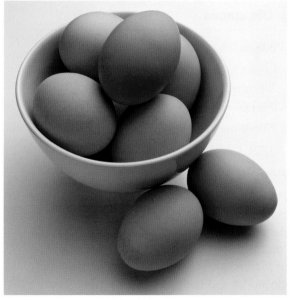

Pregnant women should avoid raw eggs

Teenagers need to have a good nutritionally balanced diet. Girls need to make sure that they are getting enough iron in their diet to help with the effects of puberty.

Vegetarians and vegans

Vegetarians generally do not eat meat, fish or any food products made from meat or fish. Some vegetarians do not eat eggs. Vegetarians have a lower risk of heart disease, stroke, diabetes, gallstones, kidney stones and colon cancer than people who eat meat. They are also less likely to be overweight or have raised cholesterol levels.

Vegans are vegetarians who also do not eat eggs or milk, or anything containing eggs or milk. They may also not consume animal products such as honey, and may refuse to use products made from leather.

A vegetarian or vegan diet may be followed for ethical reasons, certain religions (such as Hindus) usually follow a vegetarian diet, or it may be followed for health reasons.

The elderly

As we get older our bodies start to slow down and our appetite will get smaller. However, elderly people still need a nutritionally balanced diet to stay healthy.

Life stages
Babies
Children
Teenagers
Pregnant women
Elderly people

People who are ill

People who are ill, at home or in hospital, need balanced meals with plenty of the nutrients they need to help them recover. Good nutritional food is part of the healing process. In the days of Florence Nightingale hospital wards were closed for two hours a day while patients ate their nutritious meals. No doctor was allowed in the wards at mealtimes. Florence Nightingale saw food as medicine.

ACTIVITY

Produce a chart listing the food that you can use when preparing food for special diets.

Other reasons for special diets

Many people require special diets for various reasons, such as:

- health (diabetes, obesity, heart disease)
- allergies
- religious or moral beliefs.

Allergies and intolerances

Some people may be intolerant of or allergic to some types of food, so caterers must tell customers what is in the dishes on the menu.

Food allergies are a type of intolerance where the body's immune system sees harmless food as harmful and this causes an allergic reaction. Some food allergies can cause something called anaphylactic shock, which makes the throat and mouth swell, making it difficult to swallow or breathe. They can also cause skin reactions, nausea, vomiting and unconsciousness. Some allergic reactions can be fatal.

An **allergy** involves the immune system reacting to or rejecting certain foods or ingredients. **Food intolerance** does not involve the immune system, but it does cause a reaction to some foods.

Foods that sometimes cause an allergic reaction include:

- milk
- dairy products
- fish
- shellfish
- eggs
- nuts (particularly peanuts, cashew nuts, pecans, Brazil nuts, walnuts).

Gluten-free diet

A gluten-free diet is essential for people who have Coeliac disease, a condition where gluten causes the immune system to produce antibodies that attack the lining of the intestines.

Gluten is a mixture of proteins found in some cereals, particularly wheat. A gluten-free diet is not the same as a wheat-free diet, and some gluten-free foods are not wheat free.

Diabetes

Everything we eat is broken down into sugars in our body, but different foods break down at different speeds. People with diabetes need to pay attention to what they eat and when, to control their blood sugar.

The ideal diabetic meal will be balanced, with a variety of foods, in an appropriate portion size. The details will vary depending on the person, their level of physical activity and the type of diabetes that they have. There are some detailed suggestions at www.diabeticdietfordiabetes.com.

Religion-based diets

- Jewish: do not eat pork or pork products, shellfish or eels. Meat and milk are not eaten together. Meat must be kosher (killed according to Jewish custom and rules).
- Muslim: animals for meat must be slaughtered according to custom (halal). No shellfish or alcohol is consumed.
- Hindu: strict Hindus will not eat meat, fish or eggs. Those following a less strict regime will still not eat beef.
- Rastafarian: are often vegetarian. Even if they are not vegetarian, they will not eat any processed food, eels, tea, coffee or alcohol.

Moral beliefs

Some people choose special diets based on their moral beliefs, for example, some people do not eat meat because they do not believe in killing animals. Some who do eat meat will only buy meat from certain sources, which state that the animals have been ethically reared, free to roam, and humanely killed.

The chef's role – good practice

Chefs have a vital role in making healthy eating an exciting reality for us all. Customer trends show that many people are looking for healthier options on menus, particularly if they eat away from home every day. Healthy eating is one of the major consumer trends to emerge over the past decade and is an important commercial opportunity for caterers across the UK. This is not a passing fad; healthy eating is here to stay. Some sectors of catering have strict requirements relating to health and nutrition. For example, by law, school caterers have to provide meals that meet a minimum nutritional standard. Often there are health-related specifications for workplace catering contracts because employers feel they have a commitment to the health of their staff.

Chefs can be highly influential in the area of healthy eating. The amounts and proportions of the ingredients used, plus the way they are

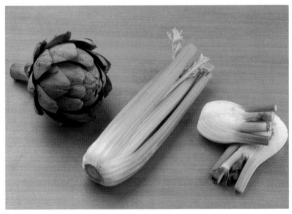

Chefs look for ways to make healthy eating exciting

cooked and served, can make an enormous difference to the nutritional content of a dish or meal. Research has shown that the most effective approach to healthy catering is to make small changes to popular dishes. This may involve the following measures:

- Making small changes in portion size, or adding a bread roll or jacket potato to a meal. Adding bread or potato to a meal means that there is more starch in proportion to fat (effectively diluting the fat).
- Making adjustments to preparation and cookery methods, such as trimming all the fat off meat, 'dry frying' and not adding butter to cooked vegetables.
- Making slight modifications to recipes for composite dishes (dishes made from several different ingredients). For instance, a pizza could be made with a thicker base, adding mushrooms and roasted peppers, and topping it with less mozzarella but adding a sprinkling of Parmesan for flavour. Instead of adding salt, rely on the Parmesan, black pepper and chopped oregano to add flavour.

This is where chefs are vital in developing healthier recipes that work. The skill is in deciding when and where dishes can be modified without losing quality. Some highly traditional dishes are best left alone, while subtle changes can be made to others without losing their texture, appearance or flavour. The 'healthy eating tips' throughout the recipe sections can help in making some of these changes.

In summary, the key to healthier catering is to:

- make small changes to best-selling items
- increase the amount of starchy foods
- increase the amount of fruit and vegetables
- increase the fibre content of dishes where it is practical and acceptable
- reduce fat in traditional recipes
- change the type of fat used
- select healthier ways to prepare dishes, and be adventurous
- be moderate in the use of sugar and salt.

Moderate: Average; within reasonable limits, without being excessive.

ACTIVITY

Choose two special diets and design a three-course meal to meet the needs of each.

Test yourself

1 When looking at nutrition, the components of food are divided into six main nutrient groups. What are they?
2 Dietary fibre cannot be digested so why is it needed in the diet?
3 What are amino acids and why are they important?
4 It is considered that there is too much fat in the average UK diet. Give three reasons why too much fat should be avoided.
5 Vitamin A in the diet is essential for good health. Name five foods that are sources of vitamin A.
6 Why is vitamin C (ascorbic acid) needed in the diet?
7 How many portions of fruit/vegetables is it recommended to eat in a day? Suggest what these could be; include portion sizes.
8 What is meant by 'an allergy?' What is anaphylactic shock?
9 Which religious/cultural diets forbid the eating of pork and pork products?
10 Suggest three ways that chefs can make the food they cook healthier.

5 Catering operations, costs and menu planning

In this chapter you will learn how to:

1. understand the organisation of kitchens, including:
- the importance of layout and workflow
- job roles, the staffing hierarchy and the partie system

2. know how to plan and prepare menus:
- the factors to be considered
- the technical terminology used

3. understand basic costs and apply basic calculations, including:
- using calculator and manual methods
- gross and net profit
- the factors which must be monitored to control food costs and profit
- calculating the food cost of dishes and determining the food cost per portion
- determining selling prices at specific percentages of gross and net profit.

The organisation of the kitchen

Effective organisation will help a kitchen to run efficiently. An efficiently run kitchen will prepare and cook the right amount of high-quality food for the required number of people, on time, making the most effective use of staff, ingredients and equipment.

Menus and the systems

Regardless of the size of the organisation, the most important factors in its success will be the menu and the systems used to prepare and present the food.

A kitchen with a large brigade of chefs can offer an extensive menu as long as the majority of the *mise en place* (preparation prior to service) is carried out during the day. The food can be kept refrigerated until it is needed at service time. If an establishment has a finishing kitchen, the final preparation and presentation of many foods (fish, meat, vegetables, potatoes, pasta and eggs) can be completed quickly and efficiently (by sautéing, grilling, deep frying, and so on) just before they are served, so the dishes are served to the customer quickly and freshly cooked. The design of the finishing kitchen is important and needs to include refrigerated cabinets for holding perishable foods, adequate cooking facilities and bain-marie space for holding sauces, etc.

Restaurants that provide a limited menu, such as steak houses, can employ fewer staff to cope with large numbers of customers, if they are organised well. The required standard can still be reached because few skills are needed. Nevertheless, whether producing grilled steaks or pancakes, the staff have to be organised and work in a systematic way so that the flow of work is smooth.

Other types of establishment, such as schools, hospitals, airlines and department stores, also have to produce large amounts of food to be served at the same time. In order to achieve this, the catering staff have to be well organised, and supplied with large-scale preparation and production equipment and the means to finish dishes quickly. There has to be a good system in place for the preparation–production–freezing or chilling–reheat cycle, so that staff can simply reheat or finish the foods just before service. It is essential that very high standards of hygiene are maintained in situations that use a system of deep freezing or chilling and reheating.

Organisation and layout of the kitchen

As the costs of space, equipment, fuel, maintenance and labour are continually going up, considerable time, thought and planning must be given to the organisation and layout of kitchen systems. The requirements of the kitchen have to be clearly identified with regard to the type of food that is to be prepared, cooked and served. The working areas and the different types of equipment available must be thought through carefully, and the organisation of the kitchen personnel must be planned.

In the late nineteenth century, when labour was relatively cheap, skilled and plentiful, the public wanted elaborate and extensive menus. In response to this, Auguste Escoffier, one of the most respected chefs of his era, devised what is known as the *partie* system, in which different sections of the kitchen were delegated to carry out specific jobs, such as preparing or cooking the fish, meat or vegetables. This system is still used in many establishments today. The number of *parties* (different areas) required, and the number of staff in each, will depend on the size of the establishment.

With a sound knowledge of fresh, part-prepared and ready prepared foods, together with an understanding of kitchen equipment and planning, a kitchen can be organised economically and efficiently. Even with two similar kitchens, the internal organisation is likely to vary, as each person in charge will have their own way of running their kitchen. However, everyone working in the system should know what he or she has to do, and how and when to do it.

The kitchen organisation will vary according to the size and type of establishment. Obviously the organisation of a kitchen with 100 chefs preparing banquets for up to 1000 people and a lunch and dinner service for 300 customers with an à la carte menu and floor service, will be quite different from that of a small restaurant serving 30 table d'hôte lunches, or a full-view coffee shop, a speciality restaurant with a busy turnover or a hospital kitchen.

 ACTIVITY

Describe in a sentence why a kitchen needs to be well organised.

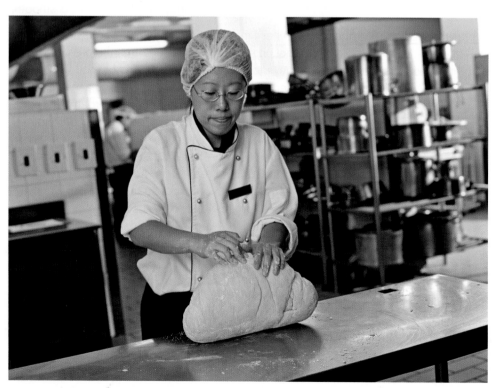

A tidy and organised kitchen promotes efficiency and good hygiene

Staffing hierarchy and good working relationships

Teamwork is essential to develop good working relationships and improve efficiency and productivity.

The organisation of the staffing hierarchy depends on the establishment. A large hotel or restaurant will have a head chef or executive head chef with one or two sous chefs, who deputise for the head chef. They may also run a department – for example, the pastry chef may also be the sectional chef, chef de partie and one of the sous chefs.

The chef de partie is in charge of a section such as sauces or vegetables. There may also be a demi chef de partie, who works on the opposite shift to the chef de partie. There will also be a number of assistant chefs (e.g. commis chefs), and there could be apprentices and trainees. The latter will move from section to section to complete their training.

Kitchen porters will also be employed, and in large establishments a kitchen clerk or personal assistant to the chef will be employed to assist with paperwork.

In other establishments, such as hospitals and centralised kitchens, a kitchen manager will take charge of the kitchen and have a number of cooks

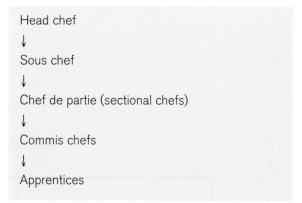

Head chef
↓
Sous chef
↓
Chef de partie (sectional chefs)
↓
Commis chefs
↓
Apprentices

and kitchen assistants working under them. A centralised kitchen is one that serves a number of different outlets, and the food is transported to these outlets usually chilled or frozen. Each outlet will have a satellite or finishing kitchen where the food is finished and made ready to serve to the customer.

Today, kitchens are organised in many different ways but, in each case, a senior member of staff will be responsible for the smooth operation of the kitchen. This person must have leadership skills, human resource management skills and detailed product knowledge. In order to achieve an efficient and effective system that satisfies customers' needs, it is important to work as a team and develop good working relationships in the kitchen

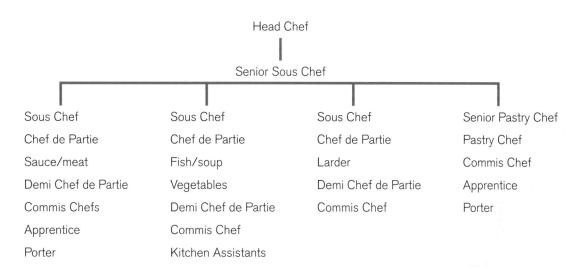

Head Chef

Senior Sous Chef

Sous Chef	Sous Chef	Sous Chef	Senior Pastry Chef
Chef de Partie	Chef de Partie	Chef de Partie	Pastry Chef
Sauce/meat	Fish/soup	Larder	Commis Chef
Demi Chef de Partie	Vegetables	Demi Chef de Partie	Apprentice
Commis Chefs	Demi Chef de Partie	Commis Chef	Porter
Apprentice	Commis Chef		
Porter	Kitchen Assistants		

Example of a kitchen brigade for a 4-star deluxe hotel: 300 rooms, 1 fine-dining restaurant (50 covers), 1 brasserie restaurant (80 covers), banqueting (up to 200 covers)

and with the food service staff. This will also contribute to high staff morale and will improve the productivity of staff.

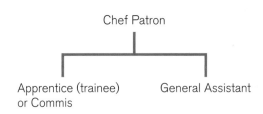

Example of a kitchen brigade for a 30-seater restaurant

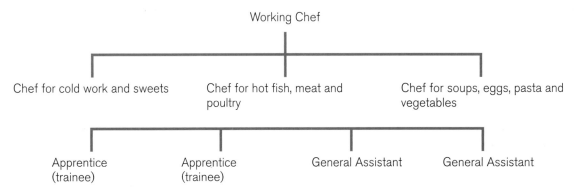

Example of a kitchen brigade for a restaurant kitchen serving 60–80 meals a day

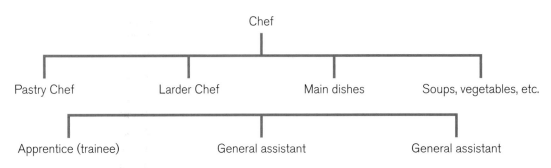

Example of a kitchen brigade for an industrial catering kitchen

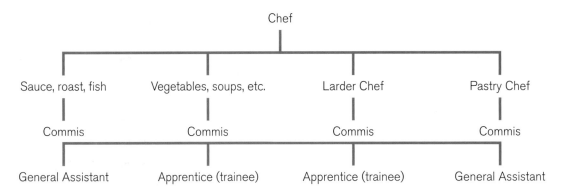

Example of a kitchen brigade for the kitchen of a commercial hotel or restaurant

Head chef: has overall responsibility for the organisation and management of the kitchen, including staffing, training, menus, budget control and sourcing of food.

Sous chef: is the deputy to the head chef and would take overall responsibility in the head chef's absence. The sous chef may also have specific areas of responsibility, such as food safety, health and safety, quality control or training of staff.

Chef de partie: is in charge of a specific section within the kitchen, such as meat, vegetables or fish. There may be a demi chef de partie working on an opposite shift and covering days off. Commis chefs and apprentices usually work with these chefs in different sections.

Commis chef: is the junior chef in the kitchen and works under overall supervision of the sous chef. A commis chef will work around the various kitchen sections.

Apprentice: is similar to a commis chef and will complete similar tasks but is usually on a planned programme of learning, often managed by a college or training provider.

 ACTIVITY

1 How can the layout of the kitchen you work in be improved?

2 Think of a successful team. Say why you think it is successful and what you could learn from this team's success.

Planning a kitchen

Different establishments will have different requirements for their kitchens. The most important factor to consider is the menu that is going to be offered, which will determine the amount of space and type of equipment you will need (known as operational requirements) in order to produce the food the customers are going to buy.

Equipment and layout

Properly planned layouts with adequate equipment, tools and materials to do the job are essential if practical work is to be carried out efficiently. If equipment is in the right place then work will proceed smoothly and in the proper sequence, without back-tracking or criss-crossing. Work surfaces, sinks, stores and refrigerators should be within easy reach in order to avoid unnecessary walking.

Food deliveries should have a separate entrance because of the risk of contamination. It is also a good idea to have a separate staff entrance to the kitchen and, for food safety reasons, it is essential

to have separate changing facilities for employees wherever possible – they should not have to use customer facilities.

The layout of the preparation areas (for vegetables, meat, poultry, dairy products, etc.) is also important. In large catering establishments the preparation areas will be zoned to assist with the workflow. The flow of work through the kitchen and serving areas is essential to the smooth running of any operation. Where possible, the layout of the kitchen should focus on a linear workflow.

Effective workflow will:

- help to establish good communication between departments
- improve efficiency
- improve the quality of the finished product
- reduce the risk of accidents
- promote good health and safety and food safety,

all of which will provide a better service to customers.

Table 5.1 An example of a job description: senior sous chef

Reporting to head chef

The senior sous chef position reports to the head chef and is responsible for the day-to-day kitchen operation, overseeing the stores, preparation and production areas. The position involves supervising and managing the kitchen staff, with direct responsibility for rostering and scheduling production. In the absence of the head chef, the senior sous chef will be required to take on the duties of the head chef and to attend senior management meetings in his or her absence.

Duties

- Monitor and check stores operation
- Train new and existing staff in health and safety, HACCP (hazard analysis critical and control point), etc.
- Chair the Kitchen Health and Safety Committee
- Develop new menus and concepts together with senior management
- Schedule and maintain accurate records of staff absences
- Maintain accurate kitchen records
- Be responsible for the overall cleanliness of the kitchen operation
- Assist in the production of management reports
- Establish an effective and efficient team
- Assist with the overall establishment and monitoring of budget
- Roster all kitchen staff

Conditions

- Grade 3 management spine
- Private health insurance
- Five-day week
- 20 days' holiday
- Profit-share scheme after one year's service

Personal specification: senior sous chef

Qualifications

Level 3 /Level 4 qualification

Experience

Five years' experience in four- and five-star hotel kitchens; restaurant and banqueting experience

Skills

- Proficiency in culinary arts
- Microsoft Excel, Access, Word
- Operation of inventory control software
- Written and oral communication skills
- Team-building skills

Knowledge

- Current health and safety legislation
- Food hygiene
- HACCP
- Risk assessment
- Production systems
- Current technology

Other attributes

- Honesty
- Reliability
- Attention to detail
- Initiative
- Accuracy

Essential

- Basic computer skills
- High degree of culinary skills
- Good communication skills
- Supervisory and leadership skills

Desirable

- Knowledge of employment law
- Public relations profile

Kitchen layout

Remember:

- health and safety
- food safety
- time and motion (workflow).

Other factors to consider

Chefs and managers are often asked to assist in the design of food service systems. There are various factors that influence the planning and design of a kitchen, including:

- the size and extent of the menu and the market it serves
- services – gas, electricity and water
- labour – skill level of staff

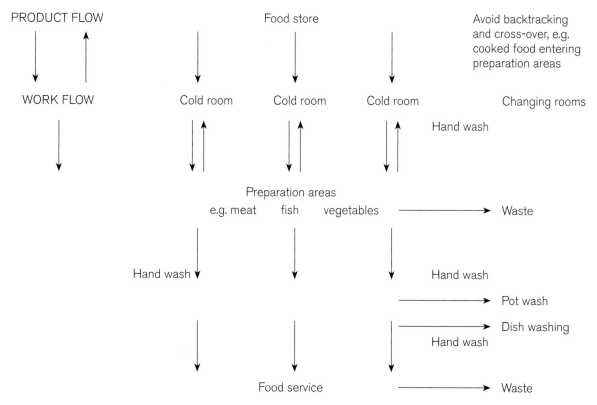

Example of linear workflow

- amount of capital expenditure, costs
- use of prepared convenience foods
- types of equipment available
- hygiene and the Food Safety Acts and Regulations (see Chapter 2)
- design and decor
- multi-usage requirements.

The size and extent of the menu

If possible all designs should be market-led. Before a kitchen is planned, the management must know its goals and objectives – what it is aiming to achieve. In other words, what market is it aiming at (e.g. fine dining, gastro pub), what style of operation is it going to run (e.g. traditional, modern contemporary, silver service, plate service) and what type of food and prices will the customers expect? Management will have found out answers to these questions by carrying out market research, and this will determine the menu. They also need to know the number of customers they intend to cater for at each service.

Services

The designer must know, when planning the layout of the kitchen, where the services (gas, electricity, water) are located. The designer must make sure that the layout of the kitchen uses the services in the most efficient way.

Labour and skill level

How many and what kind of people does the company intend to employ? This will have an effect on the technology and equipment that is installed. For example, will they employ fewer, unspecialised staff and a lot of pre-prepared food, or more skilled people and a traditional *partie* system that makes dishes with entirely fresh ingredients. Whichever system they choose will affect the overall kitchen design.

Amount of capital expenditure

There will be a detailed budget for most kitchen designs. It is not always possible, and is not a good idea, to design a kitchen and then worry about how much it will cost. The money available (the finance) will very often determine the overall design.

Because space is at a premium (property is expensive and the best use possible needs to be made of the space), kitchens are generally becoming smaller. Equipment is therefore being designed to cater for this trend, becoming more modular and streamlined and generally able to fit into less space. Equipment is also being designed to be easy to use, maintain and clean, because labour is a significant cost and the best use needs to be made of people's time.

Use of prepared convenience foods

A kitchen preparing a fast-food menu using prepared convenience food will be planned and equipped very differently from an à la carte or cook–chill kitchen. Certain factors must be taken into consideration:

- Will sweets and pastries be made?
- Will there be a need for a larder or a butcher?
- Will fresh or frozen food be used, or a combination of both?

Types of equipment available

The type, amount and size of the equipment will depend on the type of menu being provided. The equipment must be located in the right place. When planning a kitchen, standard symbols are used for the different equipment. A scale design can be produced on squared paper and these symbols can be included to show where each piece of equipment will be located. Hand-washing facilities and storage of cleaning equipment should also be included. Computer-aided design (CAD) is now often used to do this.

Not only should the equipment be suitably situated, it should also be the right weight – it is important that it can be used without overtiring the user.

Kitchen equipment manufacturers and gas and electricity suppliers can provide technical details for equipment, such as output and size.

 ACTIVITY

List the four pieces of large equipment you would expect to find in most commercial kitchens.

Hygiene and the Food Safety Act 1990/91/95

The design and construction of the kitchen must comply with the Food Safety Act 1990/91/95 and Food Hygiene Regulations 2006. The basic layout and construction should allow enough space for all food-handling areas, and associated areas for equipment. There should be enough room for the work to be carried out safely, and for frequent cleaning of the different areas and equipment.

Design and decor

The trend towards providing more attractive eating places (which can be seen in particular in many of

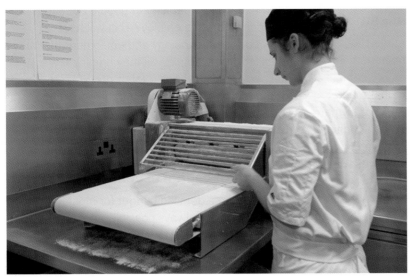

The type and location of equipment should be considered when planning a kitchen

the chain and franchise operators), has also had an effect on kitchen planning and design. One trend has been to bring the kitchen area totally or partially into view, with back-bar equipment – for example, grills or griddles may be in full public view and food prepared on them to order.

Future trends in design and decor will be affected by:
- changes in technology
- social changes in eating habits
- lifestyle changes.

While there will be a continuing demand for the traditional heavy-duty type of equipment found in larger hotels and restaurant kitchens, the constant need to change and update the design and decor of modern restaurants means that the equipment's life is generally shorter – reduced perhaps from ten years to seven or five, or even less – to cope with the rate of change and redevelopment. This has resulted in the design of catering equipment generally being improved.

Multi-usage requirements

The need for round-the-clock catering, such as in hospitals, factories where shift work takes place, the police and armed forces, has forced

kitchen planners to consider how kitchens can be used efficiently outside peak times. As a result, equipment is being made more adaptable and flexible, so that whole sections of the kitchen can be closed down when they are not in use, which means that savings can be made on heating, lighting and maintenance.

When planning a kitchen, it is important to consider the following:
- What type of customers do you want to attract?
- What type of food do you want to serve?
- Will your menu be à la carte, table d'hôte, a combination of both, or will it be self-service?
- Will you organise the kitchen based on the traditional *partie* system?
- Does the design comply with food safety law and health and safety regulations?

You must remember that whatever systems you choose, good communication between all departments in the kitchen and restaurant is important in order to improve efficiency.

 ACTIVITY

What is meant by good communication?

 Kitchen design

Kitchens must be designed so that they can be managed easily. Managers must have easy access to the areas under their control and must have a clear view of the areas they have to supervise. For reasons of efficiency and hygiene, large kitchens should have different working areas for different processes. The following factors must be taken into consideration:

- Product – how and where the different processes are carried out (raw materials to finished product), e.g. raw food should be prepared and stored in different areas from cooked food.
- Personnel – how people move within the kitchen, e.g. staff working in dirty areas (areas

of contamination) should not enter areas of finished product, or where blast-chilling is taking place.
- Containers/equipment/utensils – equipment should, where possible, be separated out into specific process areas, e.g. pastry equipment should not leave the pastry area, equipment and containers used for preparing and storing raw food should be washed and stored in the raw food area, chopping boards and other small equipment used for raw preparation should not be allowed to enter the cooking areas.
- Refuse – rubbish must be kept in an appropriate area and should not have to pass through other areas to get to its storage destination.

Product and workflow

Each section should be subdivided into high-risk and contaminated sections.

- High-risk food which is likely to be contaminated easily while it is being prepared, e.g. ready-to-eat foods such as soups and sauces, cooked meat and desserts.
- Food that may be already contaminated when it arrives, before processing, e.g. unprepared vegetables, raw meat.

Back-tracking or crossover of materials and products must be avoided. Food preparation rooms should be planned so that the flow of work to process the food allows it to be moved through the premises, from the point of delivery to the point of sale or service, with the minimum of obstruction. The various processes should be separated as far as possible, and food intended for sale should not cross paths with waste food or refuse. Staff time is valuable, so a design that reduces wasteful journeys is efficient and cost-effective.

The overall sequence of receiving, storing, preparing, holding, serving and clearing should involve:

- minimum movement
- minimal back-tracking
- maximum use of space

- maximum use of equipment with minimum time and effort.

Working areas

A good receiving area needs to be designed for easy delivery of supplies. Storage facilities should be located nearby, in a suitable position for the food to be distributed to preparation and production areas.

The size and style of the menu and the ability of the staff will determine the number of preparation and production areas necessary and their layout. A straight-line layout would be suitable for a snack bar, while an island layout would be more suitable for a hotel restaurant.

Food safety must also be considered. There should be room to access all kitchen equipment so that it can be cleaned thoroughly, and there should be room for all used equipment from the dining area to be cleared, cleaned and stored. Still room facilities (e.g. for storing preserves and cakes) may also be required. Sufficient handwashing facilities for staff must also be provided

Kitchens can be divided into sections based on the process involved. For example:

- **dry areas** – for storage
- **wet areas** – for fish preparation, vegetable preparation, butchery, cold preparation

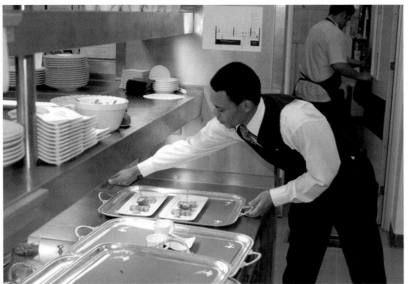

Good kitchen design will consider the flow of the food through the preparation and service areas

- **hot wet areas** – for boiling, poaching, steaming; equipment needed will include atmospheric steamers, bratt pans, pressure steamers, steam jacketed boilers, combination oven
- **hot dry areas** – for frying, roasting, grilling; equipment needed will include cool zone fryers, salamanders, pressure fryers, induction cookers, bratt pans, halogen cookers, roasting ovens, microwave, charcoal grills, cook and hold ovens
- **dirty areas** – for refuse, pot wash areas, plate wash; equipment needed will include compactors, dishwashers, refuse storage units, glass washers, pot wash machines.

Preparation areas

The various preparation processes require different areas depending on what food is involved. In a vegetable preparation area, water from the sinks and dirt from the vegetables are going to accumulate, so adequate facilities for drainage should be provided. Pastry preparation, on the other hand, involves mainly dry processes.

Whatever the processes, there are certain basic rules that can be applied to make working conditions easier and help to ensure that food hygiene regulations are complied with.

Proper design and layout of the preparation area can make a major contribution to good food safety. Staff generally respond to good working conditions by taking more of a pride in themselves, in their work and in their working environment.

Adequate workspace must be provided for each process and every effort must be made to separate dirty and clean processes.

Vegetable preparation and wash-up areas should be separate from the actual food preparation and service areas. The layout must ensure a continuous workflow in one direction in order to avoid crossover of foods and cross-contamination. The staff should not get in each other's way by having to cross each other's paths more than is absolutely necessary.

Actual worktop areas should be big enough for the preparation processes that will be done on them, and should be designed so that the food handler has all the necessary equipment and utensils close to hand.

The cooking area

Because 'raw materials' enter the cooking section from the main preparation areas (vegetables, meat and fish, dry goods), this section will be designed so that the flow movement continues through to the servery. So, for example, roasting ovens are best located close to the meat preparation area, and steamers next to the vegetable preparation area.

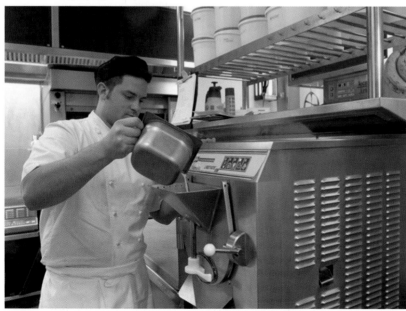

A chef making ice cream in the pastry section

However, layout is not just a question of choosing and positioning equipment; it also depends on the management policy regarding the use of prepared foods and the operating cycle. Obviously the cooking area should not be used by other staff to cross to another section of the kitchen or to get to the service area. The layout should be planned so that raw foodstuffs arrive at one point, are processed in the cooking section and then despatched to the servery. There should be a distinct progression in one direction.

> The **operating cycle** is the numbers of meals you are serving, which meal you are serving (breakfast, lunch or dinner) and the number of days a week you are open. So it is about the frequency of the operation.

As with other areas, the cooking section should be designed with a view to making maximum use of the available space with as little effort as possible.

Maintenance and cleaning

Planning and equipping a kitchen is an expensive investment, so to avoid any action by the Environmental Health Officer, efficient, regular cleaning and maintenance is essential. (For example, the kitchens at the Dorchester hotel are swept during the day, given soap/detergent and water treatment after service, and any spillages cleaned up immediately. At night, contractors clean the ceilings, floors and walls.)

In most cases, throughout the industry, companies are trying to reduce labour costs while maintaining or enhancing the meal experience for the customer. Some trends that will affect the design of kitchens are as follows:

- Hotels: there is greater use of buffet and self-assisted service units.
- Banqueting: there is a move towards plated service, with less traditional silver service.
- Fast food: new concepts are coming onto the market, with more specialised chicken and seafood courts, more choices in ethnic food.
- Roadside provision: there is an increasing number of operations and partnerships with service station companies. Basic grill menus are now enhanced by factory-produced à la carte items.
- Food courts: development has slowed down; there are minor changes all the time; most food courts offer an 'all day' menu. Restaurant Associates (Compass) are introducing food courts into hotels.
- Restaurants/hotels: there is less emphasis on luxury-end, five-star experience.
- Theme restaurants: will continue to improve and multiply.
- Hospitals: there is greater emphasis on bought-in freezer and chilled foods, meaning less on-site preparation and cooking. Some hospitals operate their own cook/chill or cook/freeze systems. Many hospitals now have food courts occupied by well-known high street names as franchises, such as Pizza Hut or Burger King.
- Industrial: there are more zero-subsidy staff restaurants, increased self-service for all items. The introduction of cashless systems will enable multi-tenant office buildings to offer varying subsidy levels.
- Prisons and other institutions: little if any change; may follow hospitals by buying in more pre-prepared food; may receive foods from multi-outlet central production units, tied in with schools, meals-on-wheels provision, etc.
- University/colleges: greater move towards providing food courts; more snack bars and coffee shops. There is evidence of more small 'satellite' outlets around the buildings rather than large refectories or cafeterias.

> **Self-service** is when the customers serve themselves from a self-service counter or buffet.
>
> Self-assisted service is when there is someone on duty to help the customer choose and, in some cases, there will be a section on a buffet where a chef will be cooking fresh items such as stirfry, omelettes, waffles, pancakes. Here the guest is helped to choose and will take the finished item to their table. This is also known as theatre cookery.

Zero-subsidy: No financial contribution or benefit. A 'zero-subsidy' staff restaurant is one in which the business does not contribute to the costs of the staff restaurant to allow its staff to purchase meals at a discounted rate. Instead, staff are expected to pay the full cost of anything they buy.

Planning and preparing menus for catering operations

As you have already learned, planning the menu is one of the most essential elements in designing and costing the operations of a catering establishment.

Evolution – the historical development of menus

Initially, menus were simply lists of food. Menus as we know them today came into use early in the nineteenth century, and courses began to be formulated. For special occasions as many as seven courses might be served, e.g. hors d'oeuvres, soup, fish, entrée, sorbet, roast, sweet, savoury.

With the formulation of menus, artistry and flair began to influence the various ways of cooking, and dishes were created after 'the style of' (e.g. à la Française) and/or given the names of important people for whom they had been created (e.g. peach Melba, a simple dish of poached fresh peach, vanilla ice cream and fresh raspberry purée created by Escoffier at the Savoy for Dame Nellie Melba, the famous opera singer).

As the twentieth century advanced, and people travelled more and settled around the world, styles of food and service from a wide variety of nations began to be introduced, resulting in the large number of ethnic dishes and ethnic restaurants that abound today.

Rapid air transport made it possible for foods from all corners of the globe to be available which, together with domestic and European produce, gives those who compose menus a tremendous range of choice.

Eating at work, at school, in hospitals and institutions led to a need for healthy, budget-conscious food.

The importance of the menu (a means of communication)

Essential considerations prior to planning a menu are:

- **Competition:** be aware of any competition in the locality, including prices and quality. It may be wiser to produce a menu that is quite different from those of competitors.
- **Location:** study the area in which your establishment is situated and the potential target market of customers.
- **Analysis:** analyse the type of people you are planning to cater for (e.g. office workers in the city requiring quick service or holidaymakers in a seaside resort).
- **Outdoor catering:** are there opportunities for outdoor catering or takeaway food?
- **Estimated customer spend per head:** this is important when catering, for example, for hospital staff and patients, children in schools, workers in industry. Whatever level of catering, a golden rule should be 'offer value for money'.
- **Modern trends in food fashions:** these should be considered alongside popular traditional dishes.
- **Range of dishes and pricing structure:** decide what you are going to offer and at what price. Will you price each dish separately, or offer set two- or three-course menus? Or a combination of both?
- **Space and equipment in the kitchens:** this will influence the composition of the menu (e.g. avoiding overloading the deep fryer, salamanders or steamers).

- **Number and capability of staff:** overstretched staff can easily reduce the standard of production envisaged and the quality of individual dishes.
- **Availability of supplies and reliability of suppliers:** consider issues such as seasonal foods and storage space.
- **Food allergies** (see Chapter 4).
- **Cost factor:** these are crucial if an establishment is to be profitable. Costing is essential for the success of any menu. Modern computer techniques can analyse costs swiftly and on a daily basis.

Types of menu

The main types of menu in use are:

- **Table d'hôte or set-price menu:** a menu forming a meal, usually of two or three courses at a set price. A choice of dishes may be offered at all courses.
- **À la carte:** a menu with all the dishes individually priced. Customers can therefore compile their own menu, which may be one, two or more courses. A true à la carte dish should be cooked to order and the customer should be prepared to wait.
- **Special party or function menus:** menus for banquets or functions of all kinds.
- **Ethnic or speciality menus:** these can be set-price menus or with dishes individually priced, specialising in the food of a particular country (or religion) or in a specialised food itself, e.g. ethnic (Chinese, Indian, kosher, African-Caribbean, Greek), speciality (steak, fish, pasta, vegetarian, pancakes).
- **Hospital menus:** these usually take the form of a menu card given to the patient the day before service so that his or her preferences can be ticked. Both National Health Service and private hospitals cater for vegetarians and also for religious requirements.
- **Menus for people at work:** these vary in standard and extent from one employer to another due to company policy on the welfare of their staff and workforce. There may also be a call-order à la carte selection charged at a higher price. The food will be varied with 'traditional' British and some ethnic and vegetarian dishes. Menus may consist of soup, main course with vegetables, followed by desserts and yoghurts. According to the policy of the management and employee requirements, there will very often be a salad bar and healthy-eating dishes included on the menu. Many companies now also serve breakfasts in their staff restaurants. When there is a captive clientele who face the same surroundings daily and meet the same people, then no matter how long the menu cycle or how pleasant the people, or how nice the decor, boredom is bound to set in and staff then long for a change of scene. So, a chef or manager needs to vary the menu constantly to encourage customers to patronise the establishment rather than going off the premises to eat. The decor and layout of the staff restaurant plays a very important part in satisfying the customer's needs. The facilities should be relaxing and comfortable so that he or she feels that the restaurant is not a continuation of the workplace. Employees who are happy, well nourished and know that the company has their interests and welfare at heart will tend to be well motivated and work better.
- **Menus for children:** in schools there is an emphasis on healthy eating and a balanced diet, particularly in boarding schools. Those areas with children of various cultural and religious backgrounds have appropriate items available on the menu. Many establishments provide special children's menus that concentrate on favourite foods and offer suitably sized portions.

Considerations when deciding which type of menu is appropriate:

- types of customers
- pricing
- staff available to produce and serve the menu
- waste control
- portion control.

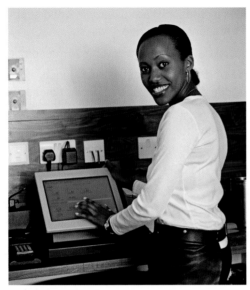

Consider how many service staff are available

Cyclical menus

These are menus that are compiled to cover a given period of time: one month, three months, etc. They consist of a number of set menus for a particular establishment, such as an industrial catering restaurant, cafeteria, canteen, directors' dining room, hospital or college refectory. At the end of each period the menu cycle starts again, thus overcoming the need to keep compiling new ones. The length of the cycle is determined by management policy, by the time of the year and by the different foods available. These menus must be monitored carefully to take account of changes in customer requirements and any variations in weather conditions that are likely to affect demand for certain dishes. If cyclical menus are designed to remain in operation for long periods of time, then they must be compiled carefully so that they do not have to be changed too drastically during operation.

Advantages:

- Cyclical menus save time by removing the daily or weekly task of compiling menus, although they may require slight alterations for the next period.
- When used in association with cook–freeze operations, it is possible to produce the entire number of portions of each item to last the whole cycle, once it has been determined that the standardised recipes are correct.

- They give greater efficiency in time and labour.
- They can cut down on the number of commodities held in stock, and can assist in planning storage requirements.

Disadvantages:

- When used in establishments with a captive clientele, the cycle has to be long enough for customers not to get bored with the repetition of dishes.
- The caterer cannot easily take advantage of 'good buys' offered by suppliers on a daily or weekly basis, unless such items are required for the cyclical menu.

 ACTIVITY

Design a cyclical menu for two weeks at a family holiday centre.

Pre-planned and pre-designed menus

Before selecting the dishes that he or she prefers, the caterer should consider what the customer likes, and the effect of these dishes upon the meal as a whole.

Advantages:

- Pre-planned or pre-designed menus enable the caterer to ensure that good menu planning is practised.
- Menus that are planned and costed in advance allow banqueting managers to quote prices instantly to a customer.
- Menus can be planned to take into account the availability of kitchen and service equipment, without placing unnecessary strain on it.
- The quality of food is likely to be higher if kitchen staff are preparing dishes they are familiar with and have prepared a number of times before.
- There is likely to be less waste.

Disadvantages:

- Pre-planned and pre-designed menus may be too limited to appeal to a wide range of customers.

- They may reduce job satisfaction for staff who have to prepare the same menus repeatedly.
- They may limit the chef's creativity and originality.

The structure of menus

Length

The number of dishes on a menu should offer the customer an interesting and varied choice. In general, it is better to offer fewer dishes of good standard than a long list of mediocre quality.

Design

This should complement the image of the dining room and be designed to allow for changes, which may be daily, weekly, monthly, etc. An insert for dishes of the day/week gives the customer added interest.

Language

Accuracy in dish description helps the customer to identify the food they wish to choose. Avoid over-elaboration and using flowery words. Wherever possible, use English language. If a foreign dish name is used then follow it with a simple, clear English version.

Factors to consider when planning a menu

Presentation

Ensure that the menu is presented in a sensible and welcoming way so that the customer is put at ease and relaxed. An offhand, brusque presentation (written or oral) can be off-putting and lower expectations of the meal.

Planning

Consider the following:

- type and size of establishment – pub, school, hospital, restaurant, etc.
- customer profile – different kinds of people have differing likes and dislikes
- special requirements – kosher, halal.
- time of the year – certain dishes acceptable in summer may not be so in winter

- foods in season – are usually in good supply and reasonable in price
- special days – Christmas, Shrove Tuesday, etc.
- time of day – breakfast, brunch, lunch, tea, high tea, dinner, supper, snack, special function
- price range – charge a fair price and ensure good value for money; customer satisfaction can lead to recommendation and repeat business
- number of courses
- sequence of courses
- use menu language that customers understand
- sensible nutritional balance
- no unnecessary repetition of ingredients
- no unnecessary repetition of flavours and colours
- be aware of the Trade Descriptions Act 1968 – 'Any person who in the course of a trade or business: applies a false trade description to any goods or supplies or offers to supply any goods to which a false trade description is applied shall be guilty of an offence.'

> **Mediocre:** Only of average, or middling quality; not very good.
> **Brusque:** Abrupt, rude or rough.

Consumer protection

There is a whole range of laws concerned with consumer protection. Some are concerned with health and safety, and some are concerned with economic protection.

Fundamentally, however, all consumer protection starts with the basic contractor. If a supplier does not supply what a consumer has contracted to purchase (e.g. if a menu says that something is 'fresh' or 'free range', if the customer is served something that is not 'fresh' or 'free range'), the supplier may be in breach of contract. However, breach of contract cases can be difficult to prove.

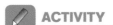 **ACTIVITY**

Suggest two types of menu that reflect religious beliefs.

Breakfast menus

Breakfast menus can be compiled from the following foods and can be offered as continental, table d'hôte, à la carte or buffet. For buffet service customers can self-serve the main items they require with assistance from counter hands. Ideally, eggs should be freshly cooked to order.

- Fruits, fruit juices, stewed fruit, yoghurts, cereals (porridge, etc.
- Eggs: fried, boiled, poached, scrambled; omelettes with bacon or tomatoes, mushrooms or sauté potatoes.
- Fish: kippers, smoked haddock, kedgeree.
- Meats (hot): fried or grilled bacon, sausages, kidneys, with tomatoes, mushrooms or sauté potatoes, potato cakes.
- Meats (cold): ham, bacon, pressed beef with sauté potatoes.
- Preserves: marmalade (orange, lemon, grapefruit, ginger), jams, honey.
- Beverages: tea, coffee, chocolate.
- Bread: rolls, croissants, brioche, toast, pancakes, waffles.

Points to consider when compiling a breakfast menu:

- It is usual to offer three of the courses previously mentioned: fruit, yoghurt or cereals; fish, eggs or meat; preserves, bread, coffee or tea.
- As large a choice as possible should be offered, depending on the size of the establishment, bearing in mind that it is better to offer a smaller number of well-prepared dishes than a large number of hurriedly prepared ones.
- A choice of plain foods, such as boiled eggs or poached haddock, should be available for people who may not require a fried breakfast.

- Buffet breakfast offers a choice of as many breakfast foods as is both practical and economic. It can be planned on a self-service basis or part self-service and assisted service (e.g. hot drinks and freshly cooked eggs prepared to order).

CONTINENTAL BREAKFAST £20.00

Freshly squeezed juices

Traditional Scottish porridge with milk or water,
topped with your choice of seasonal fruits, East London honey or brown sugar

Freshly baked croissants, Danish pastries, muffins, breads and toast
with butter, preserves, marmalade and honey

A selection from our breakfast buffet

Selection of coffee, tea or herbal infusions

TRADITIONAL FULL ENGLISH BREAKFAST £27.00

Freshly squeezed juices

Freshly baked croissants, Danish pastries, muffins, breads and toast
with butter, preserves, marmalade and honey

A selection from our breakfast buffet

Two free-range Burford Brown eggs cooked to your liking with grilled bacon,
sausage, black pudding, tomato, mushroom and baked beans

Coffee, tea or herbal infusions

A LA CARTE BREAKFAST

Freshly squeezed juices £5.00

Basket of pastries £6.50

Brown's bacon butty £8.25

Drop scones with seasonal fruit compote £6.75

De Beauvoir smoked salmon 'Hix cure' with scrambled Burford Brown eggs £13.50

Orkney kippers with lemon butter £12.75

Kedgeree £11.50

Omelette with your choice of filling £8.75

Fried duck's eggs with brown shrimps and sea purslane £9.75

Two soft-boiled Gladys May duck's eggs with sourdough soldiers £7.50

Eggs Benedict £8.25 / £12.50

Bubble and squeak with fried Burford Brown egg £11.75

Cumbrian black pudding hash with pan-fried Burford Brown eggs £8.50

Coffee, tea or herbal infusions £4.90

Any of the above may be included as part of the full English breakfast

BROWN'S HOTEL
LONDON

Sample continental, English and à la carte breakfast menu

Luncheon and dinner menus

Types of menu:

- A set-price one-, two- or three-course menu, ideally with a choice at each course.
- A list of well-varied dishes, each priced individually so that the customer can make up his or her own menu of whatever number of dishes they require.
- Buffet, which may be all cold or hot dishes, or a combination of both, either to be served or organised on a self-service basis. Depending on the time of year and location, barbecue dishes can be considered.
- Special party, which may be either: set menu with no choice; set menu with a limited choice, such as soup or melon, main course, choice of two sweets; served or self-service buffet.

Tea menus

These vary considerably, depending on the type of establishment, and could include, for example:

- assorted sandwiches
- bread and butter (white, brown, fruit loaf)
- assorted jams
- scones with clotted cream, pastries, gâteaux
- tea (Indian, China, iced, fruit, herb).

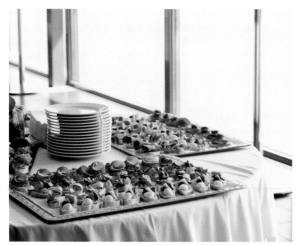

A buffet table at a function

Commercial hotels, tea rooms, public restaurants and staff dining rooms may offer simple snacks, cooked meals and high teas. For example:

- assorted sandwiches
- buttered buns, scones, cakes, Scotch pancakes, waffles, sausage rolls, assorted bread and butter, various jams, toasted teacakes, scones, crumpets, buns
- eggs (boiled, poached, fried, omelettes)
- fried fish, grilled meats, roast poultry
- cold meats and salads
- assorted pastries, gâteaux
- various ices, coupes, sundaes
- tea, orange and lemon squash.

Light buffets (including cocktail parties)

Light buffets can include:

- hot savoury pastry patties of, for example, lobster, chicken, crab, salmon, mushrooms, ham
- hot chipolatas; chicken livers, wrapped in bacon and skewered
- bite-sized items – quiche and pizza; hamburgers; meatballs with savoury sauce or dip; scampi or fried fish goujons with tartare sauce
- savoury finger toast to include any of the cold canapés; these may also be prepared on biscuits or shaped pieces of pastry
- game chips, gaufrette potatoes, fried fish balls, celery stalks spread with cheese
- sandwiches; bridge rolls, open or closed but always small
- fresh dates stuffed with cream cheese; crudités with mayonnaise and cardamom dip; tuna and chive catherine wheels; crab claws with garlic dip; smoked salmon pin wheels; choux puffs with Camembert
- sweets (e.g. trifles, charlottes, bavarois, fruit salad, gâteaux).

For fork buffets, all food must be prepared in a way that enables it to be eaten with a fork or spoon.

Fast-food menus

Although some people are scornful of the items on this type of menu, calling them 'junk food', nevertheless their popularity and success is proven by the fact that, starting with the original McDonald's, which opened in Chicago in 1955, there are now many thousands of outlets worldwide. McDonald's offers customers a nutrition guide to its products, as well as information for diabetes sufferers.

There are now many more well-known fast-food brands operating successfully in the UK.

Banquet menus

Banquets often serve a set menu of three or more courses, often to large numbers of people.

When compiling banquet menus, consider the following points:

- The food, which will possibly be for a large number of people, must be dressed in such a way that it can be served fairly quickly. Heavily garnished dishes should be avoided.
- If a large number of dishes have to be dressed at the same time, certain foods deteriorate

quickly and will not stand storage, even for a short time, in a hot place.

A normal menu is used, bearing in mind the number of people involved. It is not usual to serve farinaceous (e.g. pasta, noodles, rice) dishes, eggs, stews or savouries. A luncheon menu could be drawn from the following and would usually consist of three courses. Dinner menus, depending on the occasion, generally consist of three to five courses.

- **First course:** soup, cocktail (fruit or shellfish), hors d'oeuvres (assorted or single item), a small salad.
- **Second course:** fish, usually poached, steamed, roasted or grilled fillets with a sauce.
- **Third course:** meat, poultry or game, hot or cold, but not a stew or made-up dish; vegetables and potatoes or a salad would be served.
- **Fourth course:** if the function is being held during the asparagus season, then either hot or cold asparagus with a suitable sauce may be served as a course on its own.
- **Fifth course:** sweet, hot or cold, and/or cheese and biscuits.

Food purchasing

Once a menu is planned, a number of activities must occur to bring it into reality. One of the first and most important stages is to purchase and receive the required materials. Skilful purchasing with good receiving can help to make the best of a good menu. There are six important steps to remember:

1. Know the market.
2. Design the purchase procedures.
3. Determine purchasing needs.
4. Receive and check the goods.
5. Establish and use specifications.
6. Evaluate the purchasing task.

Knowing the market

Since markets vary considerably, to do a good job of purchasing a buyer must know the characteristics of each market.

A market is a place where buying and selling takes place. This could be done using the telephone, on a street corner, in a retail or wholesale establishment, or at an auction.

It is important that a food and beverage purchaser knows certain things about the items they plan to buy, such as:

- where they are grown
- seasons of production
- approximate costs

- conditions of supply and demand
- laws and regulations governing the market and the products
- marketing agents and their services
- processing
- storage requirements
- commodity and product, class and grade.

The buyer

This is the key person who makes decisions regarding quality, amounts, price and what will satisfy the customers but also make a profit. The wisdom of the buyer's decisions will be reflected in the success or failure of the operation. The buyer must not only be knowledgeable about the products, but must have the necessary skills to deal with sales people, suppliers and other market agents. The buyer must be prepared for hard and often aggressive negotiations.

The responsibility for buying varies from company to company according to size and management policy. Buying may be the responsibility of the chef, manager, storekeeper, buyer or buying department.

A buyer must have knowledge of the internal organisation of the company, especially the operational needs, and be able to obtain the products needed at a competitive price. Buyers must also acquaint themselves with the procedures of production and how these items are going to be used in the production operations (how they are going to be prepared and cooked), in order that the right item is purchased. For example, the item required may not always have to be of prime quality, e.g. tomatoes for use in soups and sauces.

A buyer must also be able to make good use of market conditions. For example, if there is a glut of fresh salmon at low cost, has the organisation the facility to make use of extra salmon purchases? Is there sufficient freezer space? Can the chef make use of salmon by creating a demand on the menu?

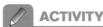 **ACTIVITY**

What qualities does a buyer have to have in order to be successful?

Buying methods

These depend on the type of market and the kind of operation. Purchasing procedures can be formal or informal. Both have advantages and disadvantages.

- **Informal buying** usually involves oral negotiations, talking directly to sales people, face to face or using the telephone. Informal methods are suitable for casual buying, where the amount involved is not large, and speed and simplicity are desirable. They vary according to market conditions – prices and supply tend to fluctuate more than with formal methods.
- **Formal buying**, known as competitive buying, involves giving suppliers written specifications quantity needed. Negotiations are normally written. Formal contracts are best for large quantities purchased over a long period of time; prices do not vary much during a year once the basic price has been established.

Selecting suppliers

Selecting suppliers is an important part of the purchasing process. First, think about how a supplier will be able to meet the needs of your operation. Consider:

- price
- delivery
- quality/standards.

Information on suppliers can be obtained from other purchasers. Visits to suppliers' establishments are to be encouraged. When interviewing prospective suppliers, you need to question how reliable a supplier will be under competition and how stable under varying market conditions.

Principles of purchasing

A menu dictates what an operation needs. Based on this, the buyer searches for a market that can supply these requirements. Once the right market is found, the buyer must investigate the various products available. The right product must be obtained – it must be suitable for the item or dish required and of the quality desired by the establishment. Other factors that might affect production needs include:

- type and image of the establishment
- style of operation and system of service
- occasion for which the item is needed
- amount of storage available (dry, refrigerated or frozen)
- finance available and supply policies of the organisation
- availability, seasonality, price trends and supply.

The skill of the employees, catering assistants and chefs must also be taken into account, as well as condition and the processing method and the storage life of the product.

Three types of product

The main products that an establishment purchases can be divided into three types:

1. **Perishable:** products that do not stay fresh for very long, such as fresh fruit and vegetables, dairy products, meat and fish; prices and suppliers may vary; informal methods of buying are frequently used; perishables should be purchased to meet menu needs for a short period only.
2. **Staple:** supplies that are canned, bottled, dehydrated or frozen; formal or informal purchasing may be used; because items are staple and can be stored easily, bid buying is frequently used to take advantage of the favourable prices available when purchasing large quantities.
3. **Daily use needs:** daily use or contract items are delivered frequently to match usage; stocks are kept up to the particular level and supply is automatic; supplies may arrive daily, several

times a week, weekly or less often; most items are perishable, therefore supplies must not be excessive but only sufficient to get through to the next delivery.

Buying tips

The following is a list of suggestions to assist the buyer.

- Learn about all commodities, both fresh and convenience, to be purchased. Keep your knowledge up to date.
- Be aware of the different types and qualities of each commodity that is available.
- When buying fresh commodities, be aware of part-prepared and ready-prepared items available on the market.
- Keep a sharp eye on price variations. Buy at the best price that will ensure the required quality and also make a profit. The cheapest item may prove to be the most expensive if lots of it ends up being wasted. When possible, order by number and weight. For example, 20 kg plaice could be 80 × 250 g plaice, 40 × 500 g plaice, 20 × 1 kg plaice. It could also be 20 kg total weight of various sizes, which makes it difficult to control portion sizes. Some suppliers (e.g. butchers, fishmongers) may offer a portion-control service by selling the required number of a given weight of certain cuts, for example, 100 × 150 g sirloin steaks, 25 kg prepared stewing beef, 200 × 100 g pieces of turbot fillet, 500 × 100 g plaice fillets.
- Organise an efficient system of ordering, keeping copies of all orders for cross-checking, whether orders are given in writing, in person or by telephone.
- Compare purchasing by retail, wholesale and contract procedures to ensure the best method is selected for your particular organisation.
- Explore all possible suppliers: local or markets, town or country, small or large.
- Keep the number of suppliers to a minimum. At the same time, have at least two suppliers for every group of commodities, when possible. This should help to keep the suppliers' prices and terms competitive.

- Issue all orders to suppliers fairly, allowing enough time for the order to be delivered on time.
- Request price lists as often as possible and compare prices continually to make sure that you buy at a good market price.
- Buy perishable goods when they are in full season as this gives the best value at the cheapest price. To help with purchasing the correct quantities, it is useful to compile a purchasing chart for 100 covers from which items can be divided or multiplied according to requirement. An indication of quality standards can also be incorporated in a chart of this kind.
- Deliveries must all be checked against the orders given, for quantity, quality and price. If any goods delivered are below an acceptable standard they must be returned, either for replacement or credit.
- Containers can account for large sums of money. Ensure that all containers are correctly stored, returned to the suppliers where possible and the proper credit given.
- All invoices must be checked for quantities and prices.
- All statements must be checked against invoices and passed swiftly to the office so that payment can be made on time, to ensure maximum discount on purchases.

- Develop good relations with trade representatives (sales people) because much useful up-to-date information can be gained from them.
- Keep up-to-date trade catalogues, visit trade exhibitions, survey new equipment and continually review the space, services and systems in use. Always be on the lookout for ways to increase efficiency.
- Organise a testing panel occasionally to keep up to date with new commodities and new products coming on to the market.
- Consider how computer applications might help the operation.
- Study weekly fresh food price lists.

> The people on a **testing panel** look at the quality of the produce, the potential portion control and yield, and will taste the products for flavour.

> **Yield:** What is produced or generated. In a restaurant this may refer to how many portions or what size of portion can be made from a certain quantity of produce.

Portion control – controlling waste and costs

Portion control means controlling the size or quantity of food served to each customer. The amount of food allowed depends on the three following considerations.

1. **The type of customer or establishment:** there will obviously be a difference in the size of portions served, such as to those working in heavy industry or to female clerical workers. In a restaurant offering a three-course table d'hôte menu for £X, including salmon, the size of the portion would naturally be smaller than in a luxury restaurant charging £X for the salmon on an à la carte menu.

2. **The quality of the food:** better-quality food usually yields a greater number of portions than poor-quality food: low-quality stewing beef often needs so much trimming that it is difficult to get six portions to the kilogramme, and the time and labour involved also loses money. On the other hand, good-quality stewing beef will often give eight portions to the kilo, with much less time and labour required for preparation, and more customer satisfaction.

3. **The buying price of the food:** this should correspond to the quality of the food if the person responsible for buying has bought

wisely. A good buyer will ensure that the price paid for any item of food is equivalent to the quality – in other words, a good price should mean good quality, which should mean a good yield, and so help to establish sound portion control. If, on the other hand, an inefficient buyer has paid a high price for food of indifferent quality then it will be difficult to get a fair number of portions, the selling price necessary to make the required profit will be too high and customer satisfaction can be affected.

Portion control should be closely linked with the buying of the food; without a good knowledge of the food bought it is difficult to state fairly how many portions should be obtained from it. To develop a sound system of portion control, each establishment (or type of establishment) needs individual consideration. A golden rule should be: 'a fair portion for a fair price'.

Conveniently portioned items are available, such as individual sachets of sugar, jams, sauce, salt and pepper, individual cartons of milk and cream, and individual butter and margarine portions. These make planning easier and create less waste but are expensive compared to non-portioned commodities.

Standard purchasing specifications

Standard purchasing specifications are drawn up for every item to be purchased, describing exactly what is required. It includes various criteria related to quality, grade, weight, size and method of preparation, if required (such as washed and selected potatoes for baking). Other information might include variety, maturity, age, colour, shape and so on.

Once an accurate specification is approved, it will be referred to every time the item is delivered. A copy is often given to the supplier and the storekeeper, who then know exactly what is needed.

These purchasing specifications (known as primary specifications) will help with the formulation of standardised recipes and assist in the costing and control procedures. Commodities that can be specified include the following:

- grown (primary): butcher's meat; fresh fish; fresh fruit and vegetables; milk and eggs
- manufactured (secondary): bakery goods; dairy products
- processed (tertiary): frozen foods including meat, fish and fruit and vegetables; dried goods; canned goods.

So, any food product can have a specification attached to it. However, the primary specifications focus on raw materials, ensuring that they are of the required quality. Without good quality raw materials, secondary or tertiary specifications are useless. For example, to specify a frozen apple pie, this product would use:

- a primary specification for the apple
- a secondary specification for the pastry
- a tertiary specification for the process (freezing).

But, no matter how good the secondary or tertiary specifications, if the apples used in the beginning are not of a very high quality, the whole product will not be of a good quality.

Example of a standard purchasing specification for tomatoes

- Commodity: round tomatoes.
- Size: 50 g (2oz) 47–57 mm diameter.
- Quality: firm, well formed, good red colour, with stalk attached.
- Origin: Dutch, available March–November.
- Class/grade: super class A.
- Weight: 6 kg (13 lb) net per box.
- Count: 90–100 per box.
- Quote: per box/tray.
- Packaging: loose in wooden tray, covered in plastic.
- Delivery: day following order.
- Storage: temperature 10–13°C (50–55°F) at a relative humidity of 75–80%.

Note: avoid storage with cucumbers and aubergines.

For most perishable items, a daily or monthly quotation system is more common than entering into a long-term contract. This is essentially a short-term contract that is regularly reviewed to ensure that a competitive situation is maintained.

The standard recipe

The standard recipe is a written formula for producing a food item of a specified quality and quantity for use in a particular establishment. It should show the precise quantities and qualities of the ingredients, together with the sequence of preparation and service. It enables the establishment to have greater control over cost and quantity.

The objective of a standard recipe is to predetermine the following:

- the quantities and qualities of ingredients to be used, stating the purchase specification
- the amount (number of portions) a recipe should make.

Accurate weighing and measuring

It is important that, when designing standardised recipes, the correct weights and measures are recorded, to achieve consistency, so no matter who prepares the dish the same standard portion size and quality is achieved.

Each recipe should tell you the following:

- the ingredients to be used
- the exact amounts of ingredients required
- how the dish is prepared
- how the dish is cooked
- the number of portions it will produce (yield).

Always read through the recipe carefully and check that you:

1. have the right ingredients and equipment

2. have the correct weights

3. have enough time to prepare the dish.

To facilitate menu planning, purchasing and internal requisitioning, food preparation and production, and portion control:

- know the food cost per portion
- know the nutritional value of a particular dish.

The standard recipe will also help new staff in the preparation and production of standard products, which can be made easier by using photographs or drawings illustrating the finished product.

Cost control

It is important to know the exact cost of each process and every item produced, so a system of cost analysis and cost information is essential.

Cost analysis: The process of breaking down the costs of an operation into all its separate parts so that it is possible to look at the exact cost of each process and every item produced, and judge the efficiency and cost effectiveness of each.

The advantages of an efficient costing system are as follows.

- It tells you the net profit made by each section of the organisation and shows the cost of each meal produced.

- It will reveal possible ways to economise and can result in a more effective use of stores, labour, materials, and so on.
- Costing provides the information necessary to develop a sound pricing policy.
- Cost records help to provide speedy quotations for all special functions, such as parties, wedding receptions, and so on.
- It enables the caterer to keep to a budget.

No one costing system will automatically suit every catering business, but the following guidelines may be helpful.

- The cooperation of all departments is essential.
- The costing system should be adapted to

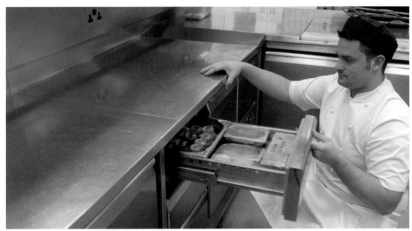

Labour means the cost of employing staff

the business, not vice versa. If the accepted procedure in an establishment is altered to fit a costing system then there is danger of causing resentment among staff and as a result losing their cooperation.

● Clear instructions in writing must be given to staff who are required to keep records.

The system must be made as simple as possible so that the amount of clerical work required is kept to a minimum. An efficient mechanical calculator or computer should be provided to save time and effort.

To calculate the total cost of any one item or meal provided it is necessary to analyse the total expenditure under several headings. Basically the total cost of each item consists of the following three main elements.

1. **Food and materials costs:** these are known as variable costs because the level will vary according to the volume of business. In an operation that uses part-time or extra staff for special occasions, the money paid to these staff also comes under variable costs; by comparison, salaries and wages paid regularly to permanent staff are fixed costs.

2. **Labour costs and overheads:** regular charges come under the heading of fixed costs, which include labour and overheads. Labour costs in the majority of operations fall into two categories:

   • direct labour cost, which is salaries and wages paid to staff such as chefs, waiters, bar staff, housekeepers, chambermaids, which can be allocated to income from food, drink and accommodation sales

   • indirect labour cost, which would include salaries and wages paid, for example, to managers, office staff and maintenance staff who work for all departments (so their labour cost should be charged to all departments).

Overheads consist of rent, rates, heating, lighting and equipment.

3. **Cleaning materials:** this is an important group of essential items that is often overlooked when costing. There are over 60 different items that come under this heading, and approximately 24 of these may be required for an average catering establishment. These may include: brooms, brushes, buckets, cloths, drain rods, dusters, mops, sponges, squeegees, scrubbing/polishing machines, suction/vacuum cleaners, wet and wet/dry suction cleaners, scouring pads, detergents, disinfectants, dustbin powder, washing-up liquids, fly sprays, sacks, scourers, steel wool, soap, soda, and so on. It is important to understand the cost of these materials and to ensure that an allowance is made for them under the heading of 'overheads'.

Overheads:

Maintenance

Gas

Electricity

Sundry expenses

Gross profit

Gross profit (or kitchen profit) is the difference between the cost of an item and the price it is sold at. If gross profit is set as a fixed percentage mark-up, the food cost of each dish is calculated and a fixed gross profit (e.g. 100 per cent) is added. So, if the food costs £2 it is sold for £4. It is usual to express each element of cost as a percentage of the selling price. This enables the caterer to control profits.

Net profit

Net profit is the difference between the selling price of the food (sales) and total cost of the product (food, labour and overheads). This box shows an example:

If the selling price of a dish is expressed as 100% (the total amount received from its sale), it can be broken down into the amount of money spent on food items and the gross profit. This can be expressed in percentages as shown below.

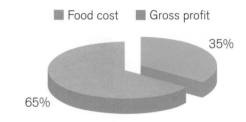

■ Food cost ■ Gross profit

35%

65%

Sales − food cost = gross profit (kitchen profit)
Sales − total cost = net profit
Food cost + gross profit = sales
Example   Food sales for 1 week = £25,000
           Food cost for 1 week = £12,000
           Labour and overheads for 1 week = £9,000
           Total costs for 1 week = £21,000
           Gross profit (kitchen profit) = £13,000
           Net profit = £4,000
Food sales − food cost   £25,000 − £12,000 = £13,000 (gross profit)
Food sales − net profit   £25,000 − £4,000 = £21,000 (total costs)
Food cost + gross profit   £12,000 + £15,000 = £25,000 (food sales)
Profit is always expressed as a percentage of the selling price.
Therefore the percentage profit for the week is:
Net profit ÷ sales × 100 = £4000 × 100 ÷ 25,000 = 16%

A breakdown reveals the figures shown in Table 5.2.

Table 5.2 Example breakdown

	Costs	Percentage of sales (%)
Food cost	£12,000	44
Labour	£6,000	25
Overheads	£3,000	18
Total costs	**£21,000**	
Sales	£25,000	
Net profit	£4,000	13

This can also be presented in monetary terms, as shown in the following diagram, if the dish was sold at £10.00, for example.

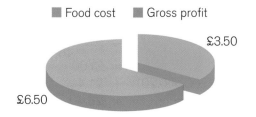

■ Food cost   ■ Gross profit

£3.50

£6.50

Calculating the selling price

If food costs come to £3.50, to calculate the selling price on the basis of a 65% gross profit, the following calculation can be used.

$$\frac{3.50 \text{ (food costs)}}{35 \text{ (food cost as a \% of the sale)}} \times 100 = £10.00$$

This calculation brings the food cost to 1% of the selling price before multiplying by 100 to bring the selling price to 100%.

To demonstrate this further, if the gross profit requirement was raised to 75%, this would reduce the food cost as a percentage of the selling price to 25%. Therefore the selling price would have to be higher if the food cost remained at £3.50.

$$\frac{3.50 \text{ (food costs)}}{25 \text{ (food cost as a \% of the sale)}} \times 100 = £14.00$$

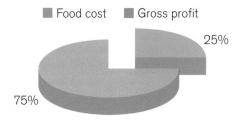

■ Food cost   ■ Gross profit

25%

75%

The percentages still add up to 100%, but the proportion spent on food is smaller in terms of the selling price. The diagrams illustrate the breakdown on this basis.

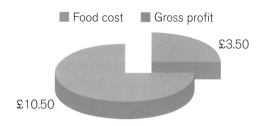

■ Food cost   ■ Gross profit

£3.50

£10.50

To check that this is correct, the following calculation can be applied.

$$\frac{14.00 \text{ (selling price)}}{100 \text{ (brings 14.00 down to 1\%)}} \times 25 = £13.50$$

(brings up to 25%)

.... and

$$\frac{14.00 \text{ (selling price)}}{100 \text{ (brings 14.00 down to 1\%)}} \times 75 = £10.50$$

(brings up to 75%)

£11.50 (75%) + £3.50 (25%) = £14.00 (100%)

If the restaurant served 1000 meals then the average amount spent by each customer would be:

$$\frac{\text{Total sales £25,000}}{\text{Number of customers 1000}} = £25.00$$

As the percentage composition of sales for a month is now known, the average price of a meal for that period can be further analysed:

Average price of a meal = £25.00 = 100%
                            25p = 1%

which means that the customer's contribution towards:

Food cost	= 25 × 48 = £12.00
Labour	= 25 × 24 = £6.00
Overheads	= 25 × 12 = £3.00
Net profit	= 25 × 16 = £4.00
Average price of meal	= £25.00

A rule that can be applied to calculate the food cost price of a dish is: let the cost price of the dish equal 40 per cent and fix the selling price at 100 per cent.

Cost of dish = 400p = 40%

Selling price = 400 × 100 ÷ 40 = £10.00

Selling the dish at £10, making 60 per cent gross profit above the cost price, would be known as 40 per cent food cost. For example:

Sirloin steak (250 g)
250 g entrecote steak at £10.00 a kg = £2.50

To fix the selling price at 40% food cost =
2.50 × 100 ÷ 40 = £6.25

If food costing is controlled accurately, the food cost of particular items on the menu and the total expenditure on food over a given period can be worked out. Finding the food costs helps to control costs, prices and profits.

An efficient food cost system will show up any bad buying and inefficient storing, and should help to prevent waste and pilfering. This can help the caterer to run an efficient business, and enable her or him to give the customer value for money.

The caterer who gives the customer value for money together with the desired type of food is well on the way to being successful.

Example

If a dish costs £2.80 to produce, what should its selling price be to achieve 60 per cent profit on sales?

Gross profit 60%, food costs 40%

$$\text{Selling price} = \frac{£2.80 \times 100}{40}$$
$$= £7.00$$

Add VAT (£7.00 × 0.20) + £1.40
Final selling price = £8.40

Example

If a dish costs £2.80 to produce, what should its selling price be to make a 200 per cent profit on cost?

Gross profit 200%, food costs 100%

$$\text{Cost price} = \frac{£2.80 \times (200 + 100)}{100}$$

Add VAT (£8.40 × 0.20) + £1.68
Final selling price = £8.88

ACTIVITY

If a dish costs £3.00 to produce, what should the selling price be to achieve a 70 per cent profit on sales?

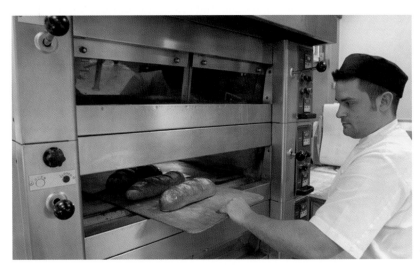

What does each loaf cost to produce?

Table 5.3 Food costings

Food cost (%)	To find the selling price multiply the cost price of the food by:	If the cost price of food is £4, the selling price is:	If the cost price is £1.20, the selling price is:	Gross profit (%)
60	1.66	£6.64	£1.92	40
55	1.75	£7.00	£2.04	45
50	2	£8.00	£2.40	50
45	2.22	£8.88	£2.64	55
40	2.5	£10.00	£2.88	60
33.3	3	£12.00	£3.60	66.6

Food costs and operational control

As food is expensive, efficient stock control levels are essential to help the profitability of the business. The main difficulties of controlling food are as follows.

- Food prices fluctuate frequently because of inflation and falls in demand and supply, through poor harvests, bad weather conditions, and so on.
- Transport costs rise due to wage demands and the cost of petrol and diesel.
- Fuel costs rise, which affects food companies' and producers' costs.
- Any food subsidies imposed by governments could be removed.
- Changes occur in the amount demanded by the customer; increased advertising increases demand; changes in taste and fashion influence demand from one product to another.

Media focus on certain products that are labelled healthy or unhealthy will affect demand, e.g. butter being high in saturated fats, sunflower margarine being high in polyunsaturates. TV cookery programmes and celebrity chefs can make certain dishes and ingredients more popular.

Changes in operational control may also be seen with the increasing emphasis on food traceability, local sourcing and reduction in food miles.

Each establishment should devise its own control system to suit its own needs. Factors that affect a control system are:

- regular changes in the menu
- menus with a large number of dishes
- dishes with a large number of ingredients
- problems in assessing customer demand
- difficulties in not adhering to or operating standardised recipes
- raw materials purchased incorrectly.

Factors assisting a control system include:

- menu remains constant (e.g. McDonald's, Harvester, Pizza Hut, Burger King)

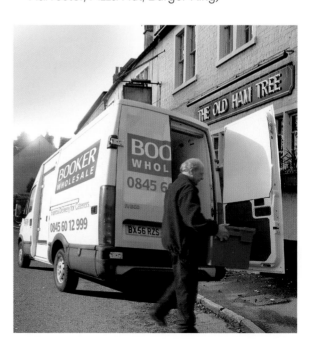

- standardised recipes and purchasing specifications are used
- menu has a limited number of dishes.

Stocktaking is therefore easier and costing is more accurate.

In order to carry out a control system, food stocks must be secure, refrigerators and deep freezers should be kept locked, portion control must be accurate. A book-keeping system must be developed to monitor the daily operation.

Test yourself

1 In the nineteenth century, who devised the system of kitchen organisation referred to as the 'partie' system?
2 What is the usual role of a chef de partie? Give examples.
3 Suggest three considerations you would need to make when planning a kitchen.
4 Why is good kitchen workflow considered to be very important?
5 When planning a menu for a new city centre restaurant, suggest four considerations that need to be made.
6 When a menu is described as table d'hote what does this mean?
7 In relation to food, what is formal/competitive buying?
8 Describe what is meant by 'portion control' and give three examples of how this may be done.
9 Give an example of 'variable costs' in a hospitality business.
10 What is the name given to the profit made by a business after all the costs such as food, labour and overheads have been taken out?

6 Applying workplace skills

In this chapter you will learn how to:

1. work effectively with customers and colleagues:
- maintain a professional personal appearance
- use correct procedures and good practice
- communicate and work with others effectively to meet targets
- identify and solve problems

2. be able to prepare for a job application:
- produce a Curriculum Vitae and covering letter
- demonstrate a variety of interview skills

3. produce a plan to develop your skills:
- produce and use a personal development plan
- set and work towards a target to develop a skill.

Professional presentation

In the hospitality industry it is important to be smart and to wear the appropriate clothing for the job, whether this is chefs' whites or a doorman's uniform. You must present a well-groomed appearance and wear smart clean clothing that is in good repair.

Employers want people with the right attitude, who are able to show initiative, be punctual, flexible and dependable. They want people who can organise themselves, communicate and manage their time effectively.

Punctual: On time.

Reasons for presenting a professional image

Presenting a professional image is important for your own personal pride and confidence, to promote you and the job role, adding status and commanding respect. It is also necessary to be clean and tidy to comply with health and safety and food safety legislation. Image can also be

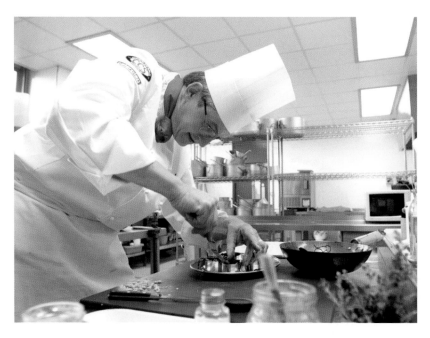

It is important to be smartly dressed in the appropriate clothing

used to match branding (e.g. uniforms) and to meet job requirements (e.g. wearing chefs' whites for cooking; wearing a smart suit when working front of house).

The way you carry out the job and are able to use the appropriate skills (see the next section) is also part of your personal presentation. Good presentation, both front and back of house, helps increase customer satisfaction, improves business, and improves staff morale and staff satisfaction, leading to happy customers and increased profits. These, in turn, enhance the reputation of the establishment.

Professional presentation and clothing

Being smart and wearing the correct clothing is an important part of working in the hospitality industry. All the clothing you wear must be smart, clean and in good repair. Your hair must be short or tied back neatly and you should be

Professional presentation includes:
- behaviour
- attitude
- conduct
- standards
- punctuality
- dependability.

These demonstrate your personal pride and develop your confidence.

A good attitude helps promote health and safety and food safety.

Professional presentation and attitude provide good role models.

clean shaven or have a neat beard/moustache. You should always wear the correct uniform in the kitchen. You must change your chefs' or cooks' uniform regularly (at least every day) and you should never wear the uniform outside the working premises as this is unhygienic. Bacteria from outside can be carried on the uniform into the kitchen and may cause harm.

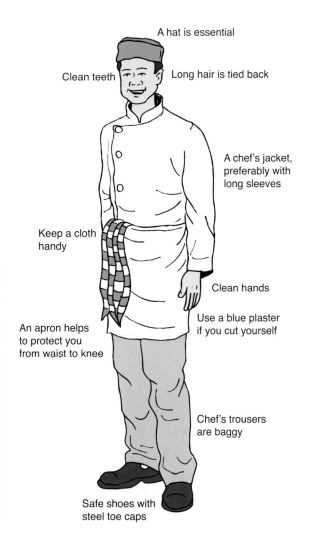

A hat is essential

Clean teeth

Long hair is tied back

A chef's jacket, preferably with long sleeves

Keep a cloth handy

Clean hands

An apron helps to protect you from waist to knee

Use a blue plaster if you cut yourself

Chef's trousers are baggy

Safe shoes with steel toe caps

Workplace skills

Some of the most important skills required in the workplace are forecasting, planning, organising, commanding, coordinating and controlling. We will take a brief look at each of these below.

Forecasting

Forecasting is the ability to plan ahead, in order to foresee possible and probable actions and allow for them. For example, if the chef de partie knows that the following day is their assistant's day off, she or he can look ahead and plan accordingly. Forecasting requires good judgement acquired from previous knowledge and experience.

Planning

From forecasting comes planning: how many meals to prepare; how much to have in stock (in case the forecast is completely accurate); how many staff will be needed, which staff and when; are the staff capable of what is required of them?

Organising

In the hospitality industry, organisational skills are applied to food, equipment and staff. Organising in this context consists of ensuring that what is wanted is where it is wanted, when it is wanted, in the right amount and at the right time. Organisation involves the production of duty rotas and training programmes, as well as cleaning schedules.

Commanding

This means giving instructions to staff on how, what and where. This means that orders have to be given, and a certain degree of order and discipline must be maintained.

Coordinating

Coordinating is the skill that is used to get staff to cooperate and work together – to coordinate the work of each section. Different tasks also need to be coordinated to allow for smooth running of the kitchen and completion of work on time. This coordination is essential to the success of any organisation in the hospitality industry.

Controlling

This involves the skills needed to control the whole operation in order to monitor and improve performance. It would include:

- checking that staff are on time
- checking that standards are maintained
- checking quality
- checking quantity

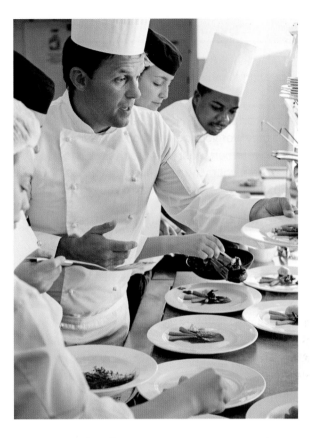

- ensuring that there is no unnecessary waste
- checking equipment
- monitoring and checking hygiene standards
- monitoring and checking cleaning.

Having a professional attitude and developing a professional organisation promotes the organisation: as customers gain confidence in the business and the staff it employs, it develops a good reputation. If the business has a good reputation this boosts staff morale – if staff have confidence in the business, this has a positive effect on profits.

Customer care

You should always:

- put the customer first
- make the customer feel good
- make the customer feel comfortable
- make the customer feel important
- make the customer want to return to your restaurant or establishment.

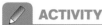
ACTIVITY

Name the skills your team will need when catering for an event of your own choice.

It is important that you treat all customers equally, as if they were special, but you must also learn to adjust your behaviour to suit certain customers. Give them your time and full attention. Use body language to put customers at ease.

Defining standards of performance

The starting point is to consider carefully what should happen at each of the points of contact a customer might have with the restaurant. This can become a checklist, as in the following example.

- A customer enters the restaurant or service area:

  (a) The entrance should be clean and tidy.

  (b) The doors could be marked 'Welcome'.

- The customer is then greeted by the head waiter, restaurant manager or receptionist:

  (a) reception area is clean and tidy, perhaps decorated with fresh flowers

  (b) menu sample and drinks list on display

  (c) all staff smartly dressed and well groomed

  (d) staff smile when greeting customers

  (e) if possible head waiter, restaurant manager or receptionist uses customer's name

  (f) customer is escorted to the table, assisted into their seat

  (g) if there is any delay, staff apologise and an explanation is given to the customer

  (h) waiter introduces him/herself to the customer.

- At the end of the meal, the head waiter or restaurant manager escorts the customer to the door, smiles and exchanges pleasantries: 'good day'/'good night'.

Measuring and monitoring performance

The defined standards of performance must be set, then monitored and measured, for example: the telephone must be answered within 3 rings; the customer's order must be taken within 5 minutes of them being seated; the pastry chef will prepare a certain number of desserts for every service. You need to measure success in terms of your promises to customers, for example: customers can park their car easily; there is sufficient choice on the menu for customers; there is always a vegetarian choice; they will be served

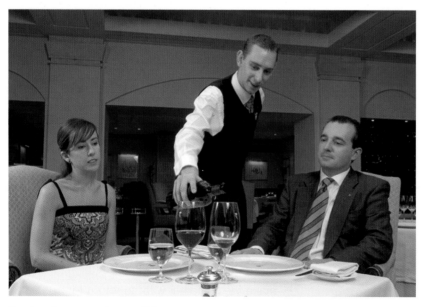

Good customer care is essential

with their choice of starter within 10 minutes of arriving. Measuring the right thing helps staff understand what is important to customers and how to act accordingly, for example: customers want staff to be able to explain the menu to them; they want to feel welcome and special; they want staff to attend to their needs and not be ignored.

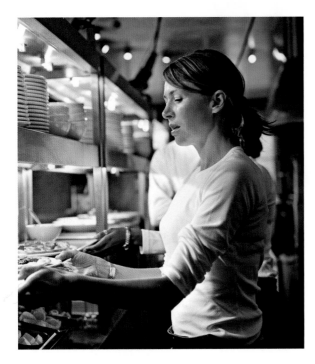

Staff who look after customers and provide the service and care they expect, deserve to be rewarded. Good positive feedback to staff is important. You may:

- just say 'well done', which goes a long way
- pay a bonus
- give an extra increase on their annual pay rise
- give a promotion.

Attitude and behaviour

If a customer is rude or aggressive to a member of the waiting staff (e.g. blames a waiter for the chef's mistake), the waiter should not be rude or aggressive in return. If the waiter can use his/her skills to remain calm and patient, the customer will often apologise for their anger. Behaviour is a choice; choose behaviour that is appropriate to the customer and the situation.

When dealing with customers, behaviour should be:

- professional
- understanding – customers in a restaurant want a service and are paying for it; learn to understand their needs
- patient – learn to be patient with all customers
- enthusiastic – enthusiasm can be contagious
- confident – confidence can increase a potential customer's trust in you
- welcoming – this can satisfy a customer's basic human desire to feel liked and be approved of
- helpful – customers warm to helpful staff
- polite – good manners are always welcomed
- caring – make each customer feel special.

If customers complain or they are unhappy about anything that is served to them, they should be encouraged to inform the member of staff who served them. This will give the establishment the opportunity to rectify the fault immediately. Ask them about their eating experience; this information will be vital for future planning. Treat customer complaints seriously. It may be appropriate to offer free drinks or a reduction on the bill. Show them empathy, use the appropriate body language, show concern, sympathise. Always apologise. If you handle the complaint well you will make the customer feel important. Remember that customer care = happy customers = profit = jobs.

Empathy: Being able to put yourself in someone else's shoes; understanding and sharing someone else's feelings.

Meeting targets

Many hospitality establishments set targets. These are usually sales targets and operational targets that relate to budgets, cost control, staffing, and so on.

In some companies individuals are given their own individual targets to achieve. Outside the workplace you may also set your own personal targets. These could be focused on your health, fitness or, say, reducing your consumption of

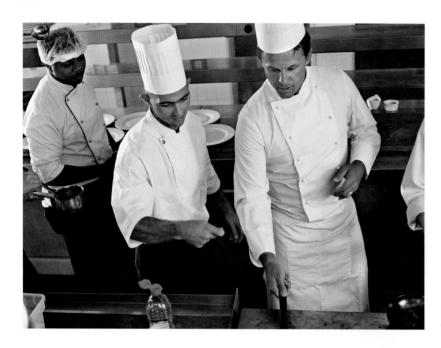

It is important to develop good working relationships

alcohol. Other targets might relate to your own personal career development: you may wish to take additional qualifications to improve your career prospects. To achieve this you may need to seek guidance and take corrective action if you find you are not meeting your targets.

ACTIVITY

What workplace skills do you need to demonstrate to an employer?

Working with colleagues

It is important to develop good working relationships with your colleagues, work as a team and be supportive of each other. Seek guidance from other team members and your line manager. Identify role models.

In some cases, it may be necessary to develop a work plan for the day and for the week. Discuss the rotas and work schedule, who will cover which tasks and what needs to be done. Discuss targets and outcomes. Evaluate your performance and the team's performance. This can be done in an informal way, or formally through a team meeting. Identify how the team and your performance are being measured.

Applying for a job

When applying for a job you will usually be asked to supply various documents and letters and then, if the first stage of your application is successful, you will be asked to go for an interview.

Producing a CV

When you apply for a job you will probably be asked to send in a current CV (curriculum vitae).

This requires you to list all your educational qualifications and work history, your interests and other activities you participate in. Employers will generally want to know where you have demonstrated certain skills, how you have dealt with certain situations in the workplace and whether you carry out any voluntary work.

When preparing a CV, you should also bear in mind the following points:

- All your work experience and work placements should be included in the CV.
- Always keep your CV up to date and keep track of all your experience, jobs, dates of employment, employers, and competitions you have entered and won (that are relevant to the employment you are seeking).
- Always check spelling, layout and punctuation.
- Always update your personal records.
- As you develop your career, personal qualities and skills, write a short profile about yourself.
- Write down what inspires you and how you use existing skills.
- Specify what your long-term goals are, as well as your immediate goals and targets.

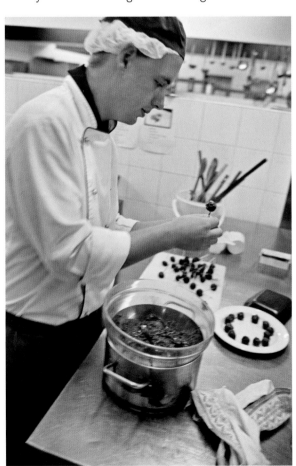

Present your work experience and skills in your CV and covering letter

- Identify ways of broadening your outlook, your range of skills, and your ability to deal with a range of different people, personalities and cultural diversity.

Producing a covering letter

A covering letter introduces you to the company; it explains why you are suitable for the job on offer, and the skills and qualities you can bring to it. In some cases, it may also give you an opportunity to say how you would be able to contribute positively to the establishment and organisation as a whole. The letter will usually accompany a copy of your CV.

Interview techniques

First impressions are important. Always prepare thoroughly for an interview. Good preparation will help to ensure that you are in control of the interview.

When preparing for an interview, you should also bear in mind the following points:

- Prepare any questions in advance.
- Consider how you are going to introduce yourself at the start of the interview.
- Make sure you are well groomed, smart and look professional.
- It is sometimes useful to practise interviews beforehand – this is known as role play.
- Before the interview, plan the journey and work out the travelling time – allow yourself plenty of time to get there so you do not feel rushed.

At the interview, always maintain eye contact with the interviewer and smile occasionally. Be confident and polite. Think about the questions you are asked before you answer them. Be clear and concise. If you do not understand a question, ask for it to be clarified.

When the interview is over, reflect on your performance. If you are unsuccessful, ask for feedback and learn from the experience. Think about how you might improve in the future.

Personal presentation for interview

Create a good first impression.

Use the correct vocabulary.

Make sure you research the job you are applying for.

Know the questions you are going to ask.

Demonstrate good communication skills.

Show that you understand the importance of time management.

Always learn from your experience:

Always ask for feedback from any interview or job application.

Assess your skills.

How could you improve?

What did you do well?

Personal development plans

It is necessary to evaluate and check your progress from time to time. Feedback from your peers and managers is a useful way of evaluating your performance. Keeping records (e.g. personal development plans) as a way of checking your progress is also an important way of referring back to your targets and thinking about the final outcome.

So, the key stages of monitoring performance to see if it meets targets are:

- work plans (e.g. personal development plans) – seeking guidance
- targets – evaluating them, taking corrective action if necessary
- outcome – must be measurable in order to know if it has been achieved.

Gathering information on your learning journey to improve your workplace skills is useful so that, once you have achieved a successful outcome, you can use that information to inform and help others, disseminating it as necessary.

Having a personal development plan will help you identify targets and timescales to improve your skills and advance your career for personal and professional success. The next step is to identify which skills you need to develop further, and ways you could do this.

Disseminating: Spreading out or scattering; broadcasting. 'Disseminating information' means communicating it to other people, or letting other people know.

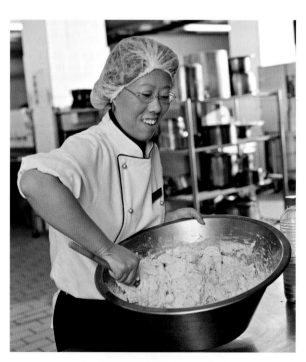

Check your progress as you improve your skills

Table 6.1 Skills for success: an example of a useful template for recording skills acquisition

Knowledge, skills, qualities and experience	Already experienced	Want to know more	Want to develop further	Order of importance
Craft skills				
Knife skills				
Culinary skills				
Kitchen skills				
Pastry skills				
Larder skills				
Restaurant skills				
Managing your time				
Identifying barriers to personal success				
Being able to reflect positively				
Knowing what kind of career you want				
Preparing good job applications				
Writing good covering letters				
Writing a good, attractive CV				
Understanding what is required to be successful				
Teambuilding skills				
Developing professional relationships				
Being assertive				
Dealing with difficult people				
Developing confidence				
Dealing with basic problem-solving				
Being self-motivated				
Evaluating personal competitiveness				

Knowing effective interview techniques				
Preparing for an interview				
Developing personal records				
Recording evidence				

Table 6.2 Personal targets

	Target 1	Target 2	Target 3
What is the target?			
The importance of the skill and why you need it.			
How you will achieve this skill and what support and guidance you will need.			
Evidence that you have achieved your aim.			

Table 6.3 Action plan for personal development

Target	Steps to take in milestones	What indicates successful completion	Start date	Target completion date	Done
1	a				
	b				
	c				
2	a				
	b				
	c				

Your personal development plan will help you to evaluate your performance feedback from your mentor, manager or tutor, and will help you to improve your own performance. The plan will help you to achieve your aims and become successful – to be where you want to be and who you want to be.

Test yourself ● ● ● ● ● ● ● ● ● ● ● ● ● ●

1 List six rules chefs should follow in regard to smart and hygienic kitchen uniform.

2 Controlling is very much part of a head chef's role. Suggest six areas of control a chef would need to manage.

3 With regard to customer care what are the positive points that would make a customer want to return to a restaurant?

4 Setting targets for yourself is a good way to monitor progress and achievement. When working in a kitchen or restaurant suggest three targets you may set for yourself.
How would you know when they had been achieved?

5 Give some examples of positive behaviour when dealing with customers.

6 Give an example of 'planning' in a large kitchen area.

7 When you are part of a kitchen team why is it important to be:
● Punctual
● Flexible
● Dependable?

8 What is a CV? What is the main information that needs to go on a CV?

9 If you have a job interview it is necessary to be prepared in advance. Suggest four ways that you can prepare for an interview.

10 How could a personal development plan help you to progress in your career?

● ●

7 Methods of cookery

In this chapter you will learn how to:

1. demonstrate a knowledge of the various methods of cookery, including:
- boiling, poaching and steaming
- stewing, casseroling and braising
- baking and roasting
- grilling and barbecuing
- shallow and deep frying

2. understand which method is most suitable for different types of food.

Cooking methods

The method chosen to cook various foods will greatly influence the finished product. Different foods can be cooked in different ways to:

- make food easy to digest and safe to eat.
- make food pleasant to eat, with an agreeable flavour
- add the required colour and variety of colour
- give food a good texture – tender, slightly firm, crisp, depending on the food
- give variety to our menus and our diets.

The different methods also have specific purposes and advantages.

It is important to think about health and safety when you are cooking. In the following sections you will find safety advice for each method of cookery. All the equipment used for cookery needs to be cleaned and maintained carefully. See Chapter 2 for more information.

What happens when food is cooked?

Heat can be applied directly to food, by **dry heat**, or by placing food in a hot cooking medium (e.g. water, stock, fat) (**moist heat**).

This can take place in three ways, by **convection**, **conduction** and **radiation**. Each of these is explained below. In practice, most cooking uses a combination of all three. For example, a basic sponge is cooked by heat reflecting from the oven walls (radiation), heat circulating in the air within the oven (convection) and heat transferred from the cake tin to the cake mixture (conduction).

Convection

Convection occurs when a liquid or gas is heated causing hot air to rise and cooler air to sink, distributing the heat through the liquid or gas and into the food.

- **Boiling food:** the water is gradually heated by convection currents from the heat source and the hot water transfers heat to the food.
- **Baking in an oven:** the heat generated in the oven is transferred to the food.

Conduction

In conduction, heat passes through one solid to another. This can only be done with materials that are good conductors of heat, such as metals. The food needs to be in direct contact with a heated item in order to cook.

An example of cooking by conduction is food in direct contact with a griddle.

Radiation

Heat is transferred directly to food by electromagnetic waves, such as microwaves or infrared waves. These waves first heat the food and then cook it. Any object that is in the path of the waves, such as a salamander, will also become hot.

Examples of cooking by radiation include grilling, toasting, barbecue and microwaving.

The effect of cooking on food

In the process of cooking, heat affects the nutrients in food. These effects lead to changes in texture, appearance and flavour of the food.

Protein

Heat causes protein in liquids to coagulate (set or solidify). Examples in cookery include:

- Egg white: it thickens, becoming opaque and then firm, when it is cooked.
- Gluten (wheat protein) in bread forms the crust on a loaf.
- Coatings on fried food (e.g. batter, breadcrumbs): these also contain gluten, which coagulates.

If protein is heated too much, it will become hard, tough, shrunken and unpalatable. Syneresis results from over-coagulated egg protein, which pushes out moisture; this can be seen in over-cooked scrambled egg.

Carbohydrates

Starches and sugars react differently to dry and moist heat, as shown in Table 7.1.

Fat

Fats melt into oils when heated. Water is given off with a bubbling noise. When all the water is gone, a faint blue haze appears; the fat itself will not evaporate. If the fat is heated even more, it will smoke and burn, giving an unpleasant smell caused by fatty acids. Fats within foods can cause a change in texture and flavour when heated: for example, melted cheese.

Vitamins

There will be some loss of water-soluble vitamins B and C when food is cooked in liquid, such as boiling. Some of the vitamins may also be lost through high temperatures, exposure to oxygen and enzyme action.

Vitamins in the A, D, E and K groups are not water soluble, so they will survive cooking in water; they are also not usually destroyed by heat.

To avoid loss of water-soluble vitamins:

- Do not prepare vegetables too far in advance and do not soak them in water.

Table 7.1 How carbohydrates react to heat

	Starch	Sugar
Moist heat	Starch grains soften and swell. Near boiling point, the cellulose framework bursts, releasing the starch, which thickens the liquid.	Sugar dissolves in water. When heated it becomes syrup. Eventually it colours, then caramelises. Finally it will turn to carbon and ash.
Dry heat	Starch changes from creamy white to brown. It gives off water when heated. Starch on the surface of food changes to dextrin, a sugar – e.g. bread becoming toast. When overheated, starch will carbonise and burn.	Sugar caramelises quickly and then burns.

- Cook vegetables in small quantities and as quickly as possible.
- Cover them with a lid during cooking, to minimise oxidation.
- Use foods that are as fresh as possible; do not store them for longer than necessary.
- Put green vegetables into boiling water to allow for rapid cooking.

Boiling, poaching and steaming

Table 7.2 explains the differences between boiling, poaching and steaming. It will help you to choose which method to use for a particular dish.

⚠ HEALTH AND SAFETY

- When you are boiling, poaching or steaming, you are dealing with large amounts of hot or boiling water; work safely to avoid accidents.
- When a pot of hot liquid is on the stove, make sure that the handle is turned in, so it is less likely to be knocked over; avoid carrying containers of very hot water from one place to another.

Table 7.2 Boiling, poaching and steaming

	Boiling	Poaching	Steaming
What exactly does it mean?	Food is immersed in liquid at 100°C. The temperature is then reduced slightly and maintained at the **simmering** point where the liquid is just moving.	Food is cooked in a liquid that is just below boiling point.	Food is cooked under pressure in the steam produced by a boiling liquid.
Why use this method?	A healthy method of cookery: • It does not use any fat. • When done properly, it will keep the flavour and nutritional value is retained in the food but care must be taken not to lose water-soluble vitamins (see above). Some foods may also be parboiled (partly boiled) and then finished using another method of cookery.	A gentle method, suitable for delicate foods such as eggs and fish. Used to cook food so that it is very tender and easy to digest.	Steaming keeps most of the nutrients in the food. It is gentle, so it prevents the food from becoming too saturated with water.
What happens to the food as it is cooked?	Gentle boiling helps to break down the tough fibres of certain foods. When boiling meats, some of the meat extracts dissolve in the cooking liquid (see below).	Poaching helps to tenderise the food and improve the texture.	Steamed food will not take on any colour. The texture will vary according to the type of food, type of steamer and level of heat. Steamed sponges and puddings are lighter in texture.

	Boiling	Poaching	Steaming
Is it economical? Does it save on labour?	Older, tougher, cheaper joints of meat and poultry can be made tasty and tender. It is an economical way of cooking as it uses minimal fuel. It is labour saving, as boiling food needs little attention.	Poaching is economical as poaching does not require excessive heat and most foods cook quickly.	It is labour saving and suitable for cooking large quantities of food at one time, e.g. in schools. Smaller quantities can be economically cooked in a multi-tiered steamer on a stove top.
How does it affect nutrition?	Water-soluble vitamins, such as Vitamins B and C, can be lost through excessive boiling.	A healthy method using water (or another liquid) without adding fats.	Steamed food tends to retain its nutritional value.
Other advantages	Nutritious, well-flavoured stock can be produced from the cooking liquor.	A quick, easy, uncomplicated cooking method.	It makes some foods lighter and easy to digest. Low-pressure steaming reduces the risk of overcooking, which can cause food to over-soften. High-pressure steaming enables food to be cooked or reheated quickly.

Boiling

There are two ways of boiling, as described in Table 7.3.

Principles of boiling
http://bit.ly/A9UsQR

Follow these guidelines when boiling food:

- Ensure that all pieces of food going into the same pan are of a similar size or density so they need the same cooking time.
- Foods that require different cooking times should not be cooked together. For example, the cooking time of potato is longer than that of cauliflower. It is important to be familiar with the cooking times of different vegetables for this reason. Choose pans that are the right size to allow for the food and the boiling water.
- Use enough water to entirely cover the food throughout its cooking time. Use minimal amounts of water for green vegetables.
- Make sure that there is enough boiling liquid

in the pan before you add the food to avoid lowering the temperature. This helps maintain the vitamins and the colour of green vegetables.

- With meat and stock, skim the surface of the liquid regularly during the cooking.
- Simmer rather than boil vigorously so that less water evaporates, and the food will not shrink too much or break up.

There are also guidelines for boiling certain foods:

- When you make stock, bring the ingredients to the boil from a cold start and skim off surface scum regularly.
- Pasta should not be overcooked but left slightly firm (called *al dente*).
- Meat and poultry should be well cooked and tender.
- Vegetables should not be overcooked but left slightly crisp.
- Tough meat must be cooked *slowly* so that there is time for the connective tissue to change into gelatine. This dissolves in the cooking liquid and the fibres in the meat are released, making the meat tender. If this all happens too

Table 7.3 Methods of boiling

Method of boiling	What is it used for?
Place the food in boiling liquid. The liquid will stop boiling when you put the food in, so heat it up to bring it back to boiling. Then reduce the heat so that the liquid just bubbles gently (**simmering**) and cooks the food.	• Cooking green vegetables – to retain maximum colour and nutritional value (when boiled for the shortest possible time). • Rice and pasta.
Cover food with cold liquid. Heat it up and bring it to the boil, then reduce the heat to allow the food to simmer.	• Meat – to tenderise the fibrous structure. • Root, pulses and other vegetables. • Vegetable soups – to extract the starch. • Stocks – to extract flavour from the ingredients.

fast, the meat will be tough and stringy. Gentle heat will allow the protein to coagulate without hardening.

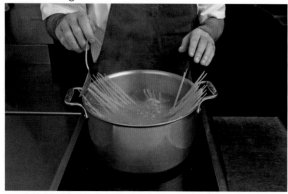
Boiling spaghetti

Poaching

A poaching medium is the liquid in which the food is cooked. As well as water, different liquids can be used for specific dishes. Milk can be used to poach fish and also meringue for desserts. Suitable stocks can be used for fish or chicken and a court bouillon for fish. Fruit can be poached in a stock syrup or in a fruit juice.

 HEALTH AND SAFETY

- When you place food into boiling or poaching liquid, lower it in gently so that the liquid does not splash up and scald you.

- Make sure that the cooking pot is large enough, to avoid boiling water being splashed over the edge.

- When removing the lid from the cooking pot, tilt it away from your face to avoid burns from the steam.

A well-flavoured sauce can be made with the cooking liquid, such as from the milk in which fish is poached.

For most foods, heat the poaching liquid first. When it reaches the right temperature just below boiling, lower the prepared food into the barely simmering liquid and allow it to cook in the gentle heat. The temperature must be controlled: there should be no sign of the liquid moving, except for the occasional bubble rising to the surface.

There are two ways of poaching: shallow and deep.

Shallow poaching

Foods such as cuts of fish and chicken are poached in a small amount of liquid and covered with silicone paper. Keep the liquid just below boiling point. A way to control the temperature when shallow poaching is to bring the liquid to the boil on top of the stove, place the food in the liquid, cover it and complete the cooking in a moderately hot oven, approximately 180°C.

Principles of poaching
http://bit.ly/wutwTE

Deep poaching

Poach eggs in approximately 8 cm of gently simmering water; a little acid such as vinegar may be added to stabilise the proteins and give the eggs a good shape. You can also deep poach whole fish (e.g. salmon), cuts of fish on or off the bone (e.g. turbot, cod and salmon), and whole chicken. All of these should be completely covered with the poaching liquid.

> **Note:** when eggs are cooked in individual shallow metal pans over boiling water, this is actually steaming rather than poaching.

Time the cooking correctly to ensure the quality of the finished dish, retention of nutrients and for food safety reasons (for example, undercooked chicken can cause food poisoning). The time and temperature needed to cook the food correctly will vary slightly for different types of food.

Foods usually retain their shape during poaching, but they may look a little pale after cooking.

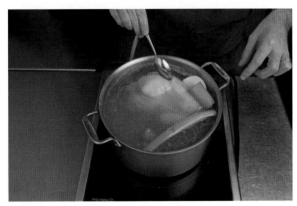

Poaching a chicken

 HEALTH AND SAFETY

When straining foods from boiling and simmering liquids do so carefully.

Steaming

Principles of atmospheric steaming
http://bit.ly/ykv2E7

There are three main methods of steaming.

1. **Atmospheric steaming** – This is done in an atmospheric steamer, a closed 'oven' heated by steam generated from water boiling at the bottom. Food in the steamer is heated by direct conduction from contact with the steam. For small quantities, atmospheric steaming may be done by placing in a perforated, covered container above a saucepan of boiling water. The steam from the boiling water rises into the container above and cooks the food.

2. **High-pressure steaming** – this is done in high-pressure steamers working like pressure cookers. Steam in the cooking chamber builds up pressure: high pressure produces higher temperatures, which makes the food cook faster. A safety valve is used to control the pressure with maximum pressures pre-set. High-pressure steamers are also used for 'batch' cooking, where small quantities of vegetables are cooked frequently throughout the service. This means the vegetables are always freshly cooked, keep their colour, flavour and nutritional content.

3. **Combination steaming** – this is done in a combination ('combi') oven. Dry heat and steam are combined in the oven, adding a little moisture to the food as it cooks. As water vapour is added to a convection oven that uses a fan, the steam is distributed evenly and quickly. Although still only at 100°C, it will cook the food more quickly than in a conventional oven.

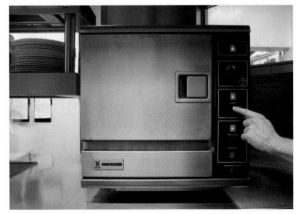

A commercial, pressureless steamer

When using steamers, timing and temperature are very important to make sure that the food is correctly cooked.

- Food cooks much faster in high-pressure steamers and therefore it can overcook very quickly.

- When you are using a high-pressure steamer, wait until the pressure gauge shows that it has reached the correct pressure before you open the door very carefully, allowing some steam to escape before you place the food in the steamer. This means that the steamer will be at the correct cooking temperature, and the food will cook efficiently.

- Cooking times will vary according to the equipment used, and the food to be steamed. It is essential that manufacturers' instructions are followed correctly.

The following notes apply to particular steamed dishes:

- The natural juices that result from steaming fish can be served with the fish or used to make the accompanying sauce.

- For meat or sweet steamed puddings, grease the basin before filling it. Make sure it is covered with greased greaseproof or silicone paper and foil to prevent moisture getting in and making the pudding soggy.

Steamers need to be cleaned and maintained, according to these guidelines:

- Before use, check that the steamer is clean and safe to use. Report any fault immediately.

- Steamer trays and runners should be washed in hot detergent water, rinsed and dried. Where applicable, drain, clean and refill the water-generating chamber. Door controls should be lightly greased occasionally. Leave the door slightly open to allow air to circulate when the steamer is not in use.

- Clean metal steamer trays and containers thoroughly using hot detergent water, rinse, then dry with kitchen paper/clean cloth.

⚠ HEALTH AND SAFETY

The steam in steamers can be very dangerous as it is extremely hot and can cause serious burns and scalds. To avoid injuring yourself:

- Make sure you are trained in how to use steamers and use them with great care.

- Check the pressure in high-pressure steamers continually.

- Allow the pressure to return to the correct level before opening doors or removing pressure-cooker lids.

- Allow time for the pressure to return to normal before opening commercial steamers. Then stand well away from the door as you open it, to avoid the full impact of the escaping steam.

Stewing/casseroling and braising

Stewing/casseroling and braising are slow, gentle methods of cookery using moist heat (see Table 7.4).

Stewing/casseroling

Principles of making a stew
http://bit.ly/yap1Ot

- **Stewing:** meat and vegetables are usually seared in hot oil/fat then placed in a saucepan and covered with liquid (water or stock). The liquid is brought to the boil, then turned down to a low simmer. A lid is placed on the pan and the food is left to cook slowly on the hob.

- **Casseroling:** this is the same process as cooking a stew, but in the oven. The term 'casserole' refers to both the cooking pot and the finished dish. Casserole dishes are usually deep and ovenproof with handles and tight-fitting lids. They can be made of glass, metal, ceramic or any other heatproof material. Cassrole ingredients may also include pulses and rice. A topping of cheese or breadcrumbs may also be added for texture and flavour.

The liquid for the stew should relate to the type of food you are cooking.

- For fruit, the liquid is usually fruit juice or syrup.

- For vegetables, use vegetable stock.

Table 7.4 Stewing and braising

	Stewing/casseroling	Braising
What exactly does it mean?	The food is completely covered by a liquid. Both the food and the sauce are served together. **Stews** are usually cooked on top of the stove. **Casseroles** are cooked in the oven. These methods use less liquid and a cooking temperature about 5°C lower than for boiling. Smaller pieces of meat are used than in braising, and therefore take less time.	A method of cooking larger pieces of food. The food is only half covered with liquid and can be cooked on the stovetop or in the oven. The food is cooked very slowly in a pan with a tightly fitted lid, using low temperatures. A combination of steaming and stewing cooks the food. Meat is usually cooked in very large pieces and carved before serving.
What foods are cooked in this way?	• Meat • Poultry • Vegetables • Fruit	• Whole joints or large pieces of meat • Tougher cuts of meat • Poultry and poultry cuts, such as turkey breast • Vegetables, sometimes with fillings (e.g. cabbage stuffed with rice) • Furred game, such as hare and rabbit • Most feathered game, such as pheasant, duck and goose
Why use this method?	• To cook cheaper cuts of meat and poultry in a way that makes them tender and palatable as well as producing a wall-flavoured sauce • To give a rich flavour to the food.	• To enhance the flavour and texture of food • To tenderise some tougher joints of meat
What happens to the food as it is cooked?	As the meat cooks slowly in gentle heat, the collagen (the protein in the connective tissue) changes into gelatine so the meat becomes tender. Protein coagulates without becoming tough. Flavours from the meat are released into the liquid, and flavours from the liquid and flavourings are absorbed by the meat. When fruit is stewed, pectin (a setting agent) is released into the cooking liquid, thickening it slightly and giving it flavour.	Braising breaks down the tissue fibre in certain meat, which softens it and makes it tender and edible. The collagen (the protein in the connective tissue) in meat changes into gelatine so that meat becomes tender. Cooking food in the braising liquid also improves the texture. Flavours from the meat are released into the liquid, and flavours from the liquid and other ingredients are absorbed by the meat.
Is it economical? Does it save on labour?	Stewing makes tougher cuts of meat and poultry tender and palatable. Usually, everything in a stew can be eaten so there is very little waste. Stews and casseroles are labour saving because foods can be cooked in bulk and do not need much attention.	Tougher, less expensive meats and poultry can be used.
How does it affect nutrition?	Some nutrients can escape from the food during cooking and will stay in the liquid. This means that nutrients are not lost, but become part of the sauce.	
Other advantages	If cooked correctly, very little liquid will evaporate, leaving sufficient sauce to serve up as part of the stew. The food does not shrink much and keeps its flavour. Stews reheat easily. The tough cuts of meat that can be stewed have lots of flavour.	Maximum flavour is retained.

- For meat, chicken and fish use meat, chicken and fish stock, respectively.
- Alcohol, such as wine or sherry, may be added to the liquid for flavour, especially when stewing red meat.

Sufficient liquid needs to be added to the stew to allow for evaporation.

Method

The process of stewing can be seen in some of the recipes in Chapter 10.

The stewing liquid may be **thickened:**

- by adding a thickening agent, such as flour, before cooking begins (for example, in blanquette)
- by adding a thickening agent later in the cooking process (for example, *beurre manié*, i.e. equal quantities of butter and flour kneaded together and added in small amounts)
- as a result of the cooking process reducing the liquid (for example, brown stew)
- as a result of the unpassed ingredients of the stew (such as potatoes in Irish stew).

However, stews should not be over-thickened and the sauce should stay light. Adjust the consistency at the end of cooking if necessary by adding more liquid or more thickening agent.

Good stews are cooked slowly, so it is important to control the temperature properly. The liquid should barely simmer (approximately 82°C). If cooking in the oven, the ideal temperature is 170°C. Cooking too fast or too hot will make the food tough, dry or stringy.

Use a tight-fitting lid to keep in the steam. This helps to keep the temperature correct and reduces evaporation.

Do not overcook stews as this:

- causes too much liquid to evaporate
- causes the food to break up
- causes the food to lose its colour
- spoils the flavour.

Expensive, tender cuts of meat are not suitable

for a stew: the meat will dry out during the long cooking process.

 HEALTH AND SAFETY

- Place large pots of stew on the stovetop carefully, to avoid splashing or spilling the liquid.
- Take cure when stirring a stew/casserole to avoid the risk of burns and scalds.
- When you lift the lid from the pan, lift it away from you to avoid burning yourself on the steam.
- If you are using Bratt pans, be very careful when stirring the large quantity of hot, semi-liquid food.

Braising

 Principles of braising
http://bit.ly/ykXwNB

There are two methods of braising:

- **Brown braising** (for joints and cuts of meat): the meat is marinated, and may be larded (covered in strips of fatty bacon), before being cooked following the method given below.
- **White braising** (for vegetables, such as celery or cabbage, and sweetbreads): the food is blanched and refreshed instead of being browned before braising; the cooking liquid is a white stock.

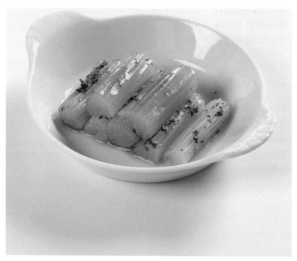

Braised celery (recipe available on Dynamic Learning)

Foods should be braised in an appropriate liquid, such as:

- vegetable stock or vegetable juice, for vegetables
- stock, water, wine or beer for meat.

The process of braising is as follows:

1. Seal and brown the meat in a pan on the stove, or in a hot oven; for white braising, blanch and refresh the food.
2. Place a layer of mirepoix or root vegetables in the base of the pan.
3. Place the food to be braised on top of the vegetables. They will protect it from contact with the base of the pan.
4. Add braising liquor to the pan, so that it half covers the food.
5. Cover the pan with a heavy, tightly fitting lid. This will keep the moisture in the pan and create steam around the food.
6. If you are braising in the oven, set the temperature at about 150°C.
7. Baste the food occasionally with the braising liquor. If you are braising a joint to be served whole, remove the lid three-quarters of the way through cooking, and then baste the joint frequently to give it a glaze.

8. The length of time for braising depends on the type, amount and size of the food. To check that meat is done, insert a metal skewer into it: if there is only slight resistance, the meat is cooked.
9. Strain off the cooking liquid. If braising vegetables, discard the liquid: it will have taken on strong flavours. For other foods, the liquid can be used to make a sauce using one of the following methods:

- Heat the liquid and allow it to reduce.
- Thicken the liquid with a thickening agent: cornflour, arrowroot or *beurre manié*.
- If the liquid is already too thick, add some stock to thin it.

 HEALTH AND SAFETY

- During cooking, the pan and its contents become extremely hot. Use thick, dry oven cloths whenever you remove the pot from the oven or lift the lid.
- The contents of the pan can become extremely hot, so take great care to lift the lid away from you to avoid burns and take care to prevent splashing yourself with hot liquid.

Baking and roasting

Baking and roasting are usually done in an oven, but food can also be roasted on a rotating spit. Low-temperature roasting is done in an oven, but this needs to be carefully controlled, and checked with a digital thermometer (food probe).

Table 7.5 Baking and roasting

	Baking	**Roasting**	**Low-temperature roasting**
What exactly does it mean?	Food is cooked in an oven using dry heat. The steam that is generated plays an important part in the process.	Food is cooked in dry heat with added fat or oil. Roasting can be done on a spit (by radiant heat) or in an oven with one of the following: • applied dry heat • forced-air convected heat • convected heat combined with microwave energy.	Food is cooked in the oven at a lower temperature than for traditional roasting. Before roasting, the meat is browned all over in a frying pan over a high heat, with a little oil brushed over the lean surfaces.

	Baking	Roasting	Low-temperature roasting
Why use this method?	Baking can give foods an appealing colour and texture. It is a traditional and accepted best method for some foods, e.g. bread.	Roasting can make good-quality meat and poultry tender and succulent. Roasting gives a distinctive finish to food, e.g. roast beef or roast potatoes.	It will keep meat tender, as long as the oven temperature is strictly controlled. Most boneless cuts of meat are suitable for this method.
What happens to the food as it is cooked?	All products that are baked contain water. When heated, this will start to evaporate, creating steam. To ensure that the food is baked, not steamed, it must be evenly spaced in order to bake efficiently. Certain ingredients, such as yeast and baking powder, are affected by heat, which chemically changes them, giving the raw structure of many foods (e.g. pastry) an edible texture.	When roasting begins, the oven is very hot. This seals the surface protein of the food, keeping food moist and adding flavour and colour. Once the food is lightly browned, the oven temperature is reduced so that the inside of the food cooks without the surface becoming hard. During cooking, the product must be basted regularly with fat or oil and cooking juices; this helps to keep the food moist and caramelises the finished product.	The meat cooks slowly until the core reaches a certain temperature. The fibrous structure of the meat is tenderised and the texture changes. Thicker cuts will take longer to roast. Meat that has a covering of fat will shrink during cooking and yield fewer portions.
Is it economical? **Does it save on labour?**	Bulk and batch cooking is possible, with products cooked uniformly and all to the same colour. Using full (not over full) baking trays and all the oven shelves will save time and energy.	It is economical as roasting is a simple, uncomplicated method of cooking that does not require multiple ingredients. It is labour saving as a large number of meals can be produced relatively quickly and easily with minimal attention.	Cheaper cuts of meat (e.g. pork belly) can be used, because this method will tenderise them. Slow roasting uses more energy than the traditional method, because it takes longer.
Other advantages	Suitable for a wide variety of foods. Baked products are appetising: they look and smell good. Ovens have effective manual or automatic temperature controls.	Continual basting with meat juices gives a distinctive flavour. Meat juices from the joint can also be used for gravy. Ovens have effective manual or automatic temperature controls. Transparent doors make it possible to check on food during cooking. Spit roasting can be a visual process for customers.	Gives a better yield (more portions) than traditional roasting.

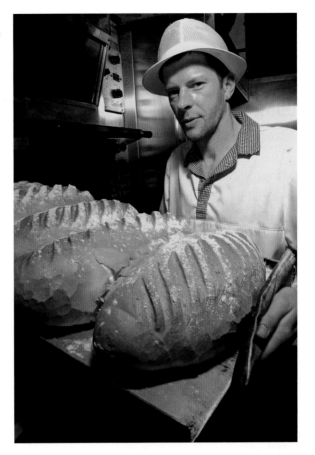

⚠ **HEALTH AND SAFETY**

- When removing trays from the oven, use thick, dry oven cloths to protect your hands.

- Do not overload baking or roasting trays or use trays of food that are too heavy to lift easily.

- Open the oven door slowly – there is likely to be a lot of steam present, which can cause burns.

Baking

There are three methods of baking, as shown in Table 7.6.

When baking and roasting it is important to use the oven correctly:

- The oven must always be **preheated** to the required temperature before putting in any food, thus allowing it to start cooking at the correct temperature.

- Only open the oven door when it is essential. The temperature inside will fall, the product can be spoiled, for example Yorkshire puddings.

- When batches of food are being cooked, allow 'recovery time' for the oven to return to the correct temperature. When chilled or frozen items go into an oven 'recovery time' will be longer.

- In general-purpose ovens, the top part of the oven is the hottest. Position the oven shelves to suit the requirements of the food being cooked. In convection ovens, heat is even throughout the oven.

- Use baking trays that remain level within the oven. Foods will bake unevenly and liquids will spill if the tray is not level.

Table 7.6 Methods of baking

Method	How it works	What it is used for
Dry baking in a preheated oven	The water in the food creates steam. This combines with the oven heat to cook the food.	Cakes, pastry, jacket potatoes
Baking with increased humidity	A bowl of water is placed in the oven, or steam is injected, to increase the humidity. This increases the water content and improves the eating quality of the food.	Bread Principles of baking and bread-making http://bit.ly/xZ76JY
Baking with heat modification: placing the container of food into a **bain marie** (tray of water) within the oven	The water modifies the heat that reaches the food. The food cooks more slowly and does not overheat.	Baked egg custard (the slower cooking prevents it from over-cooking)

Roasting

Principles of roasting
http://bit.ly/z6HCDN

Follow these guidelines when roasting food:

- Use the oven temperature and shelf settings given in the recipe.
- Adjust the cooking time according to the weight of the food (see Table 7.7 for the cooking times for various meats).
- The shape, type, bone proportion and quality of the food will also affect the cooking time.
- The centre of meat must reach a certain temperature (see Table 7.8). Use a meat thermometer or probe to check the temperature.

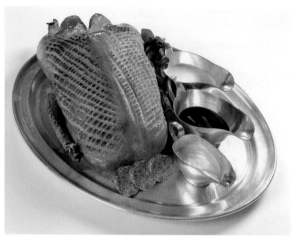

Roast goose (recipe available on Dynamic Learning)

⚠ HEALTH AND SAFETY

When basting a joint, or removing it from the oven, be very careful. Hot fat around the joint could burn or scald you if it splashes. Do not have too much fat in the roasting tray.

Table 7.7 Approximate cooking times, according to weight

Meat	Degree of cooking	Approximate cooking time
Beef	Underdone (medium)	15 minutes per ½ kg, plus 15 minutes over
	Well done	20 minutes per ½ kg, plus 20 minutes over
Lamb	Cooked pink	15 minutes per ½ kg, plus 15 minutes over
	Cooked through	20 minutes per ½ kg, plus 20 minutes over
Mutton	Cooked through	20 minutes per ½ kg, plus 20 minutes over
Veal	Cooked through	20 minutes per ½ kg, plus 25 minutes over
Pork	Cooked through	25 minutes per ½ kg, plus 25 minutes over

For food safety reasons joints of meat that have been boned and rolled or processed in any way should not be left underdone in the centre.

Table 7.8 Internal core temperatures

Meat	Core temperature
Beef (rare)	45–47°C
Beef (medium)	50–52°C
Beef (well done)	64–70°C
Lamb	55°C
Pork	60–65°C
Veal	60°C
Venison	60°C

Grilling and barbecuing

Grilling is a fast method of cookery using radiant heat. It is also known as broiling. There are four ways of grilling, as described in Table 7.9.

Grilling is only suitable for best-quality, tender meat. Inferior meat will become tough and hard to eat after grilling.

Grilling is also useful for some vegetables.

- Fierce heat reaches the surface of the food. This rapidly coagulates and seals the surface protein, helping to keep meat moist and add good colour and flavour.
- As long as the food is not pierced, meat will retain more juices when grilled than in any other method of cookery.
- The food cooks quickly, so the maximum nutrients and flavour are retained.

Meat can be grilled to various degrees of cooking. To judge how well cooked the meat is, press it and look at the colour of the juices:

- red and bloody juice: rare meat
- reddish pink juice: underdone (medium) meat
- pink juice: just done meat
- clear juice: well-done meat.

Table 7.9 Methods of grilling

	Equipment	Method
Grilling over heat Principles of grilling http://bit.ly/yywpge	Grills/griddles heated from below (under-fired grills) by charcoal, gas or electricity	Grill bars are preheated and greased so that food will not stick to them. Food starts on the hottest part of the grill, and is then moved to a cooler part. Cooking time varies according to the thickness of the food and the heat of the grill. The bars char the food to give a distinctive flavour and appearance; food is turned so that both sides are charred.
Barbecuing	A grill over a fierce heat fuelled by gas, charcoal or wood	As above. If using solid fuel, allow the flames and smoke to die down before placing food on the bars – otherwise the food will be tainted. Food may be marinated before cooking or brushed with barbecue sauce during cooking.
Grilling under heat	Salamander (over-fired grill)	The salamander is preheated and the bars are greased. Food items that would break up easily, such as fish, can be held in a double-sided wire grid with a hinge and a handle; this should be greased. Also used for browning, gratinating or glazing some dishes.
Grilling between heat	Electrically heated grill bars or plates	Food is grilled between the grill bars or plates.

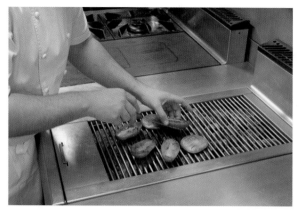

Using an under-fired grill

The advantages of grilling are that:

- it is a fast method and food can be cooked quickly to order
- food is visible during cooking, which helps the chef to keep control
- grills can be used in view of the customer
- grilled food has a distinctive appearance and flavour.

Follow these guidelines when grilling food:

- Small, thin items must be cooked quickly.
- Cook all items as quickly as possible; the slower they cook, the dryer they will become.
- Oil the bars and baste the food to prevent dryness.

⚠ **HEALTH AND SAFETY**

- Use tongs, slices or palette knives to turn or lift food: tongs for heavier items (e.g. steaks), slices for lighter or delicate items (e.g. fish).
- When reaching over to food at the back of the grill/barbecue, remember that heat is coming up from below: be careful not to burn your arm.
- If food is marinated in oil, drain it well before cooking, as excess oil could catch fire on the grill.

Shallow and deep frying

Table 7.10 explains the differences between shallow and deep frying.

Shallow frying

There are four methods of shallow frying, as shown in Table 7.11.

Table 7.10 Shallow and deep frying

	Shallow frying	Deep frying
What exactly does it mean?	Cooking food in a small amount of preheated fat or oil. Food can be fried in a shallow pan or on a flat surface (griddle plate).	Small pieces of food are completely immersed in hot fat or oil. The heat from the fat/oil penetrates into the food (by convection) as well as cooking the surface (by conduction). This is classified as a dry method of cookery, because no liquid is used and it has a drying effect on food; moisture in the oil is driven off as visible bubbles.
Why use this method?	To brown food and give a distinctive flavour.	To give food a golden-brown colour and a crisp texture.

	Shallow frying	Deep frying
What happens to the food as it is cooked?	A high temperature is used, so the surface protein of the food coagulates almost instantly. This means that moisture is retained. The food absorbs some of the frying medium (fat or oil).	Some foods are precooked (e.g. fishcakes). Deep frying them seals the surface coating by coagulating the protein in the coating; it also reheats the interior. Uncoated foods (e.g. chipped potatoes) are cooked in the oil: they can absorb a large amount of the fat, which changes the texture and nutritional content.
Is it economical? **Does it save on labour?**	Shallow frying/pan frying can be a quick method of cookery, especially for tender, small cuts of meats and fish. It is most suitable for short order and à la carte service.	Food can be partially cooked (**blanched**) and then finished in hot oil later: this saves time during busy service, and also gives a good crisp quality to chips.
How does it affect nutrition?	Some of the fat or oil is absorbed by the food during cooking: this changes the nutritional content.	
Other advantages	A very quick method of cookery, suitable for prime cuts of meat, poultry, fish and also some vegetables.	A quick and easy method of cookery. A wide variety of foods can be deep fried. Coated foods are sealed quickly, so the insides do not become greasy.

Table 7.11 Methods of shallow frying

	Method	What is it used for?
Shallow fry	Food is cooked with a small amount of fat or oil, in a frying pan or sauté pan. The presentation side of the food (the side that will be facing up) is fried first – it will look better, because the fat/oil is clean at this stage. The food is then turned so that the other side cooks and changes colour.	Small cuts of fish, meat or poultry Small whole fish (up to 400 g) Eggs Pancakes Some vegetables
Sauté	As for shallow frying (above), but with one of the following variations: 1. The food is tossed in the fat/oil until golden brown and cooked. 2. After cooking, the food is removed from the pan. The fat is discarded and then the pan is deglazed with stock or wine. This forms part of the sauce.	Sliced/chopped potatoes, onions or other vegetables such as mushrooms or courgettes Tender cuts of meat or poultry, tender offal
Griddle	Food is cooked on a griddle (a solid metal plate) which has been lightly oiled and preheated. Food is turned frequently during cooking.	Hamburgers, bacon or sausages Sliced onions and tomatoes Pancakes (turned once) Some fish
Stir fry	Food is fast-fried in a wok or frying pan with a little fat or oil.	Vegetables Strips of meat, fish or poultry Noodles

Principles of shallow frying
http://bit.ly/x4E2br

Follow these guidelines when shallow frying food:

- Select the correct type and size of pan. If the pan is too small, food will not brown evenly and may break up; if too large, the parts of the pan not covered by food will burn, and this will spoil the flavour of the food being cooked.
- Control the temperature carefully – it should be very hot to start with, then reduced.
- Clean frying pans after every use.
- When shallow frying continuously over a busy period, work in an organised and systematic way.

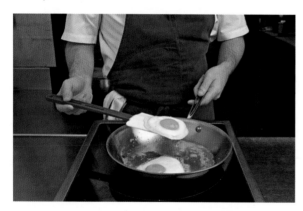

When shallow frying in butter, it is best to use **clarified butter**. This has had impurities removed and can be heated to a higher temperature without burning. To make it:

1. Melt the butter, which will separate into fat and liquid.

> ⚠ **HEALTH AND SAFETY**
>
> - Keep sleeves rolled down, as splashing hot fat/oil could burn the forearm.
> - Add food to the pan carefully, away from you, to reduce splashing.
> - Use a thick, clean, dry cloth when handling pans.
> - Move pans carefully to avoid spilling fat/oil onto the stove.

2. Strain off the fat carefully, leaving behind the liquid. This is the clarified butter.

Deep frying

Principles of deep frying
http://bit.ly/zcs2Pl

Many foods can be deep fried, including:

- small pieces of lean meat
- chicken
- whole or filleted fish
- cheese
- vegetables
- prepared items such as fishcakes, fritters, samosas or spring rolls.

Conventional deep-fried foods, except potatoes, are coated in order to:

- protect the surface of the food from intense heat and from fat/oil penetrating the food
- prevent moisture and nutrients from escaping
- modify the rapid penetration of the intense heat.

The most common coatings are:

- milk and flour
- flour/egg/breadcrumbs
- batter
- pastry.

Crumbed food should be chilled before frying: this helps to keep the crumbs attached. Immediately before cooking, shake off any excess crumbs and pat the surface to make sure the coating is in contact with the food.

Battered food should be allowed to drain before cooking, so that there is no excess batter. It needs to be lowered carefully into the hot fat.

The purpose of the fat/oil in deep frying is to achieve the distinctive texture and flavour of deep-fried food. The type of fat/oil used depends on the food being cooked, the temperature required and the flavours desired. Suitable fats are:

- oils (soya, vegetable, sunflower, etc.)
- clarified butter (but remember this may burn at a much lower temperature than oil)
- animal fats, e.g. lard
- a mixture of oil and clarified butter.

If solid fat is used, it needs to melt in the fryer at a low temperature (so that it does not burn), before being brought up to a frying temperature.

Method

The process for deep frying food is as follows:

1. Cut the food into small pieces of uniform size.
2. Coat the food (see above).
3. Fill the fryer or cooking pot with oil or fat. Commercial fryers usually have a mark showing the required fat/oil level: it is dangerous to overfill them. Any other pot or fryer should be filled between half and two-thirds full.
4. Preheat the fat/oil to the correct temperature, normally between 175°C and 195°C. It is best to use a thermostatically controlled fryer. As the fat/oil gets close to this temperature, it will become quite still, with a little haze above it. (If it gets a little too hot, it may catch fire, so take care.)
5. Place the food carefully into the fat/oil when the temperature is correct (a frying basket may be used).
6. Fry until cooked and golden brown.
7. Food can be turned with a spider (a wide, shallow mesh spoon with a long handle) during cooking, to help it cook evenly.
8. Remove and drain well before serving.

Timing and temperature are very important. Thicker pieces of food need to cook for longer without becoming over-coloured, so the fat/oil should be at a lower temperature. The smaller the pieces of food, the hotter the fat/oil and the shorter the cooking time.

The recommended temperature also varies depending on the fat/oil used. Most are used at 180°C but pure vegetable oil and dripping may be used at 170°C and olive oil at 175°C.

Smoking point occurs when oil is overheated: between 165°C and 224°C, depending on the type of oil. **Flashpoint** is the point when oil catches on fire: between 270°C and 324°C for vegetable oils. Always check oil packaging for temperature advice.

Follow these guidelines when deep frying food:

- Make sure that the fat/oil is hot enough before adding food. If it is too cool, the food will absorb extra fat/oil, making it greasy and unpalatable.
- Make sure that the fat/oil is not *too* hot. If it is, the surface of the food will burn, but the inside will stay raw. The food will become dry and tough.
- Never allow the fat/oil to smoke: this gives food a bad taste and smell as well as being dangerous as 'flashpoint' temperatures are close.
- If the fat starts to foam when food is added, lift out the food and allow the temperature to adjust.
- Do not deep fry too much food at once: it is better to fry food in batches. Adding too much food at once reduces the temperature drastically. If necessary, remove excess food from the fat/oil.
- When frying continuous batches of food, allow the temperature of the fat/oil to recover after each batch, before adding the next one. If this is not done, the food will be pale and soggy.
- Serve food as soon as possible after frying or it will lose its crisp texture.
- During cooking, skim off crumbs regularly using a spider. The fat/oil will last longer if this is done. (Crumbs build up and cause the fat/oil to go off, giving it a rancid taste.)
- Do not deep fry fatty foods, or add wet foods to the fryer.
- Any strongly flavoured food should be fried in a separate fryer from other foods, or be the last thing fried before the fat/oil is discarded. This is because the fat/oil will take on flavours from the food.
- Small, thin pieces of food can be deep fried from frozen. Fry frozen food in smaller

quantities, as it will bring down the temperature of the fat/oil.

- Turn down the temperature of the fryer during quiet periods, to save on fuel.

When you have finished frying:

- Allow the fat/oil to cool then strain it, so that there are no food particles present next time it is heated up.

- Cover the fat/oil while the fryer is not in use, so that it does not oxidise (the oxygen in the air can turn the oil or fat rancid).

Some commercial fryers have a 'cool zone'. This is a section at the base where crumbs and food particles are collected, so that they do not overcook in the oil. These crumbs must be removed when the fat is cool.

 HEALTH AND SAFETY

Deep frying can be very dangerous. Hot fat/oil can cause serious burns.

- Only use a deep fryer after proper training.

- Use a thermostatically controlled fryer with fat/oil-level indicators rather than heating oil on a stove.

- Never leave the fryer unattended. Keep a close eye on the temperature and do not let it get too hot: never let fat/oil reach its smoke point. If it is smoking, it is very close to its flashpoint and could catch fire.

- If a fryer catches fire, switch off and cover with a lid if possible so that the fire does not get any more oxygen. Fire extinguishing equipment should be kept near the fryer. (Wet chemical extinguisher or fire blanket.) Only use these if you have been trained in their use and never use any other type of fire extinguisher on a fryer fire.

- Make sure you know how to put out a fat fire. **Remember:** oil and water do not mix. If fat catches fire, cover the pot with a lid so that the fire does not get any more oxygen. Then use the correct fire extinguisher or a fire blanket: use them correctly.

- Stand back when placing food into hot fat and avoid putting your face, arms or hands over the fryer.

- Do not move a pan of hot fat/oil, leave it where it is until cool.

- Avoid sudden movements around fryers and do not drop anything into the hot fat/oil.

Other methods of cooking

Table 7.12 explains three methods of cooking: pot roasting, tandoori cooking and paper bag cooking.

Table 7.12 Pot roasting, tandoori and paper bag cooking

	Pot roasting (*poêlé*)	Tandoori cooking	Paper bag cooking (*en papillotte*)
What exactly does it mean?	Cooking food on a bed of root vegetables in a covered pan.	Cooking by dry heat at up to 375°C in a clay oven (**tandoor**). The heat source is at the base of the oven, but the clay radiates heat evenly throughout. Food is placed in vertically; no oil or fat is used. Naan (traditional Indian flat bread) is placed on the inside wall of the oven to cook.	Food is tightly sealed in oiled greaseproof paper or foil so that no steam escapes during cooking. The bags are tightly sealed, placed on a lightly greased tray and cooked in a hot oven. Food is served in the bag, to be opened by or in front of the customer.
Why use this method?	It retains the maximum flavour of all ingredients.	The cooking process and the marinade (if used) give a distinctive flavour. Food cooks quickly.	Maximum flavour and nutritional value are retained.
Preparing food for cooking	The meat is coated generously with oil or butter before the pan is covered.	Food may be marinated for between 20 minutes and two hours before cooking. It may also be brushed with marinade during cooking.	Thick items (e.g. red mullet) should be partly and quickly precooked, usually by grilling or shallow frying.
Using herbs and spices	Mix herbs with the bed of root vegetables. These can be used with a good stock as a base for the sauce.	Marinades may include onions, garlic, herbs, spices and oil, yoghurt, wine or lemon juice. A red colouring agent may be used. Marinating tenderises the food.	Finely cut vegetables, herbs and spices may be placed in the bag.
Other guidelines	Use a pan of the correct size for the food to be cooked.	If a tandoor is not available, an oven, grill rotisserie or barbecue can be used, following the principles of tandoori cooking. In this case, the spices must be cooked briefly over a fierce heat before they are added to the marinade.	

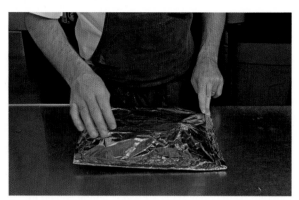

Sealing a parcel for cooking en papillotte

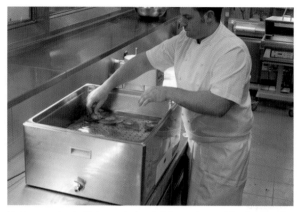

Using a water bath to cook food; this equipment is also used for sous vide cooking

Table 7.13 describes sous vide and microwave cooking and explains their advantages and disadvantages.

Sous vide

Sous vide was developed by George Pralus at the Restaurant Troisgros in Roanne, France, in 1967. It is a technique that must be managed carefully, as there are some food safety risks. The key problems are:

- It is impossible to smell vacuum packaged food and judge whether it is fresh.
- It is impossible to check the core temperature of food that is hermetically sealed in a package.

Vacuum packaging prevents **aerobic bacteria** from growing on the food. However, some bacteria are of a different type: **anaerobic**. These multiply where there is an absence of oxygen, such as inside a vacuum pouch.

Sous vide uses relatively low temperatures, and anaerobic bacteria can thrive in these conditions.

To reduce the risk of food poisoning, follow these guidelines:

- Use the freshest, highest-quality ingredients in sous vide packages. Fresh ingredients will have fewer bacteria to start with.
- Calibrate equipment every day.
- Check all seals and packages for leaks.
- Raw packages must not be kept for more than *two days* before they are pasteurised.
- Pasteurisation must take place above 55°C.

- Packages must be cooled to below 3°C within *two hours* of being pasteurised.
- Store packages below 3°C, in covered containers.
- Label packages with the date and time of packaging, pasteurisation and expiration.
- Use packages by the expiry date or discard them.

Sous vide is widely used by industrial food producers: they can package food with a minimum of processing, and it will retain its flavour, texture and size.

Fresh sous vide is also used in some restaurants, mostly at the 'high end'. The technique is less popular in the majority of restaurant kitchens because of the cost of the equipment and complexity of the technique.

Microwave cooking

Microwaves are similar to the waves that carry television signals, but are at a higher frequency.

Follow these guidelines when using a microwave oven:

- Use glass, china or plastic containers for food. Do *not* use metal unless the oven is a special model that can heat metal without any damage.
- For the best results, use round, shallow containers with straight sides.
- Keep food level; do not pile it up in mounds.
- Leave enough space in the container to allow the food to be stirred.

Table 7.13 Sous vide and microwave cooking

	Sous vide	Microwave cooking
What exactly does it mean?	A professional cooking method in which food is vacuum-sealed and cooked in plastic pouches	Cooking, defrosting or reheating food using electromagnetic waves (microwaves).
Why use this method?	It extends the useable shelf life of food. The final product retains its texture, flavour and appearance.	It is quick and convenient way of defrosting/heating/cooking food.
What happens to the food as it is cooked?	It is pasteurised by being heated in a water bath to 75°C and then quickly cooled below 3°C: this process slows the multiplication of bacteria. It is stored chilled: the plastic barrier means that the food oxidises less, and there is less contact with possible contaminants. When required, the packet of food is reheated in a water bath.	The microwaves penetrate 5 cm from each side into the food. They agitate molecules of water and particles of food, making them move around. This causes friction among the particles, which generates heat to cook the food.
Is it economical? **Does it save on labour?**	Excellent for efficiency. Single servings of meals can be prepared one or two days in advance, and can be retrieved and heated quickly when needed; unused portions can be kept. Standardised recipes may be used, ensuring quality regardless of individuals' cooking skills. Several meals can be pasteurised or regenerated in the same water bath, reducing the amount of pot washing. Traditional heat methods are not used, reducing kitchen temperatures and the cost of cooling.	It can be up to 70 per cent faster than other cooking methods, and it enables fast defrosting. It is economical on fuel. Food can also be cooked in the serving dish, which reduces the amount of dish washing. Hot meals can be available all day, and can even be self-service, keeping costs down but customers satisfied.
How does it affect nutrition?	Certain nutrients such as vitamins can be lost by this method of cookery but others, such as water-soluble vitamins, may be retained.	Food is cooked very quickly, so nutrients and flavour are retained.
Other advantages		Minimises shrinkage and drying out of food.
Disadvantages	There are some food safety issues (see below).	Not suitable for some foods and some types of container such as metal. Microwave ovens are quite small and so only small quantities can be cooked. Food is not browned unless the microwave has a browning element.

- Cover most foods during cooking, e.g. with microwave clingfilm. This helps the food cook quickly and stay moist. It also prevents splashing and condensation in the oven, and so reduces the cleaning needed after cooking.

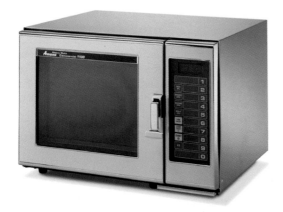

The time needed to cook food in a microwave varies depending on several factors, including the size and shape of the food. Bear these points in mind when microwaving food:

- Some foods, and some container materials, absorb energy faster than others – this means they will heat up more quickly.
- Food with a high water content will cook more quickly than dry food.
- The colder the food is to start with, the longer it will take to heat up.
- The denser the food is, the longer it will take to heat up. Turn dense foods (e.g. corn on the cob) during cooking.
- Thick or deep food is more difficult to heat through, because microwaves only penetrate 5 cm from each side of the food.
- The weight or quantity of food in the oven will affect the cooking time necessary.
- Because of all these factors, the shape of the food (e.g. a liquid could be in a tall container or a low flat one) also affects the cooking time.
- Even-shaped items of food will cook uniformly throughout. If items are an uneven shape, arrange them with the thickest part at the outside of the dish.

If there is a large quantity of food, or it is very dense or frozen, it is a good idea to heat it in stages, with rest intervals in between.

Microwave ovens tend to cook more round the edges of the food than in the middle. This means that food should be stirred during cooking, if possible, so that all the food cooks evenly. If dishes cannot be stirred, try the following alternatives:

- Rotate the dish by a quarter turn three times during cooking.
- If the edges of the food are cooked but the centre is still raw, place small pieces of microwave clingfilm over the parts that are cooked.
- Use even-shaped containers and arrange food in the containers to a uniform thickness, no more than 5 cm.
- Arrange small items or dishes in a circle. Turn each one during cooking, even if the oven has a turntable.

In general, it is better to undercook food than to overcook it. Once food is overcooked, there is nothing you can do, but undercooked food can

⚠ **HEALTH AND SAFETY**

- Follow manufacturer's instructions.
- Do not run a microwave oven when it is empty.
- Remember to pierce foods that may burst and cover foods that may splatter.
- Remove clingfilm covers carefully from hot dishes. Pull the clingfilm towards you, so that the steam escapes in the other direction and does not scald you.
- Microwavable plastic pouches need to be cut open after cooking. They will be hot and soft: handle them with care. Put the pouch on a plate before cutting it open.
- Microwave ovens should be inspected regularly.
- If the door seal is damaged, do not use the microwave. Report this to your employer or lecturer.

be cooked a little more. Consider leaving food slightly undercooked if it is going to be reheated. However, high-risk foods such as meat and poultry must reach the correct core temperature when they are cooked *and* when they are reheated: *use a thermometer to check.*

Table 7.14 Microwaving different foods

Food	Issues	Guidance for microwaving
Whole potatoes, tomatoes, peppers, unpeeled apples	Pressure may build up inside the item until it bursts.	Pierce or score the skin before cooking – this will release pressure.
Eggs	Eggs in their shells will burst in the microwave.	Never cook eggs in their shells Poached or fried eggs (in a browning dish) can be cooked in the microwave: the yolk must be lightly pricked to release pressure. Scrambled eggs can be cooked, but remove them before they are done and let them stand – they will finish cooking and turn creamy.
Deep-fried food	It is impossible to deep fry in a microwave, because you cannot control the temperature of the fat.	Microwave breadcrumbed fish in a tablespoon of oil – this will be similar to deep-fried fish.
Yorkshire puddings, choux pastry	It is impossible to maintain a soft interior with a crispy crust.	Cannot be cooked in the microwave.
Meringue		Meringue toppings (e.g. lemon meringue pie) can be cooked in the microwave.
Kidney, liver	Thin membranes on the food may split with a popping sound during cooking.	The dish should be lightly covered to prevent spattering; the popping sound is not a problem.
Food with bones	Bones act as tunnels, storing up pressure, and the food around the bone pops and spits.	
Poultry with skin	Skin may split with a popping sound during cooking.	
Fish	It is easy to overcook.	Stop cooking before the fish is done. Let it stand – it will finish cooking and change from opaque to flaky.
Joints of meat or chicken	These are large and dense.	Allow to stand for 10–15 minutes after microwaving. The food will continue to cook and heat will spread evenly throughout the food.
Moist food, e.g. stew		Cover the food, e.g. with loose clingfilm. If there is a large proportion of liquid, stir during cooking – only cover three-quarters of the dish, so that you can stir through the gap.
Food containing sugar	Sugar heats slowly at first, then suddenly becomes very hot very quickly, especially if it is dissolved in liquid. It attracts microwaves.	Do not microwave these foods for too long: the sugar will burn.
Food that should have a crispy finish		Fat attracts microwaves, so brush food with fat or oil to make the surface crispy when cooked.

Test yourself • • • • • • • • • • • • • • • •

1 When cooking the transfer of heat to food can take place in three different ways. What are they?

2 When heated by moist methods what happens to:

   (a) Starches

   (b) Sugars?

3 Vitamin C (ascorbic acid) can very easily be lost in cooking. How could you stop this from happening?

4 What are the differences between: boiling, poaching and simmering?

5 What is the difference between atmospheric steaming and high-pressure steaming?

6 Which types of meat are most suitable for stewing and why? Apart from meat, which other foods can be stewed?

7 When roasting meat why is it basted throughout its cooking time?

8 What is meant by baking with 'increased humidity'?

9 There are four ways that food can be shallow fried. What are they? Suggest a type of food for each.

10 Producing food by sous vide methods has increased in popularity but if not done properly there can be food safety risks. Suggest five ways that food safety problems can be avoided when using sous vide.

• •

8 Prepare and cook stock, soups and sauces

In this chapter you will learn how to:

1. prepare and cook stocks, soups and sauces:

- using equipment correctly
- demonstrating safe and hygienic practices
- preparing ingredients
- finishing soups and sauces
- applying quality points and evaluate the finished product

2. You should have the knowledge to:

- identify different types, quality points and purposes of stock, soup and sauce
- cook, chill and store products correctly
- state and explain the cooking times for different stocks
- identify accompaniments for soup
- identify sauce and dish combinations.

No.	Recipe title	Page no.
Stocks		
7	Crab stock	161
6	Fish stock	161
4	Lamb jus	159
5	Reduced veal stock for sauce	160
3	White chicken stock	159
1	White or brown stock	158
2	White vegetable stock	158
Soups		
12	Asparagus soup (*crème d'asperges*)	168
9	Carrot and butterbean soup	162
10	Chicken soup (*crème de volaille/crème reine*)	163
19	Chive and potato soup (*vichyssoise*)	171
14	Cream of spinach and celery soup	167
20	Gazpacho	172
15	Minestrone soup	167
11	Mushroom soup (*crème de champignons*)	164
18	New England clam chowder	170
16	Paysanne soup (*potage*)	169
22	Potato and watercress soup (*purée cressonnière*)	173
17	Prawn bisque	169
8	Pumpkin velouté	162
23	Red lentil soup	174
24	Roasted red pepper and tomato soup	174
26	Scotch broth	176
13	Tomato soup (*crème de tomates fraiche*)	166
25	Vegetable and barley soup	175
21	Vegetable soup (*purée de légumes*)	172

No.	Recipe title	Page no.
Sauces		
52	Andalusian sauce (*sauce andalouse*)	190
57	Apple sauce	192
64	Avocado and coriander salsa	195
60	Balsamic vinegar and olive oil dressing	193
76	Basil oil	201
71	Béarnaise sauce	199
41	Béchamel	184
27	Beef jus	176
33	Brown onion sauce (*sauce lyonnaise*)	180
40	Butter sauce (*beurre blanc*)	183
31	Chasseur sauce (*sauce chasseur*)	179
28	Chicken jus	177
	Choron sauce	199
78	Compound butter sauces	202
58	Cranberry and orange dressing for duck	192
46	Fish velouté	187
	Foyot or valoise sauce	199
51	Green sauce (*sauce verte*)	190
72	Herb oil	200
70	Hollandaise sauce (*sauce hollandaise*)	198
61	Horseradish sauce (*sauce raifort*)	194
32	Italian sauce (*sauce italienne*)	179
73	Lemon oil	200
30	Madeira sauce (*sauce Madère*)	178
48	Mayonnaise sauce	188
74	Mint oil	201
56	Mint sauce	192
69	Mixed pickle	198
42	Mornay sauce	185

No.	Recipe title	Page no.
47	Mushroom sauce	187
	Paloise sauce	200
44	Parsley sauce	186
65	Pear chutney	196
67	Pesto	197
34	Piquant sauce (*sauce piquante*)	180
29	Red wine jus	177
38	Reduction of stock (glaze)	182
37	Reduction of wine, stock and cream	182
50	Remoulade sauce (*sauce remoulade*)	189
35	Robert sauce (*sauce Robert*)	180
63	Salsa verde	195
45	*Sauce suprême*	186

No.	Recipe title	Page no.
54	Shellfish cocktail sauce	191
43	Soubise sauce	185
39	Sweet and sour sauce	183
68	Tapenade	197
49	Tartare sauce (*sauce tartare*)	189
53	Thousand Island dressing	190
62	Tomato and cucumber salsa	194
66	Tomato chutney	196
36	Tomato sauce (*sauce tomate*)	181
55	Tomato vinaigrette	191
75	Vanilla oil	201
77	Walnut oil	201
59	Yoghurt and cucumber raita	193

Health, safety and hygiene

For information on maintaining a safe and secure working environment, a professional and hygienic appearance, clean food production areas, equipment and utensils, and food hygiene, please refer to Chapters 2 and 3. Additional health and safety points are as follows.

- After stock, sauces, gravies and soups have been rapidly cooled, they should be stored in a refrigerator at a temperature below 5°C.
- If they are to be deep-frozen they should be labelled and dated, and stored below −20°C to −18°C.
- When taken from storage they must be boiled for at least 2 minutes before being used.
- They must not be reheated more than once.
- Ideally, stocks should be made fresh daily and discarded at the end of the day.
- Stocks can easily become contaminated and a risk to health, so be sure to use good ingredients and hygienic methods of preparation.
- Never store a stock, sauce, gravy or soup above eye level as someone could accidentally spill the contents over themselves if they don't see it.

Stocks

Stock is the basis of all meat sauces, soups and purées. It is really just the juice of meat extracted by long and gentle simmering, or the infusion/transfer of flavour from an ingredient such as bones, vegetables or shellfish. When making stock, remember that the object is to draw the goodness out of the materials and into the liquor, giving it the right flavour and nutrients for the end product, whether it is a soup, sauce or perhaps a reduction.

Stock is a liquid that contains some of the soluble nutrients and flavours of food that are extracted by prolonged and gentle simmering (with the exception of fish stock). This liquid is the foundation of many important kitchen preparations, including soups, sauces and gravies, so you should take great care when preparing them. Stocks, bouillons and nages should not be seen as a way to use up any vegetables and meat trimmings that happen to be left over. The type and quality of ingredients you use are important – respect is the greatest ingredient you can put into a stock.

> A nage is a well-seasoned stock (e.g. mushroom nage is a well-seasoned mushroom stock) usually used for cooking seafood, to enhance the flavours.

Key points to remember when making stocks

- Unsound meat or bones and decaying vegetables will give stock an unpleasant flavour and cause it to deteriorate quickly.
- Scum should be removed from the top of the stock as it cooks. If it is not removed it will boil into the stock and spoil the colour and flavour.
- Fat should also be skimmed off, otherwise the stock will taste greasy.
- Stock should always simmer gently; if it is allowed to boil quickly, it will evaporate and go cloudy/milky.
- Salt should not be added to stock.
- When making chicken stock, the bones will need to be soaked first to remove the blood that is in the cavity.
- If stock is going to be kept, strain it and cool quickly, then place it in the refrigerator.

Soups

Although you will need experience to perfect your soup making, the basic principles are quite simple to follow.

Most soup making begins by preparing a stock (see above). Stock can come in as many variations as there are meats (e.g. chicken, beef, turkey, veal, fish, lobster) and as vegetable stock.

The underlying flavours of a broth's foundation ingredients are enhanced by the herbs and seasonings that are added to it. In many cases,

you will begin this flavour base by cooking several flavourful and aromatic ingredients in a little fat or oil. For most soups these ingredients will be a combination of onion, garlic, leeks and carrots (this is called a mirepoix) or aromats.

Meat, fish, vegetables, fruits, seasonings, fats like butter or cream, and vegetables or dried pulses can then be added in countless variations to create the wealth of soups available today.

Health-conscious eaters should look for clear soups containing vegetables, beans and lean protein like chicken, fish or lean beef. Italian minestrone, bouillabaisse and gazpacho are excellent choices, and cream-based soups can often be adapted to fit a more healthy menu.

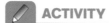

ACTIVITY

1   Name four purée soups.

2   Name two national soups.

3   Name two alternatives to cream when finishing a soup.

4   At what temperature should hot soup be served?

5   Name traditional soups served cold.

Sauces

Preparing and cooking sauces

A sauce is a liquid that has been thickened by either:

- *beurre manié* (kneaded butter)
- egg yolks
- roux (a fat and flour mixture)
- cornflour, arrowroot or starch
- cream and/or butter added to reduced stock
- rice (in the case of some shellfish bisques)
- reducing cooking liquor or stock.

We will take a closer look at some of these below.

All sauces should be smooth, should look glossy, have a definite flavour and be a light texture; use the thickening medium in moderation.

Beurre manié

Beurre manié, a paste made from equal quantities of soft butter and flour, is used chiefly for fish sauces. It is added to a simmering liquid, which should be whisked continuously to prevent it becoming lumpy.

Egg yolks

Using egg yolks for thickening is commonly known in the trade as a liaison and is traditionally used to thicken a classic velouté (see recipes 45, 46 and 47). Egg yolks and cream are mixed together and added to the sauce/velouté off the boil. It is essential to keep stirring the sauce once you have added the eggs, otherwise the eggs will curdle. Once the sauce/velouté is thickened it must be removed and served immediately. *Do not allow the liquid to boil or simmer.*

Egg yolks are used in mayonnaise, hollandaise and custard sauces. Refer to the appropriate recipe, though, as the yolks are used in a different way for each sauce.

Roux

A roux is a combination of fat and flour, which are cooked together. There are three degrees to which a roux may be cooked (white, blond and brown) and one 'modern' approach known as 'continental' roux style (see below). Liquid is then added to the cooked mixture to make the sauce.

Never add a boiling liquid to a hot roux, as you may be scalded by the steam that is produced, and the sauce may become lumpy.

Do not allow a roux sauce to stand over a moderate heat for any length of time as it may become thin due to a chemical change (dextrinisation) in the flour.

White roux

This is used for white (béchamel) sauce and soups. Cook equal quantities of margarine or butter and flour together for a few minutes, without colouring, until the mixture is a sandy texture. Alternatively, use polyunsaturated vegetable margarine or make a roux with vegetable oil, using equal quantities of oil to flour. This does give a slack roux but means the liquid can be incorporated easily.

Blond roux

This is used for veloutés, tomato sauce and soups. Cook equal quantities of margarine, butter or vegetable oil and flour for longer than a white roux, without colouring, until it is a sandy texture.

Making a blond roux and a velouté
http://bit.ly/weUClc

Brown roux

This was traditionally used for brown (espagnole) sauce and soups and is slightly browned in the roux-making process by cooking the fat and flour mixture for a bit longer than in the other methods.

Continental roux

This is a very easy and straightforward thickening agent that can be frozen and used as a quick thickener during service or at the last minute.

Mix equal quantities of flour and vegetable oil together to a paste and place in the oven at 140°C. Cook the mixture, mixing it in on itself continually until a biscuit texture is achieved. Remove and allow to cool to room temperature. When it is cool enough to handle, form it into a sausage shape using a double layer of cling film. Chill, then freeze.

To use, remove it from the freezer and shave a little off the end of the log. Whisk it into the boiling sauce (as the flour is already cooked it is not necessary to add it slowly to prevent lumping as this will not occur). Once the desired thickness has been achieved, pass the sauce (strain it) and serve.

Cornflour, arrowroot or starch

Cornflour, arrowroot or starch (such as potato starch) is used for thickening gravy and sauces. These are diluted with water, stock or milk, then stirred into the boiling liquid, which is allowed to reboil for a few minutes and is then strained. For large-scale cooking and economy, flour may be used.

Other sauces

- Vegetables or fruit purées are known as a cullis (coulis). No other thickening agent is used.
- Blood was traditionally used in recipes such as jugged hare, but is used rarely today.
- Cooking liquor from certain dishes and/or stock can be reduced to give a light sauce.

Thickening sauces with sauce flour

Sauce flour is a specially milled flour that does not need to have any fat added to it to prevent it from going lumpy. Sauces may be thickened using this flour. It is useful when making low-fat sauces.

Test yourself

1 List the ingredients for brown beef stock.
2 Name suitable pulses that can be made into a soup.
3 How does béarnaise sauce differ from hollandaise sauce?
4 Name two derivatives of béchamel.
5 How would you rectify a curdled mayonnaise?

1 White or brown stock

cal	kcal	fat	sat fat	carb	sugar	protein	fibre
4 KJ	1 kcal	0.0 g	0.0 g	0.2 g	0.0 g	0.0 g	0.0 g

For white stock

1 Chop the bones into small pieces, and remove any fat or marrow.
2 Place the bones in a large stock pot, cover with cold water and bring to the boil.
3 Drain. Wash off the bones under cold water, then clean the pot.
4 Return the bones to the cleaned pot, add fresh water and reboil.
5 Skim as and when required, wipe around inside the pot and simmer gently.
6 After 2 hours, add the washed, peeled whole vegetables, bouquet garni and peppercorns.
7 Simmer for 6–8 hours. Skim, strain and, if to be kept, cool quickly and refrigerate.

For brown stock

1 Chop the beef bones and brown well on all sides by placing in a roasting tin in the oven, or carefully brown in a little fat in a frying pan.
2 Drain any fat and place the bones in a stock pot.
3 Brown any sediment in the bottom of the tray, deglaze (swill out) with ½ litre of boiling water, simmer for a few minutes and add to the bones.

	4 litres
raw meaty bones	1 kg
water	4 litres
onion, carrot, celery, leek	400 g
bouquet garni	1
peppercorns	8

4 Add the cold water, bring to the boil and skim. Simmer for 2 hours.
5 Wash, peel and roughly cut the vegetables, fry in a little fat until brown, strain and add to the bones.
6 Add the bouquet garni and peppercorns.
7 Simmer for 6–8 hours. Skim and strain.

> A few squashed tomatoes and washed mushroom trimmings can also be added to improve flavour, as can a calf's foot and/or a knuckle of bacon. If bacon is used, dishes made with the stock will not be suitable for some religious diets.

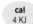

Making brown stock
http://bit.ly/A6F9q4

2 White vegetable stock

cal	kcal	fat	sat fat	carb	sugar	protein	fibre
4 KJ	1 kcal	0.0 g	0.0 g	0.2 g	0.2 g	0.0 g	0.0 g

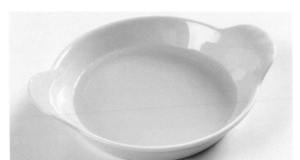

	10 portions
onions	250 g
carrots	250 g
celery	250 g
leeks	250 g
water	4 litres

1 Roughly chop all the vegetables.
2 Place all the ingredients into a saucepan, add the water, bring to the boil.
3 Allow to simmer for approximately 1 hour.
4 Skim if necessary. Strain and use.

3 White chicken stock

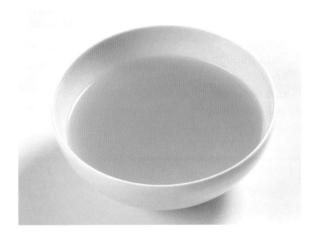

1 Remove any excess fat from the chicken carcasses and wash off under cold water.
2 Place all the bones into a pot that will hold all the ingredients, leaving 5 cm at the top to skim.
3 Add all the other ingredients and cold water, and bring to a simmer; immediately skim all the fat that rises to the surface.
4 Turn the heat off and allow the bones and vegetables to sink. Once this has happened, turn the heat back on, skim and bring to just under a simmer, making as little movement as possible to create more of an infusion than a stock. Skim continuously.
5 Leave to simmer for 2 hours then pass through a fine sieve into a clean pan; reduce down rapidly, until you have about 4 litres remaining.

	Makes 4 litres
chicken carcass/wings	5 kg
onions, peeled	1 ½
carrots, peeled	2
cloves of garlic, crushed	2
leeks, washed and blemishes removed	1
celery sticks	2
bay leaf	1
sprigs of thyme, small	1
whole white peppercorns	5 g
water, cold	7 litres

4 Lamb jus

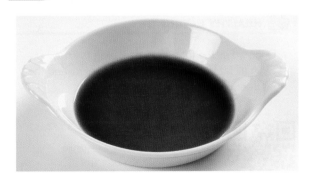

	Makes 1 litre
thyme	50 g
bay leaves, fresh	2
garlic	1 bulb
red wine	500 ml
lamb bones	1 kg
veal bones	½ kg
white onions, peeled	3
large carrots, peeled	4
celery sticks	3
leeks	2
tomato purée	3 tbsp
water	approx. 3 litres

1 Pre-heat the oven to 175°C. Place the herbs, garlic and wine in a large, deep container. Place all the bones on to a roasting rack on top of the container of herbs and wine, and roast in the oven for 50–60 minutes. When the bones are completely roasted and have taken on a dark golden-brown appearance, remove from oven.

2 Place all the ingredients in a large pot and cover with cold water. Put the pot onto the heat and bring to the simmer; immediately skim all fat that rises to the surface.

3 Turn the heat off and allow the bones and vegetables to sink. Once this has happened, turn the heat back on and bring to just under a simmer, making as little movement as possible to create more of an infusion than a stock. Simmer for 6 hours, skimming regularly.

4 Pass through a fine sieve, place in the blast chiller until cold and then in the refrigerator overnight. Next day, reduce down rapidly, until you have about 1 litre remaining.

5 Reduced veal stock for sauce

cal	kcal	fat	sat fat	carb	sugar	protein	fibre
8 KJ	2 kcal	0.0 g	0.0 g	0.5 g	0.4 g	0.0 g	0.0 g

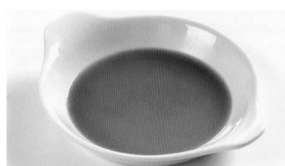

1 Brown the chopped bones on a roasting tray in the oven.

2 Place the browned bones in a stock pot, cover with cold water and bring to simmering point.

3 Roughly chop the carrots, onions and celery. Using the same roasting tray and the fat from the bones, brown them off.

4 Drain off the fat, add the vegetables to the stock and deglaze the tray.

5 Add the quartered tomatoes, chopped mushrooms, bouquet garni and garlic (if desired). Simmer gently for 4–5 hours. Skim frequently.

6 Strain the stock into a clean pan and reduce until a light consistency is achieved.

	4 litres
veal bones	4 kg
water	4 litres
carrots	400 g
onions	200 g
celery	100 g
tomatoes	1 kg
mushrooms	200 g
bouquet garni	1 large
unpeeled cloves of garlic (optional)	4

 HEALTHY EATING TIP

- Drain off all the fat before deglazing the tray. Skim all fat from the stock as it simmers, and the fat from the finished product.

You will find this reduced veal stock, or jus lié (a veal stock that has been lightly thickened with arrowroot), used in many recipes today. These stocks have replaced the traditional demi-glace, which was made by simmering a brown espagnole sauce with brown stock. Demi-glace is not used very much in modern kitchens.

Making a reduced stock and jus-lié
http://bit.ly/AxlTyH

6   Fish stock (*fumet de poisson*)

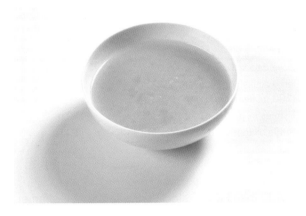

	4 litres
butter or oil	50 g
onions, sliced	200 g
white fish bones (preferably sole, whiting or turbot)	2 kg
lemon, juice of	½
bay leaf	1
parsley stalks	
water	4½ litres

1 Melt the butter, or heat the oil in a thick-bottomed pan.

2 Add the onions, the well-washed fish bones and the remainder of the ingredients except the water.

3 Cover the ingredients with greaseproof paper and a lid, and sweat (cook gently without colouring) for 5 minutes.

4 Add the water, bring to the boil, skim and simmer for 20 minutes, then strain.

Making fish stock
http://bit.ly/xzrbyn

Cooking the stock for longer than 20 minutes will spoil the flavour.

7   Crab stock

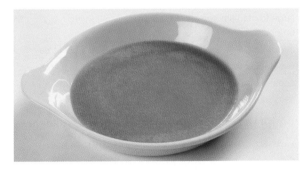

	Makes 2 litres (when reduced)
crab shells, smashed	2 kg
prawns, with shells still on	1.5 kg
corn oil	50 ml
brandy (optional)	200 ml
Pernod (optional)	100 ml
carrots, peeled and chopped for mirepoix	250 g
leeks, prepared and chopped for mirepoix	250 g
celery, chopped for mirepoix	150 g
garlic cloves, smashed	2
shallot, peeled and sliced	180 g
tomato paste	150 ml
fish stock	2.5 litres
small sprig of thyme	
bay leaf	1

1 Roast the shells in the oil and deglaze with the brandy and Pernod (or, if not using these, some of the stock).

2 In a separate pan, roast the vegetables, then add the tomato paste, stock and herbs, add the roasted shells and the prawns, and simmer for 20 minutes.

3 Turn off the heat and allow to infuse for 30 minutes. Pass, and reduce by half. The stock is now ready for use.

8 Pumpkin velouté

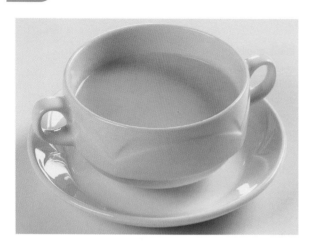

	4 portions	10 portions
shallots, sliced	1	3
butter	50 g	125 g
clove garlic, sliced (optional)	½	1
large squash or pumpkin (300 g), flesh diced	1	2
Parmesan, grated	30 g	70 g
truffle oil (optional)	1 tbsp	2 tbsp
salt, pepper		
chicken stock	600 ml	1 ½ litres

1 Sweat the shallots in butter, without colour, until cooked and soft.

2 Add the garlic, pumpkin, Parmesan and truffle oil. Correct the seasoning and cook for 5 minutes.

3 Add the chicken stock, bring to the boil, simmer for 5 minutes.

4 Blitz in a liquidiser, pass, correct the seasoning, then blast chill if to be stored.

Serve immediately.

9 Carrot and butterbean soup

cal	kcal	fat	sat fat	carb	sugar	protein	fibre	salt
891 KJ	213 kcal	5.9 g	0.7 g	33.4 g	19.3 g	8.5 g	8.1 g	8.1 g

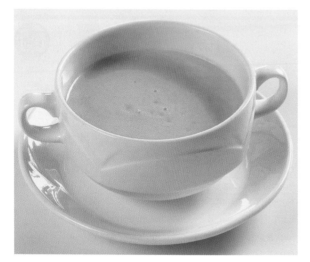

	4 portions	10 portions
onions, peeled and chopped	1	2
cloves of garlic, chopped	2	5
sunflower oil	15 ml	35 ml
large to medium carrots, brunoise	6	15
carrot juice	500 ml	1 ¼ litres
vegetable stock	500 ml	1 ¼ litres
cooked butter beans	400 g	1 kg
seasoning		

1 Cook the onion and garlic in the oil for a few minutes, without colour, then add the carrots and stir well.

2 Add the carrot juice and vegetable stock. Bring to the boil, turn down to a simmer and cook for about 15 minutes until the carrot is cooked through.

3 Add the beans and cook for a further 5 minutes or so until they are heated through.

4 Liquidise in a food processor until smooth; check seasoning.

Serve immediately.

Chef's tip

With any soup recipe, it is important to simmer the soup gently. Do not let it boil vigorously, because too much water will evaporate. If the soup has boiled, add more stock or water to make up for this.

10 Chicken soup *(crème de volaille or crème reine)*

cal	kcal	fat	sat fat	carb	sugar	protein	fibre
836 KJ	199 kcal	13.6 g	6.2 g	14.0 g	4.2 g	5.9 g	1.0 g

*

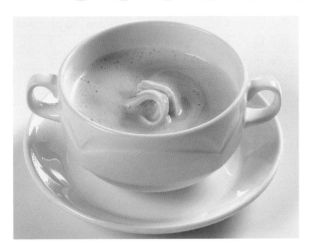

	4 portions	10 portions
onion, leek and celery	100 g	250 g
butter, margarine or oil	50 g	125 g
flour	50 g	125 g
chicken stock	1 litre	2½ litres
bouquet garni		
salt, pepper		
milk or cream	250 ml or 125 ml	625 ml or 300 ml
cooked strips of chicken (garnish)	25 g	60 g

1 Gently cook the sliced onions, leek and celery in a thick-bottomed pan, in the butter, margarine or oil, without colouring.

2 Mix in the flour; cook over a gentle heat to a sandy texture without colouring.

3 Cool slightly; gradually mix in the hot stock. Stir to the boil.

4 Add the bouquet garni and season.

5 Simmer for 30–45 minutes; skim when necessary. Remove the bouquet garni.

6 Liquidise or pass firmly through a fine strainer.

7 Return to a clean pan, reboil and finish with milk or cream; correct the seasoning.

8 Add the chicken garnish and serve.

HEALTHY EATING TIP

- Use soft margarine or sunflower/olive oil in place of the butter.

- Use the minimum amount of salt.

- The least fatty option is to use semi-skimmed milk and yoghurt or fromage frais in place of the cream.

Natural yoghurt, skimmed milk or non-dairy cream may be used in place of dairy cream. Add cooked small pasta or sliced mushrooms for variations.

* Using hard margarine

11 Mushroom soup *(crème de champignons)*

cal	kcal	fat	sat fat	carb	sugar	protein	fibre
712 KJ	170 kcal	11.8 g	5.2 g	12.6 g	3.0 g	3.8 g	1.6 g *

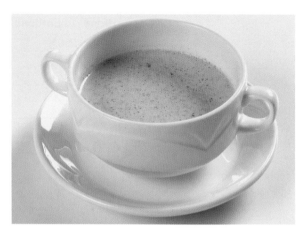

	4 portions	10 portions
onion, leek and celery, sliced	100 g	250 g
butter, margarine or oil	50 g	125 g
flour	50 g	125 g
white stock (preferably chicken)	1 litre	2½ litre
white mushrooms	200 g	500 g
bouquet garni		
salt, pepper		
milk (or cream)	125 ml or 60 ml cream	300 ml or 150 ml cream

1 Gently cook the sliced onions, leek and celery in the butter, margarine or oil in a thick-bottomed pan without colouring.

2 Mix in the flour and cook over a gentle heat to a sandy texture without colouring.

3 Remove from the heat and cool slightly.

4 Gradually mix in the hot stock. Stir to the boil.

5 Add the well-washed, chopped mushrooms, the bouquet garni and season.

6 Simmer for 30–45 minutes. Skim when needed.

7 Remove the bouquet garni. Pass through a sieve or liquidise.

8 Pass through a medium strainer. Return to a clean saucepan.

9 Reboil, correct the seasoning and consistency; add the milk or cream.

Natural yoghurt, skimmed milk or non-dairy cream may be used in place of dairy cream. A garnish of thinly sliced mushrooms may be added. Wild mushrooms may also be used.

HEALTHY EATING TIP

- Use soft margarine or sunflower/olive oil in place of the butter.

- Use the minimum amount of salt.

- The least fatty option is to use semi-skimmed milk and yoghurt or fromage frais in place of the cream.

* Using hard margarine

Making a cream soup
http://bit.ly/wsAsgc

12 Asparagus soup (crème d'asperges)

cal	kcal	fat	sat fat	carb	sugar	protein	fibre
151 KJ	361 kcal	25.3 g	11.9 g	27.1 g	8.1 g	7.7 g	2.5 g

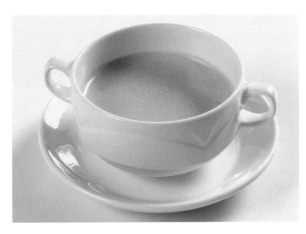

	4 portions	10 portions
onion, sliced	50 g	125 g
celery, sliced	50 g	125 g
butter, oil or margarine	50 g	125 g
flour	50 g	125 g
white stock (preferably chicken)	1 litre	2½ litres
asparagus stalk trimmings	200 g	500 g
or		
tin of asparagus	150 g	325 g
bouquet garni		
salt, pepper		
milk or cream	250 ml or 125 ml	625 ml or 300 ml

1 Gently sweat the onions and celery, without colouring, in the butter or margarine.

2 Remove from the heat, mix in the flour, return to a low heat and cook out, without colouring, for a few minutes. Cool.

3 Gradually add the hot stock. Stir to the boil.

4 Add the well-washed asparagus trimmings, or the tin of asparagus, and bouquet garni. Season.

5 Simmer for 30–40 minutes, then remove bouquet garni.

6 Liquidise and pass through a strainer.

7 Return to a clean pan, reboil, correct seasoning and consistency.

8 Add the milk or cream and serve.

See the note in recipe 10 for more ideas.

 HEALTHY EATING TIP

- Use an unsaturated oil (sunflower/olive) to lightly oil the pan. Drain off any excess after the frying is complete and skim the fat from the finished dish.

- Season with the minimum amount of salt.

- Milk with a little cornflour can be added to achieve the desired consistency.

* Using hard margarine. Using butter, 1 portion provides: 919 kJ/223 kcal Energy; 13.1 g Fat; 8.0 g Sat Fat; 18.9 g Carb; 8.8 g Sugar; 8.4 g Protein; 2.5 g Fibre

13 Tomato soup (crème de tomates fraiche)

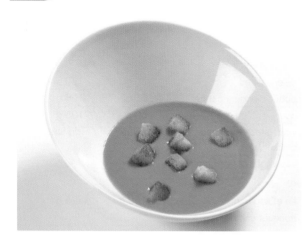

	4 portions	10 portions
butter, margarine or oil	50 g	125 g
bacon trimmings, optional	25 g	60 g
onion, diced	100 g	250 g
carrot, diced	100 g	250 g
flour	50 g	125 g
fresh fully ripe tomatoes	1 kg	2½ kg
stock	1 litre	2½ litres
bouquet garni		
salt, pepper		
Croutons		
slice stale bread	1	3
butter	50 g	125 g

1 Melt the butter, margarine or oil in a thick-bottomed pan.

2 Add the bacon, onion and carrot (mirepoix) and brown lightly.

3 Mix in the flour and cook to a sandy texture.

4 Gradually add the hot stock.

5 Stir to the boil.

6 Remove the eyes from the tomatoes, wash them well, and squeeze them into the soup after it has come to the boil.

7 If colour is lacking, add a little tomato purée soon after the soup comes to the boil.

8 Add the bouquet garni, season lightly.

9 Simmer for approximately 1 hour. Skim when required.

10 Remove the bouquet garni and mirepoix.

11 Liquidise or pass firmly through a sieve, then through a conical strainer.

12 Return to a clean pan, correct the seasoning and consistency. Bring to the boil.

13 Serve fried or toasted croutons separately.

> Flour may be omitted from recipe if a thinner soup is required.

 HEALTHY EATING TIP

- Use soft margarine or sunflower/olive oil in place of the butter.

- Serve with toasted croutons.

- Use the minimum amount of salt – there is plenty in the bacon.

14 Cream of spinach and celery soup

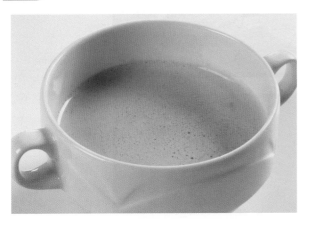

	4 portions	10 portions
shallots, peeled and chopped (small mirepoix)	2	5
leeks, washed and chopped (small mirepoix)	1	2
cloves of garlic, peeled and chopped	5	7
corn oil	2 tbsp	5 tbsp
celery sticks, washed and chopped (small mirepoix)	4	10
flour	15 g	35 g
fresh spinach, well washed	500 g	1¼ kg
soya milk	600 ml	1½ litres
vegetable stock (see recipe 2)	600 ml	1½ litres
salt, to taste		

1 Cook the shallots, leeks and garlic in the oil for a few minutes, without colour.

2 Add the celery and cook for another few minutes until starting to soften.

3 Add the flour and mix well, then throw in the spinach and mix around. Add the soya milk and vegetable stock slowly, ensuring there are no lumps.

4 Stir continuously, bring to a simmer, then switch off and remove from heat. Cover and leave for a few minutes.

5 Blend until smooth in a food processor. Check seasoning and serve.

ASSESSMENT

15 Minestrone soup

| cal 1115 KJ | kcal 265 kcal | fat 22.9 g | sat fat 5.8 g | carb 11.9 g | sugar 4.2 g | protein 3.8 g | fibre 4.1 g | * |

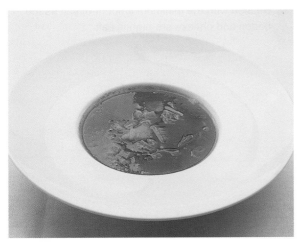

	4 portions	10 portions
mixed vegetables (onion, leek, celery, carrot, turnip, cabbage)	300 g	750 g
butter, margarine or oil	50 g	125 g
white stock or water	½ litre	2 litres
bouquet garni		
salt, pepper		
peas	25 g	60 g
French beans	25 g	60 g
spaghetti	25 g	60 g
potatoes	50 g	125 g
tomato purée	1 tsp	3 tsp
tomatoes, skinned, deseeded, diced	100 g	250 g
fat bacon	optional		
chopped parsley		50 g	125 g
clove garlic		1	2½

1 Cut the peeled and washed mixed vegetables into paysanne.

2 Cook slowly without colour in the oil or fat in the pan with a lid on.

3 Add the stock, bouquet garni and seasoning; simmer for approximately 20 minutes.

4 Add the peas and the beans cut into diamonds and simmer for 10 minutes.

5 Add the spaghetti in 2 cm lengths, the potatoes cut into paysanne, the tomato purée and the tomatoes, and simmer gently until all the vegetables are cooked.

6 Meanwhile finely chop the fat bacon, parsley and garlic, and form into a paste.

7 Mould the paste into pellets the size of a pea and drop into the boiling soup.

8 Remove the bouquet garni, correct the seasoning.

9 Serve grated Parmesan cheese and thin toasted flute (French loaf) slices separately.

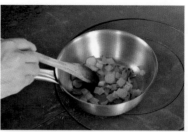

Fry or sweat the vegetables

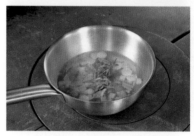

Simmer the ingredients in the stock

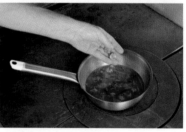

Add the pellets of paste to the soup

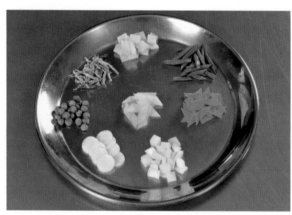

Vegetables chopped into paysanne

* Using sunflower oil

HEALTHY EATING TIP

- Use an unsaturated oil (sunflower or olive) to lightly oil the pan. Drain off any excess after the frying is complete and skim the fat from the finished dish.

- Season with the minimum amount of salt as the bacon and cheese are high in salt.

16 Paysanne soup *(potage)*

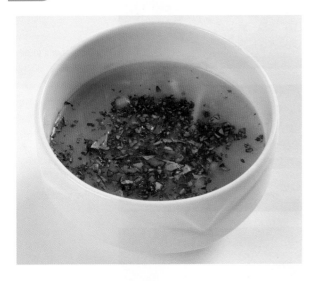

	4 portions	10 portions
chicken or vegetable stock	1 litre	2½ litres
diced streaky bacon (optional)	50 g	125 g
celery sticks	50 g	125 g
onion	100 g	250 g
carrots	100 g	250 g
turnips	50 g	125 g
leeks	50 g	125 g
cabbage (optional)	50 g	125 g
potatoes	100 g	250 g
butter, margarine or oil	50 g	125 g
chopped parsley, chopped basil		

1 Cut the celery, onion, carrots, leeks, cabbage and potatoes into paysanne.

2 In a suitable saucepan, add the butter, margarine or oil. Fry the streaky bacon until lightly cooked.

3 Add the onion, leeks and celery and sweat for 2–3 minutes.

4 Add the rest of the vegetables.

5 Add the stock. Bring to the boil. Simmer until all the vegetables are cooked.

6 The soup may be finished with 125 ml boiled milk (300 ml for 10 portions).

7 Sprinkle on the chopped parsley and basil.

> Diced tomato concassé may also be added: 50 g for 4 portions, 125 g for 10.

17 Prawn bisque

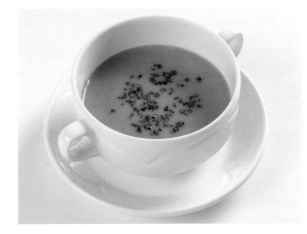

	4 portions	10 portions
oil	50 ml	125 ml
butter	30 g	75 g
unshelled prawns,	250 g	625 g
flour	20 g	50 g
tomato purée	1 tbsp	2 tbsp
shellfish nage	1 litre	2½ litres
fish stock	150 ml	375 ml
whipping cream	120 ml	300 ml
dry sherry	75 ml	180 ml
paprika, pinch		
seasoning		
chopped chives		

1 Heat the oil and the butter. Add the prawns and cook for 3–4 minutes on a moderately high heat.

2 Sprinkle in the flour and cook for a further 2–3 minutes.

3 Add the tomato purée and cook for a further 2 minutes.

4 Meanwhile, bring the nage up to a simmer and, once the tomato purée has been cooked in, slowly add to the prawn mix, being mindful that you have formed a roux; stir in the fish stock to prevent lumping.

5 Once all the stock has been added, bring to the boil and simmer for 3–4 minutes.

6 Pass through a fine sieve, return the shells to the pan and pound to extract more flavour and more colour.

7 Pour over the fish stock, bring to the boil, then pass this back onto the already passed soup.

8 Bring to the boil, add the cream and sherry, correct the seasoning and served with chopped chives.

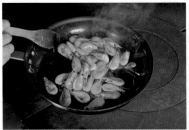

Fry the prawns in oil and butter

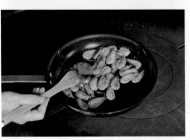

Add the tomato paste

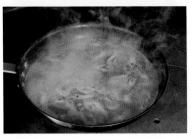

Allow the soup to simmer (step 5 in the recipe)

18 New England clam chowder

cal 1109 KJ	kcal 269 kcal	fat 14.9 g	sat fat 7.7 g	carb 24.5 g	sugar 2.5 g	protein 14.9 g	fibre 1.8 g	

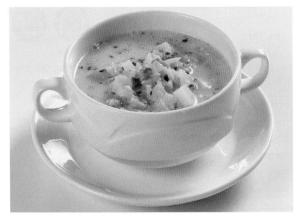

	8 portions
salt pork, cut into ½ cm dice	100 g
onion, finely chopped	100 g
cold water	625 ml
potatoes, cut into ½ cm dice	1 kg
fresh trimmed clams, or 2 × 200 g tins, and their juices	400 g
cream	375 ml
thyme, crushed or chopped	1/8 tsp
salt, white pepper	
butter	25 g
paprika	

1 Dry-fry the pork in a thick-bottomed saucepan for about 3 minutes, stirring constantly until a thin film of fat covers the bottom of the pan.

2 Stir in the chopped onion and cook gently until a light golden brown.

3 Add the water and potatoes, bring to the boil and simmer gently until the potatoes are cooked but not mushy.

4 Add the chopped clams and their juice, the cream and thyme, and heat until almost boiling. Season with salt and pepper.

5 Correct the seasoning, stir in the softened butter and serve, dusting each soup bowl with a little paprika.

> The traditional accompaniment is salted cracker biscuits. An obvious variation would be to use scallops in place of clams.

* Using bacon or salt pork

---

19 Chive and potato soup (*vichyssoise*)

cal	kcal	fat	sat fat	carb	sugar	protein	fibre
949 KJ	228 kcal	15.0 g	9.3 g	20.3 g	3.2 g	4.1 g	1.8 g

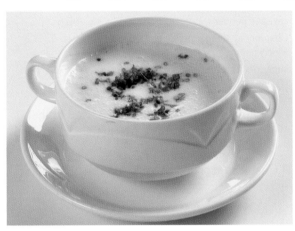

	4 portions	10 portions
butter, margarine or oil	25 g	60 g
onions, peeled, washed and sliced	50 g	125 g
white of leek, washed and sliced	50 g	125 g
potatoes, peeled, washed and sliced	400 g	1½ kg
white stock	1 litre	2½ litres
bouquet garni		
salt, pepper		
cream	125–250 ml	500 ml
chives, chopped		

1 Melt the butter, margarine or oil in a thick-bottomed pan.

2 Add the onion and leek, cook for a few minutes without colour, with the lid on.

3 Add the stock, potatoes and bouquet garni. Season.

4 Simmer for approximately 30 minutes. Remove the bouquet garni, skim.

5 Liquidise or pass the soup firmly through a sieve, then through a medium conical strainer.

6 Return to a clean pan and reboil; correct the seasoning and consistency, skim off any fat.

7 Finish with cream and garnish with chopped chives, either raw or cooked in a little butter. Usually served chilled.

🍎 HEALTHY EATING TIP

- Use an unsaturated oil (sunflower or olive). Lightly oil the pan and drain off any excess after the frying is complete.

- Season with the minimum amount of salt.

- Try using natural yoghurt or fromage frais to finish the soup.

* Using 200 ml single cream

20   Gazpacho

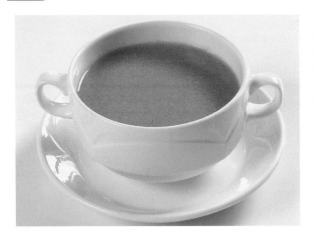

	4 portions	10 portions
plum tomatoes, ripe	2½ kg	6.25 kg
white onion, roughly chopped	1	2
cucumber, peeled and roughly chopped	1	2
garlic clove, crushed	½	1
red peppers, peeled and deseeded	550 g	1.3 kg
salt	40 g	80 g
cayenne pepper	2 g	5 g
Chardonnay vinegar or white wine vinegar	6 g	15 g
sugar (to taste, depending on season)	30 g	75 g

1 Mix all the ingredients together and leave to marinate overnight in the fridge.

2 Next day, blitz the ingredients in a food processor and strain through a chinois.

3 Discard the remaining pulp into a colander lined with muslin (this is to catch the extra juices that will come from the pulp).

4 The juices from the pulp can be used to thin out the gazpacho until it reaches the correct consistency.

5 Check seasoning. Store in the refrigerator.

21   Vegetable soup (purée de légumes)

cal	kcal	fat	sat fat	carb	sugar	protein	fibre
1105 KJ	263 kcal	20.7 g	11.1 g	17.2 g	3.7 g	3.1 g	2.8 g

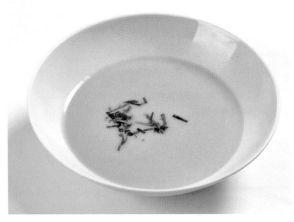

	4 portions	10 portions
mixed vegetables (onion, carrot, turnip, leek, celery)	300 g	1 kg
butter, margarine or oil	50 g	125 g
flour	25 g	60 g
white stock	1 litre	2½ litres
potatoes, sliced	100 g	300 g
bouquet garni		
salt, pepper		
Croutons		
slice stale bread	1	3
butter	50 g	125 g

1 Peel, wash and slice all the vegetables (except the potatoes).

2 Cook gently in the butter or margarine in a covered pan, without colouring.

3 Mix in the flour and cook slowly for a few minutes without colouring; cool slightly.

4 Mix in the hot stock. Stir and bring to the boil.

5 Add the sliced potatoes and bouquet garni. Season. Simmer for 30–45 minutes; skim when necessary. Remove the bouquet garni.

6 Liquidise or pass through a sieve and then through a medium strainer.

7 Return to a clean pan and reboil; correct the seasoning and the consistency.

8 Serve with croutons separately.

 HEALTHY EATING TIP

- Use soft margarine or sunflower/olive oil in place of the butter.

- Serve with toasted croutons and the minimum amount of salt.

* Using hard margarine

Making a purée soup
http://bit.ly/zp7WTh

---

22 | **Potato and watercress soup (*purée cressonnière*)**

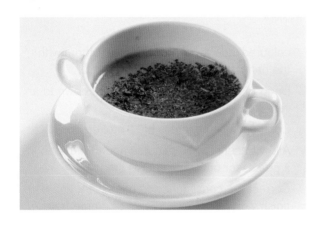

	4 portions	10 portions
butter, margarine or oil	25 g	60 g
onion	50 g	125 g
white of leek	50 g	125 g
white stock or water	1 litre	2½ litres
peeled potatoes	400 g	1½ kg
watercress	small bunch	small bunch
bouquet garni		
salt, pepper		
parsley, chopped		
Croutons		
slice stale bread	1	3
butter, margarine or oil	50 g	125 g

1 Pick off 12 neat leaves of watercress, plunge into a small pan of boiling water for 1–2 seconds. Refresh under cold water immediately; these leaves are to garnish the finished soup.

2 Melt the butter or margarine in a thick-bottomed pan.

3 Add the peeled and washed sliced onion and leek, cook for a few minutes without colour with the lid on.

4 Add the stock, the peeled, washed and sliced potatoes, the rest of the watercress, including the stalks, and the bouquet garni. Season.

5 Simmer for approximately 30 minutes. Remove the bouquet garni, skim off all fat.

6 Liquidise or pass the soup firmly through a sieve then pass through a medium conical strainer.

7 Return to a clean pan, reboil, correct the seasoning and consistency, and serve.

8 Garnish with blanched watercress, chopped or whole. Serve fried or toasted croutons separately.

23 Red lentil soup

cal	kcal	fat	sat fat	carb	sugar	protein	fibre	salt
1807 KJ	432 kcal	71.4 g	43.9 g	6.7 g	1.5 g	5.3 g	1.5 g	2.2 g

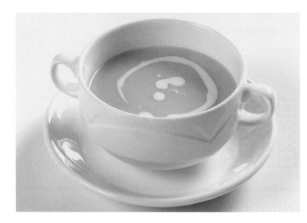

	approximately 10 portions
For the ham hock	
ham hock (800 g)	1
onion, peeled	½
whole carrot, peeled	1
For the soup	
baby shallots	3
leek	½
stick celery	½
oil	100 ml
red lentils	500 g
cooking liquid from the hock	
milk, cream or crème fraiche	300 ml

1 Place the ham hock, onion and carrot in a pan and cover with about 3 litres of water.

2 Bring to the boil and then turn down to a slow simmer. (When the hock is cooked, the centre bone will slide out in one smooth motion.)

3 Slice the shallots, leek and celery into 1 cm dice.

4 Heat a pan with about 100 ml of oil, add the vegetables and cook until they are slightly coloured; add the lentils and cover them with the ham stock.

5 Bring to the boil, then turn the heat down to a very slow simmer.

6 Cook until all the lentils have broken down.

7 Allow to cool for 10 minutes and then purée in a processor or liquidiser until smooth.

8 Correct the consistency as necessary, and finish with boiled milk, cream or crème fraiche.

24 Roasted red pepper and tomato soup

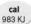

cal	kcal	fat	sat fat	carb	sugar	protein	fibre	salt
983 KJ	235 kcal	16.8 g	7.1 g	18.3 g	16.4 g	3.6 g	4.5 g	2.1 g

	4 portions	10 portions
red peppers	4	10
plum tomatoes	400 g	1.25 kg
oil, butter or margarine	50 g	125 g
onion, chopped	100 g	250 g
carrot	100 g	250 g
stock	500 ml	1.5 litres
crème fraiche	2 tbsp	5 tbsp
basil	25 g	75 g

1 Core and deseed the peppers, and halve the tomatoes.

2 Lightly sprinkle with oil, and place on a tray into a hot oven or under a grill until the pepper skins are blackened.

3 Allow the peppers to cool in a plastic bag.

4 Remove the skins and slice the flesh.

5 Place the fat or oil in a pan, add the onions and carrots and fry gently for five minutes.

6 Add the stock, peppers and tomatoes, and bring to the boil.

7 Simmer for 30 minutes, correct the seasoning and blend in a food processor until smooth.

8 Add crème fraiche and basil leaves torn into pieces, and serve with croutons.

ASSESSMENT

25 Vegetable and barley soup

	4 portions	10 portions
corn oil	50 ml	125 ml
onions, finely diced	1	2
leeks, cut into rounds	1	2
carrots, peeled and roughly chopped	2	3
celery sticks, cut into ½ cm dice	2	3
cloves of garlic, crushed	2	4
large potatoes, peeled and cut into ½ cm dice	3	7
pearl barley (cooked)	150 g	375 g
vegetable stock	1½ litres	3¾ litres
head of Swiss chard, washed and shredded (including stalks)	1	2
seasoning		

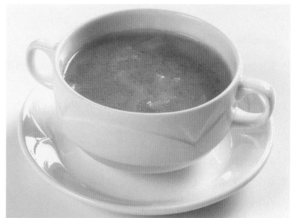

1 Heat the oil in a pan large enough to hold all the ingredients.

2 Place the onions, leeks, carrots and celery in the oil and cook until slightly golden.

3 Add the garlic and cook for a further 2 minutes. Add the potato and cook for a further 2 minutes.

4 Add the barley and vegetable stock. Bring to the boil, then simmer for 15 minutes, until the potatoes are just soft.

5 Stir in the Swiss chard and cook for a further 2 minutes.

6 Check the seasoning, correct if necessary then serve.

26 | Scotch broth

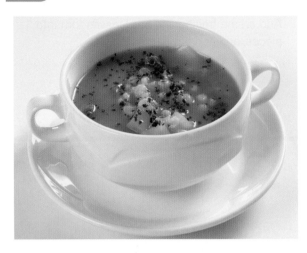

	4 portions	10 portions
lean beef, lamb or mutton	200 g	500 g
beef stock	1 litre	2½ litres
barley	25 g	60 g
vegetables (carrot, turnip, leek, celery, onion), chopped	200 g	500 g
bouquet garni		
salt, pepper		
chopped parsley		

1 Place the beef, free from fat, in a saucepan and cover with cold water.

2 Bring to the boil, then immediately wash off under running water.

3 Clean the pan, replace the meat, cover with cold water, bring to the boil and skim.

4 Add the washed barley, simmer for 1 hour.

5 Add the vegetables, bouquet garni and seasoning.

6 Skim when necessary; simmer for approximately 30 minutes, until tender.

7 Remove the meat, allow to cool and cut from the bone, remove all fat and cut the meat into neat dice the same size as the vegetables; return to the broth.

8 Correct the seasoning, skim off all the fat, add the chopped parsley and serve.

HEALTHY EATING TIP

- Remove all fat from the meat and skim any fat from the finished dish.
- Use only a small amount of salt.
- There are lots of healthy vegetables in this dish and the addition of a large bread roll will increase the starchy carbohydrate.

27 | Beef jus

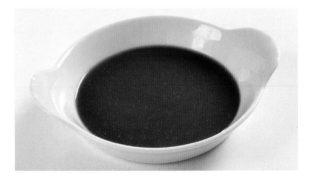

	approx. 1 litre
mushrooms, finely sliced	750 g
butter	100 g
shallots, finely sliced	350 g
beef trim, diced	350 g
sherry vinegar	100 ml
red wine	700 ml
chicken stock	500 ml
beef stock	1 litre

1 Caramelise the mushrooms in foaming butter, strain, then put aside in pan.

2 Caramelise the shallots in foaming butter, strain, then put aside in pan.

3 In another pan, caramelise the beef trim until golden brown.

4 Place the mushrooms, shallots and beef trim in one of the pans. Deglaze the other two pans with the vinegar, add to the pan with the beef, shallots and mushrooms in it.

5 In a separate pan, reduce the wine by half and add to the main pan.

6 Add the stock and jus, then reduce to sauce consistency.

7 Pass through a sieve, then chill and store until needed

28 Chicken jus

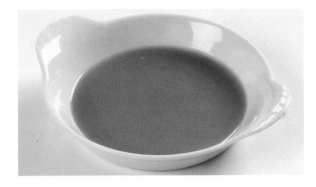

	approx. 1 litre
chicken stock	600 ml
lamb jus	600 ml
chicken wings, chopped small	300 g
vegetable oil	60 ml
shallots, sliced	100 g
butter	50 g
tomatoes, chopped	200 g
white wine vinegar	40 ml
red wine vinegar	75 ml
tarragon	3 g
chervil	3 g

1 Put the jus and stock in a pan and reduce to 1 litre.

2 Roast the chicken wings in oil until slightly golden.

3 Add the shallots and butter, and cook until lightly browned (do not allow the butter to burn).

4 Strain off the butter and return the bones to the pan; deglaze with the vinegar and add tomatoes.

5 Ensure the bottom of the pan is clean. Add the reduced stock/jus and simmer for 15 minutes.

6 Pass through a sieve, then reduce to sauce consistency.

7 Remove from the heat and infuse with the aromats for 5 minutes.

8 Pass through a chinois and then muslin cloth.

29 Red wine jus

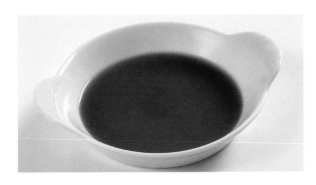

	approx. 1 litre
shallots, sliced	150 g
butter	50 g
garlic, halved	10 g
Cabernet Sauvignon vinegar or other wine vinegar	100 ml
red wine	500 ml
chicken stock	700 ml
lamb or beef jus	500 ml
bay leaves	2
sprig of thyme	1

1 Caramelise the shallots in foaming butter until golden, adding the garlic at the end.

2 Strain through a colander and then put back into the pan and deglaze with the vinegar.

3 Reduce the red wine by half along with the stock and jus, at the same time as colouring the shallots.

4 When everything is done, combine and simmer for 20 minutes.

5 Pass through a sieve and reduce to sauce consistency.

6 Infuse the aromats for 5 minutes.

7 Pass through muslin cloth and store until needed.

30 Madeira sauce (sauce Madère)

cal 43 KJ	kcal 10 kcal	fat 0.1 g	sat fat 0.0 g	carb 1.6 g	sugar 1.2 g	protein 0.3 g	fibre 0.4 g

    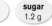

	4 portions	10 portions
demi-glace, jus-lié or reduced stock	250 ml	625 ml
Madeira wine	2 tbsp	5 tbsp
butter	25 g	60 g

1 Boil the demi-glace, jus-lié or stock in a small sauteuse.

2 Add the Madeira; reboil. Correct the seasoning.

3 Pass through a fine conical strainer. Gradually mix in the butter.

> May be served with braised ox tongue or ham. Dry sherry or port wine may be substituted for Madeira and the sauce renamed accordingly.

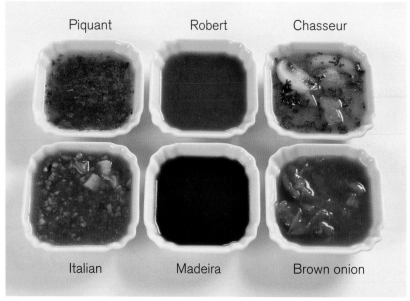

Piquant   Robert   Chasseur

Italian   Madeira   Brown onion

Recipes 30 to 35

31 Chasseur sauce *(sauce chasseur)*

cal	kcal	fat	sat fat	carb	sugar	protein	fibre
227 KJ	55 kcal	5.3 g	2.5 g	1.4 g	1.2 g	0.5 g	0.5 g

	4 portions	10 portions
butter, margarine or oil	25 g	60 g
shallots, chopped	10 g	25 g
garlic clove, chopped (optional)	1	1
button mushrooms, sliced	50 g	125 g
white wine (dry)	60 ml	150 ml
tomatoes, skinned, deseeded, diced	100 g	250 g
demi-glace, jus-lié or reduced stock	250 ml	625 ml
parsley and tarragon, chopped		

1 Melt the butter in a small sauteuse.

2 Add the shallots and cook gently for 2–3 minutes without colour.

3 Add the garlic and the mushrooms, cover and cook gently for 2–3 minutes.

4 Strain off the fat.

5 Add the wine and reduce by half. Add the tomatoes.

6 Add the demi-glace, jus-lié or stock; simmer for 5–10 minutes.

7 Correct the seasoning. Add the tarragon and parsley.

8 May be served with fried steaks, chops, chicken, etc.

 HEALTHY EATING TIP

- Use an unsaturated oil (sunflower or olive). Lightly oil the pan and drain off any excess after the frying is complete. Skim the fat from the finished dish.

- Season with the minimum amount of salt.

32 Italian sauce *(sauce italienne)*

cal	kcal	fat	sat fat	carb	sugar	protein	fibre
258 KJ	63 kcal	5.6 g	2.6 g	1.3 g	1.2 g	1.8 g	0.4 g

	4 portions	10 portions
margarine, oil or butter	25 g	60 g
shallots, chopped	10 g	25 g
mushrooms, chopped	50 g	125 g
demi-glace, jus-lié or reduced stock	250 ml	625 ml
lean ham, chopped	25 g	60 g
tomatoes, skinned, de-seeded, diced	100 g	250 g
parsley, chervil and tarragon, chopped		

1 Melt the fat or oil in a small sauteuse.

2 To make a duxelle, add the shallots and cook gently for 2–3 minutes, then add the mushrooms and cook gently for a further 2–3 minutes.

3 Add the demi-glace, jus-lié or stock, ham and tomatoes.

4 Simmer for 5–10 minutes. Correct the seasoning. Add the chopped herbs.

Usually served with fried cuts of veal, lamb or chicken.

 HEALTHY EATING TIP

- Use an unsaturated oil (sunflower or olive). Lightly oil the pan and drain off any excess after the frying is complete.

- Trim as much fat as possible from the ham.

- The ham is salty, so do not add more salt; flavour will come from the herbs.

- Skim all fat from the finished sauce.

33 Brown onion sauce (sauce lyonnaise)

cal	kcal	fat	sat fat	carb	sugar	protein	fibre
240 KJ	58 kcal	5.2 g	2.5 g	2.3 g	1.7 g	0.3 g	0.4 g

	4 portions	10 portions
margarine, oil or butter	25 g	60 g
onions, sliced	100 g	250 g
vinegar	2 tbsp	5 tbsp
demi-glace, jus-lié or reduced stock	250 ml	625 ml

1 Melt the fat or oil in a sauteuse.
2 Add the onions, cover with a lid.
3 Cook gently until tender.
4 Remove the lid and colour lightly.
5 Add the vinegar and completely reduce.
6 Add the demi-glace, jus or stock; simmer for 5–10 minutes.

7 Skim and correct the seasoning.

May be served with burgers, fried liver or sausages.

HEALTHY EATING TIP

- Use an unsaturated oil (sunflower or olive). Lightly oil the pan and drain off any excess after the frying is complete. Skim the fat from the finished dish.

- Season with the minimum amount of salt.

34 Piquant sauce (sauce piquante)

cal	kcal	fat	sat fat	carb	sugar	protein	fibre
197 KJ	48 kcal	5.1 g	3.3 g	0.3 g	0.3 g	0.0 g	0.0 g

	4 portions	10 portions
vinegar	60 ml	150 ml
shallots, chopped	50 g	125 g
demi-glace, jus-lié or reduced stock	250 ml	625 ml
gherkins, chopped	25 g	60 g
capers, chopped	10 g	25 g
chervil, tarragon and parsley, chopped	½ tbsp	1½ tbsp

1 Place the vinegar and shallots in a small sauteuse and reduce by half.
2 Add the demi-glace, jus or stock; simmer for 15–20 minutes.
3 Add the rest of the ingredients. Skim and correct the seasoning.

May be served with made-up dishes, sausages and grilled meats.

35 Robert sauce (sauce Robert)

cal	kcal	fat	sat fat	carb	sugar	protein	fibre
229 KJ	56 kcal	2.6 g	1.0 g	7.2 g	6.8 g	0.6 g	0.2 g

	4 portions	10 portions
margarine, oil or butter	20 g	50 g
onions, finely chopped	10 g	25 g
vinegar	60 ml	150 ml
demi-glace, jus-lié or reduced stock	250 ml	625 ml
English or continental mustard	½ tsp	1¼ tsp
caster sugar	1 level tbsp	2½ level tbsp

1 Melt the fat or oil in a small sauteuse. Add the onions.
2 Cook gently without colour. Add the vinegar and reduce completely.
3 Add the demi-glace, jus or stock; simmer for 5–10 minutes.
4 Remove from the heat and add the mustard diluted with a little water and the sugar; do not boil. Skim and correct the seasoning.

May be served with fried sausages and burgers, or grilled pork chops.

HEALTHY EATING TIP

- Use an unsaturated oil (sunflower or olive). Lightly oil the pan and drain off any excess after the frying is complete. Skim the fat from the finished dish.

- Season with the minimum amount of salt.

36 Tomato sauce *(sauce tomate)*

cal	kcal	fat	sat fat	carb	sugar	protein	fibre
931 KJ	221 kcal	12.5 g	5.1 g	20.2 g	11.5 g	8.5 g	2.9 g

*

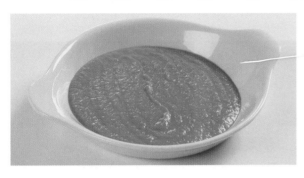

	4 portions	10 portions
margarine, butter or oil	10 g	25 g
onions (for mirepoix)	50 g	125 g
carrots (for mirepoix)	50 g	125 g
celery (for mirepoix)	25 g	60 g
bay leaf (for mirepoix)	1	3
bacon scraps (optional)	10 g	25 g
flour	10 g	25 g
tomato purée	50 g	125 g
stock	375 ml	1 litre
clove garlic	½	2
salt, pepper		

1 Melt the fat or oil in a small sauteuse.

2 Add the vegetables and herbs (mirepoix) and bacon scraps, and brown slightly.

3 Mix in the flour and cook to a sandy texture. Allow to colour slightly.

4 Mix in the tomato purée; allow to cool.

5 Gradually add the boiling stock; stir to the boil.

6 Add the garlic, season. Simmer for 1 hour.

7 Correct the seasoning and cool.

8 Pass through a fine conical strainer.

This sauce has many uses, served with pasta, eggs, fish, meats, and so on. The amount of tomato purée used may need to vary according to its strength. The sauce can also be made without using flour by adding 400 g of fresh, fully ripe tomatoes or an equivalent tin of tomatoes for 4 portions.

* Using hard margarine, for 4 portions. Using butter, this recipe provides for 4 portions: 936 kJ/223 kcal Energy; 12.6 g Fat; 6.7 g Sat Fat; 20.2 g Carb; 11.5 g Sugar; 8.5 g Protein; 2.9 g Fibre

37 Reduction of wine, stock and cream

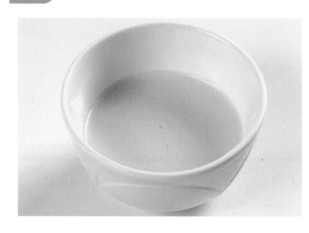

	approx. 250 ml
white or brown stock	500 ml
white wine	125 ml
double or whipping cream	125 ml

1 Place the stock and white wine in a suitable saucepan.

2 Reduce by at least two thirds and finish with cream.

Chef's tip
Reduce the stock and wine to a slightly syrupy consistency.

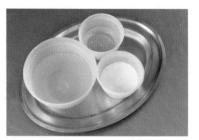

Measure out all the ingredients

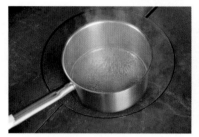

Reduce the wine and stock

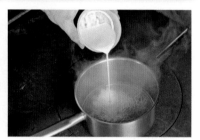

Add the cream

38 Reduction of stock (glaze)

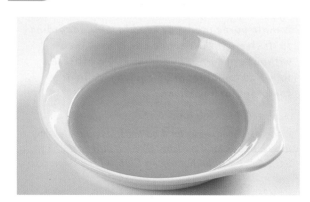

A glaze is a stock, fond or nage that has been reduced: that is, much of the water content is removed by boiling. The solid content, and all the flavour, stays in the glaze.

Any kind of stock can be used, but it is important to be careful if using meat stock. Meat stock contains collagen; if the stock is cooked at boiling temperature, there will be a lot of collagen in the glaze. This means the sauce will become thick more quickly than non-meat glazes. It will then be impossible to reduce it any more without burning it.

Glazes have a strong flavour and contain a lot of salt, so only use small amounts.

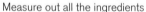

39 Sweet and sour sauce

cal	kcal	fat	sat fat	carb	sugar	protein	fibre
877 KJ	207 kcal	0.0 g	0.0 g	49.3 g	48.9 g	1.1 g	0.3 g

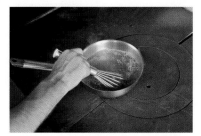

	4 portions	10 portions
white vinegar	375 ml	1 litre
brown sugar	150 g	375 g
tomato ketchup	125 ml	300 ml
soy sauce	1 tbsp	2½ tbsp
seasoning		

1 Boil the vinegar and sugar in a suitable pan.

2 Add the tomato ketchup, Worcester sauce and seasoning.

3 Simmer for a few minutes then use as required. This sauce may also be lightly thickened with cornflour or another thickening agent.

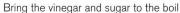

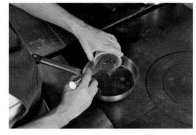

Bring the vinegar and sugar to the boil

Add the Worcester sauce, and then the other ingredients

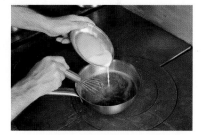

Add a thickener, if required

40 Butter sauce *(beurre blanc)*

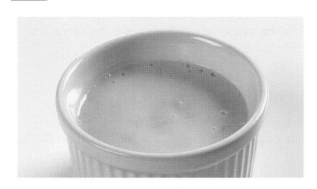

	4 portions	10 portions
water	125 ml	300 ml
wine vinegar	125 ml	300 ml
shallots, finely chopped	50 g	125 g
unsalted butter	200 g	500 g
lemon juice	1 tsp	2½ tsp
salt, pepper		

3 Whisk in the lemon juice, season lightly and keep warm in a bain-marie.

Try something different

The sauce may be strained if desired. Variations include adding freshly shredded sorrel or spinach, blanched fine julienne of lemon or lime, or chopped fresh herbs.

1 Reduce the water, vinegar and shallots in a thick-bottomed pan to approximately 62 ml, and allow to cool slightly. (Pass if required.)

2 Gradually whisk in the butter in small amounts, whisking continually until the mixture becomes creamy.

Chef's tips

Once butter is added to a sauce, the sauce must not re-boil, because it will split.

The butter should be cold and sliced/cubed when it is mounted (monté) into the sauce, and the sauce should be kept moving to create a wave, skimming layers of the butter into the sauce.

HEALTHY EATING TIP

- Use the minimum amount of salt.
- Do not use too much sauce with fish dishes.

41 Béchamel (basic white sauce)

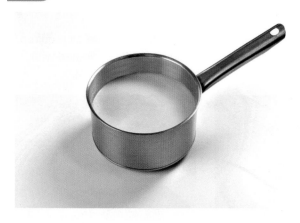

	1 litre	4½ litres
margarine, butter or oil	100 g	400 g
flour	100 g	400 g
milk, warmed	1 litre	4½ litres
onion studded with cloves	1	2–3

1 Melt the fat in a thick-bottomed pan.

2 Mix in the flour with a wooden or heat-proof plastic spoon.

3 Cook for a few minutes, stirring frequently. As you are making a white roux, do not allow the mixture to colour.

4 Remove the pan from the heat to allow the roux to cool.

5 Return the pan to the stove and, over a low heat, gradually mix the milk into the roux.

6 Add the studded onion.

7 Allow the mixture to simmer gently for 30 minutes, stirring frequently to make sure the sauce does not burn on the bottom.

8 Remove the onion and pass the sauce through a conical strainer.

To prevent a skin from forming, brush the surface with melted butter. When ready to use, stir this into the sauce. Alternatively, cover the sauce with clingfilm or greaseproof paper.

42 Mornay sauce

	500 ml
milk	500 ml
sauce flour	40 g
grated cheese	50 g
egg yolk	1

1 The milk may be first infused with a studded onion clouté, carrot and a bouquet garni. Allow to cool.

2 Place the milk in a suitable saucepan, gradually whisk in the sauce flour. Bring slowly to the boil until the sauce has thickened.

3 Mix in the cheese and egg yolk when the sauce is boiling.

4 Remove from the heat. Strain if necessary.

5 Do not allow the sauce to reboil at any time.

Alternatively, use 500 ml of béchamel (recipe 41) and begin at step 3.

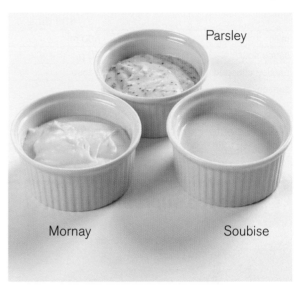

Recipes 42 to 44

 HEALTHY EATING TIP

- Try using yoghurt or fromage frais.
- Add a little cornflour prior to heating to stabilise the sauce.

43 Soubise sauce

	500 ml
onion, chopped or diced	100 g
milk	500 ml
sauce flour	40 g
seasoning	

1 Cook the onions without colouring them, either by boiling or sweating in butter.

2 The milk may be first infused with a studded onion clouté, carrot and a bouquet garni. Allow to cool.

3 Place the milk in a suitable saucepan, gradually whisk in the sauce flour. Bring slowly to the boil until the sauce has thickened.

4 Add the onions, season, simmer for approximately 5–10 minutes.

5 Blitz well (using a hand-held liquidiser). Pass through a strainer.

Alternatively, use 500 ml of béchamel (recipe 41), prepare the onions at step 1 and then proceed to step 4.

44 Parsley sauce

	500 ml
milk	500 ml
sauce flour	40 g
parsley, chopped	1 tbsp
seasoning	

1 The milk may be first infused with a studded onion clouté, carrot and a bouquet garni. Allow to cool.

2 Place the milk in a suitable saucepan, gradually whisk in the sauce flour. Bring slowly to the boil until the sauce has thickened.

3 Add the parsley. Season, simmer for approximately 5–10 minutes. Use as required.

Alternatively, use 500 ml of béchamel (recipe 41) and begin at step 3.

45 *Sauce suprême*

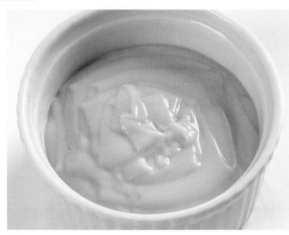

A basic suprême sauce which needs to be thinned with stock and cream

	4 portions	10 portions
margarine, butter or oil	100 g	400 g
flour	100 g	400 g
stock (chicken, veal, fish, mutton) as required	1 litre	4½ litres
mushroom trimmings	25 g	60 g
egg yolk	1	2
cream	60 ml	150 ml
lemon juice	2–3 drops	5–6 drops

1 Melt the fat or oil in a thick-bottomed pan.

2 Add the flour and mix in.

3 Cook out to a sandy texture over gentle heat without colouring.

4 Allow the roux to cool.

5 Gradually add the boiling stock.

6 Stir until smooth and boiling.

7 Add the mushroom trimmings. Allow to simmer for approximately 1 hour.

8 Pass it through a fine conical strainer.

9 Finish with a liaison of the egg yolk, cream and lemon juice.

Serve immediately; do not reboil.

The traditional stock for this recipe is good chicken stock.

46 Fish velouté

cal	kcal	fat	sat fat	carb	sugar	protein	fibre
4805 KJ	1144 kcal	90.4 g	39.0 g	77.8 g	1.6 g	9.5 g	3.6 g

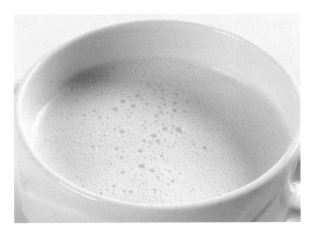

	1 litre	2½ litres
margarine or butter	100 g	250 g
flour	100 g	250 g
fish stock	1 litre	2½ litres

This will give a thick sauce that can be thinned down with the cooking liquor from the fish for which the sauce is intended.

 HEALTHY EATING TIP

- Make sure all the fat has been skimmed from the stock before adding it to the roux.

1 Prepare a blond roux using the margarine or butter and flour.

2 Gradually add the stock, stirring continuously until boiling point is reached.

3 Simmer for approximately 1 hour.

4 Pass through a fine conical strainer.

47 Mushroom sauce

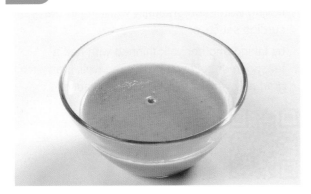

	1 litre	4½ litres
margarine, butter or oil	100 g	400 g
flour	100 g	400 g
stock (chicken, veal, fish, mutton) as required	1 litre	4½ litres
mushroom trimmings	50 g	225 g
white button mushrooms, well-washed, sliced, sweated	200 g	900 g
cream	120 ml	540 ml
egg yolk	2	9
lemon juice	1 tsp	4 tsp

1 Melt the fat or oil in a thick-bottomed pan.

2 Add the flour and mix in.

3 Cook out to a sandy texture over gentle heat without colouring.

4 Allow the roux to cool.

5 Gradually add the boiling stock.

6 Stir until smooth and boiling.

7 Add the mushrooms and trimmings. Allow to simmer for approximately 1 hour.

8 Pass it through a fine conical strainer.

9 Simmer for 10 minutes, then add the egg yolk, cream and lemon juice.

Serve immediately; do not reboil.

48 Mayonnaise sauce

cal	kcal	fat	sat fat	carb	sugar	protein	fibre
10030 KJ	2388 kcal	26.2 g	38.9 g	0.3 g	0.1 g	6.8 g	0.0 g

*

	8 portions
egg yolks, pasteurised	2
vinegar	2 tsp
salt, ground white pepper	
English or continental mustard	1/8 tsp
corn oil or other vegetable oil	250 ml
boiling water	1 tsp (approx.)

1 Place the yolks, vinegar and seasoning in a bowl and whisk well.

2 Gradually pour on the oil very slowly, whisking continuously.

3 Add the boiling water, whisking well. Correct the seasoning.

Chef's tip

Gradually adding the oil to the beaten egg yolks forms an emulsion.

Notes: This is a basic cold sauce and has a wide variety of uses, particularly in hors d'oeuvre dishes. It should always be available on any cold buffet. Because of the risk of salmonella food poisoning, it is strongly recommended that pasteurised egg yolks are used.

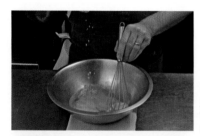

Beat the egg yolks and mix in the vinegar and seasoning

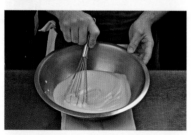

Begin whisking in the oil

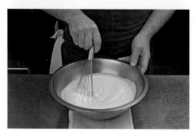

Gradually add more oil

If, during the making of the sauce, it should become too thick, then a little vinegar or water may be added. Mayonnaise will turn or curdle for several reasons:

- if the oil is added too quickly
- if the oil is too cold
- if the sauce is insufficiently whisked
- if the yolk is stale and therefore weak.

The method used to rethicken a turned mayonnaise is either:

- by taking a clean basin, adding 1 teaspoon boiling water and gradually whisking in the curdled sauce, or
- by taking another yolk thinned with half a teaspoon of cold water whisked well, then gradually whisking in the curdled sauce.

Making mayonnaise
http://bit.ly/xx315t

* For 8 portions

49 Tartare sauce *(sauce tartare)*

cal	kcal	fat	sat fat	carb	sugar	protein	fibre
938 KJ	228 kcal	24.8 g	3.6 g	0.3 g	0.3 g	0.7 g	0.1 g

	8 portions
mayonnaise	250 ml
capers, chopped	25 g
gherkins	50 g
sprig of parsley, chopped	

Combine all the ingredients.

This sauce is usually served with deep-fried fish.

Chef's tip

Finely chop the gherkins and capers, and use a blender, to give the desired texture and consistency.

HEALTHY EATING TIP

- Proportionally reduce the fat by adding some low-fat yoghurt.

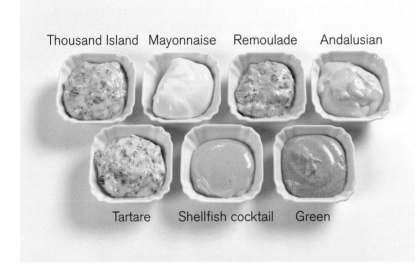

Thousand Island   Mayonnaise   Remoulade   Andalusian

Tartare   Shellfish cocktail   Green

Recipes 48 to 54

50 Remoulade sauce *(sauce remoulade)*

cal	kcal	fat	sat fat	carb	sugar	protein	fibre
938 KJ	228 kcal	24.8 g	3.6 g	0.3 g	0.3 g	0.8 g	0.1 g

Prepare as for tartare sauce (recipe 49), adding 1 teaspoon of anchovy essence and mixing thoroughly. Makes 1/8 litre.

* Using gherkins

This sauce may be served with fried fish. It can also be mixed with a fine julienne of celeriac to make an accompaniment to cold meats, terrines, etc.

51 Green sauce (*sauce verte*)

	8 portions
spinach, tarragon, chervil, chives, watercress	50 g
mayonnaise	250 ml

1 Pick, wash, blanch and refresh the green leaves. Squeeze dry.
2 Pass through a very fine sieve. Mix with the mayonnaise.

May be served with cold salmon or salmon trout (sea trout).

52 Andalusian sauce (*sauce andalouse*)

Take ¼ litre of mayonnaise and add 2 tbsp tomato juice or ketchup and 1 tbsp pepper cut into julienne. Makes ¼ litre. May be served with cold salads.

Chef's tip
For Andalusian sauce, Thousand Island dressing, green sauce and other similar recipes, use a blender to achieve the desired texture and flavour.

53 Thousand Island dressing

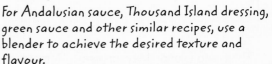

cal	kcal	fat	sat fat	carb	sugar	protein	fibre
15055 KJ	3584 kcal	387.0 g	56.5 g	10.2 g	9.8 g	16.1 g	1.8 g

*

	4–6 portions
salt, pepper	
Tabasco	3–4 drops
vinegar	125 ml
oil	375 ml
red pepper, chopped	50 g
green pepper, chopped	50 g
parsley, chopped	
hard-boiled eggs, sieved	2
tomato ketchup (optional)	2 tbsp

1 Place the salt, pepper, Tabasco and vinegar in a basin.
2 Mix well. Mix in the oil.
3 Add the chopped peppers and parsley.
4 Mix in the sieved hard-boiled eggs.
5 Mix in ketchup if desired.

* For 4–6 portions

54 Shellfish cocktail sauce

cal	kcal	fat	sat fat	carb	sugar	protein	fibre
889 KJ	216 kcal	22.7 g	14.2 g	1.9 g	1.9 g	1.2 g	0.1 g

Method 1

	4 portions	10 portions
egg yolk, pasteurised ⚠	1	3
vinegar	1 tsp	2½ tsp
salt, pepper, mustard		
olive oil or sunflower oil	5 tbsp	8 tbsp
tomato juice or ketchup to taste		
Worcester sauce (optional)	2–3 drops	6–8 drops

1 Make the mayonnaise with the egg yolk, vinegar, seasonings and oil.

2 Combine with the tomato juice and Worcester sauce (if using).

🍎 **HEALTHY EATING TIP**

- Keep added salt to a minimum.

- Extend the high-fat mayonnaise with low-fat yoghurt to proportionally reduce the fat content.

Method 2

	4 portions	10 portions
lightly whipped cream or unsweetened non-dairy cream	5 tbsp	12 tbsp
tomato juice or ketchup to taste	3 tbsp	8 tbsp
salt, pepper		
lemon juice		a few drops

1 Mix all the ingredients together.

Fresh or tinned tomato juice, or diluted tomato ketchup, may be used for both the above methods, but the use of tinned tomato purée gives an unpleasant flavour.

55 Tomato vinaigrette

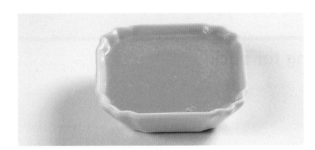

	4 portions	10 portions
tomatoes	200 g	500 g
caster sugar	½ tsp	1¼ tbsp
white wine vinegar	1 tbsp	2½ tsp
extra virgin olive oil	3 tbsp	8 tbsp
seasoning		

1 Blanch and deseed the tomatoes; purée in a food processor.

2 Add the sugar, vinegar, olive oil and seasoning; whisk well to emulsify.

3 The vinaigrette should be smooth.

56 Mint sauce

cal	kcal	fat	sat fat	carb	sugar	protein	fibre
204 KJ	49 kcal	0.0 g	0.0 g	11.3 g	11.3 g	1.5 g	1.8 g

*

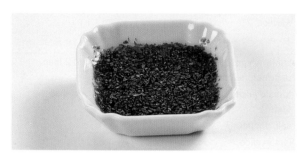

	8 portions
mint	2–3 tbsp
caster sugar	1 tsp
vinegar	125 ml

Serve with roast lamb. A less acid sauce can be produced by dissolving the sugar in 125 ml boiling water and, when cold, adding the chopped mint and 1–2 tablespoon vinegar to taste.

1 Chop the washed, picked mint and mix with the sugar.

2 Place in a china basin and add the vinegar.

3 If the vinegar is too sharp, dilute it with a little water.

* For 8 portions

57 Apple sauce

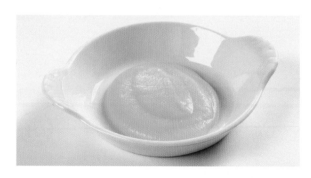

cooking apples	400 g
sugar	50 g
margarine or butter	25 g

1 Peel, core and wash the apples.

2 Place with other ingredients in a covered pan and cook gently to a purée.

3 Pass through a sieve or liquidise.

58 Cranberry and orange dressing for duck

cal	kcal	fat	sat fat	carb	sugar	protein	fibre
398 KJ	93 kcal	0.2 g	0.0 g	22.7 g	22.7 g	1.3 g	4.2 g

*

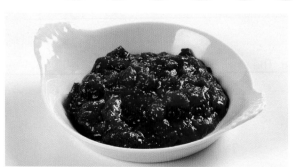

	4 portions	10 portions
cranberries	400 g	1 kg
granulated sugar	50 g	125 g
red wine	125 ml	250 ml
red wine vinegar	2 tbsp	5 tbsp
orange zest and juice	2	4

1 Place the cranberries in a suitable saucepan with the rest of the ingredients.

2 Bring to the boil and simmer gently for approximately 1 hour, stirring from time to time.

3 Remove from the heat and leave to cool. Use as required.

The dressing may also be liquidised if a smooth texture is required.

---

59 Yoghurt and cucumber raita

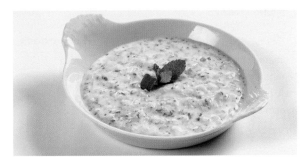

	4 portions
cucumbers	2
salt	
spring onions, chopped	2 tbsp
yoghurt	500 ml
cumin seeds	1 ½ tsp
lemon juice	1
fresh coriander or mint, chopped	

1 Peel the cucumbers, halve them lengthways and remove the seeds. Cut into small dice.

2 Sprinkle the dice with salt and leave for 15 minutes, then drain away the liquid and rinse the cucumbers quickly in cold water. Drain well.

3 Combine the onion, yoghurt and lemon juice; taste to see if more salt is required.

4 Roast the cumin seeds in a dry pan, shaking the pan or stirring constantly until brown.

5 Bruise or crush the seeds and sprinkle over the yoghurt mixture.

6 Serve chilled, garnished with mint and coriander.

This is a dish from Punjab, northern India. Serve as an accompaniment to curry.

Chef's tip
Sprinkling the cucumber with salt removes the juices, which are hard to digest. Remember to wash off the salt before use.

---

60 Balsamic vinegar and olive oil dressing

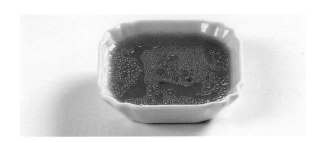

water	62 ml
olive oil	250 ml
balsamic vinegar	62 ml
sherry vinegar	2 tbsp
caster sugar	½ tsp
seasoning	

Whisk all ingredients together. Correct the seasoning.

The amount of balsamic vinegar needed will depend on its quality, age, etc. Add more or less as required.

Chef's tip

This dressing works well because it is not an emulsion. The oil and vinegar provide a stark contrast and can be stirred just before serving.

61 Horseradish sauce (*sauce raifort*)

cal	kcal	fat	sat fat	carb	sugar	protein	fibre
1807 KJ	430 kcal	43.8 g	27.8 g	6.0 g	5.0 g	3.6 g	2.1 g

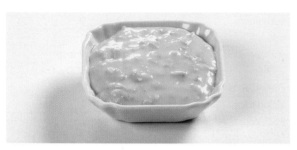

	8 portions
horseradish	25 g
vinegar or lemon juice	1 tbsp
salt, pepper	
cream or crème fraiche, lightly whipped	125 ml

1 Wash, peel and rewash the horseradish. Grate finely.
2 Mix all the ingredients together.

Serve with roast beef, smoked trout, eel or halibut.

* For 8 portions

Chef's tip

It is essential to blend the ingredients without over-mixing them, in order to get a good flavour.

62 Tomato and cucumber salsa

cal	kcal	fat	sat fat	carb	sugar	protein	fibre
202 KJ	49 kcal	4.3 g	0.7 g	2.0 g	2.0 g	0.6 g	0.7 g

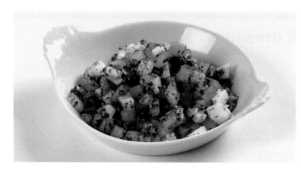

	8 portions
ripe, chopped tomatoes	400 g
cucumber, chopped	½
spring onions	6
fresh basil, chopped	1 tbsp
fresh parsley, chopped	1 tbsp
olive oil	3 tbsp
lemon or lime (juice of)	1
salt and pepper	

1 In a large bowl, mix all the ingredients together.
2 Correct seasoning and serve.

- Rely on the herbs for flavour, with the minimum amount of salt.

- Extra vegetables can be added and the salsa used liberally with grilled fish or chicken. Rice could be served or the salsa used to fill a tortilla.

> This recipe may be varied by using any chopped salad ingredients and fresh herbs (e.g. tarragon, chervil). Do not be afraid to experiment.

63 Salsa verde

cal	kcal	fat	sat fat	carb	sugar	protein	fibre
281 KJ	69 kcal	7.5 g	1.1 g	0.2 g	0.1 g	0.1 g	0.0 g

*

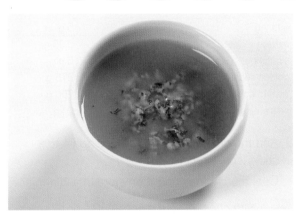

		8 portions
mint	⎱ coarsely chopped	1 tbsp
parsley		3 tbsp
capers		3
garlic clove (optional)	⎰	1
Dijon mustard		1 tsp
lemon juice		½
extra virgin olive oil		120 ml
salt		

In a large bowl, mix all the ingredients together and check the seasoning. Serve with grilled fish.

* Per tablespoon

64 Avocado and coriander salsa

cal	kcal	fat	sat fat	carb	sugar	protein	fibre
361 KJ	87 kcal	8.6 g	1.4 g	1.8 g	1.4 g	0.8 g	1.0 g

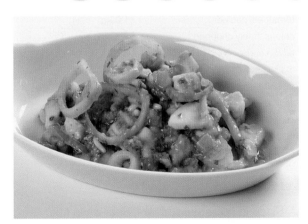

ripe avocado, peeled and diced	1
ripe tomatoes, peeled, deseeded and diced	3
shallot, peeled and cut into rings	1
fresh coriander, chopped	1 tsp
pine kernels, toasted	10 g
cucumber, diced	25 g
lemon or lime (juice)	1
virgin olive oil	3 tbsp
salt and pepper to taste	

- Although avocado is rich in fat, it is unsaturated fat and therefore healthier.

- Try using the salsa to fill a tortilla, and add grilled fish or chicken to make a healthy meal.

In a large bowl, mix all the ingredients together, check seasoning and serve.

Use with cold dishes such as salads or terrinnes.

Try something different

- Peeled, de-stoned, diced mango in place of avocado
- 1 tsp finely chopped garlic or garlic juice
- 1 tsp finely chopped red chilli
- 1 tbsp of finely chopped lemon grass
- 25 g chopped red onion in place of shallot

65 Pear chutney

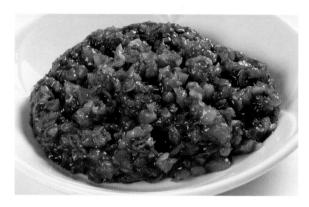

Makes approx. 5 kg	
white wine vinegar	900 g
demerara sugar	900 g
ginger, brunoise	125 g
onion, diced	375 g
nutmeg	5 g
saffron	0.25 g
cinnamon	5 g
golden sultanas	375 g
tomato concassée	750 g
pears, diced	2 kg

1 Make a thick syrup with the white wine vinegar and the sugar.
2 Add the ginger, onion, nutmeg, saffron, cinnamon, sultanas and concassée, and reduce to a thick syrup.
3 Add the diced pears and reduce again to a sticky consistency.
4 Cool the chutney and then store in a kilner jar.

Serve with cheese, cold meats, pâtés or terrines.

66 Tomato chutney

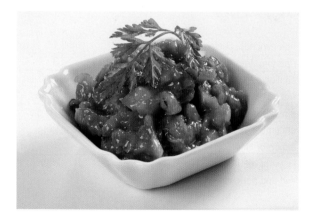

	Makes 1 litre
tomatoes, peeled	1.5 kg
onions, finely chopped	450 g
brown sugar	300 g
malt vinegar	375 ml
mustard powder	1½ tsp
cayenne pepper	½ tsp
coarse salt	2 tsp
mild curry powder	1 tbsp

1 Peel and coarsely chop the tomatoes, then combine with the remaining ingredients in a large heavy-duty saucepan.
2 Stir over heat without boiling until the sugar dissolves. Simmer uncovered, stirring occasionally until the mixture thickens (about 1½ hours).
3 Place in hot, sterilised jars. Seal while hot.

Serve with cheese, cold meats or terrines.

Chef's tip
Blend the ingredients to make a good chutney.

67 Pesto

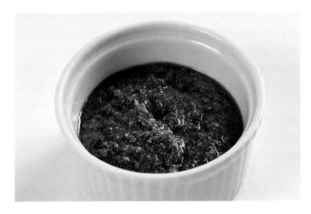

	4 portions	10 portions
fresh basil leaves	4 small	
bunches	10 small bunches	
garlic clove, chopped	1	2–3
salt, to taste		
pine nuts, lightly toasted	1 tbsp	2½ tbsp
Parmesan cheese, grated	2 tbsp	5 tbsp
extra virgin olive oil		

Pesto is a green basil sauce used in some pasta dishes, salads and fish dishes.

1 Put the basil leaves, garlic, salt and pine nuts into a mortar (or use a food processor) and pound into a smooth paste.

2 Place in a bowl, mix in the cheese and sufficient olive oil to make a sauce-like consistency.

68 Tapenade

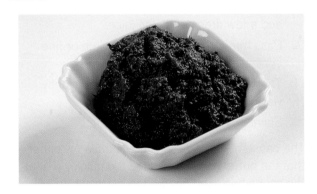

Tapenade is a Provençale dish consisting of puréed or finely chopped black olives, capers, anchovies and olive oil. It may also contain garlic, herbs, tuna, lemon juice or brandy. Its name comes from the Provençale word for capers: *tapeno*. It is popular in the South of France, where it is generally eaten as an hors d'oeuvre, spread on toast.

1 Mix all the ingredients together, adding the olive oil to make a paste.

2 For a smoother texture, place garlic, lemon juice, capers and anchovies into a food processor and process until a smooth texture. Add the olives and parsley, and sufficient oil to form a smooth paste.

3 Season, if required.

4 Garnish with a sprinkle of roast cumin and chopped red chilli.

5 Serve chilled.

69 Mixed pickle

For the spiced vinegar

vinegar	1 litre
blade mace	5 g
allspice	5 g
cloves	5 g
stick cinnamon	5 g
peppercorns	6
root ginger (for hot pickle)	5 g

To make the spiced vinegar:

1 Tie the spices in muslin, place them in a covered pan with the vinegar and heat slowly to boiling point.

2 Remove from the heat and stand for 2 hours, then remove the bag.

Prepare the vegetables, with the exception of the marrow (see note for suggested vegetables to use), and soak them in brine for 24 hours. Peel the marrow, remove the seeds and cut into small squares, sprinkle and salt, and let it stand for 12 hours. Drain the vegetables, pack them into jars, and cover with cold spiced vinegar. Cover the jars and allow the pickle to mature for at least a month before use.

The following make a good mixture: cauliflower, cucumber, green tomatoes, onions and marrow.

70 Hollandaise sauce (*sauce hollandaise*)

cal	kcal	fat	sat fat	carb	sugar	protein	fibre
6789 KJ	1616 kcal	176.2 g	107.9 g	0.1 g	0.1 g	7.3 g	0.0 g

	4 portions	10 portions
crushed peppercorn reduction (optional)	6	15
vinegar	1 tbsp	2½ tbsp
pasteurised egg yolks	2	5
butter or good-quality oil	200 g	500 g
salt, cayenne, to taste		

1 Place the peppercorns and vinegar in a small sauteuse or stainless steel pan and reduce to one-third. Strain off.

2 Add 1 tbsp cold water; allow to cool.

3 Mix in the yolks with a whisk.

4 Return to a gentle heat and, whisking continuously, cook to a sabayon (this means cooking of the yolks to a thickened consistency, like cream, that will show the mark of the whisk).

5 Remove from the heat and cool slightly.

6 Whisk the melted warm butter in gradually, until thoroughly combined.

7 Correct the seasoning. If reduction is not used, add a few drops of lemon juice.

8 Pass through a muslin, tammy cloth or fine conical strainer.

9 The sauce should be kept at only a slightly warm temperature until served.

10 Serve in a slightly warm sauceboat.

The cause of hollandaise sauce curdling is either that the butter has been added too quickly or that the sauce has been heated too much, which will cause the albumen in the eggs to harden, shrink and separate from the liquid.

Should the sauce curdle, place a teaspoon of boiling water in a clean sauteuse and gradually whisk in the curdled sauce. If this fails to reconstitute the sauce, then place an egg yolk in a clean sauteuse with 1 dessertspoon of water. Whisk lightly over a gentle heat until slightly thickened. Remove from the heat and gradually add the curdled sauce, whisking continuously. To stabilise the sauce during service, 60 ml thick béchamel sauce (recipe 41) may be added before straining.

 To reduce the risk of salmonella infection, pasteurised egg yolks should be used. Do not keep the sauce for longer than 2 hours before discarding. This applies to all egg-based sauces.

Served with hot fish (e.g. salmon, trout, turbot) and vegetables (e.g. asparagus, cauliflower, broccoli).

Variations (e.g. béarnaise) can be found in recipe 71.

 HEALTHY EATING TIP

- This recipe is obviously high in saturated fat (butter, egg yolk).
- Add the minimum of salt and consider it to be a treat.
- The fat is proportionally reduced when served with grilled or baked fish and plenty of potatoes and other vegetables.

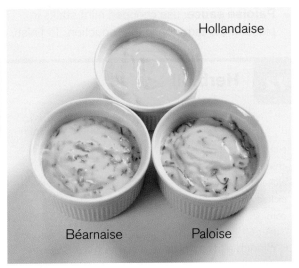

Hollandaise

Béarnaise   Paloise

Recipes 70 and 71

* For four portions

Making hollandaise sauce
http://bit.ly/wvtR4Q

---

71 Béarnaise sauce

	Makes 500 g
shallots, chopped	50 g
tarragon	10 g
peppercorns, crushed	12
white wine vinegar	3 tbsp
pasteurised egg yolks	6
melted butter	325 g
salt and cayenne pepper	
chervil and tarragon to finish, chopped	

1 Place the shallots, tarragon, peppercorns and vinegar in a small pan and reduce to one-third.

2 Add 1 tablespoon of cold water and allow to cool. Add the egg yolks.

3 Put on a bain-marie and whisk continuously to a sabayon consistency.

4 Remove from the heat and gradually whisk in the melted butter.

5 Add seasoning. Pass through muslin or a fine chinois.

6 To finish, add the chopped chervil and tarragon.

7 Store in an appropriate container at room temperature.

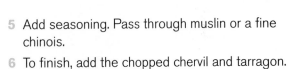 Note: Egg-based sauces should not be kept warm for more than 2 hours. After this time, they should be thrown away, but are best made fresh to order.

Variations

- **Choron sauce**: 200 g tomato concassée, well dried. Do not add the chopped tarragon and chervil to finish.

- **Foyot or valois sauce**: 25 g warm meat glaze.

- **Paloise sauce**: use chopped mint stalks in place of the tarragon in the reduction. To finish, add chopped mint instead of the chervil and tarragon.

72 Herb oil

	Makes 200 ml
picked flat leaf parsley	25 g
chives	10 g
picked basil leaves	10 g
picked spinach	100 g
corn oil	250 ml

1 Blanch all the herbs and spinach for 1½ minutes.

2 Drain well, place with the oil in a liquidiser and blitz for 2½ minutes. Pass and decant when rested.

Note: Uses include salads, salmon micuit and other fish dishes.

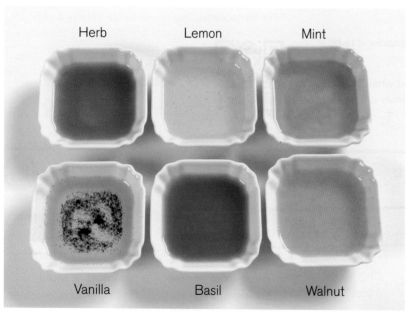

Herb   Lemon   Mint

Vanilla   Basil   Walnut

Flavoured oils (recipes 72 to 77)

73 Lemon oil

	Makes 250 ml
lemons, rind (with no pith – the whitish layer between skin and fruit)	3
lemon grass stick, cut lengthways and chopped into 2 cm strips	1
grapeseed oil	250 ml
olive oil	2 tbsp

1 Place all the ingredients into a food processor and pulse the mix until the lemon peel and grass are approximately 3 mm thick.

2 Allow to stand for two days. Decant and store in the fridge until ready for use (or you could freeze for longer if you wish).

Use to dress salads or cold meats, for marinating fish or to finish fish dishes.

74 Mint oil

	Makes 150 ml
mint	100 g
vegetable oil	150 ml
salt	½ tsp

1 Blanch the mint for 30 seconds.
2 Refresh and squeeze the water out.
3 Place in a blender and slowly add the oil.
4 Allow to settle overnight and decant into bottles.

Uses include lamb dishes, salads and fish dishes.

75 Vanilla oil

	Makes 200 ml
vegetable oil	200 ml
vanilla pods, whole	5
vanilla pods, used	2
vanilla extract	50 ml

1 Warm the oil to around 60°C; add the vanilla in its various forms and infuse, scraping all the seeds into the oil. Store in a plastic bottle.
2 Uses include salads, salmon micuit and other fish dishes.

76 Basil oil

	Makes 200 ml
fresh basil	25 g
vegetable oil	200 ml
salt, to taste	
mill pepper	

Note: Basil extract can be used in place of fresh basil; 50 g of grated Parmesan or Gorgonzola cheese may also be added to the basil oil.

1 Blanch and refresh the basil; purée with the oil.
2 Allow to settle overnight and decant.
3 Store in bottles with a sprig of blanched basil.

77 Walnut oil

	Makes 500 ml
olive or walnut oil	500 ml
walnuts, finely crushed	75 g
Parmesan cheese	75 g
salt, to taste	
mill pepper	

1 Mix all the ingredients together and bottle until required.

78 Compound butter sauces

Compound butters are made by mixing the flavouring ingredients into softened butter, which can then be shaped into a roll 2 cm in diameter, placed in wet greaseproof paper or foil, hardened in a refrigerator and cut into ½ cm slices when required.

- *Parsley butter:* chopped parsley and lemon juice.
- *Herb butter:* mixed herbs (chives, tarragon, fennel, dill) and lemon juice.
- *Chive butter:* chopped chives and lemon juice.
- *Garlic butter:* garlic juice and chopped parsley or herbs.
- *Anchovy butter:* few drops anchovy essence.
- *Shrimp butter:* finely chopped or pounded shrimps.
- *Garlic:* mashed to a paste.
- *Mustard:* continental-type mustard.
- *Liver pâté:* mashed to a paste.

Compound butters are served with grilled and some fried fish, and with grilled meats.

9 Prepare and cook fruit and vegetables

In this chapter you will learn how to:

1. prepare and cook fruits and vegetables:

- using equipment correctly to peel, wash and cut fruits and vegetables
- cooking, assembling, holding and serving fruit and vegetable dishes in a safe and hygienic way
- storing prepared vegetables before or after cooking, if appropriate

2. you should have the knowledge to:

- identify commonly used fruits and vegetables, their classifications and seasons
- check the quality of fruits and vegetables
- identify correct methods for storing, preparing, cooking and preserving fruits and vegetables
- identify additions, preparations, cooking liquids, sauces and garnishes.

No.	Recipe title	Page no.
Fruit		
2	Avocado pear (*l'avocat*)	219
6	Caribbean fruit curry	222
	Florida cocktail	218
3	Fresh fruit salad	220
4	Fruit cocktail	220
1	Grapefruit (*pamplemousse*)	218
	Grapefruit and orange cocktail	218
	Mango	221
	Orange cocktail	218
5	Tropical fruit plate	221
	Additional recipes using fruit are provided in Chapters 14 and 15.	
Potatoes		
10	Baked jacket potatoes (*pommes au four*)	225
	Château potatoes (*pommes château*)	230
11	Croquette potatoes (*pommes croquettes*)	225
17	Delmonico potatoes (*pommes Delmonico*)	229
8	Duchess potatoes (basic recipe) (*pommes duchesse*)	223
14	Fondant potatoes (*pommes fondants*)	227
15	Fried or chipped potatoes (*pommes frites*)	227
23	Hash brown potatoes	232
21	Macaire potatoes (*pommes Macaire*)	231
9	Mashed potatoes (*pommes purée*)	224
18	Parmentier potatoes (*pommes parmentier*)	229

No.	Recipe title	Page no.
7	Parsley potatoes (*pommes persillées*)	223
22	Potatoes cooked in milk with cheese (*gratin dauphinoise*)	231
12	Potatoes with bacon and onions (*pommes au lard*)	226
20	Roast potatoes (*pommes rôties*)	230
13	Sauté potatoes (*pommes au sautées*)	226
16	Sauté potatoes with onions (*pommes lyonnaise*)	228
19	Swiss potato cakes (*rösti*)	229
Vegetables		
56	Alu-chole (vegetarian curry)	249
46	Asparagus points or tips (*pointes d'asperges*)	244
48	Asparagus wrapped in puff pastry with Gruyère	245
69	Basic tomato preparation (*tomate concassée*)	257
24	Braised onions (*oignons braisés*)	232
29	Braised red cabbage (*choux à la flamande*)	235
34	Broad beans (*fèves*)	237
31	Broccoli	236
64	Buttered celeriac, turnips or swedes	255
25	Caramelised button onions	233
50	Cauliflower au gratin (*chou-fleur mornay*)	246
51	Cauliflower polonaise (*chou-fleur polonaise*)	247
55	Chinese vegetables and noodles	248
60	Coleslaw	252
36	Corn on the cob (*maïs*)	238
42	Courgette and potato cakes with mint and feta cheese	242

54	Deep-fried sea weed	248
40	Deep-fried courgettes (*courgettes frites*)	240
43	Fettuccini of courgette with chopped basil and balsamic vinegar	243
47	Globe artichokes (*artichauts en branche*)	245
67	Goats' cheese and beetroot tarts, with salad of rocket	256
62	Golden beetroot with Parmesan	254
61	Greek-style mushrooms (*champignons à la grecque*)	253
33	Ladies' fingers (okra) in cream sauce (*okra à la crème*)	237
35	Mangetout	238
57	Onion bhajias	250
65	Parsnips (*panais*)	255
32	Peas French-style (*petit pois à la française*)	236
68	Pickled red cabbage	257
27	Poached fennel	234
37	Ratatouille	238
52	Roast butternut squash	247
26	Roast garlic	233
66	Salsify (*salsifi*)	256
49	Sauté of wild mushrooms	246
53	Sea kale (*chou de mer*)	247
45	Shallow-fried chicory (*endive meunière*)	244
39	Shallow-fried courgettes (*courgettes sautées*)	240

44	Spiced aubergine purée	243
30	Spinach purée (*epinards en purée*)	235
28	Stir-fried cabbage with mushrooms and beansprouts	234
38	Stuffed aubergine (*aubergine farcie*)	239
41	Stuffed tomatoes (*tomates farcies*)	241
58	Tempura	250
59	Vegetarian strudel	251
63	Vichy carrots (*carottes Vichy*)	254
Pulses		
70	Bean goulash	258
73	Dhal	260
72	Hummus (chickpea and sesame seed paste)	259
71	Mexican bean pot	259
Textured vegetable protein		
76	Barbecued tofu	262
75	Crispy deep-fried tofu	261
74	Oriental stir-fry Quorn	261
Salads		
82	Caesar salad	266
77	Haricot bean salad (*salade de haricots blancs*)	263
78	Niçoise salad	263
79	Potato salad (*salade de pommes de terre*)	264
80	Vegetable salad (Russian salad) (*salade de légumes/salade russe*)	265
81	Waldorf salad	265

Fruit

Quality requirements and purchasing points

Fresh fruit should be:

- whole and fresh looking (for maximum flavour the fruit must be ripe but not overripe)
- firm, according to type and variety
- clean, and free from traces of pesticides and fungicides
- free from external moisture
- free from any unpleasant foreign smell or taste
- free from pests or disease

- sufficiently mature; it must be capable of being handled and travelling without being damaged
- free from any defects characteristic of the variety in shape, size and colour
- free of bruising and any other damage due to weather conditions.

Soft fruits deteriorate quickly, especially if they are not sound. Take care to see that they are not damaged or overripe when purchased. Soft fruits should look fresh; there should be no signs of wilting, shrinking or mould. The colour of certain soft fruits is an indication of their ripeness (e.g. strawberries or dessert gooseberries).

Storage

Hard fruits, such as apples, should be left in boxes and kept in a cool store. Soft fruits, such as raspberries and strawberries, should be left in their punnets or baskets in a cold room. Stone fruits, such as apricots and plumbs, are best placed in trays so that any damaged fruit can be seen and discarded. Peaches and citrus fruits are left in their delivery trays or boxes. Bananas should not be stored in too cold a place because their skins will turn black.

Fruit recipes also appear in other chapters, for example in chutneys and sauces (in Chapter 8) and desserts (in Chapters 14 and 15).

Vegetables

Classification

Vegetable is a culinary term that generally refers to the edible part of a plant. The definition is traditional rather than scientific and so is not always exact. All parts of herbaceous plants (plants that have leaves and stems that die down at the end of the growing season) eaten as food by humans are normally considered to be vegetables. Although mushrooms actually belong to the biological family of fungi, they are also commonly considered to be vegetables.

In general, vegetables are thought of as being savoury, rather than sweet, although there are many exceptions (e.g. parsnips, sweet potatoes, pumpkin). Vegetables are eaten in a variety of ways, as part of main meals (served with poultry, meat or fish), as an ingredient and as snacks. Nuts, grains, herbs, spices and culinary fruits are not normally considered to be vegetables. Some vegetables are botanically (scientifically) classed as fruits, e.g. tomatoes and avocados, but both are commonly used as vegetables because they are not sweet. Since 'vegetable' is not a botanical term, there is no contradiction in referring to a plant part as a fruit when it is also considered to be a vegetable. You can find out more about sweet fruits and how to use them in cooking in chapters 14 and 15.

Vegetables can also include leaves (lettuce), stems (asparagus), roots (carrots), flowers (broccoli), bulbs (garlic), seeds (peas and beans) and botanical fruits such as cucumbers, squash, pumpkins and capsicums.

Nutritional value

The nutritional content of different types of vegetables varies considerably. With the exception of pulses, vegetables do not contain much protein or fat. They contain water-soluble vitamins like vitamin B and vitamin C, fat-soluble vitamins including vitamin A and vitamin D, as well as carbohydrates and minerals. Root vegetables contain starch or sugar for energy, a small but valuable amount of protein, some mineral salts and vitamins. They are also useful sources of cellulose (fibre) and water. Green vegetables are rich in mineral salts and vitamins, particularly vitamin C and carotene. The greener the leaf, the larger the quantity of vitamins it contains. The chief mineral salts are calcium and iron.

Fresh vegetables are important both from an economic and nutritional point of view. They are an important part of our diet, so it is essential to pay attention to quality, purchasing, storage and efficient preparation and cooking if their nutritional content is to be conserved.

Purchasing and selection

The purchasing of vegetables is affected by:

- the perishable nature of the product
- varying availability owing to seasonal fluctuations, and supply and demand
- the effects of preservation (e.g. freezing, drying, canning vegetables).

Automation: The use of machinery to do a task (e.g. packaging) automatically, removing or reducing the need for manpower.

The fact that vegetables are very perishable (do not stay fresh for very long) causes particular problems. Fresh vegetables are living organisms and will lose quality quickly if they are not properly stored and handled. Automation in harvesting and packaging procedures speeds up the handling process and helps retain quality.

Quality and purchasing points

The EU vegetable quality grading system is:

- **Extra class:** produce of the highest quality
- **Class 1:** produce of good quality
- **Class 2:** produce of reasonably good quality
- **Class 3:** produce of low market quality.

Root vegetables must be:

- clean, free from soil
- firm, not soft or spongy
- sound and free from blemishes
- of an even size and shape.

Green vegetables must be absolutely fresh and have leaves that are bright in colour, crisp and not wilted. In addition:

- cabbage and Brussels sprouts should be compact and firm
- cauliflowers should have closely grown flowers, a firm white head and not too much stalk or too many outer leaves
- peas and beans should be crisp and of medium size; pea pods should be full and beans not stringy
- blanched stems must be firm, white, crisp and free from soil.

Storage

Many root and non-root vegetables that grow underground can be stored over winter in a root cellar or other similarly cool, dark and dry place, to prevent the growth of mould, greening and sprouting. It is important to understand the properties and vulnerabilities of the particular roots to be stored (what will help them to last longer and what will damage them quickly). These vegetables can last through to early spring and be almost as nutritious as when they were fresh.

Vulnerabilities: Weaknesses; ways in which something may be exposed to injury or harm.

During storage, leafy vegetables lose moisture and vitamin C. They should be stored for as short a time as possible in a cool place in a container, such as a plastic bag or a sealed plastic container.

Storage points

- Store all vegetables in a cool, dry, well-ventilated room at an even temperature of 4–8°C, which will help to minimise spoilage. Check vegetables daily and discard any that are unsound.
- Remove root vegetables from their sacks and store in bins or racks.
- Store green vegetables on well-ventilated racks.
- Store salad vegetables in a cool place and leave in their containers.
- Store frozen vegetables at −18°C or below. Check for use-by dates, damaged packages and any signs of freezer burn.
- The fresher the vegetables, the better the flavour, so ideally they should not be stored at all. However, as storage is often necessary, then it should be for the shortest time possible.
- Green vegetables lose vitamin C quickly if they are bruised, damaged, stored for too long or overcooked.

Health, safety and hygiene

For information on maintaining a safe and secure working environment, a professional and hygienic appearance, clean food production areas, equipment and utensils, and food hygiene, please refer to Chapters 2 and 3. Additional health and safety points are as follows.

- If vegetables are stored at the incorrect temperature micro-organisms may develop.
- If vegetables are stored in damp conditions, moulds may develop.
- To prevent bacteria from raw vegetables passing on to cooked vegetables, store them in separate areas.
- Thaw out frozen vegetables correctly and *never* refreeze them once they have thawed out.

Preparing and cooking vegetable dishes

Approximate times only are given in the recipes in this chapter for cooking vegetables – quality, age, freshness and size all affect the length of cooking time required. Young, freshly picked vegetables will need to be cooked for a shorter time than vegetables that have been allowed to grow older and that may have been stored after picking.

Boiling and blanching

As a general rule, all root vegetables (except new potatoes) are put in cold salted water, which is then heated until boiling. Vegetables that grow above the ground are put directly into boiling salted water, so they are cooked for the minimum amount of time. Cooking them as quickly as possible helps them to keep their flavour, food value and colour.

Delicate vegetables – particularly green vegetables – must be blanched in salted boiling water and then refreshed in ice-cold water to stop the cooking process. The main reason for this is because, between the temperatures of 66°C and 77°C, chlorophyll (the pigment in green plants) is unstable. To keep the colour of the vegetables it is important to get through this temperature zone as quickly as possible.

Steaming and stir-frying

All vegetables cooked by boiling may also be cooked by steaming. The vegetables are prepared in exactly the same way as for boiling, then placed into steamer trays, lightly seasoned with salt and steamed under pressure. As with boiling, they should be cooked for the minimum period of time in order to conserve maximum food value and retain colour. High-speed steam cookers are ideal for this purpose and, because they cook so quickly, can be used for batch cooking (cooking in small quantities throughout the service) so that large quantities do not have to be cooked prior to service, then refreshed and reheated.

Many vegetables can be cooked from raw by stir-frying, which is a quick and nutritious method of cooking.

Pulses and lentils

Cook pulses and lentils in sparkling bottled water. The motion of the bubbles helps them to cook evenly. Also, bottled water contains less calcium than tap water. Calcium blocks the pores of pulses, causing beans to 'boil in their jackets', so the jackets burst and the pulses are less attractive and less tasty. Bottled water passes through the tiny pores and cooks the bean evenly without bursting the skin.

Cuts of vegetables

The size to which vegetables are cut may vary according to their use; however, the shape does not change.

Julienne (strips):

- Cut the vegetables into 2 cm lengths (short julienne).
- Cut the lengths into thin slices.
- Cut the slices into thin strips.
- Double the length gives a long julienne, used for garnishing (e.g. salads, meats, fish, poultry dishes).

Brunoise (small dice):

- Cut the vegetables into convenient-sized lengths.
- Cut the lengths into 2 mm slices.
- Cut the slices into 2 mm strips.
- Cut the strips into 2 mm squares.

Macédoine (½ cm dice):

- Cut the vegetables into convenient lengths.
- Cut the lengths into ½ cm slices.
- Cut the slices into ½ cm strips.
- Cut the strips into ½ cm squares.

Jardinière (batons):

- Cut the vegetables into 1½ cm lengths.
- Cut the lengths into 3 mm slices.
- Cut the slices into batons (3 × 3 × 18 mm).

Paysanne: there are at least four accepted methods of cutting paysanne. In order to cut

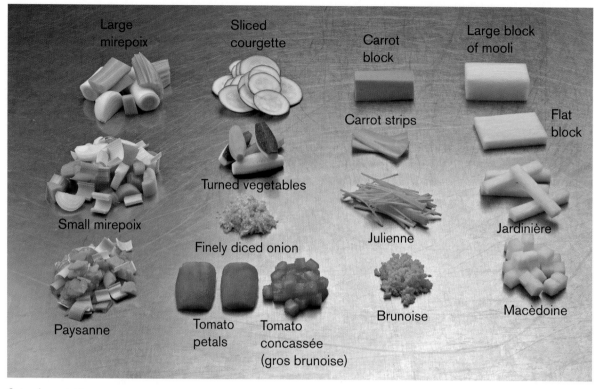

Cuts of vegetables

economically, the shape of the vegetables should dictate which method to choose. All are cut thinly. Options include:

- 1 cm sided triangles
- 1 cm sided squares
- 1 cm diameter rounds
- 1 cm diameter rough-sided rounds.

Concassée means roughly chopped (e.g. skinned and deseeded tomatoes are roughly chopped for many food preparations – see recipe 69).

Cutting vegetables into gros brunoise
http://bit.ly/ySdUEu

Cutting vegetables into macédoine
http://bit.ly/AOoPrD

Cutting vegetables into paysanne
http://bit.ly/yR3COz

Potatoes

Potatoes are tubers. A tuber is a fleshy, food-storing swelling at the tip of an underground stem of a plant. Potatoes have white, brown, purple or red skin, and white or golden flesh.

Potato varieties

Several named varieties of potato are grown in Britain and these will be available according to the season. The different varieties have differing characteristics and some are more suitable for certain methods of cooking than others (see Table 9.1).

Table 9.1 Potato varieties and recommended cooking methods

Variety	Cooking method
Cara	boil, bake, chip, wedge
Charlotte	boil, salad use
Desiree	boil, roast, bake, chip, mash, wedge
Golden Wonder	boil, roast, crisps
King Edward	boil, bake, roast, mash, chip
Maris Piper	boil, roast, bake, chip
Pink Fir Apple	boil, salad use
Premiere	boil
Record	make into crisps
Romano	boil, bake, roast, mash
Saxon	boil, bake, chip
Wilja	boil, bake, chip, mash

Common potato cooking styles

During cooking, the starch in the potato starts to absorb water and swell in size. Potatoes need to be cooked long enough for the starch to soften (gelatinise), or they will look and taste undercooked.

This section describes what happens to the potato when it is cooked in three common styles.

Baked

For the best baked potatoes, long slow cooking is best. The skin becomes very crisp and turns darker because the starch just below the skin converts to sugar, which browns in heat. Make sure you cut a slit in the potato as soon as it comes out of the oven so the inside doesn't steam, as this makes the potato a heavier consistency.

Mashed

The starch in the potatoes absorbs water and swells during the cooking process. Then, when the potato is mashed or riced, the cells break open, releasing more starch, which makes the potatoes creamy and smooth. When you boil potatoes for mashing, return them to the hot pan after draining and shake over a medium heat for 2–3 minutes to dry the potatoes. Whatever cooking method you use, add butter when you begin mashing.

The butter coats the cells and the starch so they absorb less liquid, making the potatoes fluffier and less gluey. The slower the potato is cooked the better for the starch as it has more structure in the final mixing process, allowing the potato to hold in more fat/liquid than if cooked by the more traditional quicker method.

A quick tip on the cooking of mash

Bring the potatoes up to the boil from cold as normal and boil for 2–3 minutes. Remove and rinse in cold water, then repeat the process of boiling from cold and turn the heat down to below a simmer. This will obviously take longer but will reduce the water absorption rate dramatically and help to give you fluffier mash.

Roast

Roast potatoes are simply cut into chunks and parboiled slowly until just cooked on the inside. Drain and toss in a liberal amount of olive oil or other vegetable oil and seasoning, then roast at a hot oven (220°C) for 15 minutes. Then turn the temperature down to 180°C and baste every 5 minutes to ensure a crisp coat all over. Once cooked, serve immediately, as keeping them warm for too long will cause the inside to steam, making the outside soft and leathery.

Purchasing, selection and storage

Purchasing

Inspect and select your potatoes before buying or on delivery. Choose firm, smooth ones. Avoid excessively wrinkled, withered, cracked potatoes, and do not to buy those that have a lot of sprouts or green areas.

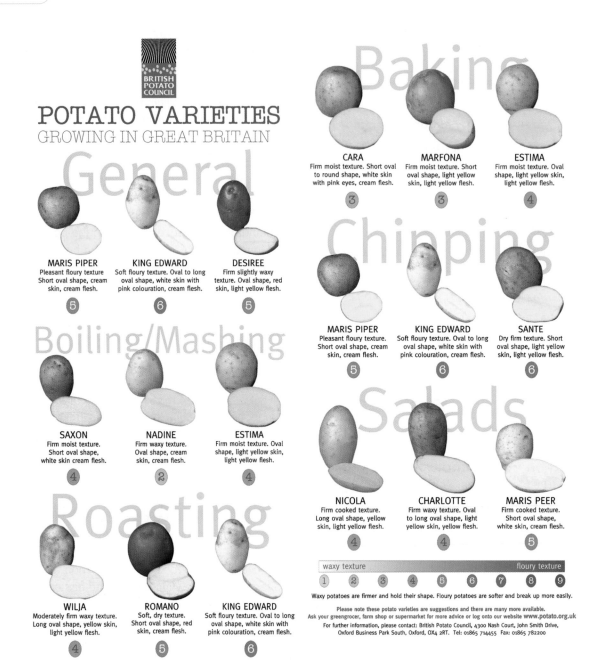

POTATO VARIETIES
GREAT BRITAIN

General

MARIS PIPER
Pleasant floury texture Short oval shape, cream skin, cream flesh.
5

KING EDWARD
Soft floury texture. Oval to long oval shape, white skin with pink colouration, cream flesh.
6

DESIREE
Firm slightly waxy texture. Oval shape, red skin, light yellow flesh.
5

Boiling/Mashing

SAXON
Firm moist texture. Short oval shape, white skin cream flesh.
4

NADINE
Firm waxy texture. Oval shape, cream skin, cream flesh.
2

ESTIMA
Firm moist texture. Oval shape, light yellow skin, light yellow flesh.
4

Roasting

WILJA
Moderately firm waxy texture. Long oval shape, yellow skin, light yellow flesh.
4

ROMANO
Soft, dry texture. Short oval shape, red skin, cream flesh.
5

KING EDWARD
Soft floury texture. Oval to long oval shape, white skin with pink colouration, cream flesh.
6

Baking

CARA
Firm moist texture. Short oval to round shape, white skin with pink eyes, cream flesh.
3

MARFONA
Firm moist texture. Short oval shape, light yellow skin, light yellow flesh.
3

ESTIMA
Oval shape, light yellow skin, light yellow flesh.
4

Chipping

MARIS PIPER
Pleasant floury texture. Short oval shape, cream skin, cream flesh.
5

KING EDWARD
Soft floury texture. Oval to long oval shape, white skin with pink colouration, cream flesh.
6

SANTE
Dry firm texture. Short oval shape, light yellow skin, light yellow flesh.
6

Salads

NICOLA
Firm cooked texture. Long oval shape, yellow skin, light yellow flesh.
4

CHARLOTTE
Firm waxy texture. Oval to long oval shape, light yellow skin, yellow flesh.
4

MARIS PEER
Firm cooked texture. Short oval shape, white skin, cream flesh.
5

waxy texture								floury texture
1	2	3	4	5	6	7	8	9

Waxy potatoes are firmer and hold their shape. Floury potatoes are softer and break up more easily.

Please note these potato varieties are suggestions and there are many more available.
Ask your greengrocer, farm shop or supermarket for more advice or log onto our website www.potato.org.uk
For further information, please contact: British Potato Council, 4300 Nash Court, John Smith Drive,
Oxford Business Park South, Oxford, OX4 2RT. Tel: 01865 714455 Fax: 01865 782200

Varieties of potato (Potato Council)

Selection

It is essential to select potatoes carefully to suit the purpose they are to be used for, as the variety chosen (see Table 9.1) will affect the end product.

Cooked potatoes may have different textures, depending on whether they are 'waxy' or 'floury' varieties. This is due to changes that happen to the potato cells during cooking. 'Waxy' potatoes are translucent and may feel moist and pasty. 'Floury' potatoes are brighter, look more grainy and feel drier. These differences affect the performance of the potato when cooked in different ways (e.g. boiling versus roasting).

Floury potatoes

Floury potatoes are especially popular in the UK. They are suitable for baking, mashing and chipping as they have a soft, dry texture when cooked. They are not suitable for boiling, however, because they tend to disintegrate. Popular varieties of floury potato include King Edward and Maris Piper.

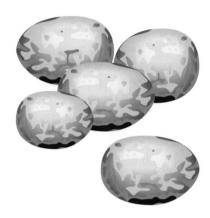

Floury potatoes

Waxy potatoes

These are more solid than floury potatoes and hold their shape when boiled, but do not mash well. They are particularly suitable for baked and layered potato dishes such as boulangère potatoes. Popular varieties include Cara and Charlotte.

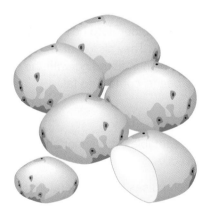

Waxy potatoes

Storage

You can store potatoes for several months without affecting their quality, but they should be stored at a constant temperature (3°C). If this is not possible, buying fresh potatoes regularly is best practice. There are three essential rules to bear in mind when storing potatoes: 'dry, dark and cool'. You should avoid light as this will cause sprouting and eventually the greening effect that contains mild toxins; if you have inadvertently purchased potatoes with this green tinge, remove the green bits and the rest of the potato is then fine to use.

Food value

Potatoes are a good source of vitamin C; they also contain iron, calcium, thiamin, nicotine acid, protein and fibre.

Yield

- ½ kg of old potatoes will yield approximately 3 portions.
- ½ kg of new potatoes will yield approximately 4 portions.
- 1½ kg of old potatoes will yield approximately 10 portions.
- 1¼ kg of new potatoes will yield approximately 10 portions.

Ready prepared potatoes

Potatoes can be bought in many convenience forms: peeled, turned, cut into various shapes for frying, or scooped into balls (Parisienne) or an olive shape.

Chips are available fresh, frozen, chilled or vacuum packed.

Frozen potatoes are available as croquettes, hash browns, sauté and roast.

Mashed potato powder is also available.

The advantages of using ready prepared potatoes are that they are labour saving and reduce wastage. However, they cost more than fresh potatoes and may not taste as good.

Pulses

The term 'pulse' refers to annual crops harvested solely for the dry grain, with between 1 and 12 grains or seeds per pod (these can be any size, shape or colour). This therefore excludes green beans and green peas, which are considered vegetable crops. Also excluded are crops that are grown mainly for their oil (oilseeds like soybeans and peanuts), and crops that are used only for sowing (e.g. clovers, alfalfa).

Pulses are important food crops because they contain a lot of protein and essential amino acids. They contain double the amount of protein found in wheat and three times that found in rice. Pulses are sometimes called 'poor man's meat'. Pulse protein is equivalent in quality to soy protein, which has been shown by the World Health Organization to be the equal of meat, milk and egg proteins.

All pulses, except for soybeans (also known as soya beans), are very similar in nutritional content. They are rich in protein, carbohydrate and fibre, and low in fat. The fat they do contain is mostly unsaturated fat. They are also important sources of some B vitamins. Fresh pulses contain vitamin C, but this reduces once they are harvested and virtually all of it is lost from dried pulses. Canned pulses, however, retain about half their vitamin C, and frozen peas will still contain about three-quarters of their vitamin C. With the exception of canned, processed peas (which have been dried before canning), canning doesn't affect protein content, eliminates the need for soaking and considerably reduces cooking time compared with dried pulses.

One advantage of dried pulses is that they store very well for long periods if kept in a dry, airtight container away from the light. However, it is best to eat them as fresh as possible. Pulses toughen when they are stored, and older ones will take longer to cook. Allow about 55 g dry weight per person – once soaked and cooked they will at least double in weight. Most dried pulses need soaking for several hours before they can be cooked; exceptions are all lentils, green and yellow split peas, black-eyed beans and mung beans.

Soaking times vary from 4–12 hours. It is usually most convenient to soak pulses overnight. Always discard the soaking water, rinse the pulses and cook them in fresh water without any salt (salt toughens the skins and makes for longer cooking). Changing the water will also help to reduce the flatulence some people suffer after eating pulses; adding of a pinch of aniseed, caraway, dill or fennel seeds is also supposed to help with this.

Soya beans should be soaked for at least 12 hours, drained and rinsed then covered with fresh water and brought to the boil. Soya beans should be boiled for the first hour of cooking. They can then be simmered for the remaining 2–3 hours that it takes to cook them.

Warning	
It is not safe to eat raw or undercooked kidney beans and soya beans.	

Food value

Pulses are a good source of protein and carbohydrate, and therefore help to provide the body with energy. They also contain iron and vitamin B, are high in fibre and, with the exception of the soya beans, contain no fat.

Storage

As with all vegetables, it is important to store pulses correctly.

- Store fresh pulses in a refrigerator at a temperature below 5°C.
- Store frozen pulses in a freezer at a temperature below −18°C.
- Store dried pulses in clean airtight containers off the floor in the dry store.
- Unpack tinned pulses and check that the tins are sound and undamaged.

Health, safety and hygiene

For information on health and safety and food hygiene, please refer to Chapters 2 and 3. Additional health and safety points for pulses are as follows.

- Always check pulses for food pests (e.g. flour moths) and any foreign matter (stones, etc.).
- When storing cooked pulses, keep them covered and in a refrigerator at a temperature below 5°C.
- To prevent risk of cross-contamination, store cooked pulses away from any raw foods.

Types of pulses

There is a huge variety of pulses available that can be used in many different ways.

Beans

- **Aduki:** small, round, deep red, shiny, nutty and sweet (the flavour used in oriental confectionery).
- **Black:** glistening black skins, creamy flesh.
- **Black-eyed:** small white beans with a savoury, creamy flavour, and with a black 'scar' where they were joined to the pod. Used a lot in American and African cooking, they are the essential ingredient in the traditional southern-style dish 'Hoppin John' – a mixture of black-eyed beans, bacon and white rice traditionally eaten on New Year's Day.
- **Broad:** also known as fava beans, strongly flavoured.
- **Borlotti:** Italian beans with a mild bittersweet flavour; they're used in regional stews and often mixed with rice, and are particularly good in soups such as minestrone and *pasta e fagioli*.
- **Butter:** also known as lima beans, available large or small.
- **Cannellini:** Italian haricot beans, slightly larger than the UK version.
- **Dutch brown:** light brown in colour.
- **Flageolet:** pale green, kidney-shaped with a delicate flavour.

- **Ful mesdames:** also known as Egyptian brown beans; small, brown and knobbly, known as the field bean in the UK.
- **Haricot:** white, smooth and oval; used for baked beans.
- **Mung beans:** small, olive green in colour, good flavour, available split, whole and skinless. Widely used sprouted for their shoots.
- **Pinto beans:** the original ingredient of Mexican refried beans; an orange-pink bean with rust-coloured specks that grows freely across Latin America and throughout the American southwest; the bean is creamy-white in colour, with a fluffy texture when cooked, and is good in soups, salads and rich stews.
- **Red kidney beans:** normally dark red-brown, this kidney-shaped bean holds its shape and colour and is therefore great in mixed bean salads and stews, including the traditional chilli con carne. Dried kidney beans need to be cooked carefully – soak for at least eight hours; after soaking, drain and rinse them, discarding the soaking water; put them into a pan with cold water to cover and bring to the boil – the beans must be boiled for 10 minutes to destroy toxins; after this, simmer until cooked (approximately 45–60 minutes). The beans should have an even, creamy texture throughout – if the centre is still hard and white, they require longer cooking.
- **Soissons:** finest haricot beans.
- **Soy:** soybeans (or soya beans) are very high in nutrients, especially protein, and they contain all the essential amino acids. They are processed into many forms: soy flour, TVP (meat substitute), tofu (curd), oils, margarine, soya milk and soy sauce.

Peas

- **Blue:** also known as marrowfat peas; pleasant flavour, floury texture, retain shape when cooked.
- **Chickpeas:** shaped like hazelnuts, they have a tasty nutty flavour when cooked. Chickpeas are used all over the world in dishes such as the Indian kabli chana or Spanish caldo gallego.

Chickpeas are a key ingredient of hummus – a traditional Greek dip of cooked chickpeas, tahini, oil and garlic. They can be bought dried and then soaked, but canned chickpeas do just as well for most recipes.

- **Split green:** a sweeter variety than the blue pea; cook to a purée easily.
- **Split yellow:** cook to a purée easily.

Both yellow and green split peas are used for vegetable purées and soups.

Lentils

Lentils, varying in size and colour, can form a nutritious basis for a meal. Larger brown or green lentils retain their shape during cooking and are particularly good in soups. Red and yellow lentils cook down well, can be puréed and are used a great deal in Indian cooking, such as in dhal. Tiny green puy lentils have a distinctive flavour and also keep their shape and colour when cooked.

- **Orange:** several types, which vary in size and shade and may be sold whole or split.
- **Green or continental:** retain shape after cooking, available in small or large varieties.
- **Yellow:** of Asian origin, often used as a dhal accompaniment to curry dishes.
- **Red:** purée easily, used for soups, stews etc.
- **Indian brown:** red lentils from which the seed coat has not been removed; they purée easily.
- **Puy:** dark French lentils, varied in size, retain their shape when cooked and are considered the best of their type.
- **Dhal:** the Hindi word for dried peas and beans.

Using pulses

Pulses are one of the most versatile commodities. They can be used extensively in a wide range of dishes. Imaginative and experimental use of different herbs, spices, flavourings and vegetables can give individual variation to the pulse recipes. Several pulse recipes are presented in this book, including recipes 69–72 in this chapter.

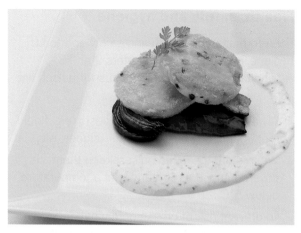

Polenta and lentil cakes with roasted vegetables, served with cucumber and yoghurt sauce (recipe available on Dynamic Learning)

> **Versatile:** Having many different uses; able to be adapted or changed for use in many different ways.

Cooking

Some pulses require pre-soaking in cold water before cooking; the soaking time will vary according the type and quality and the length of time they have been stored.

For soaking, pulses should be amply covered with cold water (they will expand gradually) and kept in a cold place. In some cases this may be for a few hours; in others it may be overnight, in which case they should be stored in the refrigerator at a temperature below 5°C. After soaking, salt should *not* be added before or during the cooking as this causes the pulses to toughen. However, salt may be added if required towards the end of the cooking process.

 ACTIVITY

1 What are pulses?
2 List three different types of pulse
3 How should pulses be stored?
4 Name two dishes in which pulses are used

The vegetarian diet

According to the Vegetarian Society, vegetarians who eat milk products and eggs enjoy excellent health. Vegetarian diets can be perfectly healthy and can meet the recommended dietary allowances for nutrients. You can get enough protein from a vegetarian diet as long as the variety of foods and the amounts consumed are adequate. Meat, fish and poultry are important sources of iron, zinc and B vitamins in most diets, and vegetarians need to pay special attention to getting enough of these nutrients.

What vegetarians need to eat every day

Here's a quick summary from the Vegetarian Society of what vegetarians need to eat every day:

- 4 or 5 servings of fruit and vegetables
- 3 or 4 servings of cereals/grains or potatoes
- 2 or 3 servings of pulses, nuts and seeds
- 2 servings of milk, cheese, eggs or soya products (e.g. tofu)
- a small amount of vegetable oil, margarine or butter
- some yeast extract that has been fortified with vitamin B12.

A guide to vegetarian proteins

Here's a quick rundown of vegetarian foods that are high in protein, as well as a few suggestions on how to make the most of them.

Dairy products

Milk

Different types of milk can be used for different dishes. There are options other than cows' milk and soya milk, a few of which are discussed below.

- **Buttermilk** is excellent in baked goods, and also as a soup and salad dressing base. It gives a rich, hearty flavour with fewer calories than milk or cream. The tangy flavour of buttermilk goes well with sweet fruits such as peaches, cherries and pears, particularly as crème fraîche. The acidic properties of buttermilk make it an effective and flavourful marinade, particularly with poultry. It is used in baked goods to help prevent the dingy greyish discolouring (caused by a chemical reaction) often found in blueberries, walnuts and other foods with a blue cast. It also helps to brown baked goods and improves texture.

- **Condensed milk** is a generic term for milk that has had 60 per cent of its water removed by evaporation. With sweetened condensed milk, great quantities of sugar are added first, accounting for 40–45 per cent of the total volume before **evaporation**. Once all the water is removed, it is a very sticky and sweet mixture. Unsweetened condensed milk, however, is simply called **evaporated milk**.

- **Goats' milk** can be an excellent alternative to cows' milk as it contains many of the same nutrients found in cows' milk. It is a very good source of calcium and protein, phosphorous, riboflavin (vitamin B2) and potassium. Perhaps the greatest benefit of goat's milk, however, is that many people who are allergic to cows' milk can drink goats' milk without risk.

Cream

There are other cream options apart from the more usual double or single varieties.

- **Soured cream** contains 18 per cent fat and is soured by adding bacteria cultures to it, which grow until the cream is both soured and thick. It is then pasteurised to stop the process.

- **Crème fraîche** is soured cream with a higher fat content.

Yoghurt

Yoghurt is a cultured milk product made from cows', ewes', goats' or buffalo milk. This means that it has been fermented with bacteria that make lactic acid, which gives the yoghurt its sour taste. It is available plain (which can be used in both sweet and savoury dishes) or in a variety of fruit flavours.

Butter

As well as being used in its more traditional form, butter can be changed to a form called **ghee** to be used in cooking. Ghee is clarified butter without any solid particles or water. It is used in India and throughout South Asia in daily cooking. A good-quality ghee adds a great aroma, flavour and taste to food. Ghee can be a great asset for people who are on a low-fat diet since even a modest quantity of ghee can add a lot of flavour to food compared with other oil or fat products.

When ghee is produced 'properly' (see page 144 for instructions on how to clarify butter), all of the water is completely evaporated from the butter. To check whether all the water has evaporated completely, pour some heated ghee onto a small piece of paper. Light the paper so that it burns. If you hear a crackling noise, this indicates the presence of water. Heat the butter some more to get rid of any remaining water. With experience you will be able to tell if ghee is 'done', by examining its smell and colour.

Ghee can also be bought ready made. It is generally available in the 'ethnic' section of any big grocery store or in any Indian/South Asian store. Be sure to buy ghee that comes from an animal such as a cow; do not buy an artificial ghee made by hydrogenating vegetable oil.

Cheese

Dairy products are an important source of calcium as well as protein, but be careful not to eat too much cheese as it has a high fat content – make sure you eat plenty of pulses too.

Vegetarian cheese made using non-animal rennet (an ingredient often used in cheese making) is now widely available, so look out for the words 'suitable for vegetarians' on the packet or, if buying from a cheese-monger, ask if it is suitable.

Meat substitutes

Textured vegetable protein (TVP)

This is a meat substitute manufactured from protein derived from wheat, oats, cottonseed, soybeans and other sources. The main source of

A note on Parmesan

Unfortunately, there is no such thing as vegetarian Parmesan, so the recipes in this chapter that use it are not, strictly speaking, truly vegetarian. Although dishes including Parmesan may be acceptable to, say, semi-vegetarians and those who prefer to avoid meat, they are not suitable for strict vegetarians. Use vegetarian Cheddar as a substitute ingredient where possible. If Parmesan is being used to garnish a finished dish, offer it separately if you can so that diners can choose for themselves whether or not they wish to add it

TVP is the soybean, because of its high protein content.

TVP is used mainly as a meat extender, to make meat go further. The TVP content can vary from 10 to 60 per cent replacement of fresh meat. Some caterers on very tight budgets use it, but it is mainly used in food manufacturing. By partially replacing the meat in certain dishes – such as casseroles, stews, pies, pasties, sausage rolls, hamburgers, meat loaf and pâté – it is possible to reduce costs, meet nutritional targets and serve food that looks acceptable.

Soya protein can also be useful in making vegetarian dishes.

Myco-protein

A meat substitute such as Quorn (see below) is produced from a plant that is a distant relative of the mushroom. This myco-protein contains protein and fibre, and is the result of a fermentation process similar to the way yoghurt is made. It may be used as an alternative to chicken or beef or in vegetarian dishes.

Quorn

Quorn is a low-fat food that can be used in a variety of dishes (e.g. oriental stir-fry). Quorn does not shrink during preparation and cooking. Quorn mince or pieces can be substituted for chicken or minced meats. Its mild savoury flavour means that it complements the herbs and spices in a recipe and it is able to absorb flavour. Frozen Quorn may be cooked straight from the freezer or may be defrosted overnight in the refrigerator. Once thawed, it must be stored in the refrigerator and used within 24 hours. A recipe for stir-fried Quorn appears later in this chapter (recipe 73). Quorn is a low-fat, high-protein food.

Other sources of protein

Eggs

There are many varieties of eggs available, including:

- hens' eggs
- quails' eggs
- ducks' eggs
- goose eggs
- turkey eggs
- gulls' eggs.

Grains, rice and cereals

There are many varieties of grains and cereals available, including:

- wheat (whole, cracked, bulgar, flakes, bran, germ, semolina, couscous)
- buckwheat
- barley
- corn (or maize – sweetcorn, popcorn, polenta)
- millet
- oats
- rye
- quinoa.

Rice

There are many varieties of rice available, including:

- white
- brown
- white and black sticky rice

- white and brown long-grain rice
- Basmati rice
- white short-grain rice (also known as pudding rice)
- Thai fragrant (or jasmine) rice
- red rice
- Italian risotto rice (Arborio, Carnaroli, Vialone Nano)
- Valencia (paella) rice
- wild rice.

Nuts

There are many varieties of nuts available, including:

- almonds
- Brazil nuts
- cashew nuts
- coconuts
- hazelnuts
- macadamia nuts
- peanuts
- pecans
- pine nuts
- pistachios
- sweet chestnuts
- walnuts.

Seeds

There are many varieties of seeds available, including:

- poppy
- pumpkin
- sesame
- sunflower
- linseeds.

Test yourself

1 Suggest types of fruit that could be included in a fruit salad.
2 Name six varieties of potato suitable for roasting and boiling.
3 Describe the following cuts of vegetables:
   Macédoine
   Jardiniere
   Julienne
   Paysanne
4 Describe the preparation and cooking of braised red cabbage.
5 List two vegetarian dishes.
6 How should fresh vegetables be stored?
7 What is meant by 'blanching' of vegetables?
8 Explain what is meant by 'textured vegetable protein'.

ACTIVITY

1 Name two fruits that are used as vegetables.
2 Name one vegetable used as a fruit.
3 List four varieties of potatoes.
4 List the importance of vegetables and fruit to the diet.

---

1 Grapefruit (*pamplemousse*)

The fruit should be peeled with a sharp knife in order to remove all the white pith and yellow skin. Cut into segments and remove all the pips. The segments and the juice should then be dressed in a cocktail glass or grapefruit coupe and chilled. A cherry may be added.

Allow ½ –1 grapefruit per head.

The common practice of sprinkling with caster sugar is incorrect, as some customers prefer their grapefruit without sugar.

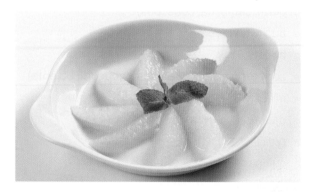

Chef's tip

Make sure all the pith is removed from the grapefruit: it tastes very bitter.

 HEALTHY EATING TIP

● This, and the following fruit dishes, contribute to the recommended five portions of fruit and vegetables per day. Include them as often as possible on the menu.

Try something different

● Grapefruit may also be served hot, sprinkled with rum and demerara sugar.
● **Grapefruit and orange cocktail**, allowing half an orange and half a grapefruit per head.
● **Orange cocktail**, using oranges in place of grapefruit.
● **Florida cocktail** – a mixture of grapefruit, orange and pineapple segments.

2 Avocado pear *(l'avocat)*

The pears must be ripe (test by pressing gently – the pear should give slightly). Allow half an avocado per portion.

1 Cut in half length-wise. Remove the stone.

2 Serve garnished with lettuce accompanied by vinaigrette or variations on vinaigrette.

Try something different

Avocado pears are sometimes filled with shrimps or crabmeat bound with a shellfish cocktail sauce or other similar fillings, and may be served hot or cold using a variety of fillings and sauces.

Avocados may also be halved lengthwise, the stone removed, the skin peeled and the flesh sliced and fanned on a plate. Garnish with a simple or composed salad.

Chef's tip

Once the avocado is open and/or peeled, it will start to discolour; to stop this from happening, brush the avocado with lemon juice.

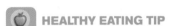 **HEALTHY EATING TIP**

- Serve with plenty of salad vegetables and bread or toast (optional butter or spread).

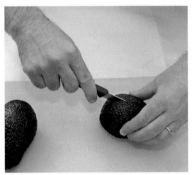

Cut the avocado in half

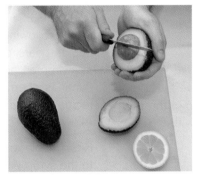

Remove the stone

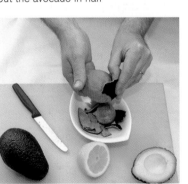

Peel the skin before slicing the avocado (if required)

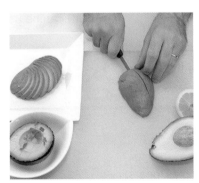

Slice the avocado

3   Fresh fruit salad *(salade de fruits)*

cal	kcal	fat	sat fat	carb	sugar	protein	fibre
493 KJ	117 kcal	0.0 g	0.0 g	30.3 g	29.5 g	0.9 g	3.0 g

	4 portions	10 portions
orange	1	2–3
dessert apple	1	2–3
dessert pear	1	2–3
cherries	50 g	125 g
grapes	50 g	125 g
banana	1	2–3
Stock syrup		
caster sugar	50 g	125 g
water	125 ml	375 ml
lemon, juice of	½	1

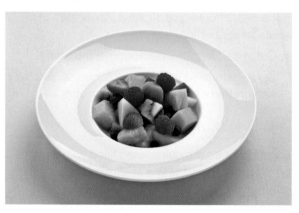

1 For the syrup, boil the sugar with the water and place in a bowl.
2 Allow to cool, add the lemon juice.
3 Peel and cut the orange into segments.
4 Quarter the apple and pear, remove the core, peel and cut each quarter into two or three slices, place in the bowl and mix with the orange.
5 Stone the cherries, leave whole.
6 Cut the grapes in half, peel if required, and remove the pips.
7 Mix carefully and place in a glass bowl in the refrigerator to chill.
8 Just before serving, peel and slice the banana and mix in.

Try something different

All the following fruits may be used: dessert apples, pears, pineapple, oranges, grapes, melon, strawberries, peaches, raspberries, apricots, bananas, cherries. Kiwi fruit, plums, mangoes (see recipe 5), pawpaws and lychees may also be used. Allow about 150 g unprepared fruit per portion.

Kirsch, Cointreau or Grand Marnier may be added to the syrup. All fruit must be ripe.

A fruit juice (e.g. apple, orange, grape or passion fruit) can be used instead of syrup.

4   Fruit cocktail

This is a mixture of fruits, such as apples, pears, pineapples, grapes and cherries, washed, peeled and cut into neat segments or dice, and added to a syrup – 100 g sugar to ¼ litre water – and the juice of half a lemon. Neatly place in cocktail glasses and chill.

Allow ½ kg unprepared fruit for four portions, 1½ kg for ten.

Variations include a tropical fruit cocktail, which uses a variety of tropical fruits, such as mango, passion fruit, lychees, pineapple and kiwi fruit.

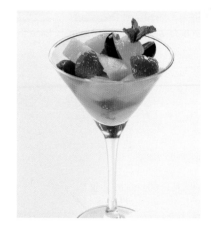

5   Tropical fruit plate

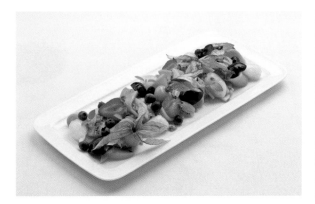

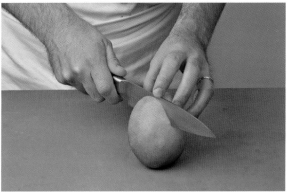

An assortment of fully ripe fruits, e.g. pineapple, papaya, mango (see photos), peeled, deseeded, cut into pieces and neatly dressed on a plate. An optional accompaniment could be yoghurt, vanilla ice cream, crème fraiche, fresh or clotted cream.

To dice a mango, first slice through it, keeping lateral to the stone

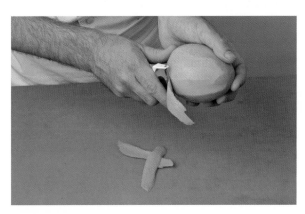

Peeling a mango

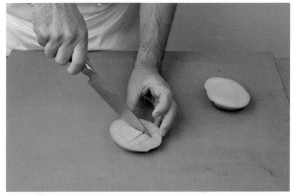

Next, score the flesh

 HEALTHY EATING TIP

- This colourful dessert helps to meet the recommended target of five portions of fruit and vegetables per day.

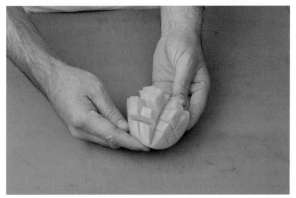

Bend out the cubes

6 Caribbean fruit curry

cal	kcal	fat	sat fat	carb	sugar	protein	fibre
1729 KJ	412 kcal	19.6 g	6.1 g	57.2 g	51.6 g	5.4 g	8.3 g

*

	4 portions	10 portions
pineapple	1 small	1 large
dessert apples	2	5
small dessert pears	2	5
mangoes	2	5
bananas	2	5
guava	1	2–3
pawpaw	1	2–3
rind and juice of lime, grated	1	2–3
onion, chopped	50 g	125 g
sunflower margarine	25 g	60 g
sunflower oil	60 ml	150 ml
Madras curry powder	50 g	125 g
wholemeal flour	25 g	60 g
ginger, freshly grated	10 g	25 g
desiccated coconut	50 g	125 g
tomato, skinned, deseeded and diced	100 g	250 g
tomato purée	25 g	60 g
yeast extract	5 g	12 g
sultanas	50 g	125 g
fruit juice	½ litre	1¼ litres
cashew nuts	50 g	125 g
single cream or smetana	60 ml	150 ml

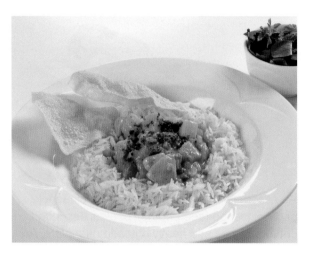

1 Skin and cut the pineapple in half, remove the tough centre. Cut into 1 cm chunks. Peel the apples and pears, remove the cores, cut into 1 cm pieces. Peel and slice the mangoes. Skin and cut the bananas into 1 cm pieces. Cut the guavas and pawpaws in half, remove the seeds, peel, dice into 1 cm pieces. Marinate the fruit in the lime juice.

2 Fry the onion in the sunflower margarine and oil until lightly brown, add the curry powder, sweat together, add the wholemeal flour and cook for 2 minutes.

3 Add the ginger, coconut, tomato concassée, tomato purée and sultanas.

4 Gradually add sufficient boiling fruit juice to make a light sauce.

5 Add yeast extract, stir well. Simmer for 10 minutes.

6 Add the sultanas, fruit juice and cashew nuts, stir carefully, allow to heat through.

7 Finish with cream or smetana.

8 Serve in a suitable dish; separately serve poppadoms, wholegrain pilaff rice and a green salad.

HEALTHY EATING TIP

- Lightly oil a well-seasoned pan with the sunflower oil to fry the onion.
- No added salt is needed.
- Try finishing the dish with low-fat yoghurt in place of the cream.
- Serve with plenty of starchy carbohydrate and salad.

* Using single cream

7 Parsley potatoes *(pommes persillées)*

cal	kcal	fat	sat fat	carb	sugar	protein	fibre	*
798 KJ	190 kcal	8.3 g	5.2 g	28.6 g	0.6 g	2.1 g	1.5 g	

1 Wash, peel and rewash the potatoes.
2 Cut or turn into even-sized pieces, allowing 2–3 pieces per portion.
3 Cook carefully in lightly salted water for approximately 20 minutes.
4 Drain well. Brush with melted butter and sprinkle with chopped parsley.

* Using 10 g butter per portion, old potatoes

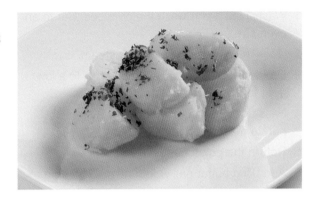

8 Duchess potatoes (basic recipe) *(pommes duchesse)*

cal	kcal	fat	sat fat	carb	sugar	protein	fibre	*
819 KJ	195 kcal	8.2 g	3.3 g	28.6 g	0.6 g	3.5 g	1.5 g	

1 Wash, peel and rewash the potatoes. Cut to an even size.
2 Cook in lightly salted water.
3 Drain off the water, cover and return to a low heat to dry out the potatoes.
4 Pass through a medium sieve or a special potato masher or mouli.
5 Place the potatoes in a clean pan.
6 Add 1 egg yolk per ½ kg and stir in vigorously with a wooden spoon.
7 Mix in 25 g butter or margarine per ½ kg. Correct the seasoning.
8 Place in a piping bag with a large star tube and pipe out into neat spirals, about 2 cm in diameter and 5 cm tall, on to a lightly greased baking sheet.
9 Place in a hot oven at 230°C for 2–3 minutes in order to firm the edges slightly.
10 Remove from the oven and brush with eggwash.
11 Brown lightly in a hot oven or under the salamander.

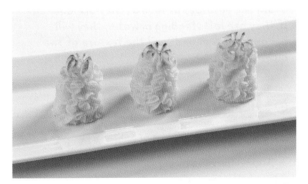

Chef's tip
At step 3, it is important to return the drained potatoes to the heat, so that they are as dry as possible.

* Using old potatoes, whole milk, hard margarine

Making duchess potatoes
http://bit.ly/zZhyQy

9 Mashed potatoes *(pommes purée)*

cal	kcal	fat	sat fat	carb	sugar	protein	fibre
763 KJ	182 kcal	7.1 g	4.4 g	29.0 g	1.1 g	2.4 g	1.5 g

*

1 Wash, peel and rewash the potatoes. Cut to an even size.

2 Cook in lightly salted water, or steam.

3 Drain off the water, cover and return to a low heat to dry out the potatoes.

4 Pass through a medium sieve or a special potato masher.

5 Return the potatoes to a clean pan.

6 Add 25 g butter per ½ kg and mix in with a wooden spoon.

7 Gradually add warm milk (30 ml), stirring continuously until a smooth creamy consistency is reached.

8 Correct the seasoning and serve.

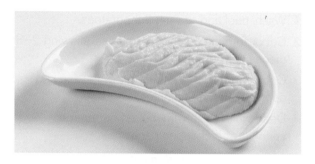

Chef's tip

Drain the potatoes as soon as they are cooked. If they are left standing in water, they will become too wet and spoil the texture of the dish.

HEALTHY EATING TIP

- Add a minimum amount of salt.
- Add a little olive oil in place of butter and semi-skimmed milk.

Try something different

Variations of mashed potatoes can be achieved by:

- dressing in a serving dish and surrounding with a cordon of fresh cream
- placing in a serving dish, sprinkling with grated cheese and melted butter, and browning under a salamander
- adding 50 g diced cooked lean ham, 25 g diced red pepper and chopped parsley
- adding lightly sweated chopped spring onions
- adding a good-quality olive oil in place of butter
- adding a little garlic juice (use a garlic press)
- adding a little fresh chopped rosemary or chives
- mixing with equal quantities of parsnip
- adding a little freshly grated horseradish or horseradish cream.

* *Using old potatoes, butter and whole milk*

10 Baked jacket potatoes (pommes au four)

cal	kcal	fat	sat fat	carb	sugar	protein	fibre	*
401 KJ	94 kcal	0.2 g	0.0 g	21.8 g	0.9 g	2.7 g	1.6 g	

1 Select good-sized potatoes; allow one potato per portion.

2 Scrub well, make a 2 mm deep incision round the potato.

3 Place the potato, on a small mound of ground (sea) salt to help keep the base dry, on a tray in a hot oven at 230–250°C for about 1 hour. Turn the potatoes over after 30 minutes.

4 Test by holding the potato in a cloth and squeezing gently; if cooked it should feel soft.

Try something different

Variations include the following.

- Split and filled with any of the following: grated cheese, minced beef or chicken, baked beans, chilli con carne, cream cheese and chives, mushrooms, bacon, ratatouille, prawns in mayonnaise, coleslaw, and so on.

- The cooked potatoes can also be cut in halves lengthwise, the potato spooned out from the skins, seasoned, mashed with butter, returned to the skins, sprinkled with grated cheese and reheated in an oven or under the grill.

* Using medium potato, 180 g analysis given per potato

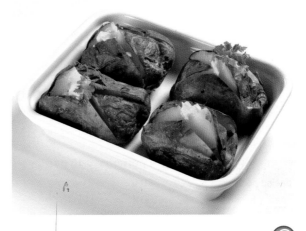

Chef's tip

Lightly scoring the potatoes will help to make sure that they cook evenly. If the potatoes are being cooked in a microwave, you must prick the skins first.

HEALTHY EATING TIP

- Oven bake without sea salt.

- Fillings based on vegetables with little or no cheese or meat make a healthy snack meal.

11 Croquette potatoes (pommes croquettes)

cal	kcal	fat	sat fat	carb	sugar	protein	fibre	*
1699 KJ	405 kcal	25.4 g	6.6 g	40.8 g	1.1 g	6.0 g	2.2 g	

1 Use a duchess mixture (see recipe 8) moulded into cylinder shapes 5 × 2 cm.

2 Pass through flour, eggwash and breadcrumbs.

3 Reshape with a palette knife and deep-fry in hot deep oil (185°C) in a frying basket.

4 When the potatoes are a golden colour, drain well and serve.

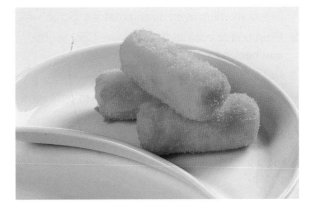

HEALTHY EATING TIP

- Add the minimum amount of salt.

- Use peanut or sunflower oil to fry the croquettes, and drain on kitchen paper.

* Using hard margarine and frying in peanut oil

---

12 Potatoes with bacon and onions (*pommes au lard*)

cal	kcal	fat	sat fat	carb	sugar	protein	fibre
836 KJ	199 kcal	10.1 g	3.8 g	22.2 g	1.8 g	6.4 g	2.5 g

	4 portions	10 portions
peeled potatoes	400 g	1¼ kg
streaky bacon (lardons)	100 g	250 g
button onions	100 g	250 g
white stock	¼ litre	600 ml
salt, pepper		
chopped parsley		

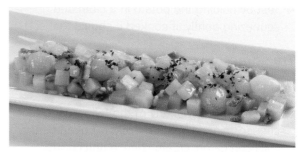

1 Cut the potatoes into 1 cm dice.

2 Cut the bacon into ½ cm lardons; lightly fry in a little fat together with the onions and brown lightly.

3 Add the potatoes, half cover with stock, season lightly with salt and pepper. Cover with a lid and cook steadily in the oven at 230–250°C for approximately 30 minutes.

4 Correct the seasoning, serve in a vegetable dish, sprinkled with chopped parsley.

* Using old potatoes

HEALTHY EATING TIP

- Dry-fry the bacon in a well-seasoned pan and drain off any excess fat.

- Add little or no salt.

---

13 Sauté potatoes (*pommes sautées*)

cal	kcal	fat	sat fat	carb	sugar	protein	fibre
1249 KJ	297 kcal	11.4 g	1.3 g	46.8 g	0.4 g	4.9 g	1.7 g

1 Select medium even-sized potatoes. Scrub well.

2 Plain boil or cook in the steamer. Cool slightly and peel.

3 Cut into 3 mm slices.

4 Toss in hot shallow oil in a frying pan until lightly coloured; season lightly with salt.

5 Serve sprinkled with chopped parsley.

Maris piper or Cara potatoes are good varieties for this dish.

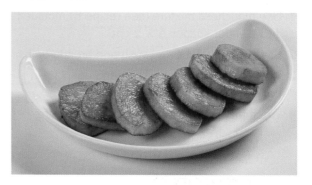

* Using old potatoes and sunflower oil

14 **Fondant potatoes *(pommes fondantes)***

cal	kcal	fat	sat fat	carb	sugar	protein	fibre
956 KJ	228 kcal	7.0 g	2.1 g	39.6 g	0.9 g	4.1 g	1.5 g

1 Select small or even-sized medium potatoes.

2 Wash, peel and rewash.

3 Turn into eight-sided barrel shapes, allowing 2–3 per portion, about 5 cm long, end diameter 1½ cm, centre diameter 2½ cm.

4 Brush with melted butter, margarine or oil.

5 Place in a pan suitable for the oven.

6 Half cover with white stock, season lightly with salt and pepper.

7 Cook in a hot oven at 230–250°C, brushing the potatoes frequently with melted butter, margarine or oil.

8 When cooked, the stock should be completely absorbed by the potatoes.

9 Brush with melted butter, margarine or oil and serve.

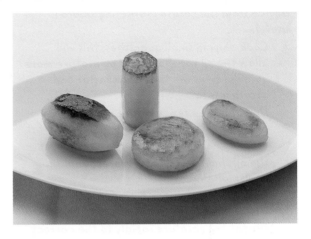

Try something different

Fondant potatoes can be lightly sprinkled with:

- thyme, rosemary or oregano (or this can be added to the stock)
- grated cheese (Gruyère and Parmesan or Cheddar)
- chicken stock in place of white stock.

Chef's tip
To give the potatoes a good glaze, use a high-quality stock and baste during cooking.

HEALTHY EATING TIP

- Use a little unsaturated oil to brush over the potatoes before and after cooking.
- No added salt is needed; rely on the stock for flavour.

* Using old potatoes and hard margarine for 1 portion (125 g raw potato)

Making fondant potatoes
http://bit.ly/yWfGg1

---

15 **Fried or chipped potatoes *(pommes frites)***

cal	kcal	fat	sat fat	carb	sugar	protein	fibre
1541 KJ	367 kcal	15.8 g	2.8 g	54.1 g	0.0 g	5.5 g	1.5 g

1 Prepare and wash the potatoes.

2 Cut into slices 1 cm thick and 5 cm long.

3 Cut the slices into strips 5 × 1 × 1 cm.

4 Wash well and dry in a cloth.

5 Cook in a frying basket without colour in moderately hot fat (165°C).

6 Drain and place on kitchen paper on trays until required.

7 When required, place in a frying pan and cook in hot fat (185°C) until crisp and golden.

8 Drain well, season lightly with salt and serve.

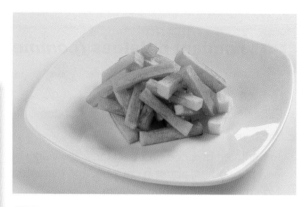

Because chips are so popular, the following advice from the Potato Marketing Board is useful.

- Cook chips in small quantities; this will allow the oil to regain its temperature more quickly; chips will then cook faster and absorb less fat.

- Do not let the temperature of the oil exceed 199°C as this will accelerate the fat breakdown.

- Use oils high in polyunsaturates for a healthier chip.

- Ideally use a separate fryer for chips and ensure that it has the capacity to raise the fat temperature rapidly to the correct degree when frying chilled or frozen chips.

- Although the majority of chipped potatoes are purchased frozen, the Potato Marketing Board recommends the following potatoes for those who prefer to make their own chips: Maris Piper, Cara, Désirée.

King Edward and Santé are also good choices.

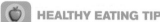 **HEALTHY EATING TIP**

- Chipped potatoes may be blanched twice, first at 140°C, followed by a re-blanch at 160°C until lightly coloured.

- For healthy eating, blanch in a steamer until just cooked, drain and dry well – final temperature 165°C.

* Using old potatoes and peanut oil

16 Sauté potatoes with onions (*pommes lyonnaise*)

1 Allow ¼ kg onion to ½ kg potatoes.

2 Shallow fry the onions slowly in 25–50 g oil, turning frequently, until tender and nicely browned; season lightly with salt.

3 Prepare sauté potatoes as for recipe 13.

4 Combine the two and toss together.

5 Serve as for sauté potatoes.

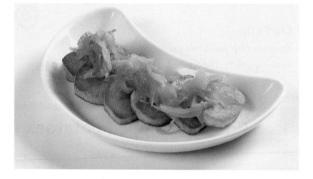

 HEALTHY EATING TIP

- Use a little hot sunflower oil to fry the potatoes.

- Add little or no salt; the customer can add more if required.

17 Delmonico potatoes *(pommes Delmonico)*

cal	kcal	fat	sat fat	carb	sugar	protein	fibre
900 KJ	214 kcal	6.3 g	3.7 g	37.5 g	2.7 g	4.4 g	2.0 g	*

1 Wash, peel and rewash the potatoes.
2 Cut into 6 mm dice.
3 Barely cover with milk, season lightly with salt and pepper and allow to cook for 30–40 minutes.
4 Place in an earthenware dish, sprinkle with breadcrumbs and melted butter, brown in the oven or under the salamander and serve.

* Using old potatoes and whole milk

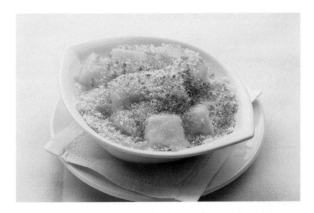

18 Parmentier potatoes *(pommes parmentier)*

cal	kcal	fat	sat fat	carb	sugar	protein	fibre
1819 KJ	433 kcal	33.5 g	6.3 g	32.8 g	0.7 g	2.3 g	1.7 g	*

½ kg will yield 2–3 portions
1 Select medium to large potatoes.
2 Wash, peel and rewash.
3 Trim on three sides and cut into 1 cm slices.
4 Cut the slices into 1 cm strips.
5 Cut the strips into 1 cm dice.
6 Wash well and dry in a cloth.
7 Cook in hot shallow oil in a frying pan until golden brown.
8 Drain, season lightly and serve sprinkled with chopped parsley.

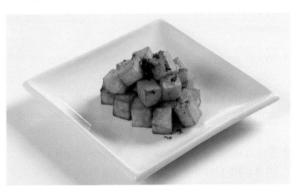

* Using peanut oil

19 Swiss potato cakes (rösti)

cal	kcal	fat	sat fat	carb	sugar	protein	fibre
700 KJ	168 kcal	10.5 g	6.5 g	17.3 g	0.7 g	2.2 g	1.3 g	*

1 Allow 100 g unpeeled potato per portion.
2 Parboil in salted water (or steam) for approximately 5 minutes.
3 Cool, then shred into large flakes on a grater.
4 For 4 portions, heat 50 g oil, butter or margarine in a frying pan.

5 Add the potatoes, and season lightly with salt and pepper.
6 Press the potato together and cook on both sides until brown and crisp.

The potato can be made in a four-portion cake or in individual rounds.

HEALTHY EATING TIP

- Lightly oil a well-seasoned pan with sunflower oil to fry the rösti.
- Use the minimum amount of salt.

Try something different

- These potato cakes may also be made from raw potatoes.
- Add sweated chopped onion.
- Add sweated lardons of bacon.

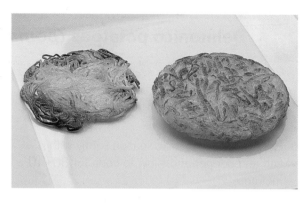

- Use 2 parts of grated potato to 1 part grated apple.

* Using butter

20 Roast potatoes *(pommes rôties)*

4 portions	
large roasting potatoes	6
dripping or 2nd-press olive oil	250 ml
seasoning	

1 Wash and peel the potatoes and cut into approx. 5 cm chunks.

2 Place in a pan of cold water, bring to the boil and cook slowly until just cooked; pre-heat the oven to 220°C.

3 Drain well. Meanwhile heat the dripping or oil in a pan, place the potatoes carefully in the roasting tray (with enough room to allow for roasting – too close together and they will steam).

4 Pour the hot oil or fat over the potatoes and place in the oven for 15 minutes.

5 After 15 minutes, reduce the heat to 180°C and baste every 5 minutes until the potatoes are golden and crisp.

6 Once cooked, serve immediately as prolonged holding will inevitably cause the inside to steam, making the outside soft and leathery.

Chef's tip
After draining the potatoes, shake them in the pan. This gives them a fluffy texture, which turns into a crisp coating when they are roasted.

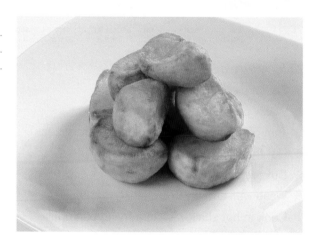

Try something different

To make château potatoes (*pommes château*):

1. Select small, even-sized potatoes and wash them.

2. Turn the potatoes into barrel-shaped pieces about the same size as fondant potatoes (recipe 14).

3. Place in a saucepan of boiling water for 2–3 minutes, then refresh immediately. Drain in a colander.

4. Finish as for roast potatoes. Use a non-stick tray, lightly oiled greaseproof paper or non-stick mat for the roasting.

21   Macaire potatoes (potato cakes) *(pommes Macaire)*

cal	kcal	fat	sat fat	carb	sugar	protein	fibre	
4392 KJ	1047 kcal	65.7 g	14.7 g	109.8 g	2.7 g	11.4 g	10.8 g	*

½ kg will yield 2–3 portions

1 Prepare and cook as for baked jacket potatoes (recipe 10).

2 Cut in halves, remove the centre with a spoon, and place in a basin.

3 Add 25 g butter per ½ kg, a little salt and milled pepper.

4 Mash and mix as lightly as possible with a fork.

5 Using a little flour, mould into a roll, then divide into pieces, allowing one or two per portion.

6 Mould into 2 cm round cakes, flour lightly.

7 Shallow-fry on both sides in very hot oil and serve.

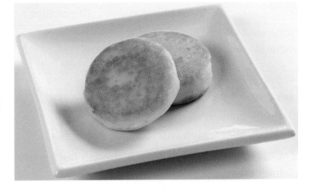

Chef's tip

Make sure the potato mixture is firm enough to be shaped, and fry the cakes in very hot oil, or they will lose their shape.

Try something different

Additions to potato cakes can include:

- chopped parsley, fresh herbs or chives, or duxelle
- cooked chopped onion
- grated cheese.

* Using hard margarine and sunflower oil

22   Potatoes cooked in milk with cheese *(gratin dauphinoise)*

cal	kcal	fat	sat fat	carb	sugar	protein	fibre
747 KJ	178 kcal	5.4 g	3.4 g	5.4 g	4.0 g	8.0 g	1.8 g

	4 portions	10 portions
potatoes	500 g	1¼ kg
milk	250 ml	600 ml
salt, pepper		
grated cheese, preferably Gruyère	50 g	125 g

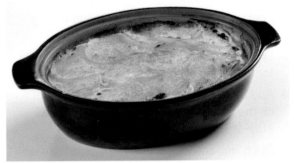

1 Slice the peeled potatoes ½ cm thick.

2 Place in an ovenproof dish and cover with milk.

3 Season, sprinkle with grated cheese and cook in a moderate oven, 190°C, until the potatoes are cooked and golden brown.

23 Hash brown potatoes

cal	kcal	fat	sat fat	carb	sugar	protein	fibre
954 KJ	228 kcal	11.3 g	5.3 g	25.8 g	0.9 g	7.1 g	2.0 g

	4 portions	10 portions
potatoes	600 g	2 kg
butter or margarine	25 g	60 g
lardons of bacon	100 g	250 g
seasoning		

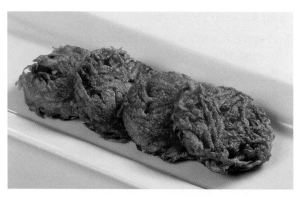

1 Wash, peel and rewash the potatoes.
2 Coarsely grate the potatoes, rewash quickly and then drain well.
3 Melt the fat in a suitable frying pan. Add the lardons of bacon, fry until crisp and brown, remove from the pan and drain.
4 Pour the fat back into the frying pan, add the grated potato and season.
5 Press down well, allow 2 cm thickness, and cook over a heat for 10–15 minutes or in a moderate oven at 190°C, until a brown crust forms on the bottom.
6 Turn out into a suitable serving dish and sprinkle with the lardons of bacon and chopped parsley.

🍎 **HEALTHY EATING TIP**

- Dry-fry the lardons in a well-seasoned pan.
- Brush a little oil over the potatoes and cook in a hot oven. Use the minimum amount of salt.

24 Braised onions (*oignons braisés*)

cal	kcal	fat	sat fat	carb	sugar	protein	fibre
245 KJ	58 kcal	0.4 g	0.1 g	10.9 g	10.4 g	3.4 g	2.8 g

1 Select medium even-sized onions; allow ½ kg per 2–3 portions.
2 Peel, wash and cook in lightly salted boiling water for 30 minutes, or steam.
3 Drain and place in a pan or casserole suitable for use in the oven.
4 Add bouquet garni, half cover with stock; put on the lid and braise gently in the oven at 180–200°C until tender.
5 Drain well and dress neatly in a vegetable dish.
6 Reduce the cooking liquor with an equal amount of jus-lié, reduced stock or demi-glace. Correct the seasoning and consistency and pass. Mask the onions and sprinkle with chopped parsley.

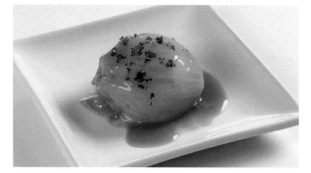

25 Caramelised button onions

butter or vegetable oil	50 g
button onions	250 g
water or brown stock	
sugar	50 g

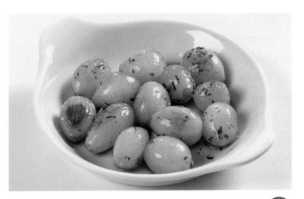

1 Place the butter or oil in a shallow pan.
2 Fry the button onions quickly to a light golden brown colour.
3 Barely cover with water or brown stock. Add the sugar. Cook the button onions until they are tender and the liquid has reduced with the sugar to a light caramel glaze. Carefully coat the onions with the glaze.

Chef's tip
The important thing is to reduce the stock and sugar until they form a light caramel syrup.

26 Roast garlic

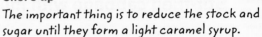

1 Peel the garlic.
2 Divide it into natural segments and place in a suitable roasting tray.
3 Sprinkle with olive oil and roast in the oven until golden brown and tender.

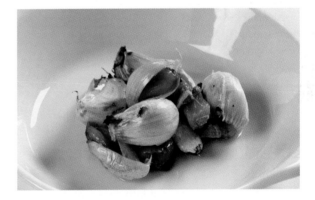

27 Poached fennel

1 Trim the fennel heads and remove any blemishes.
2 Gently place in a suitable pan of boiling stock or water.
3 Remove to the side of the stove and gently poach until tender.

Poached fennel may be served as an accompanying vegetable or used as a garnish.

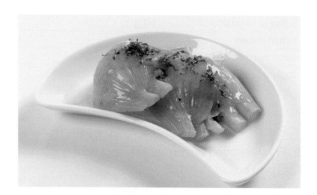

28 Stir-fried cabbage with mushrooms and beansprouts

	4 portions	10 portions
sunflower oil	2 tbsp	5 tbsp
spring cabbage or pak choi, shredded	400 g	1 kg
soy sauce	2 tbsp	5 tbsp
mushrooms	200 g	500 g
beansprouts	100 g	250 g
freshly ground pepper		

1 Heat the oil in a suitable pan (e.g. a wok).
2 Add the cabbage and stir for 2 minutes.
3 Add the soy sauce, stir well. Cook for a further minute.
4 Add the mushrooms, cut into slices, and cook for a further 2 minutes.
5 Stir in the beansprouts and cook for 1–2 minutes.
6 Stir well. Season with freshly ground pepper and serve.

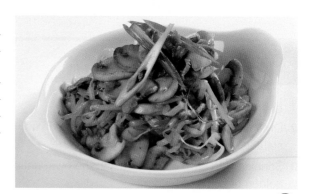

Chef's tip
The cabbage must be shredded evenly and the mushrooms cut evenly, so that they will cook evenly.

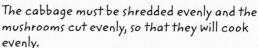 **HEALTHY EATING TIP**

- Reduce the oil by half when cooking the cabbage.
- No added salt is needed as soy sauce is used.

29   Braised red cabbage *(choux à la flamande)*

cal	kcal	fat	sat fat	carb	sugar	protein	fibre
754 KJ	180 kcal	15.2 g	8.4 g	7.8 g	7.7 g	3.4 g	3.2 g

	4 portions	10 portions
red cabbage	300 g	1 kg
salt, pepper		
butter	50 g	125 g
cooking apples	100 g	250 g
caster sugar	10 g	25 g
vinegar or red wine	125 ml	300 ml
bacon trimmings (optional)	50 g	125 g

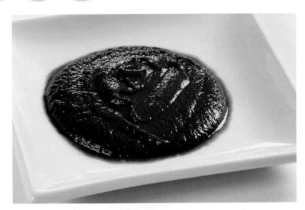

1 Quarter, trim and shred the cabbage. Wash well and drain.

2 Season lightly with salt and pepper.

3 Place in a well-buttered casserole or pan suitable for placing in the oven (not aluminium or iron, because these metals will cause a chemical reaction that will discolour the cabbage).

4 Add the peeled and cored apples. Cut into 1 cm dice and sugar.

5 Add the vinegar and bacon (if using), cover with a buttered paper and lid.

6 Cook in a moderate oven at 150–200°C for 1½ hours.

7 Remove the bacon (if used) and serve.

Other optional flavourings include 50 g sultanas, grated zest of one orange, pinch of ground cinnamon.

 HEALTHY EATING TIP

- The fat and salt content will be reduced by omitting the bacon.

30   Spinach purée *(epinards en purée)*

cal	kcal	fat	sat fat	carb	sugar	protein	fibre
588 KJ	143 kcal	11.9 g	6.7 g	3.3 g	3.1 g	5.7 g	4.2 g

½ kg will yield 2 portions.

1 Remove the stems and discard them.

2 Wash the leaves very carefully in plenty of water, several times if necessary.

3 Wilt for 2–3 minutes, taking care not to overcook.

4 Place on a tray and allow to cool.

5 Pass through a sieve or mouli, or use a food processor.

6 Reheat in 25–50 g butter, mix with a wooden spoon, correct the seasoning and serve.

Try something different

Creamed spinach purée can be made by mixing in 30 ml cream and 60 ml béchamel or natural yoghurt before serving. Serve with a border of cream. An addition would be 1 cm triangle-shaped croutons fried in butter.

Spinach may also be served with toasted pine kernels or finely chopped garlic.

* Using 25 g butter per kg

The purée shown here is quite soft. For a firmer finish, dry the spinach well before passing through the sieve.

31 Broccoli

cal	kcal	fat	sat fat	carb	sugar	protein	fibre
76 KJ	18 kcal	0.0 g	0.0 g	1.6 g	1.5 g	3.1 g	4.1 g

Cook in lightly salted water, or steam.

Green and purple broccoli need less cooking time than cauliflower. Broccoli is usually broken down into florets and requires very little cooking: once brought to the boil, 1–2 minutes should be sufficient. This leaves the broccoli slightly crisp.

Boiling vegetables
http://bit.ly/w817Pb

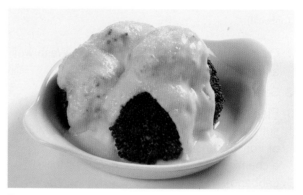

Broccoli served with hollandaise sauce

ASSESSMENT

32 Peas French-style (*petit pois à la française*)

cal	kcal	fat	sat fat	carb	sugar	protein	fibre
515 KJ	123 kcal	5.6 g	3.4 g	12.9 g	5.8 g	5.9 g	5.7 g

	4 portions	10 portions
peas (in the pod)	1 kg	2½ kg
spring or button onions	12	40
small lettuce	1	2–3
butter	25 g	60 g
salt		
caster sugar	½ tsp	1 tsp
flour	5 g	12 g

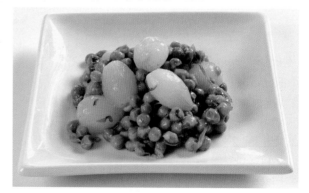

1 Shell and wash the peas and place in a sauteuse.

2 Peel and wash the onions, shred the lettuce and add to the peas with half the butter, a little salt and the sugar.

3 Barely cover with water. Cover with a lid and cook steadily, preferably in the oven, until tender.

4 Correct the seasoning.

5 Mix the remaining butter with the flour and shake into the boiling peas until thoroughly mixed; serve.

When using frozen peas, allow the onions to almost cook before adding the peas.

33 Ladies' fingers (okra) in cream sauce *(okra à la crème)*

cal	kcal	fat	sat fat	carb	sugar	protein	fibre	
928 KJ	221 kcal	20.2 g	9.8 g	5.7 g	5.7 g	4.4 g	3.2 g	*

	4 portions	10 portions
ladies' fingers (okra)	400 g	1¼ kg
butter or margarine	50 g	125 g
cream sauce	¼ litre	625 ml

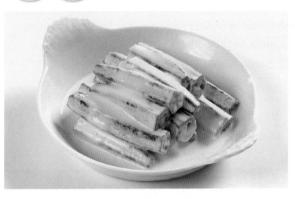

1 Top and tail the ladies' fingers.

2 Blanch in lightly salted boiling water, or steam; drain.

3 Sweat in the margarine or butter for 5–10 minutes, or until tender.

4 Carefully add the cream sauce.

5 Bring to the boil, correct the seasoning and serve in a suitable dish.

Okra may also be served brushed with butter or sprinkled with chopped parsley.

HEALTHY EATING TIP

- Use a little unsaturated oil to sweat the okra.

- Try using half cream sauce and half yoghurt, adding very little salt.

* Using hard margarine

> **Chef's tip**
> Okra can become glutinous (slimy) when it is cooked in a sauce. To avoid this, wash the okra and let it dry before cooking.

34 Broad beans *(fèves)*

cal	kcal	fat	sat fat	carb	sugar	protein	fibre	
344 KJ	81 kcal	0.6 g	0.1 g	5.0 g	0.4 g	7.9 g	6.5 g	*

½ kg will yield about 2 portions

1 Shell the beans and cook in boiling salted water for 10–15 minutes until tender. Do not overcook.

2 If the inner shells are tough, remove before serving.

Try something different

Variations include:

- brushing with butter

- brushing with butter then sprinkling with chopped parsley

- binding with ½ litre cream sauce or fresh cream.

* 100 g portion

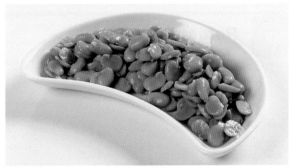

> **Chef's tip**
> The modern technique is to take the beans out of their pod and outer skin before serving – this reveals the bright green, tender beans.

35 Mangetout

½ kg of mangetout will yield 4–6 portions.

1 Top and tail, wash and drain.
2 Cook in boiling salted water for 2–3 minutes, until slightly crisp.
3 Serve whole, brushed with butter.

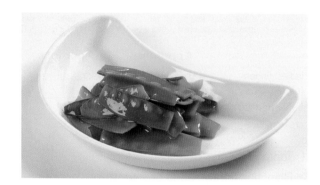

36 Corn on the cob (*maïs*)

cal	kcal	fat	sat fat	carb	sugar	protein	fibre
646 KJ	154 kcal	2.9 g	0.5 g	28.5 g	2.1 g	5.1 g	5.9 g

Allow 1 cob per portion.

1 Trim the stem.
2 Cook in lightly salted boiling water for 10–20 minutes or until the corn is tender. Do not overcook.
3 Remove the outer leaves and fibres.
4 Serve with a sauceboat of melted butter.

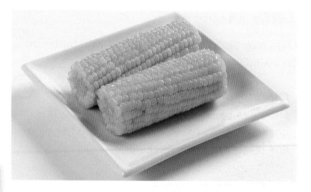

Creamed sweetcorn can be made by removing the corn from the cooked cobs, draining well and binding lightly with cream (fresh or non-dairy), béchamel sauce or yoghurt.

ASSESSMENT

37 Ratatouille

cal	kcal	fat	sat fat	carb	sugar	protein	fibre
579 KJ	138 kcal	12.6 g	1.7 g	5.2 g	4.6 g	1.3 g	2.4 g

	4 portions	10 portions
baby marrow (courgette)	200 g	500 g
aubergines	200 g	500 g
tomatoes	200 g	500 g
oil	50 ml	125 ml
onions, finely sliced	50 g	125 g

garlic clove, peeled and chopped	1	2
red peppers, diced	50 g	125 g
green peppers, diced	50 g	125 g
salt, pepper		
parsley, chopped	1 tsp	2–3 tsp

1 Trim off both ends of the marrow and aubergines.

2 Remove the skin using a peeler.

3 Cut into 3 mm slices.

4 Concassée the tomatoes (peel, remove seeds, roughly chop).

5 Place the oil in a thick-bottomed pan and add the onions.

6 Cover with a lid and allow to cook gently for 5–7 minutes without colour.

7 Add the garlic, marrow and aubergine slices, and the peppers.

8 Season lightly with salt and mill pepper.

9 Allow to cook gently for 4–5 minutes, toss occasionally and keep covered.

10 Add the tomato and continue cooking for 20–30 minutes or until tender.

11 Mix in the parsley, correct the seasoning and serve.

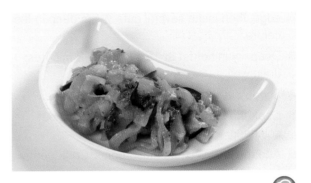

Chef's tip

The vegetables need to be cut evenly so that they will cook evenly; it also improves the texture of the dish.

 HEALTHY EATING TIP

- Use a little unsaturated oil to cook the onions.

- Use the minimum amount of salt.

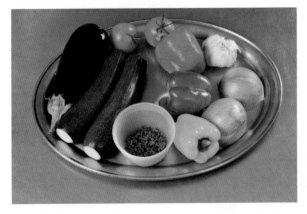

Ingredients for ratatouille

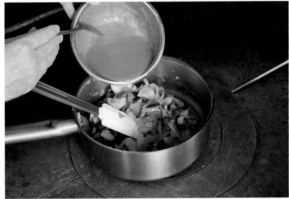

Add the tomato to the vegetables during cooking (step 10)

38 Stuffed aubergine (aubergine farcie)

	4 portions	10 portions
aubergines	2	5
shallots, chopped	10 g	25 g
oil or fat, to fry		
mushrooms	100 g	250 g
parsley, chopped		
tomato concassée	100 g	250 g
salt, pepper		
demi-glace or jus-lié	125 ml	300 ml

1 Cut the aubergines in two lengthwise.

2 With the point of a small knife, make a cut round the halves approximately ½ cm from the

edge, then make several cuts ½ cm deep in the centre.

3 Deep-fry in hot fat at 185°C for 2–3 minutes; drain well.

4 Scoop out the centre pulp and chop it finely.

5 Cook the shallots in a little oil or fat without colouring.

6 Add the well-washed mushrooms. Cook gently for a few minutes.

7 Mix in the pulp, parsley and tomato; season. Replace in the aubergine skins.

8 Sprinkle with breadcrumbs and melted butter. Brown under the salamander.

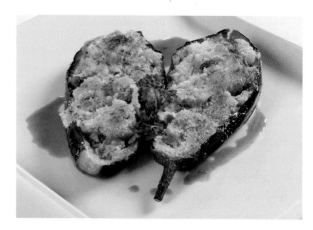

9 Serve with a cordon of demi-glace or jus-lié.

39 Shallow-fried courgettes (*courgettes sautées*)

cal	kcal	fat	sat fat	carb	sugar	protein	fibre
456 KJ	111 kcal	10.7 g	6.6 g	1.9 g	1.8 g	1.9 g	0.9 g

*

1 Wash. Top and tail, and cut into round slices 3–6 cm thick.

2 Gently fry in hot oil or butter for 2 or 3 minutes, drain and serve.

* Using butter

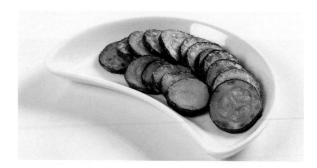

40 Deep-fried courgettes (*courgettes frites*)

cal	kcal	fat	sat fat	carb	sugar	protein	fibre
481 KJ	111 kcal	11.4 g	1.4 g	1.8 g	1.7 g	1.8 g	0.9 g

*

1 Wash. Top and tail, and cut into round slices 3–6 cm thick.

2 Pass through flour, or milk and flour, or batter, and deep-fry in hot fat at 185°C. Drain well and serve.

Chef's tip

Make sure the oil is very hot before adding the courgette. Fry it quickly and drain it before serving.

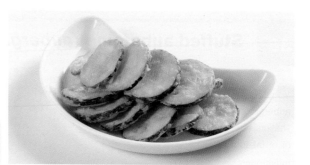

* Using vegetable oil

41 Stuffed tomatoes *(tomates farcies)*

cal	kcal	fat	sat fat	carb	sugar	protein	fibre
430 KJ	102 kcal	5.9 g	3.5 g	10.6 g	5.7 g	2.5 g	2.2 g

	4 portions	10 portions
medium-sized or plum tomatoes	8	20
Duxelle		
shallots, chopped	10 g	25 g
butter, oil or margarine	25 g	60 g
mushrooms	150 g	375 g
salt, pepper		
clove garlic, crushed (optional)	1	2–3
breadcrumbs (white or wholemeal)	25 g	60 g
parsley, chopped		

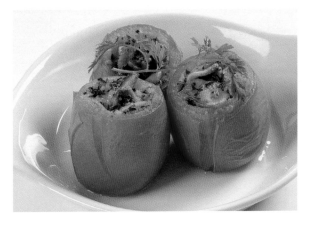

1 Wash the tomatoes, remove the eyes.

2 Remove the top quarter of each tomato with a sharp knife.

3 Carefully empty out the seeds without damaging the flesh.

4 Place on a greased baking tray.

5 Cook the shallots in a little oil, butter or margarine without colour.

6 Add the washed chopped mushrooms; season with salt and pepper; add the garlic if using. Cook for 2–3 minutes.

7 Add a little of the strained tomato juice, the breadcrumbs and the parsley; mix to a piping consistency. Correct the seasoning. At this stage, several additions may be made (e.g. chopped ham, cooked rice).

8 Place the mixture in a piping bag with a large star tube and pipe into the tomato shells. Replace the tops.

9 Brush with oil, season lightly with salt and pepper.

10 Cook in a moderate oven at 180–200°C for 4–5 minutes.

11 Serve garnished with picked parsley or fresh basil or rosemary.

 HEALTHY EATING TIP

- Use a small amount of an unsaturated oil to cook the shallots and brush over the stuffed tomatoes.

- Add the minimum amount of salt.

- Adding cooked rice to the stuffing will increase the amount of starchy carbohydrate.

42 Courgette and potato cakes with mint and feta cheese

cal	kcal	fat	sat fat	carb	sugar	protein	fibre
910 KJ	219 kcal	13.6 g	7.4 g	15.4 g	2.4 g	9.5 g	1.6 g

	6 portions
courgettes	3 large
potatoes	350 g
fresh mint, chopped	2 tbsp
spring onions, finely chopped	2
feta cheese	200 g
eggs	1
plain flour	25 g
butter	25 g
olive oil	1 tbsp
salt, pepper	

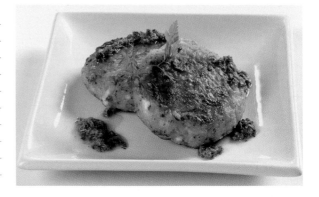

1 Lightly scrape the courgettes to remove the outside skin. Purée in a food processor. Remove, sprinkle with salt to remove the excess moisture, leave for 1 hour. Rinse under cold water, squeeze out all excess moisture, dry on a clean cloth.

2 Steam or parboil the potatoes for 8–10 minutes. Cool and peel.

3 Carefully grate the potatoes, place in a bowl, then season.

4 Add the courgettes, mint, spring onion, chopped feta cheese and the beaten egg. Mix well.

5 Divide the mixture into 6 and shape into cakes approximately 1 cm thick.

6 Dust with flour.

7 Brush the cakes with melted butter and oil, place on a baking sheet, cook in an oven at 200°C for 15 minutes; turn over and continue to cook for a further 15 minutes.

8 Serve on suitable plates garnished with fresh blanched mint leaves and green sauce (see page 190).

Chef's tip

Make sure that all excess moisture is removed from the courgettes at step 1. If they are too moist, the mixture will be difficult to handle.

HEALTHY EATING TIP

- Make sure the puréed courgettes are rinsed well to remove the added salt.

- Use a little sunflower oil to brush the cakes before cooking.

43 Fettuccini of courgette with chopped basil and balsamic vinegar

	4 portions	10 portions
large courgettes	2	5
olive oil	50 ml	125 ml
olive oil, to finish	20 ml	125 ml
balsamic vinegar, to finish	20 ml	50 ml
basil leaves, shredded	2	5

1 Slice the courgettes finely lengthwise, using a mandolin (Japanese slicer).

2 Heat the olive oil in a suitable pan. Sauté the courgette slices quickly without colour for 35 seconds.

3 Place on suitable plates. Drizzle with olive oil and balsamic vinegar, and top with shredded basil leaves.

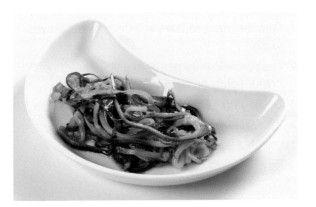

This may be served as a vegetarian starter or as a garnish for fish and meat dishes.

44 Spiced aubergine purée

	4–6 portions
diced aubergine	1 kg
salt	20 g
cumin	5 g
tomato purée	45 g
water	200 ml
rose harissa	15 g
vegetable nage	200 ml

1 Dice the aubergine and mix with the salt and cumin in a suitable bowl.

2 Allow to stand for 30 minutes.

3 Dry in a cloth and deep-fry for 10 minutes.

4 Purée with the rest of the ingredients and pass.

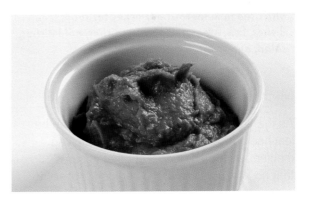

This purée can be added to rice or couscous, or used as a filling for stuffed vegetables. It can also be used as a garnish for meat dishes.

45 Shallow-fried chicory (*endive meunière*)

cal	kcal	fat	sat fat	carb	sugar	protein	fibre
484 KJ	118 kcal	12.0 g	7.3 g	4.8 g	1.3 g	0.9 g	1.5 g *

1 Trim the stem, remove any discoloured leaves, wash.

2 Drain, shallow-fry gently in a little butter and colour lightly on both sides.

3 Serve with 10 g per portion nut brown butter, lemon juice and chopped parsley.

* Using 37.5 g butter

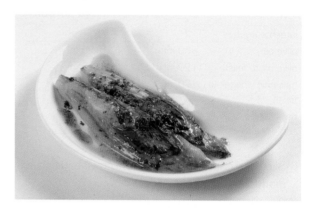

46 Asparagus points or tips (*points d'asperges*)

Note: Young thin asparagus, 50 pieces to the bundle, is known as sprew or sprue. It is prepared in the same way as asparagus except that, when it is very thin, the removal of the leaf tips is dispensed with. It may be served as a vegetable, perhaps brushed with butter. Asparagus tips are also used in numerous garnishes for soups, egg dishes, fish, meat and poultry dishes, cold dishes, salad, and so on.

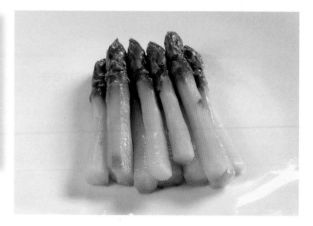

Microwaved asparagus

As the flavour of asparagus is mild and can be leached out very easily through the cooking medium, a method of cookery that ensures that no flavour is lost in the cooking process is microwaving.

To microwave, place a piece of clingfilm over a plate that will fit in the microwave and, more importantly, is microwave safe. Spread the clingfilm with a little oil and salt, evenly place the asparagus on the plate in a single layer. Cover the plate and asparagus with another piece of clingfilm, and microwave for 30 second stints until the asparagus is tender; serve immediately.

The benefit of this method is that it retains flavour and colour, and it can be cooked in minutes, as opposed to batch cooking, which will, invariably, cause the asparagus to lose flavour and colour the longer it is stored.

If larger-scale cooking is required, the more traditional method, boiling in lightly salted water, should be used: cooking, say, 100 portions of asparagus in the microwave should be avoided for obvious reasons!

47   Globe artichokes *(artichauts en branche)*

cal	kcal	fat	sat fat	carb	sugar	protein	fibre
32 KJ	8 kcal	0.0 g	0.0 g	1.4 g	1.4 g	0.6 g	0.0 g

*

1 Allow 1 artichoke per portion.

2 Cut off the stems close to the leaves.

3 Cut off about 2 cm across the tops of the leaves.

4 Trim the remainder of the leaves with scissors or a small knife.

5 Place a slice of lemon at the bottom of each artichoke.

6 Secure with string.

7 Simmer in gently boiling, lightly salted water (to which a little ascorbic acid – one vitamin C tablet – may be added) until the bottom is tender (20–30 minutes).

8 Refresh under running water until cold.

9 Remove the centre of the artichoke carefully.

10 Scrape away all the furry inside (the choke) and leave clean.

11 Replace the centre, upside down.

12 Reheat by placing in a pan of boiling salted water for 3–4 minutes.

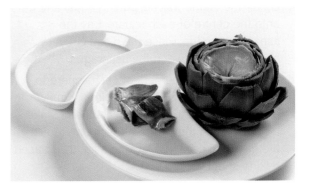

13 Drain and serve accompanied by a suitable sauce.

> Artichokes may also be served cold with vinaigrette sauce. Do not cook artichokes in an iron or aluminium pan because these metals cause a chemical reaction that will discolour them.

* Not including sauce

48   Asparagus wrapped in puff pastry with Gruyère

cal	kcal	fat	sat fat	carb	sugar	protein	fibre
2017 KJ	485 kcal	37.7 g	15.0 g	23.4 g	2.5 g	15.9 g	0.8 g

	4 portions	10 portions
Gruyère cheese	175 g	400 g
Parmesan, freshly grated	3 tbsp	7 tbsp
crème fraiche	250 ml	625 ml
puff pastry (page 490)	350 g	875 g
eggwash or milk, for brushing		
asparagus, freshly cooked	350 g	875 g
salt, pepper		
watercress, for garnish		

1 Cut the Gruyère cheese into 1 cm dice. In a suitable bowl, mix the Parmesan cheese and crème fraiche; season.

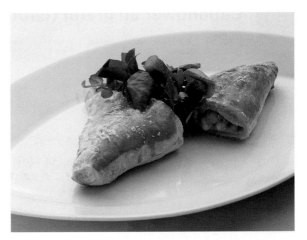

2 Roll out the puff pastry to approximately ¼ cm thick and cut into squares approximately 18 × 18 cm.

3 Brush the edges with eggwash or milk.

4 Divide the crème fraiche, putting equal amounts onto the centre of each square. Lay the asparagus on top. Place the diced Gruyère cheese firmly between the asparagus.

5 Fold the opposite corners of each square to meet in the centre, like an envelope. Firmly pinch the seams together to seal them. Make a small hole in the centre of each one to allow the steam to escape. Place on a lightly greased baking sheet.

6 Allow to relax for 20 minutes in the refrigerator. Brush with eggwash or milk, sprinkle with Parmesan.

7 Bake in a hot oven at 200°C for approximately 20–25 minutes until golden brown.

8 Serve garnished with watercress.

Chef's tip

Make sure the pastry parcels are well sealed so that the mixture does not escape during cooking.

HEALTHY EATING TIP

- The puff pastry and cheese make this dish high in fat. Serve with plenty of starchy carbohydrate to dilute it.

49 Sauté of wild mushrooms

Allow 50 g of mixed wild mushrooms per portion. Shallow fry.

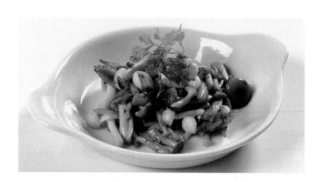

50 Cauliflower au gratin (chou-fleur mornay)

cal	kcal	fat	sat fat	carb	sugar	protein	fibre	
632 KJ	150 kcal	10.4 g	3.9 g	8.6 g	3.8 g	6.3 g	2.0 g	*

1 Cut the cooked cauliflower into four.

2 Reheat in a pan of hot salted water (chauffant), or reheat in butter in a suitable pan.

3 Place in vegetable dish or on a greased tray.

4 Coat with ¼ litre mornay sauce (see page 185).

5 Sprinkle with grated cheese.

6 Brown under the salamander and serve.

 HEALTHY EATING TIP

- No additional salt is needed as cheese is added.

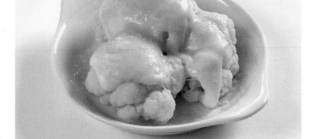

* Au gratin

51 Cauliflower polonaise *(chou-fleur polonaise)*

cal	kcal	fat	sat fat	carb	sugar	protein	fibre
575 KJ	139 kcal	11.9 g	6.9 g	4.1 g	1.9 g	4.0 g	1.7 g

1 Cut the cooked cauliflower into four. Reheat in a chauffant or in butter in a suitable pan.

2 Heat 50 g butter, add 10 g fresh breadcrumbs in a frying pan and lightly brown. Pour over the cauliflower, sprinkle with sieved hardboiled egg and chopped parsley.

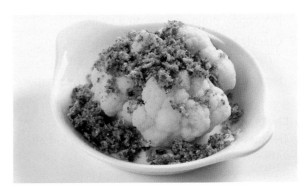

52 Roast butternut squash

1 Peel the squash and cut it into thick, even pieces.

2 Place on a lightly oiled roasting tray and roast for approximately 20–25 minutes in a hot oven, until the flesh is soft and golden brown.

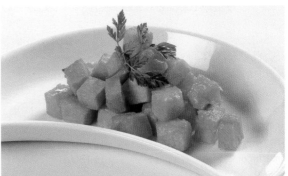

53 Sea kale *(chou de mer)*

cal	kcal	fat	sat fat	carb	sugar	protein	fibre
33 KJ	8 kcal	0.0 g	0.0 g	0.6 g	0.6 g	1.4 g	0.0 g

½ kg will yield about 3 portions.

1 Trim the roots and remove any discoloured leaves.

2 Wash well and tie into a neat bundle.

3 Cook in boiling lightly salted water for 15–20 minutes. Do not overcook.

4 Drain well, serve accompanied with a suitable sauce (e.g. melted butter, hollandaise).

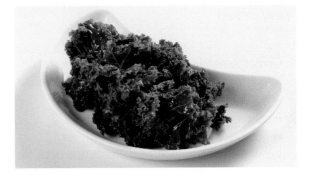

54 Deep-fried seaweed

1 Carefully pick over the seaweed. Wash and thoroughly drain and dry on a cloth.
2 Quickly fry in hot, deep fat (approximately 175–190°C).
3 Remove and drain on absorbent kitchen paper.

Chef's tip
The seaweed must be cooked quickly in hot oil, until it is crisp.

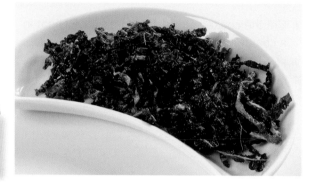

55 Chinese vegetables and noodles

cal	kcal	fat	sat fat	carb	sugar	protein	fibre
2332 KJ	554 kcal	21.6 g	1.8 g	80.6 g	5.7 g	14.3 g	1.9 g	*

	4 portions	10 portions
Chinese noodles	400 g	1¼ kg
oil	60 ml	150 ml
celery	100 g	250 g
carrot, cut in paysanne	100 g	250 g
bamboo shoots	50 g	125 g
mushrooms, finely sliced	75 g	180 g
Chinese cabbage, shredded	75 g	180 g
beansprouts	100 g	250 g
soy sauce	30 ml	75 ml
garnish (spring onions, sliced lengthways and quickly stir-fried)	4	10

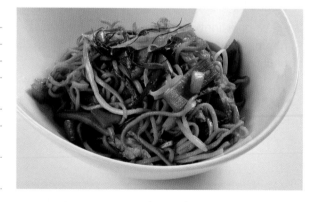

1 Cook the noodles in boiling salted water for about 5–6 minutes until *al dente*. Refresh and drain.
2 Heat the oil in a wok and stir-fry all the vegetables, except the beansprouts, for 1 minute. Then add the beansprouts and cook for a further minute.

3 Add the drained noodles, stirring well; allow to reheat through.
4 Correct the seasoning.
5 Serve in a suitable dish, garnished with the spring onions.

 HEALTHY EATING TIP

- Keep added salt to a minimum.
- Use an unsaturated oil (olive or sunflower) and reduce the quantity used.

* *Using canned bamboo shoots*

56 Alu-chole (vegetarian curry)

cal	kcal	fat	sat fat	carb	sugar	protein	fibre
1214 KJ	290 kcal	17.5 g	1.6 g	26.6 g	5.3 g	10.6 g	5.5 g

*

	4 portions	10 portions
vegetable ghee or oil	45 ml (3 tsp)	112 ml (7½ tsp)
small cinnamon sticks	4	10
bay leaves	4	10
cumin seeds	5 g (1 tsp)	12½ g (2½ tsp)
onion, finely chopped	100 g	250 g
cloves garlic, finely chopped and crushed	2	5
plum tomatoes, canned, chopped	400 g	1 kg
hot curry paste	45 ml (3 tsp)	112 ml (7½ tsp)
salt, to taste		
potatoes in 1 cm dice	100 g	250 g
water	125 ml	312 ml
chickpeas, canned, drained	400 g	1 kg
coriander leaves, chopped	50 g	125 g
tamarind sauce or lemon juice	30 g (2 tbsp)	75 g (3 tbsp)

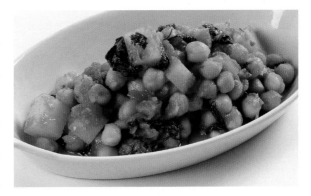

1 Heat the ghee in a suitable pan.
2 Add the cinnamon, bay leaves and cumin seeds; fry for 1 minute.
3 Add the onion and garlic. Fry until golden brown.
4 Add the chopped tomatoes, curry paste and salt, and fry for a further 2–3 minutes.
5 Stir in the potatoes and water. Bring to the boil. Cover and simmer until the potatoes are cooked.
6 Add the chickpeas; allow to heat through.
7 Stir in the coriander leaves and tamarind sauce or lemon juice; serve.

This is a dish from northern India.

Chef's tip
Fry the spices well to extract the maximum flavour from them.

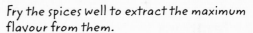
HEALTHY EATING TIP

- Use a small amount of unsaturated oil to fry the spices and onion.
- Skim the fat from the finished dish.
- No added salt is necessary.
- This can be served as a vegetarian dish with rice, or to accompany meat and chicken dishes.

* Using lemon juice and vegetable oil

57 Onion bhajias

cal	kcal	fat	sat fat	carb	sugar	protein	fibre
630 KJ	152 kcal	12.1 g	1.3 g	8.5 g	1.7 g	2.9 g	2.4 g	*

	4 portions	10 portions
bessan or gram flour	45 g (3 tbsp)	112 g (7½ tbsp)
hot curry powder	5 g (1 tsp)	12½ g (2½ tsp)
salt		
water	75 ml (5 tbsp)	187 ml (12½ tbsp)
onion, finely shredded	100 g	250 g

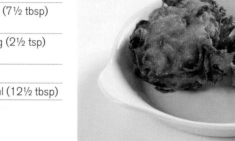

1 Mix together the flour, curry powder and salt.
2 Blend in the water carefully to form a smooth, thick batter.
3 Stir in the onion, stir well.
4 Drop the mixture off a tablespoon into deep oil at 200°C. Fry for 5–10 minutes until golden brown.
5 Drain well and serve as a snack with mango chutney as a dip.

Chef's tip
The oil must be at the correct temperature before the bhajias are fried.

HEALTHY EATING TIP

- Use the minimum amount of salt.
- Make sure the oil is hot so that less is absorbed into the surface. Drain on kitchen paper.

Reduced to half using margarine

58 Tempura

cal	kcal	fat	sat fat	carb	sugar	protein	fibre
3397 KJ	815 kcal	55.9 g	7.4 g	67.4 g	5.3 g	14.8 g	5.0 g	*

	4 portions
vegetable oil	500 ml
courgettes, sliced	2
sweet potato, scrubbed and sliced	1
green pepper, seeds removed and cut into strips	1
shiitake mushroom, stalks removed and halved if large	4
onion, sliced as half moons	1
parsley sprigs, to garnish	4
Batter (NB all ingredients must be stored in the fridge until just before mixing)	
egg yolk	1
ice-cold water	200 ml
plain flour, sifted	100 g
Tentsuyu dipping sauce (optional)	
dashi stock	200 ml

mirin	3 tbsp
soy sauce	3 tbsp
grated ginger	½ tsp

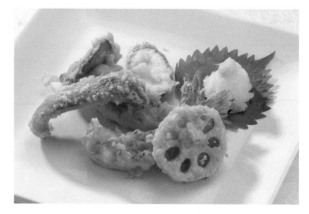

1 To prevent splattering during the frying, make sure to dry all deep-fry ingredients thoroughly first with a kitchen towel.

2 For the batter, beat the egg yolk lightly and mix with the ice-cold water.

3 Add half the flour to the egg and water mixture. Give the mixture a few strokes. Add the rest of the flour all at once. Stroke the mixture a few times with chopsticks or a fork until the ingredients are loosely combined. The batter should be very lumpy. If over-mixed, tempura will be oily and heavy.

4 Heat the oil to 160°C.

5 Dip the vegetables into the batter, a few pieces at a time. Fry until just crisp and golden (about 1½ minutes).

6 Drain the cooked vegetables on a kitchen towel.

7 Serve immediately with a pinch of salt, garnished with parsley sprigs and lemon wedges, dry-roasted salt or with Tentsuyu dipping sauce in a small bowl with grated ginger. This dish can also be served with an accompaniment of grated white radish.

8 To make the Tentsuyu sauce (if required), combine the ingredients in a small saucepan before sifting the flour; heat it through and leave to one side.

Any vegetables with a firm texture may be used for tempura.

Chef's tips

The water and other batter ingredients must be ice cold.

The batter should be lumpy to give it texture. Do not over-mix it; this will make it oily and heavy. Only fry a few pieces at once.

HEALTHY EATING TIP

- Use sunflower or groundnut oil for frying.

- Drain excess oil on kitchen paper.

---

59 Vegetarian strudel

cal	kcal	fat	sat fat	carb	sugar	protein	fibre
2117 KJ	504 kcal	27.6 g	4.0 g	54.1 g	10.5 g	14.3 g	9.7 g

*

	4 portions	10 portions
Strudel dough		
strong flour	200 g	500 g
pinch of salt		
sunflower oil	25 g	60 g
egg	1	2–3
water at 37°C	83 ml	125 ml
Filling		
large cabbage leaves	200 g	500 g
sunflower oil	4 tbsp	10 tbsp
onion, finely chopped	50 g	125 g
cloves garlic, chopped	2	5
courgettes	400 g	1 kg
carrots	200 g	500 g

	4 portions	10 portions
turnips	100 g	250 g
tomato, skinned, deseeded and diced	300 g	750 g
tomato purée	25 g	60 g
toasted sesame seeds	25 g	60 g
wholemeal breadcrumbs	50 g	125 g
fresh chopped basil	3 g	9 g
seasoning		
eggwash		

1 To make the strudel dough, sieve the flour with the salt and make a well.

2 Add the oil, egg and water, and gradually incorporate the flour to make a smooth dough; knead well.

3 Place in a basin, cover with a damp cloth; allow to relax for 3 minutes.

4 Meanwhile, prepare the filling: take the large cabbage leaves, wash and discard the tough centre stalks, blanch in boiling salted water for 2 minutes, until limp. Refresh and drain well in a clean cloth.

5 Heat the oil in a sauté pan, gently fry the onion and garlic until soft.

6 Peel and chop the courgettes into ½ cm dice, blanch and refresh. Peel and dice the carrots and turnips, blanch and refresh.

7 Place the well-drained courgettes, carrots and turnips into a basin, add the tomato concassée, tomato purée, sesame seeds, breadcrumbs and chopped basil, and mix well. Season.

8 Roll out the strudel dough to a thin rectangle, place on a clean cloth and stretch until extremely thin.

9 Lay the drained cabbage leaves on the stretched strudel dough, leaving approximately a 1 cm gap from the edge.

10 Place the filling in the centre. Eggwash the edges.

11 Fold in the longer side edges to meet in the middle. Roll up.

12 Transfer to a lightly oiled baking sheet. Brush with the sunflower oil.

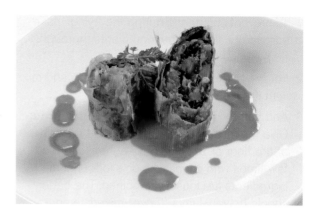

13 Bake for 40 minutes in a preheated oven at 180–200°C.

14 When cooked, serve hot, sliced on individual plates with a cordon of tomato sauce made with vegetable stock.

Chef's tip
The essential point in this recipe is to roll out and stretch the strudel dough so that it is very thin, but without breaking it.

HEALTHY EATING TIP

- Use the minimum amount of salt.
- Use a little unsaturated oil to cook the onion and garlic.

60 Coleslaw

cal	kcal	fat	sat fat	carb	sugar	protein	fibre
2514 KJ	599 kcal	59.0 g	8.8 g	11.7 g	11.4 g	5.9 g	7.2 g

	4 portions	10 portions
white or Chinese cabbage	200 g	500 g
carrot	50 g	125 g
onion (optional)	25 g	60 g
mayonnaise, natural yoghurt or fromage frais	125 ml	300 ml

1 Trim off the outside leaves of the cabbage.

2 Cut into quarters. Remove the centre stalk.

3 Wash the cabbage, shred finely and drain well.

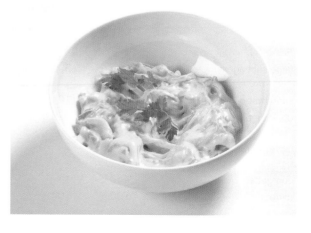

4 Mix with a fine julienne of raw carrot and shredded raw onion. To lessen the harshness of raw onion, blanch and refresh.

5 Bind with mayonnaise, natural yoghurt or vinaigrette.

Chef's tip
Cut the cabbage into fine julienne to give the coleslaw a good, even texture.

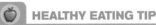
HEALTHY EATING TIP

- Replace some or all of the mayonnaise with natural yoghurt and/or fromage frais.

- Add salt sparingly.

* Using mayonnaise, for 4 portions

---

61 # Greek-style mushrooms (*champignons à la grecque*)

cal	kcal	fat	sat fat	carb	sugar	protein	fibre
587 KJ	142 kcal	15.2 g	2.2 g	0.4 g	0.3 g	1.0 g	0.6 g

	4 portions	10 portions
water	250 ml	625 ml
olive oil	60 ml	150 ml
lemon, juice of	1	1½
bay leaf	½	1
sprig of thyme		
peppercorns	6	18
coriander seeds	6	18
salt		
small white button mushrooms, cleaned	200 g	500 g

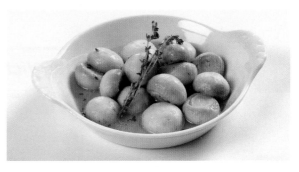

1 Combine all the ingredients except the mushrooms, to create a Greek-style cooking liquor.

2 Cook the mushrooms gently in the cooking liquor for 3 to 4 minutes.

3 Serve cold with the unstrained liquor.

Chef's tip
Simmer the vegetables carefully so that they are correctly cooked and absorb the flavours.

Try something different

Other vegetables can also be cooked in this style, using the same liquor.

- For artichokes, peel and trim 6 artichokes for 4 portions (or 15 for 10); cut the leaves short and remove the chokes. Blanch the artichokes in water with a little lemon juice for 10 minutes, refresh, then simmer in the Greek-style liquor for 15–20 minutes.

- For cauliflower, trim and wash one medium cauliflower for 4 portions (2½ for 10); break it into small sprigs about the size of cherries. Blanch the sprigs for about 5 minutes, refresh, then simmer in the Greek-style liquor for 5–10 minutes. Keep the cauliflower slightly undercooked and crisp.

62 Golden beetroot with Parmesan

	4 portions	10 portions
golden beetroot	400 g	1 kg
Parmesan, freshly grated	50 g	125 g
seasoning		

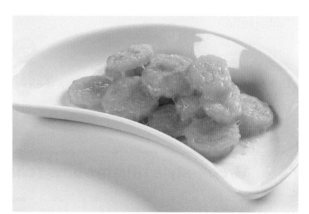

1 Peel the golden beetroot and cut into 5 mm slices. Either steam or plain boil until tender.

2 Drain well and place in a suitable serving dish. Sprinkle with Parmesan and grill under the salamander or in the oven.

63 Vichy carrots (carottes Vichy)

| cal 338 KJ | kcal 82 kcal | fat 5.4 g | sat fat 3.4 g | carb 8.0 g | sugar 7.5 g | protein 0.7 g | fibre 2.4 g | * |

     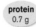

	4 portions	10 portions
carrots	400 g	1 kg
salt, pepper		
sugar		
butter	25 g	60 g
Vichy water (optional)		
parsley, chopped		

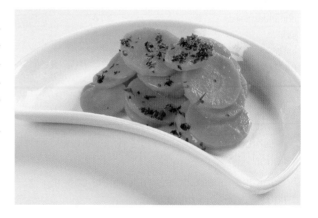

1 Peel and wash the carrots (which should not be larger than 2 cm in diameter).

2 Cut into 2 mm-thin slices on the mandolin.

3 Place in a pan with a little salt, a pinch of sugar and butter. Barely cover with Vichy water.

4 Cover with a buttered paper and allow to boil steadily in order to evaporate all the water.

5 When the water has completely evaporated, check that the carrots are cooked; if not, add a little more water and continue cooking. Do not overcook.

6 Toss the carrots over a fierce heat for 1–2 minutes in order to give them a glaze.

7 Serve sprinkled with chopped parsley.

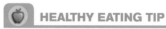 **HEALTHY EATING TIP**

● Use the minimum amount of salt.

Vichy water is water from the French town of Vichy. This dish is characterised by the glaze produced by reducing the butter and sugar.

* Using water only

64 Buttered celeriac, turnips or swedes

cal	kcal	fat	sat fat	carb	sugar	protein	fibre
253 KJ	60 kcal	5.4 g	3.3 g	2.5 g	2.5 g	0.7 g	1.9 g

	4 portions	10 portions
celeriac, turnips or swedes	400 g	1 kg
salt, sugar		
butter	25 g	60 g
parsley, chopped		

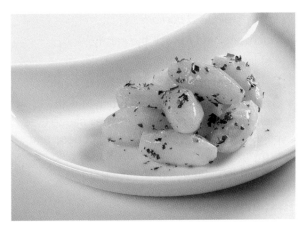

1 Peel and wash the vegetables.
2 Cut into neat pieces or turn barrel shaped.
3 Place in a pan with a little salt, a pinch of sugar and the butter. Barely cover with water.
4 Cover with a buttered paper and allow to boil steadily in order to evaporate all the water.
5 When the water has completely evaporated, check that the vegetables are cooked; if not, add a little more water and continue cooking. Do not overcook.
6 Toss the vegetables over a fierce heat for 1–2 minutes to glaze.
7 Drain well, and serve sprinkled with chopped parsley.

65 Parsnips *(panais)*

cal	kcal	fat	sat fat	carb	sugar	protein	fibre
235 KJ	56 kcal	0.0 g	0.0 g	13.5 g	2.7 g	1.3 g	2.5 g

1 Wash well. Peel the parsnips and re-wash well.
2 Cut into quarters lengthwise, remove the centre root if tough.
3 Cut into neat pieces and cook in lightly salted water until tender, or steam.
4 Drain and serve with melted butter or in a cream sauce.

Roasting

Parsnips may be roasted in the oven in a little fat (as shown here) or in with a joint, and can be cooked and prepared as a purée.

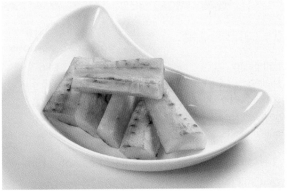

Chef's tip
For great roast parsnips, blanch them for 2 minutes, drain, then roast in hot olive oil.

66 Salsify *(salsifi)*

cal	kcal	fat	sat fat	carb	sugar	protein	fibre
76 KJ	18 kcal	0.0 g	0.0 g	2.8 g	2.8 g	1.9 g	0.0 g

½ kg will yield 2–3 portions

1 Wash, peel and rewash the salsify.

2 Cut into 5 cm lengths.

3 Cook in a blanc (see below). Do not overcook.

4 Salsify may then be served brushed with melted butter, or coated in mornay sauce (see page 185), sprinkled with grated cheese and browned under a salamander. It may also be passed through batter and deep-fried.

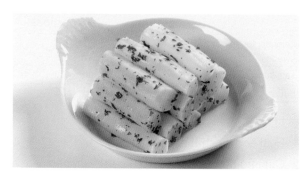

To make the blanc

	4 portions	10 portions
flour	10 g	20 g
cold water	½ litre	1 litre
salt, to taste		
lemon, juice of	½	1

1 Mix the flour and water together.

2 Add the salt and lemon juice. Pass through a strainer.

3 Place in a pan, bring to the boil, stirring continuously.

67 Goats' cheese and beetroot tarts, with salad of rocket

cal	kcal	fat	sat fat	carb	sugar	protein	fibre	salt
2377 KJ	568 kcal	37.7 g	9.0 g	43.6 g	4.5 g	18.6 g	1.8 g	1.7 g

	4 portions	10 portions
puff pastry	400 g	1 kg
shallots	150 g	375 g
cooked beetroot	200 g	500 g
goats' cheese	200 g	500 g
bunch rocket	1	2

1 Roll the puff pastry to a thickness of 3 mm.

2 Chill the rolled puff pastry for 10 minutes.

3 Finely slice the shallots and sweat down without colour.

4 Cut the puff pastry into four discs approximately 150 mm in diameter.

5 Chill the pastry discs for 10 minutes.

6 Dice the cooked beetroot into pieces 10 × 10 mm.

7 To make the tarts, place the shallots on the pastry discs.

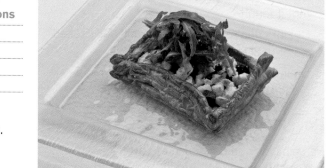

8 Cook at 180°C for 12 minutes.

9 Once cooked, remove from the oven and top with the diced beetroot and crumbled goats' cheese.

10 To finish the dish, place the tarts on plates and finish with picked rocket and vinaigrette.

68 Pickled red cabbage

Remove the outer leaves of the cabbage and shred the rest finely. Place in a deep bowl, sprinkle each layer with dry salt and leave for 24 hours. Rinse and drain, cover with spiced vinegar (see recipe for mixed pickle, page 198) and leave for a further 24 hours, mixing occasionally. Pack and cover.

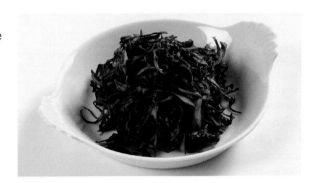

69 Basic tomato preparation (*tomate concassée*)

	4 portions	10 portions
tomatoes	400 g	1¼ kg
shallots or onions, chopped	25 g	60 g
butter, margarine or oil	25 g	60 g
salt, pepper		

1 Plunge the tomatoes into boiling water for 5–10 seconds – the riper the tomatoes, the less time is required. Refresh immediately.

2 Remove the skins, cut in halves across the tomato and remove all the seeds.

3 Roughly chop the flesh of the tomatoes.

4 Meanwhile, cook the chopped onion or shallots without colour in the oil, butter or margarine.

5 Add the tomatoes and season lightly.

6 Simmer gently on the side of the stove until the moisture is evaporated.

This is a cooked preparation that is usually included in the normal *mise-en-place* of a kitchen as it is used in a great number of dishes.

70 Bean goulash

cal	kcal	fat	sat fat	carb	sugar	protein	fibre
1728 KJ	411 kcal	17.9 g	2.7 g	50.0 g	7.3 g	17.3 g	18.5 g

	4 portions	10 portions
red kidney or haricot beans, dried	200 g	500 g
sunflower oil	60 ml	150 ml
onion, finely chopped	50 g	125 g
clove garlic, crushed	1	2–3
paprika	25 g	60 g
red peppers	2	5
green pepper	1	2–3
yellow pepper	1	2–3
button mushrooms, sliced	200 g	500 g
tomato purée	50 g	125 g
vegetable stock	750 ml	2 litre
bouquet garni		
seasoning		
small turned potatoes, cooked	8	20
parsley, chopped, to serve		

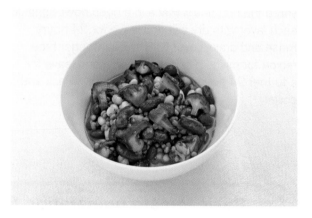

1 Soak the beans for 24 hours in cold water. Drain, place into a saucepan. Cover with cold water, bring to the boil and simmer until tender.

2 Heat the oil in a sauté pan, sweat the onion and garlic without colour for 2–3 minutes; add the paprika and sweat for a further 2–3 minutes.

3 Add the peppers, cut in halves, remove the seeds and cut into 1 cm dice. Add the button mushrooms; sweat for a further 2 minutes.

4 Add the tomato purée, vegetable stock and bouquet garni. Bring to the boil and simmer until the pepper and mushrooms are cooked.

5 Remove the bouquet garni. Add the drained cooked beans, correct the seasoning and stir.

6 Garnish with potatoes (or gnocchi) and chopped parsley.

7 Serve wholegrain pilaff or wholemeal noodles separately.

HEALTHY EATING TIP

- Use less sunflower oil to sweat the onions.
- Add a pinch of salt.
- Serve with rice or noodles and a green salad or mixed vegetables.

71 Mexican bean pot

cal	kcal	fat	sat fat	carb	sugar	protein	fibre
672 KJ	161 kcal	1.2 g	0.2 g	27.0 g	4.6 g	12.3 g	14.0 g

	4 portions	10 portions
red kidney or haricot beans, dried	300 g	1 kg
onions, finely chopped	100 g	250 g
carrots, sliced	100 g	250 g
tomato, skinned, deseeded and diced	200 g	500 g
cloves garlic, crushed and chopped	2	5
paprika	10 g	25 g
dried marjoram	3 g	9 g
small fresh chilli, finely chopped	1	2–3
small red pepper, finely diced	1	2–3
yeast extract	5 g	12 g
chives, chopped		
seasoning		

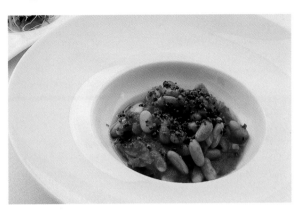

2 When three-quarters cooked, add all the other ingredients except the chopped chives.

3 Continue to simmer until all is completely cooked.

4 Serve sprinkled with chopped chives.

1 Soak the beans in cold water for 24 hours. Drain. Place into a saucepan, cover with cold water, bring to the boil and simmer gently.

 HEALTHY EATING TIP

- No added salt is needed; there is plenty in the yeast extract.
- Serve with a selection of colourful vegetables.

72 Hummus (chickpea and sesame seed paste)

cal	kcal	fat	sat fat	carb	sugar	protein	fibre
1546 KJ	367 kcal	15.3 g	2.0 g	39.2 g	3.0 g	20.9 g	1.7 g

	4 portions	10 portions
chickpeas, soaked	300 g	750 g
seasoning		
sesame seed paste (tahini)	75 g	187 g
clove garlic, crushed and chopped	1	2–3
onion, finely chopped	50 g	125 g
lemon, juice of	1	2
paprika	5 g	10 g

1 Cook the chickpeas in simmering water for 2 hours. Drain well.

2 Purée the chickpeas in a food processor, add seasoning, sesame seed paste, garlic and onion. Finish with lemon juice.

3 Place into a suitable serving dish decorated with a line of paprika.

Serve with pitta bread as a starter or as an accompaniment to main dishes.

Chef's tip
The chickpeas must be processed into a smooth paste.

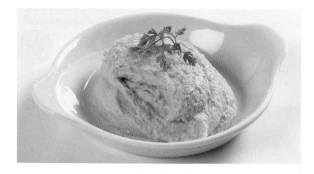

HEALTHY EATING TIP

- Use the minimum amount of salt.

- Serve with plenty of hot pitta bread and crudités to make a healthy starter.

73 Dhal

cal	kcal	fat	sat fat	carb	sugar	protein	fibre
1083 KJ	258 kcal	11.1 g	6.6 g	29.6 g	2.0 g	12.4 g	2.7 g

*

	4 portions	10 portions
lentils	200 g	500 g
turmeric	1 tsp	2½ tsp
ghee, butter or oil	50 g	125 g
onion, finely chopped	50 g	125 g
garlic clove, crushed and chopped	1	2–3
green chilli, finely chopped (optional)	1	2–3
cumin seeds	1 tsp	2½ tsp

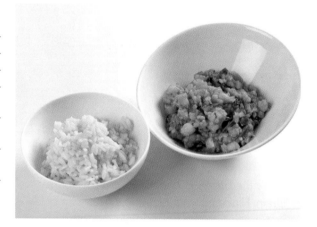

1 Place the lentils in a saucepan and cover with water. Add the turmeric, bring to the boil and gently simmer until cooked. Stir occasionally.

2 In a suitable pan, heat the fat and sweat the onion, garlic, chilli (if using) and cumin seeds. Stir into the lentils and season.

3 Serve hot to accompany other dishes. The consistency should be fairly thick but spoonable.

HEALTHY EATING TIP

- Lightly oil a pan to sweat the onion.

- This dish is high in protein and starchy carbohydrate, and low in fat. It is a very useful accompaniment for many higher-fat dishes and will help to dilute the overall fat content.

* Using butter

Dhal is made from lentils and is an important part of the basic diet for many Indian people. It can also be made using yellow split peas.

74 Oriental stir-fry Quorn

cal	kcal	fat	sat fat	carb	sugar	protein	fibre
836 KJ	200 kcal	11.8 g	1.3 g	11.6 g	7.3 g	12.7 g	5.6 g

	4 portions	10 portions
soy sauce	62 ml	156 ml
ginger, freshly grated	12 g	30 g
black pepper, to taste		
Quorn pieces, defrosted	200 g	500 g
vegetable oil	1 tbsp	3 tbsp
spring onions	8	20
red pepper, halved, deseeded and finely sliced	1	3
yellow pepper, halved, deseeded and finely sliced	1	3
green pepper, halved, deseeded and finely sliced	1	3
dry sherry	1 tbsp	3 tbsp
vegetable stock	62 ml	156 ml
sugar	¼ tsp	1 tsp
cornflour	6 g	15 g
blanched almonds or cashews	50 g	100 g

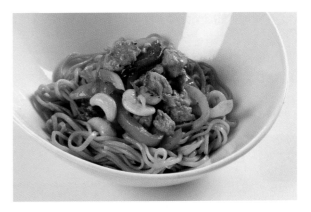

1 Prepare a marinade by mixing the soy sauce with the ginger, and season with black pepper.

2 Add the Quorn pieces, mix well and chill for 1 hour.

3 Strain the Quorn from the marinade. In a wok, add half the vegetable oil and stir-fry the Quorn quickly for approximately 4 minutes. Remove from the wok.

4 Add the remaining oil, and fry the spring onion and peppers for another 1–2 minutes.

5 Return the Quorn to the wok.

6 Add the strained marinade, sherry, stock and sugar. Bring to the boil.

7 Thicken lightly with the cornflour. Add the blanched almonds or cashews and stir gently to enable the ingredients to be covered with the sauce.

8 Serve with noodles or rice.

HEALTHY EATING TIP

- Use a little unsaturated oil to fry the Quorn, onions and peppers.

- No added salt is needed; there is plenty of flavour from the soy sauce, ginger and stock.

75 Crispy deep-fried tofu

cal	kcal	fat	sat fat	carb	sugar	protein	fibre
543 KJ	131 kcal	8.9 g	0.0 g	1.0 g	0.5 g	11.8 g	0.0 g

	4 portions	10 portions
firm tofu, cut into cubes	200g	500g

1 Coat the tofu cubes with any of the following: flour, egg and breadcrumbs; milk and flour; cornstarch; arrowroot.

2 Deep-fry the tofu at 180°C, until golden brown. Drain.

3 Serve garnished with freshly grated ginger and julienne of herbs.

4 Serve with a tomato sauce flavoured with coriander.

HEALTHY EATING TIP

- Use an unsaturated oil to fry the tofu.
- Make sure the oil is hot so that less is absorbed.
- Alternatively, try dry-frying the tofu.

* *50 g*

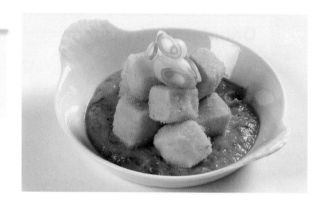

76 Barbecued tofu

cal	kcal	fat	sat fat	carb	sugar	protein	fibre
821 KJ	198 kcal	13.5 g	1.9 g	7.8 g	5.2 g	10.5 g	0.5 g

*

	4 portions	10 portions
spring onions, chopped	3	7
garlic cloves, crushed and chopped	4	10
maple syrup or honey	30 ml (2 tbsp)	75 ml (5 tbsp)
black pepper	2 g	5 g
soy sauce	60 ml (4 tbsp)	90 ml (10 tbsp)
sesame oil	30 ml (2 tbsp)	75 ml (5 tbsp)
rice wine or sake	30 ml (2 tbsp)	75 ml (5 tbsp)
toasted ground sesame seeds	1 tbsp	2½ tbsp
solid tofu, cubes	400 g	1 kg
broccoli florets	10	25

1 Mix together the chopped onions, garlic, maple syrup, pepper, soy sauce, sesame oil, rice wine or sake and the sesame seeds until thoroughly mixed.

2 Marinate the tofu in this mixture for several hours.

3 Remove the tofu from the marinade, and grill or fry it.

4 Boil the marinade and serve with the tofu in individual bowls with cooked broccoli florets.

5 Serve separately or on a bed of plain boiled or steamed fragrant Thai rice.

 HEALTHY EATING TIP

- Grill the marinated tofu and serve with fragrant Thai rice and vegetables to make an interesting vegetarian dish.

* *Using maple syrup*

77 Haricot bean salad *(salade de haricots blancs)*

cal	kcal	fat	sat fat	carb	sugar	protein	fibre
278 KJ	66 kcal	2.1 g	0.4 g	9.0 g	0.7 g	3.3 g	3.1 g

	4 portions	10 portions
haricot beans, cooked	200 g	500 g
vinaigrette	1 tbsp	2½ tbsp
parsley, chopped		
onion, chopped and blanched		
if required, or chives (optional)	15 g	40 g
salt, pepper		

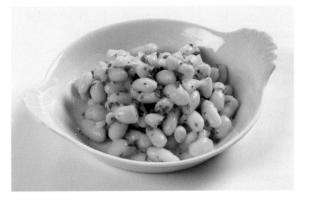

1. Combine all the ingredients.

This recipe can be used for any type of dried bean (see page 213).

Making vinaigrette
http://bit.ly/AFhvFa

HEALTHY EATING TIP

- Lightly dress with vinaigrette and add salt sparingly.

78 Niçoise salad

cal	kcal	fat	sat fat	carb	sugar	protein	fibre	
867 KJ	207 kcal	9.6 g	1.5 g	25.0 g	4.9 g	6.9 g	9.9 g	*

	4 portions	10 portions
tomatoes	100 g	250 g
French beans, cooked	200 g	500 g
diced potatoes, cooked	100 g	250 g
salt, pepper		
vinaigrette	1 tbsp	2½ tbsp
anchovy fillets	10 g	25 g
capers	5 g	12 g
stoned olives	10 g	25 g

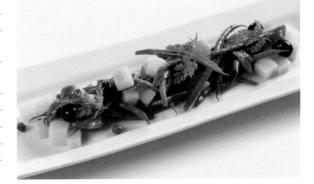

1 Peel the tomatoes, deseed and cut into neat segments.
2 Dress the beans, tomatoes and potatoes neatly.
3 Season with salt and pepper. Add the vinaigrette.
4 Decorate with anchovies, capers and olives.

HEALTHY EATING TIP

- Lightly dress with vinaigrette.
- The anchovies are high in salt, so no added salt is necessary.

* For 4 portions

79 Potato salad (*salade de pommes de terre*)

cal	kcal	fat	sat fat	carb	sugar	protein	fibre
2013 KJ	479 kcal	34.9 g	5.1 g	40.0 g	1.3 g	4.0 g	2.6 g

*

	4 portions	10 portions
potatoes, cooked	200 g	500 g
vinaigrette	1 tbsp	2½ tbsp
onion or chive (optional), chopped	10 g	25 g
mayonnaise or natural yoghurt	125 ml	300 ml
salt, pepper		
parsley or mixed fresh herbs, chopped		

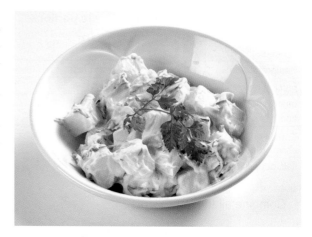

1 Cut the potatoes into ½–1 cm dice; sprinkle with vinaigrette.

2 Mix with the onion or chive, add the mayonnaise and correct the seasoning. (The onion may be blanched to reduce its harshness.)

3 Dress neatly and sprinkle with chopped parsley or herbs.

This is not usually served as a single hors d'oeuvre or main course.

Chef's tip

Mixing the potato, onion and mayonnaise gives a good flavour and texture, but be careful not to mix them too much or the potatoes will break up.

Try something different

● Potato salad can also be made by dicing raw peeled or unpeeled potato, cooking them – preferably by steaming (to retain shape) – and mixing with vinaigrette while warm.

● Variations include the addition of two chopped hard-boiled eggs, or 100 g of peeled dessert apple mixed with lemon juice, or a small bunch of picked watercress leaves.

● Potatoes may be cooked with mint and allowed to cool with the mint.

● Cooked small new potatoes can be tossed in vinaigrette with chopped fresh herbs (e.g. mint, parsley, chives).

* Using mayonnaise, for 4 portions

80 Vegetable salad (Russian salad) *(salade de légumes/salade russe)*

| cal 1566 KJ | kcal 373 kcal | fat 35.0 g | sat fat 5.2 g | carb 10.1 g | sugar 8.2 g | protein 5.0 g | fibre 11.9 g | * |

	4 portions	10 portions
carrots	100 g	250 g
turnips	50 g	125 g
French beans	50 g	125 g
peas	50 g	125 g
vinaigrette	1 tbsp	2–3 tbsp
mayonnaise or natural yoghurt	125 ml	300 ml
salt, pepper		

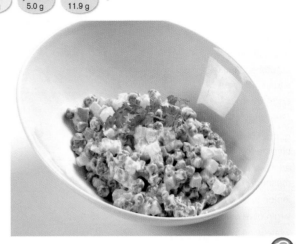

1 Peel and wash the carrots and turnips, cut into ½ cm dice or batons.
2 Cook separately in salted water, refresh and drain well.
3 Top and tail the beans, and cut into ½ cm dice; cook, refresh and drain well.
4 Cook the peas, refresh and drain well.
5 Mix all the well-drained vegetables with vinaigrette and then mayonnaise.
6 Correct the seasoning. Dress neatly.

Chef's tip
Do not overcook the vegetables, and drain them well before adding the dressing – otherwise the salad will be too wet.

HEALTHY EATING TIP

- Try half mayonnaise and half natural yoghurt.
- Season with the minimum amount of salt.

* Using mayonnaise, for 4 portions

81 Waldorf salad

1 Dice celery or celeriac and crisp russet apples.
2 Mix with shelled and peeled walnuts, and bind with mayonnaise.
3 Dress on quarters or leaves of lettuce (may also be served in hollowed-out apples).

Chef's tip
When mixing in the mayonnaise, add just enough to give the right texture and flavour.

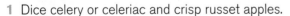

HEALTHY EATING TIP

Try using some yoghurt in place of the mayonnaise, which will proportionally reduce the fat.

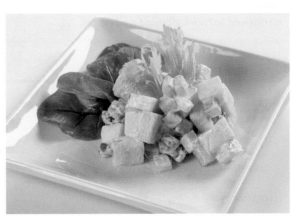

77 Caesar salad

cal	kcal	fat	sat fat	carb	sugar	protein	fibre
1494 KJ	361 kcal	32.2 g	7.9 g	5.1 g	2.0 g	12.9 g	1.2 g *

	4 portions	10 portions
cos lettuce (medium size)	2	4
croutons, 2 cm square	16	40
eggs, fresh	2	4
Dressing		
garlic, finely chopped	1 tsp	2 tsp
anchovy fillets, mashed	4	8
lemon juice	1	2
virgin olive oil	6 tbsp	15 tbsp
white wine vinegar	1 tbsp	2 tbsp
salt, black mill pepper		
To serve		
Parmesan, freshly grated	75 g	150 g

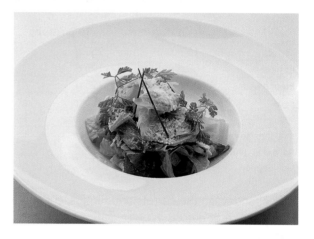

1 Separate the lettuce leaves, wash, dry thoroughly and refrigerate.

2 Lightly grill or fry (in good fresh oil) the croutons on all sides.

3 Plunge the eggs into boiling water for 1 minute, remove and set aside.

4 Break the lettuce into serving-sized pieces and place into a salad bowl.

5 Mix the dressing, break the eggs, spoon out the contents, mix with a fork, add to the dressing and mix into the salad.

6 Mix in the cheese, scatter the croutons on top and serve.

> Because the eggs are only lightly cooked, they must be perfectly fresh, and the salad must be prepared and served immediately. In the interests of food safety, the eggs are sometimes hardboiled. Alternatively the salad may be garnished with hardboiled gull's eggs. ⚠

🍎 HEALTHY EATING TIP

- No added salt is needed; anchovies and cheese are high in salt.
- Oven bake the croutons.
- Serve with fresh bread or rolls.

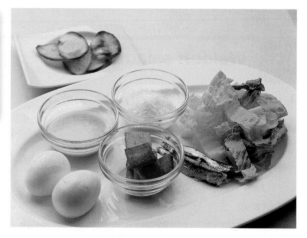

Ingredients for Caesar salad

* Using toast for croutons

In this chapter, you will learn how to:

1. prepare and cook meat and offal, including:

- select correct tools and equipment; prepare according to dish specification; use correct portions; apply flavourings; use moulds/basins or shape pastes according to recipe; and apply coatings
- undertake correct storage procedures for meat and offal
- apply appropriate cooking methods and principles; make sauces, prepare dressings, butters/oils, garnishes and apply finishing skills
- assemble dishes correctly; demonstrate safe and hygienic practices; evaluate the finished dish

2. have the knowledge to:

- identify types and quality points of meat and offal
- state the most commonly used joints and cuts of meat and offal
- identify tools and equipment used in the cooking of meat and offal
- explain cooking and preservation methods and principles for meat and offal
- explain how to know when meat and offal are cooked correctly and how to finish the dish.

Recipe number	Recipe	Page number
Beef		
7	Beef olives (paupiettes de boeuf)	296
8	Beef stroganoff (sauté de boeuf stroganoff)	297
6	Boeuf bourguignonne	294
5	Boiled silverside, carrots and dumplings	293
11	Carbonnade of beef (Belgian) (carbonnade de boeuf)	300
1	Chateaubriand with Roquefort butter	291
12	Cornish pasties	300
	Cottage pie	316
14	Goulash (Hungarian) (goulash de boeuf)	302
13	Hamburg or Vienna steak (bitok)	302
2	Roasting of beef (boeuf rôti)	291
4	Sirloin steak with red wine sauce (entrecote bordelaise)	293
10	Steak pie	299
9	Steak pudding	298
3	Yorkshire pudding	292
Lamb		
15	Best end of lamb with breadcrumbs and parsley	303
27	Braised lamb shanks with ratatouille	312
20	Breadcrumbed cutlets (côtelettes d'agneau panées)	307

Recipe number	Recipe	Page number
30	Brown lamb or mutton stew (navarin d'agneau)	314
19	Grilled cutlets (côtelettes d'agneau grilles)	306
21	Grilled loin or chump chops, or noisettes of lamb	307
31	Hot pot of lamb or mutton	315
23	Irish stew	308
25	Lamb fillets with beans and tomatoes	311
22	Lamb kebabs (shish kebab)	308
29	Mixed grill	313
16	Roast leg of lamb with mint, lemon and cumin	304
28	Roast saddle of lamb with rosemary mash	313
33	Samosas	317
32	Shepherd's pie (cottage pie)	316
18	Slow-cooked shoulder of lamb with vegetables	306
17	Stuffed roast loin of lamb	305
26	Valentine of lamb	311
24	White lamb stew (blanquette d'agneau)	310
Veal		
39	Braised shin of veal (osso buco)	323
41	Escalope of veal	325
	Escalope of veal Viennoise	325
	Escalope of veal with spaghetti and tomato sauce	325
	Fricassée de veau à l'ancienne	319

Recipe number	Recipe	Page number
32	Fricassée of veal (fricassée de veau)	319
38	Grilled veal cutlet (côte de veau grille)	322
40	Hot veal and ham pie	324
36	Roast veal four-bone rib	321
	Veal escalope Holstein	325
42	Veal escalopes with Parma ham and mozzarella cheese (involtini di vitelllo)	326
37	Veal stuffing	321
35	White stew or blanquette of veal (blanquette de veau)	320
Pork and bacon		
50	Boiled bacon (hock, collar or gammon)	332
51	Griddled gammon with apricot salsa	333
46	Pork loin chops with pesto and mozzarella	329
48	Pork escalopes	331
47	Raised pork pie/hot water paste	330
	Roast gravy	327
43	Roast leg of pork	327

Recipe number	Recipe	Page number
	Sage and onion dressing for pork	327
44	Slow roast pork belly	328
45	Spare ribs of pork in barbecue sauce	328
49	Sweet and sour pork	331
Offal and mixed meats		
55	Braised lambs' hearts (coeurs d'agneau braisés)	335
58	Braised veal sweetbreads (white) (ris de veau braisé – à blanc)	337
56	Fried lambs' liver and bacon (foie d'agneau au lard)	336
54	Grilled lambs' kidneys (rognons grillés)	335
60	Grilled veal sweetbreads	339
57	Kidney sauté (rognons sautés)	337
	Kidney sauté Turbigo	337
61	Lambs' kidneys bouchées	339
53	Oxtail with Guinness	334
52	Potted meats	333
59	Sweetbread escalope (escalope de ris de veau)	338

Meats

The structure of meat

To cook meat properly it is important to understand its structure.

- Meat is made of fibres bound together by connective tissue.
- Connective tissue is made up of elastin (yellow) and collagen (white).
- Yellow tissue needs to be removed.
- Small fibres are present in tender cuts and young animals.
- Coarser fibres are present in tougher cuts and older animals.
- Fat helps to provide flavour, and moistens meat in roasting and grilling.
- Tenderness, flavour and moistness are increased if meat is hung after slaughter and before being used.

- Storage times: beef up to 3 weeks; veal 1–3 weeks; lamb 10–15 days; pork 7–14 days.
- Hang and store meat between 18°C and 58°C.

Meat varies considerably in its fat content. The fat is found round the outside of meat, in marbling and inside the meat fibres. The visible fat (saturated) should be trimmed off as much as possible before cooking.

Lots of useful information about meat can be obtained at www.qmscotland.co.uk.

Offal and other edible parts of the carcass

Offal is the edible parts taken from the inside of a carcass of meat: liver, kidneys, heart and sweetbreads. Tripe, brains, tongue, head and oxtail are also sometimes included under this term.

Fresh offal (unfrozen) should be purchased as required and can be refrigerated under hygienic conditions at a temperature of 21°C, at a relative humidity of 90 per cent, for up to seven days. Frozen offal must be kept in a deep freeze and defrosted in a refrigerator as required.

Liver and kidney dishes may traditionally have been served undercooked or lightly cooked, but it is now advised that they are **cooked thoroughly all the way through** to avoid possible food poisoning.

Liver and kidneys

- **Calf's liver** is considered to be the most tender and tasty. It is also the most expensive.
- **Lamb's liver** is mild in flavour, light in colour and tender. **Sheep's liver**, being from an older animal, is firmer, deeper in colour and has a stronger flavour.
- **Ox** or **beef liver** is the cheapest and, if taken from an older animal, can be coarse and have a strong flavour. It is usually braised.
- **Pig's liver** has a strong, full flavour and is used mainly for pâté recipes.

Quality points:

- Liver should look fresh, moist and smooth, with a pleasant colour and no unpleasant smell.
- Liver should not be dry or contain an excessive number of tubes.

Food value: liver is a good source of protein and iron. It contains vitamins A and D, and is low in fat.

- **Lamb's kidneys** are light in colour, delicate in flavour and ideal for grilling and frying.
- **Sheep's kidneys** are darker in colour and stronger in flavour.
- **Calf's kidneys** are light in colour, delicate in flavour and used in a variety of dishes.
- **Ox kidney** is dark in colour, strong in flavour, and is either braised or used in pies and puddings (mixed with beef).
- **Pig's kidneys** are smooth, long and flat and have a strong flavour.

Quality points:

- Suet – the saturated fat in which kidneys are encased – should be left on until they are used, otherwise the kidneys will dry out. The suet should be removed when kidneys are being prepared for cooking.
- Both suet and kidneys should be moist and have no unpleasant smell.

The food value is similar to that of liver.

Hearts

- **Lamb's hearts** are small and light; they are normally served whole.
- **Sheep's hearts** are dark and solid; they can be dry and tough unless cooked carefully.
- **Ox** or **beef hearts** are dark coloured and solid, and tend to be dry and tough.
- **Calf's hearts**, coming from a younger animal, are lighter in colour and more tender.

Most hearts need slow braising to tenderise them.

Quality points: hearts should not be too fatty and should not contain too many tubes. When cut they should be moist, not sticky, and with no unpleasant smell.

Food value: hearts are a good source of protein.

Sweetbreads

These are the pancreas and thymus glands, known as heart breads and neck. The heart bread is round, plump and a better quality than the neck bread, which is long and uneven. Calf's heart bread, considered the best, weighs up to 600 g, lamb's heart bread up to 100 g.

Quality points:

- Heart and neck breads should be fleshy and a good size.
- They should be creamy white and have no unpleasant smell.

Food value: sweetbreads are an easily digested source of protein, which makes them valuable for use in special diets for people who are ill.

Tripe

Tripe is the stomach lining or white muscle of the ox, consisting of the rumen or paunch and the honeycomb tripe (considered the best); sheep tripe, darker in colour, is available in some areas.

Quality points: tripe should be fresh, with no signs of stickiness or unpleasant smell.

Food value: tripe contains protein, is low in fat and high in calcium.

Brains

Calves' brains are normally used. They must be fresh and have no unpleasant smell. They are a good source of protein, with other trace elements.

Tongues

Ox, lamb and sheep tongues are those most used in cooking. Ox tongues are usually salted then soaked before being cooked. Lamb tongues are cooked fresh.

Quality points:

- Tongues must be fresh and have no unpleasant smell.
- There should not be too much waste at the root end.

Head

Sheep's heads can be used for stock, pigs' heads for brawn (a cold meat preparation) and calves' heads for speciality dishes (e.g. calf's head vinaigrette). Heads should have plenty of flesh on them, and should be fresh; they should not be sticky or have any unpleasant smell.

Oxtail

Oxtails usually weigh 1½–2 kg; they should be lean, without much fat. There should be no sign of stickiness and no unpleasant smell.

Suet

Beef suet should be creamy-white, brittle and dry. Other meat fat should be fresh, not sticky, and with no unpleasant smell.

Marrow

Marrow comes from the bones of the leg of beef. It should be a good size, firm, creamy-white and odourless. Sliced, poached marrow may be used as a garnish for some meat dishes and savouries.

Bones

Bones must be fresh, not sticky, with no unpleasant smell, and preferably meaty as they are used for stock, the foundation for so many preparations.

Preservation of meat

Salting

Meat can be pickled in brine. This method of preservation may be applied to silverside, brisket and ox tongues. Salting is used in the production of bacon, before the sides of pork are smoked, and for hams.

Chilling

This means that meat is kept at a temperature just above freezing point in a controlled atmosphere. Chilled meat cannot be kept in the usual type of cold room for more than a few days – long enough for the meat to hang, making it more tender.

Freezing

Small carcasses, such as lamb and mutton, can be frozen; their quality is not affected by freezing. They can be kept frozen until required and then thawed out before being used. Some beef is frozen, but it is not such good quality as chilled beef.

Canning

Large quantities of meat are canned; corned beef is worth mentioning since it has a very high protein content. Pork is used for tinned luncheon meat.

Health, safety and hygiene

For information on maintaining a safe and secure working environment, a professional and hygienic appearance, clean food production areas, equipment and utensils, and food hygiene, please refer to Chapters 2 and 3. Additional health and safety points to reduce the risk of cross-contamination are as follows.

- When preparing uncooked meat or poultry, and then cooked food, or changing from one type of meat or poultry to another, equipment, working areas and utensils must be thoroughly cleaned, or changed.

- If colour-coded boards are used, it is essential to always use the correct colour-coded boards for the preparation of foods, and different ones for cooked foods.

- Store uncooked meat and poultry on trays to prevent dripping, in separate refrigerators at a temperature of 3–5°C, preferably at the lower temperature. If separate refrigerators are not available then store in separate areas within the refrigerator.

- Wash all work surfaces with a bactericidal detergent to kill bacteria. This is particularly important when handling poultry and pork.

- When using boning knives, wear a safety apron as a protection; if a great deal of boning is being done then it is also a good idea to wear protective gloves.

To maintain the quality and safety of meat and poultry dishes once cooked, it is advisable to check internal temperatures using a probe. The recommended temperatures are shown in Table 10.1.

Choosing and buying

Meat from specific parts of an animal may be cut and cooked according to local custom and, more strictly, by religious observance – especially in Jewish kosher and Islamic halal butchery, which stipulates the killing of the animal by an authorised person of the religion, total voiding of the blood by draining, soaking and salting, and the consumption of the meat within 72 hours. Kosher dietary laws further demand that only the forequarters of permitted animals – goats, sheep, deer and cattle – may be used.

Voiding: Emptying or draining away.

Meat is a natural and therefore not a uniform product, varying in quality from carcass to carcass, while flavour, texture and appearance are determined by the type of animal and the way it has been fed. Fat gives a characteristic flavour to meat and helps to keep it moist during roasting, but meat does not have to be fatty to be good quality and flavoursome. Neither is the colour of meat any guide to quality. Consumers are inclined to choose light-coloured meat – bright red beef, for example – because they think it will be fresher than an alternative dark-red piece. Freshly butchered beef is bright red because the pigment (myoglobin) in the tissues has been chemically affected by the oxygen in the air, not because the meat itself is fresh. After several hours, the colour changes to dark red or brown as the pigment is oxidised more to become metamyoglobin, so darker meat can still be fresh. The colour of fat can vary from almost pure white in lamb, to bright yellow in beef. Colour depends on the feed, on the breed and, to a certain extent, on the time of year.

The most useful guide to tenderness and quality is a knowledge of the cuts of meat and their location on the carcass. The various cuts are described under their respective headings (see below), but a few principles can be followed.

Table 10.1 Recommended internal temperatures*

Beef	rare: 45–47°C; medium 50–52°C; well done 64–70°C
Lamb	pink: 55°C; well done 62°C
Pork	60–65°C
Veal	60°C
Turkey/chicken	77°C
Duck	pink 57°C; well done 62°C

*Environmental Health Officers may require higher temperatures

- The leanest and tenderest cuts – the 'prime' cuts – come from the hindquarters.

- The parts of the animal that have had plenty of muscular exercise and where fibres have become hardened – the 'coarse' cuts – come from the neck, legs and forequarters. These provide meat for braising and stewing, and many consider them to have more flavour, although they require slow cooking to make them tender.

- The meat from young animals is generally more tender. Tenderness is a prime factor, so animals may also be injected with an enzyme such as papin before slaughter, which softens the fibres and muscles. This merely speeds up a natural and more satisfactory process, as meat contains its own enzymes that gradually break down the protein cell walls as the carcass ages.

- It is for this tenderisation process that meat is hung for 10 to 20 days in controlled conditions (temperature and humidity) before it is sold. The longer meat is aged, the more expensive it becomes, as the cost of refrigeration is high and the meat itself shrinks because of evaporation and the trimming of the outside hardened edges.

Cooking

Meat is an extremely versatile product that can be cooked in a multitude of ways, and matched with practically any vegetable, fruit or herb. The cut (e.g. shin, steak, brisket), the method of heating (e.g. roasting, braising, grilling), and the time and temperature all affect the way the meat will taste. Raw meat is difficult to chew because the muscle fibre contains an elastic protein (collagen), which is softened only by mincing – as in steak tartare – or by cooking. When you cook meat, the protein gradually coagulates as the internal temperature increases. At 77°C coagulation is complete and the protein begins to harden, so any further cooking makes the meat tougher.

Since tenderness combined with flavour is the aim in meat cookery, time and temperature are the key concerns. In principle, slow cooking retains the juices and produces a more tender result than fast cooking at high temperatures. There are, of course, occasions when high temperatures are essential: for instance, you need to grill a steak under a hot flame for a very short time in order to get a crisp, brown surface and a pink, juicy interior – using a low temperature would not give you the desired result. But in potentially tough cuts (e.g. breast of lamb), or where there is a lot of connective tissue (e.g. in neck of lamb), slower cooking converts the tissues to gelatine and helps to make the meat more tender. Meat containing bone will take longer to cook because bone is a poor conductor of heat.

Tips for cooking meat

Meat bones are useful for giving flavour to soups and stocks, especially beef bones with plenty of marrow. Veal bones are gelatinous and help to enrich and thicken soups and sauces. Fat can be rendered down for frying, or used as an ingredient (suet or lard).

With regard to cooking the meat itself:

- Tough or coarse cuts of meat should be cooked by braising, pot roasting or stewing. These longer, slower methods of cooking dissolve the collagen (one of the proteins that can make meat tough), forming gelatine and making the meat more tender and tasty

- Marinating in a suitable marinade, such as wine and wine vinegar, helps to tenderise the meat and adds flavour.

- Prime cuts, such as beef fillets, contain little collagen and do not require long cooking to tenderise the meat. Although most chefs would start the prime cuts at a high temperature for a short period, this does not always give a perfect result.

- Searing meat in hot fat or in a hot oven before roasting or stewing helps to produce a crisp exterior by coagulating the protein but does not, as is widely supposed, seal in the juices. Also, if the temperature is too high and the meat is cooked for too long, rapid evaporation of the juices and contraction of the meat will cause much of the juices and fat to be lost, making the meat tougher, drier and less tasty. This is particularly true for prime cuts, as they do not contain much fat or collagen to start with. A lower temperature and longer in the oven will produce a better result.

- Sprinkling salt on meat before cooking will also speed up the loss of moisture because salt absorbs water (it is hygroscopic).

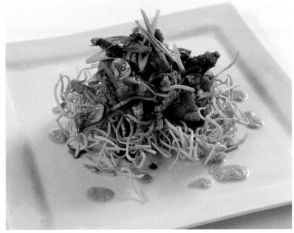

The shredded pork in this dish has been marinated before cooking (recipe available on Dynamic Learning)

Slow cooking meat

When cooking meats at low temperatures there is one obvious flaw: the meat will not be exposed to the high cooking temperatures that develop that beautiful roasted flavour. This chemical reaction of browning is called the Maillard reaction and is an extremely complicated chain of reactions that involves carbons, proteins, sulphurs, etc. One thing we do know about this reaction is that at 140°C and above, you will start to release the wonderful roasted meat flavours. Therefore, when slow-cooking meats they need to be started very quickly on a hot pan on the stove to start this Maillard reaction. In some cases you will need to return the meat quickly to the pan to re-caramelise the outside; alternatively, if the joint is dense and large, remove it from the low oven and increase the temperature to 190–200°C. When the oven is up to temperature, put the joint back in for a short while to crisp the outside. The density of the meat and size of the joint will ensure that there is very little secondary cooking or residual heat left to cook through to the core.

As already mentioned, the collagen that makes up connective tissue requires long cooking at a moderate temperature to convert it into gelatine. This provides a form of secondary or internal basting. When basting the outside of the meat, take care not to raise the internal temperature of the meat too much as this will destroy the secondary basting properties of the collagen – at temperatures above 88°C the collagen will dissolve rapidly into the braising medium, making the meat less tender and moist. Therefore, the traditional braising method of bringing a casserole to a simmer and placing it in the oven at 140°C could, in theory, make the meat dry. The more modern approach to braising is to have the cooking medium at between 80°C and 85°C, and this can be controlled best on the top of the stove. Alternatively, set your oven at 90°C (approximately) and check the cooking medium once in a while.

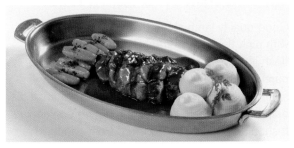

Braising is the best method of cookery for shin of beef: here it has been braised with stout, ale and honey (recipe available on Dynamic Learning)

Making braised beef
http://bit.ly/wGNSvn

When slow-cooking prime joints, the rule of thumb is to reduce the temperature of cooking as, in some cases, shrinkage can occur from 59°C, up to 65°C for sirloin of beef. A steak of sirloin beef has more collagen than a fillet (it is essentially a worked muscle group) and is generally cooked on a high heat, either roasted or pan-fried. This will make the sirloin extremely tender and moist, with a roasted outer and the flavoursome roasted meat taste that people enjoy.

An average sirloin joint for roasting can weigh from 2–5 kg whole off the bone. The method for cooking this is to seal the meat on the outside, as you would normally, place it into a pre-heated oven at 180°C, cook at 180°C for 10 minutes, then reduce the temperature to 64°C (the oven door will need to be open at this stage). Once the oven has come down to 64°C, close the door and cook for a further 1 hour 50 minutes. This will give you an extremely tender piece of sirloin.

(You will find more information about methods of cooking meat in Chapter 7 Methods of cookery.)

Lamb and mutton

Lamb is the meat from a sheep under a year old; above that age the animal is called a 'hogget' and its meat becomes mutton. The demand for lamb in preference to mutton is partly due to the fact that the lamb carcass provides smaller cuts of more tender meat. Mutton needs to be well ripened by long hanging before cooking and, as it is usually fatty, needs a good deal of trimming as well.

Good-quality lamb should have fine, white fat, with pink flesh when freshly cut; in mutton the flesh is a deeper colour. Lamb has a very thin, parchment-like covering on the carcass, known as the 'fell', which is usually left on roasts to help them maintain their shape during cooking. It should, however, be removed from chops. The flesh of a younger lamb is usually more tender. A good way to judge age is through weight – especially with legs of lamb: the highest quality weighs about 2.3 kg and never more than 4 kg. Smaller chops are also more tender and, therefore, more expensive. Mutton is rarely available to buy; when it is, it is much less expensive than lamb.

As a guide, when ordering lamb allow approximately 100 g meat off the bone per portion, and 150 g on the bone per portion. However, these weights are only approximate and will vary according to the quality of the meat and what it will be used for. For example, a chef will often cut up a carcass differently from a shop butcher because a chef needs to consider the presentation of the particular joint, while the butcher is more often concerned with being economical. In the text that follows, simple orders of dissection are given for each carcass. In general, bones only need to be removed when preparing joints, to make carving easier. The bones are used for stock and the excess fat can be rendered down for second-class dripping.

Joints, uses and weights

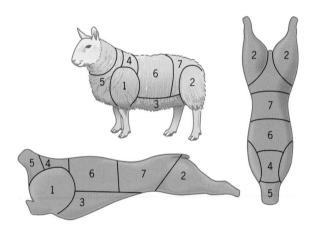

Joints of lamb (see Table 10.2)

Quality of lamb (sheep under 1 year old) and mutton

- A good-quality animal should be compact and evenly fleshed.
- The lean flesh should be firm, a pleasing dull-red colour with a fine texture or grain.
- There should be an even distribution of surface fat, which should be a hard, brittle, flaky texture and a clear white colour.
- In a young animal the bones should be pink and porous, so that when they are cut a little blood can be seen inside them. As animals grow older, their bones become hard, dense and white, and are more likely to splinter when chopped.

Table 10.2 Joints, uses and weights (numbers in left-hand column refer to the diagram on page 274)

Joint	Uses	Lamb (kg)	Mutton (kg)
whole carcass		16	25
(1) shoulder (two)	roasting, stewing	3	4½
(2) leg (two)	roasting (mutton boiled)	3½	5½
(3) breast (two)	roasting, stewing	1½	2½
(4) middle neck	stewing	2	3
(5) scrag end	stewing, broth	½	1
(6) best end rack (two)	roasting, grilling, frying	2	3
(7) saddle	roasting, grilling, frying	3½	5½
kidneys	grilling, sauté	–	–
heart	braising	–	–
liver	frying	–	–
sweetbreads	braising, frying	–	–
tongue	braising, boiling	–	–

Order of dissection of a carcass

Dissect a carcass in the following order:

1 Remove the shoulders.
2 Remove the breasts.
3 Remove the middle neck and scrag.
4 Remove the legs.
5 Divide the saddle from the best end.

Preparation of joints and cuts

The different joints and cuts need to be prepared in different ways.

Table 10.3 Common cooking methods

Saddle	roast, pot roast (poêlé)
Loin	roast
Fillet	grill, fry
Loin chop	grill, fry, stew, braise
Chump chop	grill, fry, stew, braise
Kidney	grill, sauté

Shoulder

● **Roasting:** clean and trim the knucklebone, leaving approximately 3 cm of clean bone.
● **Boning:** remove the blade bone and upper arm bone (see the diagram on the next page), then tie with string; the shoulder may be stuffed (see recipe 18) before tying.
● **Cutting for stews:** bone out the meat and cut into even 25–50 g pieces.
● **Roasting:** remove the pelvic or aitchbone; trim the knuckle, cleaning 3 cm of bone; trim off excess fat and tie with string if necessary.

Breasts

● Remove excess fat and skin.
● **Roasting:** bone; stuff and roll; tie with string.
● **Stewing:** bone and then cut into even 25–50 g pieces.

Tying butcher's knots
http://bit.ly/y1VCTX

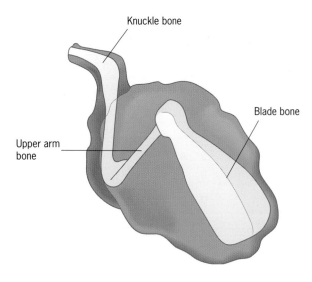

Shoulder of lamb, showing three bones

Middle neck

Stewing: remove excess fat, excess bone and gristle; cut into even 50 g pieces. When butchered correctly, this joint can give good uncovered second-class cutlets.

Scrag-end

Stewing: this can be chopped down the centre, the excess bone, fat and gristle removed, and cut into even 50 g pieces, or boned out and cut into pieces.

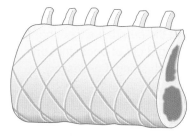

Best end (rack) of lamb

Saddle

A full saddle is illustrated on the right. For large banquets it is sometimes found better to remove the chumps and use short saddles.

Divide up the saddle as follows:

- Remove the skin, starting from head to tail and from breast to back.

- Split down the centre of the backbone to produce two loins.

Each loin can be roasted whole, boned and stuffed, or cut into loin and chump chops.

Saddle for roasting

- Skin and remove the kidney.
- Trim the excess fat and sinew.
- Cut off the flaps, leaving about 15 cm each side so that they meet in the middle under the saddle.
- Remove the aitch, or pelvic, bone.
- Score neatly and tie with string.
- For presentation the tail may be left on, protected with foil and tied back.
- The saddle can also be completely boned, stuffed and tied.

Loin

- **Roasting:** skin; remove excess fat and sinew; remove the pelvic bone; tie with string.
- **Boning and stuffing:** remove the skin, excess fat and sinew. Bone out, replace the fillet and tie with string. Season, stuff and tie.

Chops

Loin chops

- Skin the loin, remove the excess fat and sinew, then cut into chops approximately 100–150 g in weight.
- A first-class loin chop should have a piece of kidney skewered in the centre.

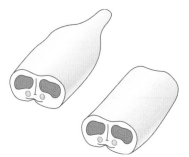

Saddle of lamb

Double loin chop (also known as a Barnsley chop)

- These are cut approximately 2 cm across a saddle on the bone.
- When trimmed they are secured with a skewer and may include a piece of kidney in the centre of each chop.

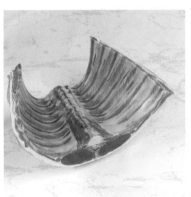

A saddle of lamb

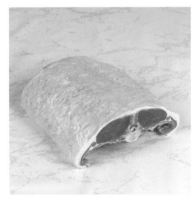

A pair of best ends of lamb

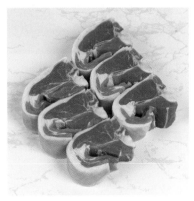

Lamb loin chops

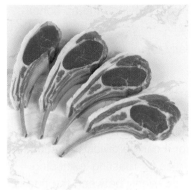

Lamb cutlets

Chump chops

- These are cut from the chump end of the loin.
- Cut into approximately 150 g chops and trim where necessary.

Noisette

- This is a cut from a boned-out loin.
- Cut slantwise into approximately 2 cm thick slices, bat out slightly and trim into a cutlet shape.

Rosette

This is a cut from a boned-out loin approximately 2 cm thick. It is shaped round and tied with string.

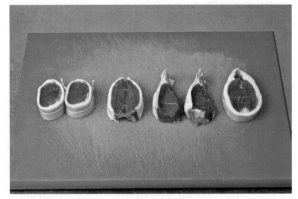

Left to right: rosette, valentine, noisette, Barnsley (double loin) chop

Best end (rack)

- Remove the skin from head to tail and from breast to back.
- Remove the sinew and the tip of the blade bone.
- Complete the preparation of the rib bones as shown in the photos opposite.

- Clean the sinew from between the rib bones and trim the bones.
- Score the fat neatly to approximately 2 mm deep.
- Trim the overall length of the rib bones to two and a half times the length of the nut of meat.

The whole joint can be **roasted** (prepare as shown in photo 6) or it can be divided into cutlets. For **cutlets**, prepare as for roasting, excluding the scoring, and divide evenly between the bones. Alternatively, the cutlets can be cut from the best end and prepared separately. A double cutlet consists of two bones, so a six-bone best end yields six single or three double cutlets.

Preparation of offal

Kidney

- **Grilling:** skin and split lengthwise three-quarters of the way through; cut out and discard the gristle, and skewer.

- **Sauté:** skin and remove the gristle. Cut slantwise into 6–8 pieces.

Hearts

Braising: remove the tubes and excess fat.

Liver

Remove skin, gristle and tubes and cut into thin slices on the slant.

Sweetbreads

- Wash well, blanch and trim.
- Soak in salted water for 2–3 hours to remove any traces of blood.

Tongue

- Remove the bone and gristle from the throat end.
- Soak in cold water for 2–4 hours. If salted, soak for 3–4 hours.

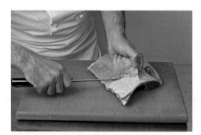

(1) To prepare best end of lamb, first remove the bark/skin, leaving as much fat as possible on the joint

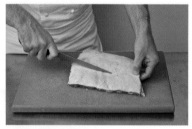

(2) Mark/score 2 cm from end of bone

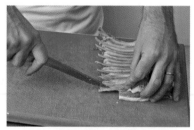

(3) Score down the middle of the back of the bone, scoring the cartilage

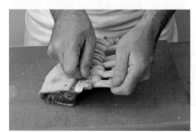

(4) Pull the skin fat and meat from the bone (to bring out the bone ends – this is an alternative to scraping them)

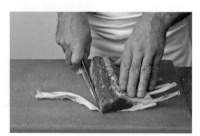

(5) Remove the elastin;

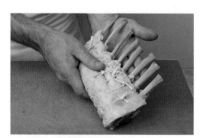

(6) Tie the joint

Beef

Butchery

A whole side (approximate weight 180 kg) is divided into the wing ribs and the fore ribs.

Hindquarter of beef

Dissection

- Remove the rump suet and kidney.
- Remove the thin flank.
- Divide the loin and rump from the leg (topside, silverside, thick flank and shin).
- Remove the fillet.
- Divide the rump from the sirloin.
- Remove the wing ribs.
- Remove the shin.
- Bone out the aitchbone.
- Divide the leg into the three remaining joints (silverside, topside and thick flank).

Preparation of joints and cuts of hindquarter

- **Shin:** bone out, remove excess sinew; cut or chop as required.

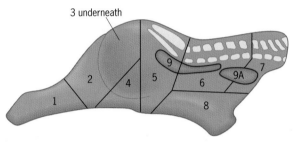

Hindquarter of beef

- **Topside:** roasting – remove excess fat, cut into joints and tie with string; braising – as for roasting; stewing – cut into dice or steaks as required.
- **Silverside:** remove the thigh bone; this joint is usually kept whole and pickled in brine prior to boning.
- **Thick flank:** as for topside.
- **Rump:** bone out; cut off the first outside slice for pies and puddings. Cut into approximately 1½ cm slices for steaks. The point steak – considered the most tender – is cut from the pointed end of the slice.

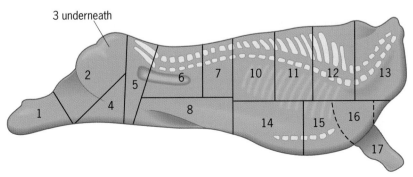

Side of beef

Table 10.4 Joints, uses and weights of the hindquarter (numbers in left-hand column refer to the diagram above)

Joint	Uses	Approx. weight (kg)
(1) shin	consommé, beef tea, stewing	7
(2) topside	braising, stewing, second-class roasting	10
(3) silverside	pickled in brine then boiled	14
(4) thick flank	braising and stewing	12
(5) rump	grilling and frying as steaks, braised in the piece	10
(6) sirloin	roasting, grilling and frying in steaks	9
(7) wing ribs	roasting, grilling and frying in steaks	5
(8) thin flank	stewing, boiling, sausages	10
(9) fillet	roasting, grilling and frying in steaks	3
fat and kidney	–	10

Forequarter of beef

Dissection

- Remove the shank.
- Divide in half down the centre.
- Take off the fore ribs.
- Divide into joints.

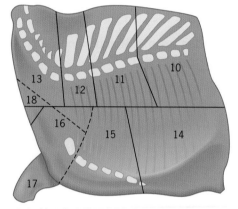

Forequarter of beef

Table 10.5 Joints, uses and weights of the forequarter (numbers in left-hand column refer to the diagram above)

Joint	Uses	Approx. weight (kg)
(10) fore rib	roasting and braising	8
(11) middle rib	roasting and braising	10
(12) chuck rib	stewing and braising	15
(13) sticking piece	stewing and sausages	9
(14) plate	stewing and sausages	10
(15) brisket	pickled in brine and boiled, pressed beef	19
(16) leg of mutton cut	braising and stewing	11
(17) shank	consommé, beef tea	6

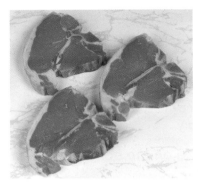

T-bone steaks

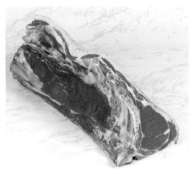

Fillet and loin of beef

Beef offal

Table 10.6 Uses of beef offal

Offal	Uses
tongue	pickled in brine, boiling, braising
heart	braising
liver	braising, frying
kidney	stewing, soup
sweetbread	braising, frying
tripe	boiling, braising
tail	braising, soup
suet	suet paste and stuffing, or rendered down for first-class dripping
bones	beef stocks

Quality of beef

- The lean meat should be bright red, with small flecks of white fat (marbled).
- The fat should be firm, brittle in texture, creamy-white in colour and odourless. Older animals and dairy breeds usually have fat that is a deeper-yellow colour.

Salting

Salting, especially of meat, is an ancient preservation technique. The salt draws out moisture and creates an environment inhospitable to bacteria. Meat is salted in cold weather so that it does not spoil while the salt takes effect.

Today, salting is still used with bacon and other pork and beef products (e.g. dried beef, corned beef (see below) and pastrami), which are made by soaking beef in a 10 per cent saltwater brine for several weeks.

Classifications and joints

Cuts of beef vary considerably, from very tender fillet steak to tough brisket or the shin, and there is a greater variety of cuts in beef than for any other type of meat. While their names may vary, there are 14 primary cuts from a side of beef, each one composed of muscle, fat, bone and connective tissue. The least developed muscles, usually from the inner areas, can be roasted or grilled, while leaner and more sinewy meat is cut from the more highly developed external muscles. Exceptions are rib and loin cuts, which come from external but basically immobile muscles.

Inhospitable: Difficult to live in, unwelcoming. An 'inhospitable environment' is one that does not support or encourage life or growth.

Immobile: Not moving or unable to move. Rib and loin cuts come from 'immobile muscles' at the top of the animal; muscles which play no part in the animal moving from one place to another.

Knowing where the cuts come from helps to decide which method of cooking to use.

Fillet

Taken from the back of the animal, this is the most tender part, cut from the centre of the sirloin. It is usually cut into steaks and can be fried or grilled.

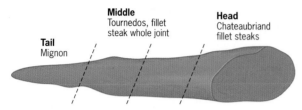

Tail
Mignon

Middle
Tournedos, fillet steak whole joint

Head
Chateaubriand fillet steaks

Cuts of fillet of beef

Sirloin

A boneless steak, which is more tender than rump, but not as tender as fillet. It is suitable for grilling or frying.

Rump

A good-quality cut, though it is less tender than fillet or sirloin. It is suitable for grilling or frying.

Rib

Sold on the bone or boned and rolled, it is suitable for roasting.

Topside

A lean, tender cut from the hindquarters, it is suitable for braising or pot roasting.

Silverside

Taken from the hindquarters, this can be pot roasted or used for traditional boiled beef.

Flank

A boneless cut from the mid-to-hindquarters; suitable for braising or stewing.

Skirt

A boneless rather gristly cut. It is usually stewed or made into mince.

Brisket

A cut from the fore end of the animal, below the shoulder. Quite a fatty joint, it is sold on or off the bone or salted. It is suitable for slow roasting.

Preparation of joints and cuts

Sirloin

- **Roasting:** carefully cut back the covering fat in one piece for approximately 10 cm. Trim off the sinew, replace the covering fat and tie with string if necessary.

Method 1: whole on the bone Aloyau de boeuf

Saw through the chine bone, lift back the covering fat in one piece for approx. 10 cm. Trim off the sinew and replace the covering fat. Tie with string if necessary. Ensure that the fillet has been removed.

Method 2: boned out

The fillet is removed and the sirloin boned out, and the sinew is removed as before. Remove the excess fat and sinew from the boned side. This joint may be roasted open, or rolled and tied with string.

- **Grilling and frying:** prepare as above and cut into steaks as required.
  - **Minute steaks:** cut into 1 cm slices, flatten with a cutlet bat dipped in water, making it as thin as possible, then trim.
  - **Sirloin steaks (entrecôte):** cut into 1 cm slices and trim (approximate weight 150 g).
  - **Double sirloin steaks:** cut into 2 cm-thick slices and trim (approximate weight 250–300 g).
  - **Porterhouse and T-bone steak:** porterhouse steaks are cut including the bone from the rib end of the sirloin; T-bone steaks are cut from the rump end of the sirloin, including the bone and fillet.

Fillet

As a fillet of beef can vary from 2½ to 4½ kg it follows that there must be considerable variation in the number of steaks obtained from it. A typical breakdown of a 3 kg fillet would be as follows.

- **Chateaubriand:** double fillet steak 3–10 cm thick, 2–4 portions. Average weight 300 g–1 kg. Cut from the head of the fillet, trim off all the nerve and leave a little fat on the steak.

- **Fillet steaks:** approximately 4 steaks of 100–150 g each, 1½–2 cm thick. These are cut as shown in the diagram above and trimmed as for chateaubriand.
- **Tournedos:** approximately 6–8 at 100 g each, 2–4 cm thick. Continue cutting down the fillet. Remove all the nerve and all the fat, and tie each tournedos with string.
- **Tail of fillet:** approximately ½ kg. Remove all fat and sinew, and slice or mince as required.
- **Whole fillet:** preparation for roasting and pot roasting (poêlé) – remove the head and tail of the fillet, leaving an even centre piece from which all the nerve and fat should be removed. This may be larded by using a larding needle to insert pieces of fatty bacon cut into long strips.

Wing rib (côte de boeuf)

This joint usually consists of the last three rib bones which, because of their curved shape, act as a natural trivet and, because of its prime quality, make it a first-class roasting joint to be served hot or cold, particularly when it is to be carved in front of the customer.

To prepare, cut seven-eighths of the way through the spine or chine bone, remove the nerve, saw through the rib bones on the underside 5–10 cm from the end. Tie firmly with string. When the joint is cooked, remove the chine bone to make the meat easier to carve.

For **thin flank**, trim off excessive fat and cut or roll as required.

Forequarter

- Fore ribs and middle ribs – prepare as for wing ribs.

- Chuck ribs, sticking piece, brisket, plate, leg of mutton cut, shank – bone out, remove excess fat and sinew, and use as required.

Beef offal

- **Tongue:** remove bone and gristle from the throat end.
- **Hearts:** remove arterial tubes and excess fat.
- **Liver:** skin, remove the gristle and cut into thin slices on the slant.
- **Kidney:** skin, remove the gristle and cut as required.
- **Sweetbreads:** soak in salted water for 2–3 hours to remove any traces of blood; wash well, trim, blanch and refresh.
- **Tripe:** wash well and soak in cold water, then cut into even pieces.
- **Tail:** cut between the natural joints, trim off excess fat. The large pieces may be split in two.

✎ ACTIVITY

1 Name two joints from a hindquarter of beef and two from a forequarter.

2 List joints from a beef carcass that are traditionally roasted.

3 What is meant by marbling?

4 A sirloin of beef may be cut into steaks. Name these steaks.

5 What is a chateaubriand?

Veal

Veal is obtained from good-quality carcasses weighing around 100 kg. This quality of veal is required for first-class cookery and is produced from calves slaughtered at between 12 and 24 weeks.

Butchery

The average weight of English or Dutch milk-fed veal calves is 18 kg. The joints of veal are as follows (the numbers refer to those used in the diagram that follows).

1	Knuckle	4	Best end	7	Scrag
2	Leg	5	Shoulder	8	Breast
3	Loin	6	Neck end		

Corresponding joints in beef

- Cushion = topside.
- Under cushion = silverside.
- Thick flank = thick flank.

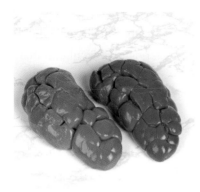

Veal kidneys

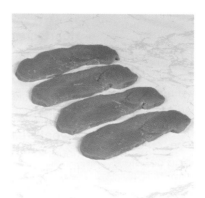

Veal escalopes

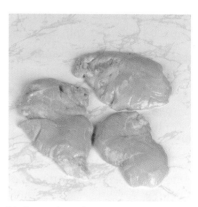

Veal sweetbreads

Table 10.7 Joints, uses and weights of veal (numbers in left-hand column refer to used in the diagram below)

Joint	Uses	Approximate weight (kg)
(1) knuckle	osso buco, sauté, stock	2
(2) leg	roasting, braising, escalopes, sauté	5
(3) loin	roasting, frying, grilling	3½
(4) best end	roasting, frying, grilling	3
(5) shoulder	braising, stewing	5
(6) neck end	stewing, sauté	2½
(7) scrag	stewing stock	1½
(8) breast	stewing, roasting	2½
kidneys	stewing (pies and puddings), sauté	–
liver	frying	–
sweetbreads	braising, frying	–
head	boiling, soup	4
brains	boiling, frying	–
bones	stock	–

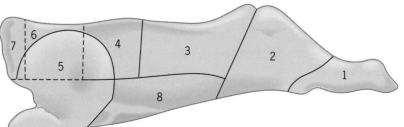

Side of veal

Order of dissection for veal

- Remove the shoulders.
- Remove the breast.
- Take off the leg.
- Divide the loin and best end from the scrag and neck end.
- Divide the loin from the best end.

Dissecting a leg of veal

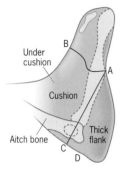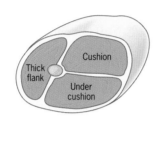

Dissection of a leg of veal

The letters refer to those in the diagram above.

1. Remove the knuckle by dividing the knee joint (A) and cut through the meat away from the cushion line (A–B).
2. Remove the aitch bone (C) at thick end of the leg, separating it at the ball and socket joint.
3. Remove all the outside skin and fat, thus exposing the natural seams. It will now be seen that the thigh bone divides the meat into two-thirds and one-third (thick flank).
4. Stand the leg on the thick flank with point D uppermost. Divide the cushion from the under cushion, following the natural seam, using the

hand and the point of a knife. Having reached the thigh bone, remove it completely.

5. When the boned leg falls open, the three joints can easily be seen joined only by membrane. Separate and trim the cushion, removing the loose flap of meat.
6. Trim the under cushion, removing the layer of thick gristle. Separate into three small joints through the natural seams. It will be seen that one of these will correspond with the round in silverside of beef.
7. Trim the thick flank by laying it on its round side and making a cut along the length about 2½ cm deep. A seam is reached and the two trimmings can be removed.
8. The anticipated yield of escalopes from this size of leg would be 62½ kg – that is, 55 kg × 100 g or 73 kg × 80 g.

Preparation of the joints and cuts of veal

Shin

- **Stewing (on the bone) (osso buco):** cut and saw into 2–4 cm thick slices through the knuckle.
- **Sauté:** bone out and trim, then cut into even 25 g pieces.

Leg

- **Braising or roasting whole:** remove the aitch bone, clean and trim 4 cm off the knuckle bone. Trim off the excess sinew.
- **Braising or roasting the nut:** remove all the sinew; if there is insufficient fat on the joint

Table 10.8 Joints of the leg (see the diagram above)

Cuts	Weight	Proportion	Uses
cushion or nut	2¾ kg	15%	escalopes, roasting, braising, sauté
under cushion or under nut	3 kg	17%	escalopes, roasting, braising, sauté
thick flank	2½ kg	14%	escalopes, roasting, braising, sauté
knuckle (whole)	2½ kg	14%	osso buco, sauté
bones (thigh and aitch)	2½ kg	14%	stock, jus-lié, sauces
usable trimmings	2 kg	11%	pies, stewing

then bard thinly (cover with bacon fat) and secure with string.

- **Escalopes:** remove all the sinew, cut against the grain into large 50–75 g slices and bat out thinly.
- **Sauté:** remove all the sinew and cut into 25 g pieces.

Loin and best end

- **Roasting:** bone out and trim the flap, roll out and secure with string. This joint may be stuffed before rolling.
- **Frying:** trim and cut into cutlets.

Shoulder

- **Braising:** bone out as for lamb; usually stuffed.
- **Stewing:** bone out, remove all the sinew and cut into 25 g pieces.

Neck end and scrag

Stewing and sautéing: bone out and remove all the sinew; cut into approximately 25 g pieces.

Breast

- **Stewing:** as for neck end.
- **Roasting:** bone out, season, stuff and roll up, then tie with string.

Kidneys

- Remove the fat and skin and cut down the middle lengthwise.
- Remove the sinew and cut into thin slices or neat dice.

Liver

Skin if possible, then remove the gristle and cut into thin slices on the slant.

Sweetbreads

- Soak in several changes of cold salted water to remove blood, which would darken the sweetbreads during cooking.
- Blanch and refresh, then peel off the membrane and connective tissues. The sweetbreads can then be pressed between two trays with a weight on top, and refrigerated.

Head

- Bone out by making a deep incision down the middle of the head to the nostrils.
- Follow the bone carefully and remove all the flesh in one piece.
- Remove the tongue.
- Wash the flesh well and keep covered in acidulated water (e.g. containing lemon juice) to keep it fresh.
- Wash off, blanch and refresh.
- Cut into 2–5 cm squares.
- Cut off the ears and trim the inside of the cheek.

Brains

- Using a chopper or saw, remove the top of the skull, making certain that the opening is large enough to remove the brain undamaged.
- Soak the brain in running cold water, then remove the membrane or skin, and wash well to remove all blood.
- Keep in cold salted water until required.

Quality of veal

- Veal is available all year round.
- The flesh should be pale pink in colour and firm in texture – not soft or flabby.
- Cut surfaces should be slightly moist, not dry.
- Bones, as in all young animals, should be pinkish white and porous, with some blood in their structure.
- The fat should be firm and pinkish white.
- The kidney should be firm and well covered with fat.

ACTIVITY

1 From which joints of veal are escalopes usually cut?

2 What is the basic difference between a blanquette of veal and a fricassee of veal?

3 What is the traditional dish produced from a knuckle of veal?

Pork and bacon

The keeping quality of pork is less than that of other meat; therefore it must be handled, prepared and cooked with great care. Pork should always be well cooked.

Butchery

The cuts of pork are as follows (the numbers refer to those used in the diagram below).

1 Leg

2 Loin

3 Spare rib

4 Belly

5 Shoulder

6 Head

When 5–6 weeks old a piglet is known as a sucking or suckling pig. Its weight is then between 5 kg and 10 kg.

Order of dissection

- Remove the head.
- Remove the trotters.
- Remove the leg.
- Remove the shoulder.
- Remove the spare ribs.
- Divide the loin from the belly.

Preparation of the joints and cuts of pork

Leg

- **Roasting:** remove the pelvic or aitch bone, trim and score the rind neatly – that is, with a sharp-pointed knife, make a series of 3 mm deep incisions approximately 2 cm apart all over the skin of the joint; trim and clean the knuckle bone.

Table 10.9 Cuts, uses and weights of pork (numbers in left-hand column refer to the diagram below)

Joint	Uses	Approximate weight (kg)
(1) leg	roasting and boiling	5
(2) loin	roasting, frying, grilling	6
(3) spare rib	roasting, pies	1½
(4) belly	pickling, boiling, stuffed, rolled and roasted	2
(5) shoulder	roasting, sausages, pies	3
(6) head (whole)	brawn	4
trotters	grilling, boiling	–
kidneys	sauté, grilling	–
liver	frying, pâté	–

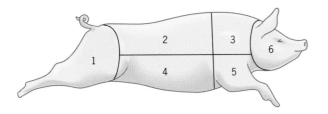

1 Leg
2 Loin
3 Spare rib of neck
4 Belly
5 Shoulder
6 Head

Pig carcass dissection

- **Boiling:** it is usual to pickle the joint either by rubbing dry salt and saltpetre into the meat or by soaking in a brine solution; then remove the pelvic bone, trim and secure with string if necessary.

Loin

- **Roasting (on the bone):** saw down the chine bone in order to facilitate carving; trim the excess fat and sinew and score the rind in the direction that the joint will be carved; season and secure with string.

- **Roasting (boned out):** remove the fillets and bone out carefully; trim off the excess fat and sinew, score the rind and neaten the flap, season, replace the filet mignon, roll up and secure the string; this joint is sometimes stuffed.

- **Grilling or frying chops:** remove the skin, excess fat and sinew, then cut and saw or chop through the loin in approximately 1 cm slices; remove the excess bone and trim neatly.

Spare rib

- **Roasting:** remove the excess fat, bone and sinew, and trim neatly.

- **Pies:** remove the excess fat and sinew, bone out and cut as required.

Belly

Remove all the small rib bones, season with salt, pepper and chopped sage, roll and secure with string. This joint may be stuffed.

Shoulder

- **Roasting:** the shoulder is usually boned out, the excess fat and sinew removed, seasoned, scored and rolled with string; it may be stuffed and can also be divided into two smaller joints.

- **Sausages and pies:** skin, bone out and remove the excess fat and sinew; cut into even pieces or mince.

Head

These are usually boned and pressed by specialist pork butchers to make a cold meat called brawn.

Trotters

Boil in water for a few minutes, scrape with the back of a knife to remove the hairs, wash off in cold water and split in half.

Kidneys

Remove the fat and skin, cut down the middle lengthwise. Remove the sinew and cut into slices or neat dice.

Liver

Skin if possible, then remove the gristle and cut into thin slices on the slant.

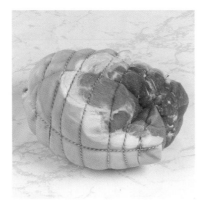

Leg of pork, boned and rolled

Boned leg of pork

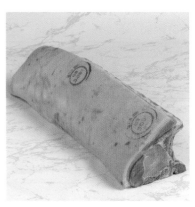

Loin of pork

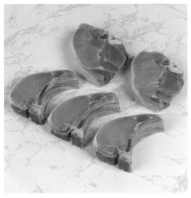

Pork chops

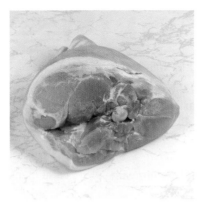

Gammon

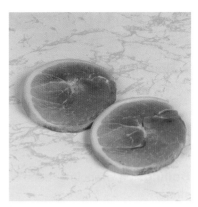

Gammon steaks

Signs of quality

- Lean flesh should be pale pink, firm and of a fine texture.
- The fat should be white, firm, smooth and not excessive.
- Bones should be small, fine and pinkish.
- The skin or rind should be smooth.

Bacon

Bacon is the cured flesh of a bacon-weight pig that is specifically reared for bacon – because its shape and size yield economic bacon joints. Bacon is cured either by dry salting and then smoking or by soaking in brine followed by smoking. Green bacon is brine-cured but not smoked; it has a milder flavour but does not keep for as long as smoked bacon.

Depending on the degree of salting during the curing process, bacon joints may need to be soaked in cold water for a few hours before being cooked.

Butchery

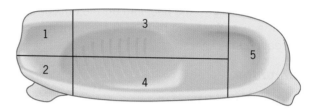

1. Collar
2. Hock
3. Back
4. Streaky
5. Gammon

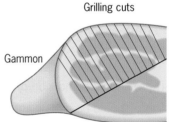

Grilling cuts

Gammon

Cuts of bacon

Table 10.10 Cuts, uses and weights of bacon (numbers in left-hand column refer to the diagram above)

Joint	Uses	Approximate weight (kg)
(1) collar	boiling, grilling	4½
(2) hock	boiling, grilling	4½
(3) back	grilling, frying	9
(4) streaky	grilling, frying	4½
(5) gammon	boiling, grilling, frying	7½

Preparation of joints and cuts

Collar

- **Boiling:** remove bone (if any) and tie with string.
- **Grilling:** remove the rind, trim off the outside surface and cut into thin slices (rashers), across the joint.

Hock

Boiling: leave whole or bone out and secure with string.

Back and streaky

- **Grilling:** remove all bones and rind, and cut into thin rashers.
- **Frying:** remove the rind, trim off the outside surface, and cut into rashers or chops of the required thickness.

Gammon

- **Grilling:** fairly thick slices are cut from the middle of the gammon; they are then trimmed and the rind removed.
- **Frying:** as for grilling.

Quality

- There should be no sign of stickiness.
- There should be a pleasant smell.
- The rind should be thin, smooth and free from wrinkles.
- The fat should be white, smooth and not excessive in proportion to the lean.
- The lean should be a deep-pink colour and firm.

Note: Do not confuse gammon with ham.

 ACTIVITY

1 What is the difference between a ham and a gammon?

2 Which part of the pig does streaky bacon come from?

3 Which joint of pork is suitable for escalopes of pork?

4 Which joint of pork is suitable for roasting?

 ACTIVITY

1 Name four types of offal.

2 Name the nutritional benefits from two types of offal.

3 List the quality points you would look for when purchasing offal.

4 Create a dish using offal suitable for an à la carte menu.

Test yourself • • • • • • • • • • • • • • •

1 Which part of the veal carcass are escalopes cut from?

2 What is a chateaubriand?

3 Which country does goulash originate from?

4 Which cut of beef are sirloin steaks cut from?

5 What is the translation for carré?

6 Where are cutlets of lamb cut from?

7 Is there a difference between cottage pie and shepherd's pie? If so, what is it?

8 Osso Bucco is produced from which cut of veal?

9 State the difference between a blanquette and fricassée.

10 What is meant by the word 'offal'?

• •

1 Chateaubriand with Roquefort butter

cal	kcal	fat	sat fat	carb	sugar	protein	fibre	salt
2368 KJ	566 kcal	43.3 g	19.9 g	0.0 g	0.0 g	44.0 g	0.0 g	0.6 g

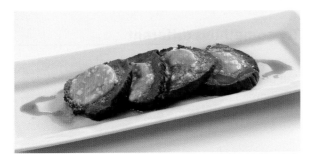

	2–3 portions
olive oil	
1 chateaubriand	500 g
salt, pepper	
Roquefort cheese	25 g
unsalted butter	40 g
ground black pepper	½ tsp

1 Heat the olive oil in a hot frying pan and brown the chateaubriand all over.

2 Season the chateaubriand and place in the oven at 190°C; the timing depends on the degree of cooking required.

3 Remove from oven, allow to rest, then carve into thick slices.

4 Mash together the Roquefort cheese, butter and black pepper. Form into a roll using aluminium foil or cling film. Refrigerate.

5 Place a slice of Roquefort and butter on each slice of chateaubriand. Serve with deep-fried potatoes and a tossed green salad.

Chef's tip
For the best texture and flavour, brown the chateaubriand all over before roasting, and leave it slightly underdone.

2 Roasting of beef *(boeuf rôti)*

cal	kcal	fat	sat fat	carb	sugar	protein	fibre
911 KJ	217 kcal	10.3 g	4.7 g	0.0 g	0.0 g	31.2 g	0.0 g

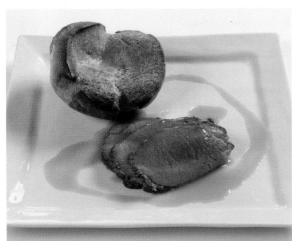

1 Season joints with salt, place on a trivet or bones in a roasting tray.

2 Place a little dripping or oil on top and cook in a hot oven at 230–250°C.

3 Baste frequently and reduce the heat gradually when necessary, as for example in the case of large joints.

4 Roasting time is approximately 15 minutes per ½ kg, plus 15 minutes.

5 To test if cooked, place on a tray and press firmly in order to see if the juices released contain any blood.

6 Beef is normally cooked underdone and a little blood should show in the juice.

7 On removing the joint from the oven, rest for 15 minutes to allow the meat to set and facilitate carving, then carve against the grain.

Suitable joints for roasting are: first class – sirloin, wing ribs, fore ribs, fillet; second class – topside, middle ribs.

Where applicable, name the origin and breed of the beef (e.g. Aberdeen Angus, Hereford) on the menu.

Roast gravy can be made when the joint is cooked and removed from the roasting tray. Serve the slices moistened with a little gravy.

Serve with Yorkshire pudding (recipe 3) (allowing 25 g flour per portion) and garnish with watercress. Serve sauceboats of gravy and horseradish sauce separately.

> **Chef's tip**
> Roast beef is usually slightly underdone, as this gives the best texture to the meat.

Making roast beef
http://bit.ly/wEdAJJ

Try something different

Some roughly chopped onion, carrot and celery can be added to the roasting tray approximately 30 minutes before the joint is cooked to give additional flavour to the gravy.

---

3   Yorkshire pudding

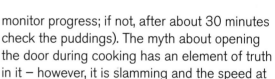

	4 portions	10 portions
flour	85 g	215 g
eggs	2	5
milk	85 ml	215 ml
water	40 ml	100 ml
dripping or oil	20 g	50 g

1 Place the flour and eggs into a mixing bowl and mix to a smooth paste.
2 Gradually add the milk and water, and place in the refrigerator for 1 hour. Pre-heat the oven to 190°C.
3 Heat the pudding trays in the oven with a little dripping or oil in each well.
4 Carefully ladle the mixture in, up to about two-thirds full.
5 Place in the oven and slowly close the door (if you have a glass-fronted door it will be easy to

monitor progress; if not, after about 30 minutes check the puddings). The myth about opening the door during cooking has an element of truth in it – however, it is slamming and the speed at which the door is opened that have most effect, so have just a small, careful peek to check and see if they are ready.

6 For the last 10 minutes of cooking, invert the puddings (take out and turn upside down in the tray) to dry out the base.
6 Serve immediately.

> **Chef's tip**
> The oven, and the oil, must be very hot before the mixture is placed into the pudding tray; if they are not hot enough, the puddings will not rise.

4 Sirloin steak with red wine sauce (*entrecôte bordelaise*)

cal	kcal	fat	sat fat	carb	sugar	protein	fibre
3013 KJ	717 kcal	62.2 g	21.6 g	6.0 g	3.0 g	26.1 g	1.4 g	*

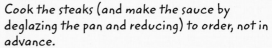

	4 portions	10 portions
butter or oil	50 g	125 g
sirloin steaks (approx. 150–200 g each)	4	10
red wine	60 ml	150 ml
red wine sauce (see page 177)	¼ litre	½ litre
parsley, chopped		

1 Heat the butter or oil in a sauté pan.
2 Lightly season the steaks on both sides with salt and pepper.
3 Fry the steaks quickly on both sides, keeping them underdone.
4 Dress the steaks on a serving dish.
5 Pour off the fat from the pan.
6 Deglaze with the red wine. Reduce by half and strain.
7 Add the red wine sauce, reboil and correct the seasoning.
8 Coat the steaks with the sauce.
9 Sprinkle with chopped parsley and serve.

Traditionally, two slices of beef bone marrow, poached in stock for 2–3 minutes, would be placed on each steak.

Chef's tip
Cook the steaks (and make the sauce by deglazing the pan and reducing) to order, not in advance.

HEALTHY EATING TIP

- Use little or no salt to season the steaks.
- Fry in a small amount of an unsaturated oil and drain off all excess fat after frying.
- Serve with plenty of boiled new potatoes or a jacket potato and a selection of vegetables.

* Using sunflower oil and 150 g raw steak per portion. Using sunflower oil and 200 g raw steak per portion provides: 3584 kJ/853 kcal Energy; 73.6 g Fat; 26.2 g Sat Fat; 6.0 g Carb; 3.0 g Sugar; 34.4 g Protein; 1.4 g Fibre

5 Boiled silverside, carrots and dumplings

cal	kcal	fat	sat fat	carb	sugar	protein	fibre
1068 KJ	254 kcal	10.1 g	4.6 g	15.5 g	5.5 g	26.3 g	2.6 g

	4 portions	10 portions
silverside, pre-soaked in brine	400 g	1¼ kg
onions	200 g	500 g
carrots	200 g	500 g
suet paste	100 g	250 g

1 Soak the meat in cold water for 1–2 hours to remove excess brine.
2 Place in a saucepan and cover with cold water, bring to the boil, skim and simmer for 45 minutes.
3 Add the whole prepared onions and carrots and simmer until cooked.

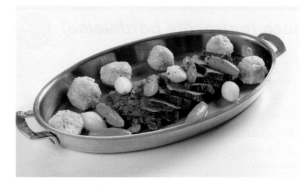

4 Divide the suet paste into even pieces and lightly mould into balls.

5 Add the dumplings and simmer for a further 15–20 minutes.

6 Serve by carving the meat across the grain, garnish with carrots, onions and dumplings, and moisten with a little of the cooking liquor.

Chef's tip

The beef is salted because this gives the desired flavour. The meat is usually salted before it is delivered to the kitchen.

A large joint of silverside is approximately 6 kg; for this size of joint, soak it overnight and allow 25 minutes per ½ kg plus 25 minutes.

 HEALTHY EATING TIP

- Adding carrots, onions, boiled potatoes and a green vegetable will give a healthy balance.

Try something different

- Herbs can be added to the dumplings.
- Boiled brisket and tongue can be served with the silverside.
- French-style boiled beef is prepared using unsalted thin flank or brisket with onions, carrots, leeks, celery, cabbage and a bouquet garni, all cooked and served together accompanied with pickled gherkins and coarse salt.

---

6 Boeuf bourguignonne

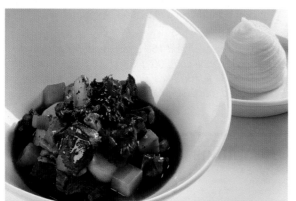

	4 portions	10 portions
Beef		
beef shin pre-soaked in red wine (see below) for 12 hours	600 g	1½ kg
olive oil	50 ml	125 ml

bottle of inexpensive red Bordeaux wine	1	2
onion	100 g	250 g
carrot	100 g	250 g
celery sticks	75 g	180 g
leek	100 g	250 g
cloves of garlic	2	5
sprig fresh thyme	1	2
bay leaf	1	2
seasoning		
veal/brown stock to cover		
Garnish		
button onions, cooked	12 (150 g)	30 (300 g)
cooked bacon lardons	150 g	300 g
button mushrooms, cooked	12 (150 g)	30 (150 g)
parsley, chopped	2 tsp	5 tsp
To finish		
mashed potato	300 g	750 g
washed, picked spinach	300 g	750 g
cooked green beans	250 g	625 g

1 Pre-heat the oven to 180°C.

2 Trim the beef shin of all fat and sinew, and cut into 2½ cm-thick rondelles.

3 Heat a little oil in a thick-bottomed pan and seal/brown the shin. Place in a large ovenproof dish.

4 Meanwhile, reduce the red wine by half.

5 Peel and trim the vegetables as appropriate, then add them to the pan that the beef has just come out of and gently brown the edges. Then place this, along with the garlic and herbs, in the ovenproof dish with the meat.

6 Add the reduced red wine to the casserole, then pour in enough stock to cover the meat and vegetables. Bring to the boil, then cook in the oven pre-heated to 180°C for 40 minutes; after that, turn the oven down to 90–95°C and cook for a further 4 hours until tender.

7 Remove from the oven and allow the meat to cool in the liquor. When cold, remove any fat. Reheat gently at the same temperature to serve.

8 Heat the garnish elements separately and sprinkle over each portion. Serve with a mound of mashed potato, wilted spinach and buttered haricots verts. Finish the whole dish with chopped parsley.

Another classic. Other joints of beef can be used here: beef or veal cheek can be used, reducing the time for the veal, or modernise the dish by using the slow-cooked fillet preparation and serving the same garnish.

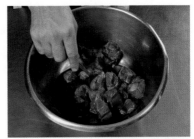

Marinate the beef

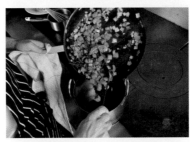

Gently brown the vegetables

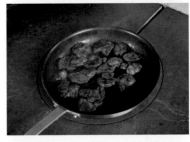

Brown the meat

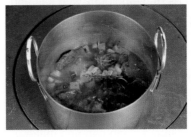

Pour in stock to cover the meat and vegetables

Chef's tip
Shallow fry the beef in hot oil to brown it all over, but do not let it boil in the oil. Then allow it to stew gently in the red wine.

7 Beef olives *(paupiettes de boeuf)*

cal	kcal	fat	sat fat	carb	sugar	protein	fibre
1134 KJ	271 kcal	13.1 g	2.6 g	13.6 g	5.0 g	25.4 g	1.5 g

*

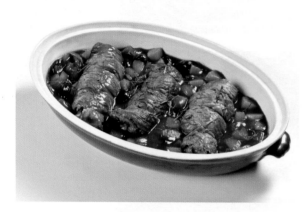

	4 portions	10 portions
Stuffing	50 g	125 g
white or wholemeal breadcrumbs	50 g	125 g
parsley, chopped	1 tbsp	3 tbsp
thyme	small pinch	small pinch
suet, prepared and chopped	5 g	25 g
onion, finely chopped and lightly sweated in oil	25 g	60 g
salt		
egg	½	1
Olives		
lean beef (topside)	400 g	1 ¼ kg
salt, pepper		
dripping or oil	35 g	100 g
carrot	100 g	250 g
onion	100 g	250 g
flour, browned in the oven	25 g	60 g
tomato purée	25 g	60 g
brown stock	500–750 ml	1 ¼–1 ½ litres
bouquet garni		

1 Combine all the stuffing ingredients and mix thoroughly.

2 Cut the meat into thin slices across the grain and bat out.

3 Trim to approximately 10 x 8 cm, chop the trimmings finely and add to the stuffing.

4 Season the slices of meat lightly with salt and pepper, and spread a quarter of the stuffing down the centre of each slice.

5 Roll up neatly and secure with string.

6 Fry off the meat to a light-brown colour, add the vegetables and continue cooking to a golden colour.

7 Drain off the fat into a clean pan and make up to 25 g fat if there is not enough (increase the amount for 10 portions). Mix in the flour.

8 Mix in the tomato purée, cool and then mix in the boiling stock.

9 Bring to the boil, skim, season and pour on to the meat.

10 Add the bouquet garni.

11 Cover and simmer gently, preferably in the oven, for approximately 1½–2 hours.

12 Remove the string from the meat.

13 Skim, correct the sauce and pass on to the meat.

Chef's tip

When you have stuffed and shaped the olives, tie them with string so that they will keep their shape during cooking

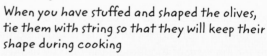

HEALTHY EATING TIP

● Use little or no salt to season the steaks.

● Fry in a small amount of an unsaturated oil and drain off all excess fat after frying.

● Serve with a large portion of potatoes and vegetables

* *Using 625 ml stock*

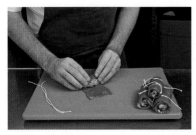

Roll the meat around the stuffing and tie the roll securely.

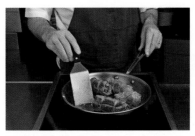

Fry the rolls to a light golden brown

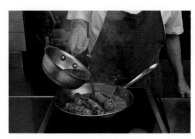

Pour the cooking liquid over the rolls

8   Beef stroganoff *(sauté de boeuf stroganoff)*

cal	kcal	fat	sat fat	carb	sugar	protein	fibre
1364 KJ	325 kcal	23.7 g	7.9 g	1.7 g	1.7 g	21.2 g	0.3 g

*

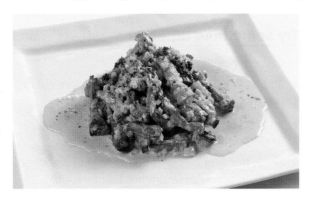

	4 portions	10 portions
fillet of beef (tail end)	400 g	1 ½ kg
butter, margarine or oil	50 g	125 g
salt, pepper		
shallots, finely chopped	25 g	60 g
dry white wine	125 ml	300 ml
cream	125 ml	300 ml
lemon, juice of	¼	½
parsley, chopped		

1. Cut the meat into strips approximately 1 x 5 cm.

2. Place the butter in a sauteuse over a fierce heat.

3. Add the beef strips, lightly season with salt and pepper, and allow to cook rapidly for a few seconds. The beef should be brown but underdone.

4. Drain the beef into a colander. Pour the butter back into the pan.

5. Add the shallots, cover with a lid and allow to cook gently until tender.

6. Drain off the fat, add the wine and reduce to one-third.

7. Add the cream and reduce by a quarter.

8. Add the lemon juice and the beef strips; do not reboil. Correct the seasoning.

9. Serve lightly sprinkled with chopped parsley. Accompany with rice pilaff (see page 421).

🍎 HEALTHY EATING TIP

- Use little or no salt to season the steaks.

- Fry in a small amount of an unsaturated oil and drain off all excess fat after frying.

- Serve with a large portion of rice and a salad.

* Using sunflower oil

9 Steak pudding

cal	kcal	fat	sat fat	carb	sugar	protein	fibre
1369 KJ	326 kcal	17.3 g	7.8 g	20.6 g	1.0 g	23.0 g	1.1 g

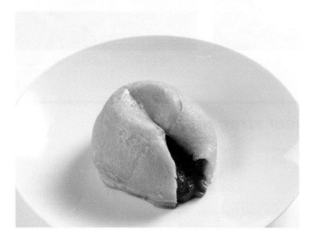

	4 portions	10 portions
suet paste	200 g	500 g
prepared stewing beef (chuck steak)	400 g	1½ kg
Worcester sauce		
parsley, chopped	1 tsp	2½ tsp
salt, pepper		
onion, chopped (optional)	50–100 g	200 g
water	125 ml approx.	300 ml approx.

1 Line a greased ½ litre basin with three-quarters of the suet paste and retain one-quarter for the top.
2 Mix all the other ingredients, except the water, together.
3 Place in the basin with the water to within 1 cm of the top.
4 Moisten the edge of the suet paste, cover with the top and seal firmly.
5 Cover with greased greaseproof paper and also, if possible, foil or a pudding cloth tied securely with string.
6 Cook in a steamer for at least 3½ hours.
7 Serve with the paper and cloth removed, clean the basin, place on a round flat dish and fasten a napkin round the basin.

Extra gravy should be served separately. If the gravy in the pudding is to be thickened, the meat can be lightly floured.

 HEALTHY EATING TIP

- Use little or no salt as the Worcester sauce contains salt.
- Trim off as much fat as possible from the raw stewing beef.
- Serve with plenty of potatoes and vegetables.

Try something different

Variations include:

- adding 50–100 g ox or sheep's kidneys cut in pieces with skin and gristle removed
- adding 50–100 g sliced or quartered mushrooms
- steak pudding can also be made with a cooked filling, in which case simmer the meat until cooked in brown stock with onions, parsley, Worcester sauce and seasoning; cool quickly and proceed as above, steaming for 1–1½ hours.

To make suet paste

	5–8 portions	10 portions
soft or self-raising flour	200 g	500 g
baking powder	10 g	25 g
salt	Pinch	Large pinch
prepared beef suet	100 g	250 g
water	125 ml	300 ml

1 Sieve the flour, baking powder and salt.
2 Mix in the suet. Make a well in the middle and pour in the water.
3 Mix lightly to a fairly stiff paste.

If the paste is heavy and soggy, the cooking temperature may be too low. If the paste is tough, it may have been handled or cooked too much.

10 Steak pie

cal	kcal	fat	sat fat	carb	sugar	protein	fibre
1442 KJ	346 kcal	22.2 g	2.9 g	13.6 g	1.8 g	24.3 g	0.4 g

*

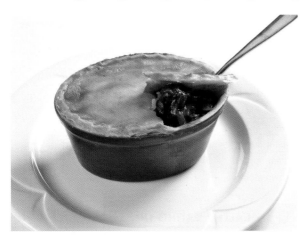

	4 portions	10 portions
prepared stewing beef (chuck steak)	400 g	1½ kg
oil or fat	50 ml	125 ml
onion, chopped (optional)	100 g	250 g
few drops Worcester sauce		
parsley, chopped	1 tsp	3 tsp
water, stock, red wine or dark beer	125 ml	300 ml
salt, pepper		
cornflour	10 g	25 g
short, puff or rough puff pastry (see pages 501 and 502)	100 g	250 g

1 Cut the meat into 2 cm strips then cut into squares.

2 Heat the oil in a frying pan until smoking, add the meat and quickly brown on all sides.

3 Drain the meat off in a colander.

4 Lightly fry the onion.

5 Place the meat, onion, Worcester sauce, parsley and the liquid in a pan, season lightly with salt and pepper.

6 Bring to the boil, skim, then allow to simmer gently until the meat is tender.

7 Dilute the cornflour with a little water, stir into the simmering mixture, reboil and correct seasoning.

8 Place the mixture into a pie dish and allow to cool.

9 Cover with the pastry, eggwash and bake at 200°C for approximately 30–45 minutes.

25–50 per cent wholemeal flour may be used in the pastry in place of plain flour.

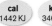 **HEALTHY EATING TIP**

- Use little or no salt as the Worcester sauce contains salt.

- Fry in a small amount of an unsaturated oil and drain off all excess fat after frying.

- There will be less fat in the dish if short paste is used.

- Serve with boiled potatoes and plenty of vegetables.

Try something different

Variations include:

- adding 50–100 g ox or sheep's kidneys with skin and gristle removed and cut into neat pieces

- adding 50–100 g sliced or quartered mushrooms

- adding 1 heaped tsp tomato purée and some mixed herbs

- in place of cornflour the meat can be tossed in flour before frying off.

* Using puff pastry (McCance data)

11 Carbonnade of beef (Belgian) (*carbonnade de boeuf*)

cal	kcal	fat	sat fat	carb	sugar	protein	fibre
1037 KJ	247 kcal	9.1 g	1.8 g	14.0 g	8.1 g	24.7 g	1.1 g

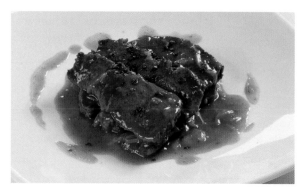

	4 portions	10 portions
lean beef (topside)	400 g	1¼ kg
salt, pepper		
flour (white or wholemeal)	25 g	60 g
dripping or oil	25 g	60 g
onions, sliced	200 g	500 g
beer	250 ml	625 ml
caster sugar	10 g	25 g
tomato purée	25 g	60 g
brown stock		

1 Cut the meat into thin slices.

2 Season with salt and pepper and pass through the flour.

3 Quickly colour on both sides in hot fat and place in a casserole.

4 Fry the onions to a light brown colour. Add to the meat.

5 Add the beer, sugar and tomato purée and sufficient brown stock to cover the meat.

6 Cover with a tight-fitting lid and simmer gently in a moderate oven at 150–200°C until the meat is tender (approx. 2 hours).

7 Skim, correct the seasoning and serve.

HEALTHY EATING TIP

- Trim off as much fat as possible before frying and drain off all surplus fat after frying.

- Use the minimum amount of salt to season the meat.

- Skim all fat from the finished sauce.

- Serve with plenty of potatoes and vegetables.

12 Cornish pasties

cal	kcal	fat	sat fat	carb	sugar	protein	fibre
1217 KJ	290 kcal	16.2 g	6.0 g	29.3 g	1.2 g	8.7 g	1.8 g

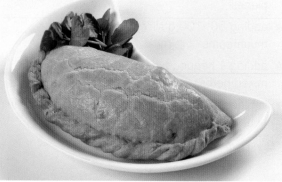

	4 portions	10 portions
short paste (see page 501)	200 g	500 g
potato (raw), finely diced	100 g	250 g
raw beef, chuck or skirt, cut in thin pieces	100 g	250 g
onion or leeks, chopped	50 g	125 g
swede (raw), finely diced (optional)	50 g	125 g
eggwash		

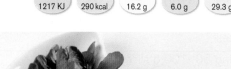

1 Roll out the short paste to 3 mm thick and cut into rounds 12 cm in diameter. Quickly brown the meat in oil, drain and cook quickly.

2 Mix the remaining ingredients together, moisten with a little water and place in the rounds in piles. Eggwash the edges.

3 Fold in half and seal; flute the edge and brush with eggwash.

4 Cook in a moderate oven at 150–200°C for ½–1 hour.

5 Serve with a suitable sauce, or hot or cold as a snack.

Chef's tip
The filling can be made from cooked meat that has been quickly chilled and held at 3°C.

HEALTHY EATING TIP

- Use the minimum amount of salt.
- Brush a little oil over the potatoes.
- Adding baked beans, tomatoes and/or mushrooms will 'dilute' the fat from the meat.
- Serve with a large portion of vegetables.

Try something different

Variations include:

- potato, onion or leek, and turnip or swede, fresh herbs
- bacon, hard-boiled eggs and leeks
- lamb, carrot and potato
- apples, cinnamon, cloves, brown sugar, cider.

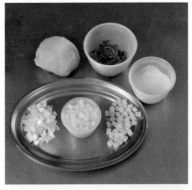

Ingredients for Cornish pasties

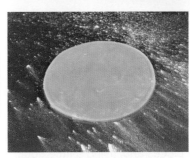

Roll out the pastry

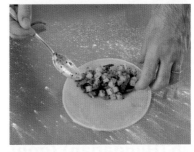

Place the filling on to the pastry

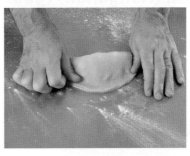

Fold the pastry over and seal the edge

13 Hamburg or Vienna steak (bitok)

   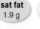 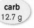

cal	kcal	fat	sat fat	carb	sugar	protein	fibre
681 KJ	162 kcal	6.7 g	1.9 g	12.7 g	1.0 g	13.8 g	1.0 g

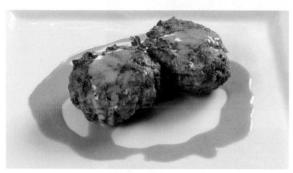

	4 portions	10 portions
onion, finely chopped	25 g	60 g
butter, margarine or oil	10 g	25 g
lean minced beef	200 g	500 g
small egg	1	2–3
breadcrumbs	100 g	250 g
cold water or milk	2 tbsp approx.	60 ml approx.

1 Cook the onion in the fat without colour, then allow to cool.

2 Add to the rest of the ingredients and mix in well.

3 Divide into even pieces and, using a little flour, make into balls, flatten and shape round.

4 Shallow-fry in hot fat on both sides, reducing the heat after the first few minutes, making certain they are cooked right through.

5 Serve with a light sauce, such as piquant sauce (page 180).

The 'steaks' may be garnished with French-fried onions and sometimes with a fried egg.

HEALTHY EATING TIP

- Use a small amount of an unsaturated oil to cook the onion and to shallow-fry the meat.
- The minced beef will produce more fat, which should be drained off.
- Serve with plenty of starchy carbohydrate and vegetables.

14 Goulash (Hungarian) (goulash de boeuf)

    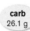

cal	kcal	fat	sat fat	carb	sugar	protein	fibre
1625 KJ	389 kcal	20.4 g	6.0 g	26.1 g	3.9 g	26.9 g	1.7 g

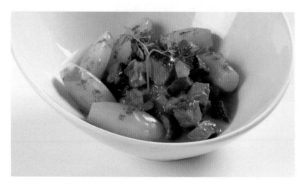

	4 portions	10 portions
prepared stewing beef	400 g	1¼ kg
lard or oil	35 g	100 g
onions, chopped	100 g	250 g
flour	25 g	60 g
paprika	10–25 g	25–60 g
tomato purée	25 g	60 g
stock or water	750 ml approx.	2 litres approx.
turned potatoes or small new potatoes	8	20
choux paste (see page 502)	125 ml	300 ml

1 Remove excess fat from the beef. Cut into 2 cm square pieces.

2 Season and fry in the hot fat until slightly coloured. Add the chopped onion.

3 Cover with a lid and sweat gently for 3 or 4 minutes.

4 Add the flour and paprika, and mix in with a wooden spoon.

5 Cook out in the oven or on top of the stove. Add the tomato purée, mix in.

6 Gradually add the stock, stir to the boil, skim, season and cover.

7 Allow to simmer, preferably in the oven, for approximately 1½–2 hours until the meat is tender.

8 Add the potatoes and check that they are covered with the sauce. (Add more stock if required.)

9 Re-cover with the lid and cook gently until the potatoes are cooked.

10 Skim, and correct the seasoning and consistency. A little cream or yoghurt may be added at the last moment.

11 Serve sprinkled with a few gnocchis made from choux paste (see page 502), reheated in hot salted water or lightly tossed in butter or margarine.

> ### HEALTHY EATING TIP
>
> - Trim off as much fat as possible before frying and drain all surplus fat after frying.
>
> - Use the minimum amount of salt to season the meat.
>
> - Skim all fat from the finished sauce.
>
> - Serve with a large side salad.

15 Best end or rack of lamb with breadcrumbs and parsley

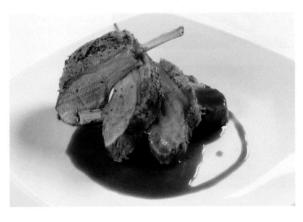

1 Roast the best end.

2 Ten minutes before cooking is completed cover the fat surface of the meat with a mixture of 25–50 g of fresh white breadcrumbs mixed with plenty of chopped parsley, an egg and 25–50 g melted butter or margarine.

3 Return to the oven to complete the cooking, browning carefully.

> **Chef's tip**
> Cook the lamb until it is pink. Carefully bind the breadcrumbs with herbs and beaten egg, so that they will hold together during cooking.

Try something different

Variations include:

- mixed fresh herbs used in addition to parsley
- finely chopped garlic added
- chopped fresh herbs, shallots and mustard.

16 Roast leg of lamb with mint, lemon and cumin

cal	kcal	fat	sat fat	carb	sugar	protein	fibre	salt
2192 KJ	524 kcal	39.1 g	13.7 g	0.3 g	0.3 g	39.7 g	0.0 g	0.3 g

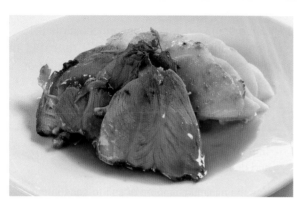

	4 portions	10 portions
mint	25 g	62.5 g
lemons, juice of	2	5
cumin	2 tsp	5 tsp
olive oil	4 tbsp	10 tbsp
leg of lamb	3.5 kg	2 x 3.5 kg

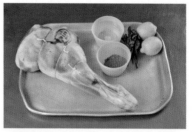

Ingredients for roast leg of lamb with mint, lemon and cumin

1 Place the mint, lemon juice, cumin and olive oil in a food processor.

2 Rub the mixture into the lamb in a suitable roasting tray.

3 Roast the lamb in the normal way.

4 Serve on a bed of boulangère potatoes or dauphinoise potatoes and a suitable green vegetable, e.g. leaf spinach with toasted pine nuts, or with a couscous salad.

Using a 225 g portion of lamb.

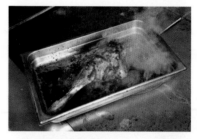

Place the leg of lamb in a roasting tray and rub with the mint and lemon mixture

Chef's tip
Carefully blend the mint, lemon juice, cumin and olive oil to give maximum flavour.

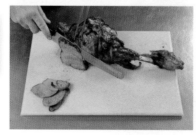

Carving a leg of lamb

17 ## Stuffed roast loin of lamb

1 Take a short loin of lamb, bone it out and lightly bat out the flaps of meat.

2 Add the stuffing, roll up the meat and tie with string. Season and smear with oil.

3 Roast in an oven at approximately 200°C for 15 minutes. Reduce the heat to 150–160°C and continue to cook. Allow 20 minutes per ½ kg of meat plus an additional 20 minutes.

Shoulder or best end of lamb may also be boned, stuffed and rolled for roasting.

To make the stuffing

	For 1 joint
Suet, chopped	50 g
Onions, chopped and cooked in a little butter or margarine without colour	50 g
Egg yolk, or small egg	1
White breadcrumbs	100 g
Pinch powdered thyme	
Pinch chopped parsley	
Salt, pepper	
Grated zest of one lemon	

Combine all the ingredients together.

 HEALTHY EATING TIP

- Use the minimum amount of salt – the herbs, pepper and lemon provide plenty of flavour.

18 Slow-cooked shoulder of lamb with vegetables

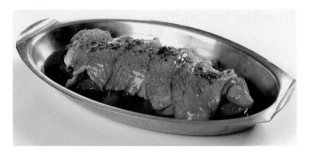

	4 portions	10 portions
boned shoulder of lamb, rolled and tied	1	3
olive oil		
salt, pepper		
rosemary	6 sprigs	18 sprigs
thyme	6 sprigs	18 sprigs
garlic, crushed and chopped	4 cloves	10 cloves
red onions, quartered	2	5
carrots, turned	3	7½
celery batons	2 sticks	5 sticks
leeks, shredded	1	3
tomatoes, halved	6	18
bay leaves, chopped	2	5
canned plum tomatoes, chopped	375 g	950 g
red wine or dry cider	½ bottle	1½ bottles

1 Rub the lamb with oil, and season with salt and pepper. Place in a suitable roasting tray and cook in an oven at 200°C for 15 minutes.

2 Remove from the oven and reduce the temperature to 140°C .

3 Add the remaining ingredients to the roasting tray.

4 Cover with a lid or aluminium foil and cook for 2½ to 3 hours (removing the foil 40 minutes before the end) until the lamb is tender and sticky.

5 Remove the herbs, then remove the lamb and allow to rest.

6 Carve the lamb and serve on top of the vegetables.

7 To make the sauce, once the vegetables are removed, reduce the cooking liquor to the required consistency. Add a tablespoon of redcurrant jelly, mix well, correct seasoning, then strain.

8 Couscous makes a good accompaniment.

19 Grilled cutlets *(côtelettes d'agneau grillées)*

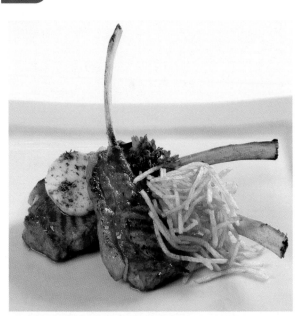

1 Season the cutlets lightly with salt and mill pepper.

2 Brush with oil or fat.

3 When cooked on the bars of the grill, place the prepared cutlet on the preheated bars that have been greased.

4 Cook for approximately 5 minutes, turn and complete the cooking.

5 When cooked under the salamander, place on a greased tray, cook for approximately 5 minutes, turn and complete the cooking.

6 Serve dressed, garnished with a deep-fried potato and watercress. A compound butter (e.g. parsley, herb or garlic) may also be served.

7 Each cutlet bone may be capped with a cutlet frill.

HEALTHY EATING TIP

- When served with boiled new potatoes and boiled or steamed vegetables, the plate of food becomes more 'balanced'.

---

20 Breadcrumbed cutlets *(côtelettes d'agneau panées)*

1 Pass the prepared and flattened cutlets through seasoned flour, eggwash and fresh white breadcrumbs. Pat firmly, then shake off surplus crumbs.

2 Shallow-fry in hot clarified butter, margarine or oil for the first few minutes; then allow to cook gently.

3 Turn, and continue cooking until a golden-brown (approx. 5 minutes each side).

4 To test if cooked, press firmly – no signs of blood should appear.

These may be served with a garnish of pasta, such as spaghetti with tomato sauce or noodles with butter or oil.

Chef's tip
Make sure the oil is hot before placing the cutlets in the pan. Placing the cutlets into cold or lukewarm oil will spoil the quality.

HEALTHY EATING TIP

- Lightly oil the pan with an unsaturated oil to fry the cutlets. Drain off any excess fat after the frying is complete.

- Serve with plenty of vegetables.

---

21 Grilled loin or chump chops, or noisettes of lamb

1 Season and shallow-fry on both sides in a sauté pan.

2 Serve with the appropriate garnish (see below) and sauce. Unless specifically stated, a jus-lié or demi-glace should be served.

Suitable garnishes

- Tomatoes filled with jardinière of vegetables and château potatoes.

- Balls of cauliflower mornay and château potatoes.

- Artichoke bottoms filled with carrot balls and noisette potatoes.

- Artichoke bottoms filled with asparagus heads and noisette potatoes.

- Artichoke bottoms filled with peas and cocotte potatoes.

Chef's tip
Cutlets, chops and noisettes should be cooked to order, not in advance.
Note: fillet of lamb should be trimmed of fat and sinew before cooking.

HEALTHY EATING TIP

- Trim off as much fat as possible before cooking.

- Grilling or braising is a healthier way of cooking.

- Add starchy carbohydrate and vegetables to proportionately reduce the amount of fat.

22   Lamb kebabs *(shish kebab)*

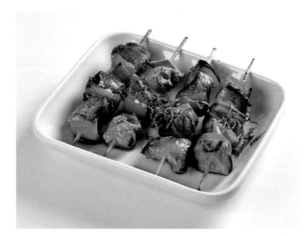

Kebabs, a dish of Turkish origin, are pieces of food impaled and cooked on skewers over a grill or barbecue. There are many variations and different flavours can be added by marinating the kebabs in oil, wine, vinegar or lemon juice with spices and herbs for 1–2 hours before cooking. Kebabs can be made using tender cuts, or mince of lamb and beef, pork, liver, kidney, bacon, ham, sausage and chicken, using either the meats individually or combining two or three. Vegetables and fruit can also be added (e.g. onion, apple, pineapple, peppers, tomatoes, aubergine). Kebabs can be made using vegetables exclusively (e.g. peppers, onion, aubergine, tomatoes). Kebabs are usually served with a pilaff rice (see page 421).

The ideal cuts of lamb are the nut of the lean meat of the loin, best end or boned-out meat from a young shoulder of lamb.

1 Cut the meat into squares and place them on skewers with squares of green pepper, tomato, onion and bay leaves in between.

2 Sprinkle with powdered thyme and cook over a hot grill.

3 Serve with pilaff rice, or with chickpeas and finely sliced raw onion.

Chef's tip
The pieces of lamb and vegetables must be cut evenly so that they will cook evenly.

Try something different

Variations include:

- miniature kebabs (one mouthful) can be made, impaled on cocktail sticks, grilled and served as a hot snack at receptions
- fish kebabs can be made using a firm fish, such as monkfish, and marinating in olive oil, lemon or lime juice, chopped fennel or dill, garlic and a dash of Tabasco or Worcester sauce.

23   Irish stew

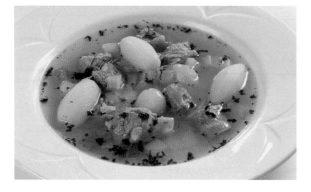

	4 portions	10 portions
stewing lamb	500 g	1½ kg
salt, pepper		
bouquet garni		
potatoes	400 g	1 kg
onions	100 g	250 g
celery	100 g	250 g
savoy cabbage	100 g	250 g
leeks	100 g	250 g
button onions	100 g	250 g
parsley, chopped		

1 Trim the meat and cut into even pieces. Blanch and refresh.

2 Place in a shallow saucepan, cover with water, bring to the boil, season with salt and skim. If tough meat is being used, allow ½–1 hour stewing time before adding any vegetables.

3 Add the bouquet garni. Turn the potatoes into barrel shapes.

4 Cut the potato trimmings, onions, celery, cabbage and leeks into small neat pieces and add to the meat; simmer for 30 minutes.

5 Add the button onions and simmer for a further 30 minutes.

6 Add the potatoes and simmer gently with a lid on the pan until cooked.

7 Correct the seasoning and skim off all fat.

8 Serve sprinkled with chopped parsley.

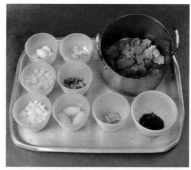

Ingredients for Irish stew

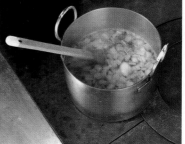

Boil the meat

Chef's tip

Keep the meat and vegetables covered with liquid during cooking, to keep the dish consistent and tasty.

Try something different

Alternatively, a more modern approach is to cook the meat for 1½–2 hours until almost tender, then add the vegetables and cook until all are tender. Optional accompaniments include Worcester sauce and/or pickled red cabbage (see page 257).

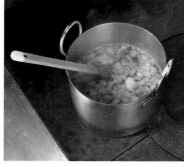

Add the vegetables

🍎 HEALTHY EATING TIP

- Trim as much fat as possible from the stewing lamb and skim all fat from the finished dish.

- Use the minimum amount of salt.

- Serve with colourful seasonal vegetables to create a 'healthy' dish.

24 White lamb stew *(blanquette d'agneau)*

cal	kcal	fat	sat fat	carb	sugar	protein	fibre
1181 KJ	283 kcal	15.5 g	7.8 g	9.2 g	3.9 g	27.3 g	0.0 g

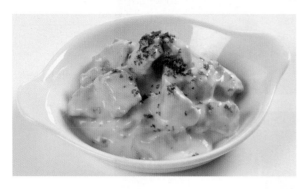

	4 portions	10 portions
stewing lamb	500 g	1½ kg
white stock	750 ml	1½ litres
onion, studded	50 g	125 g
carrot	50 g	125 g
bouquet garni		
salt, pepper		
butter, margarine or oil	25 g	60 g
flour	25 g	60 g
cream, yoghurt or quark	2–3 tbsp	5 tbsp
parsley, chopped		

1 Trim the meat and cut into even pieces. Blanch and refresh.

2 Place in a saucepan and cover with cold water.

3 Bring to the boil then place under running cold water until all the scum has been washed away.

4 Drain and place in a clean saucepan and cover with stock, bring to the boil and skim.

5 Add whole onion and carrot, and bouquet garni, season lightly with salt and simmer until tender, approximately 1–1½ hours.

6 Meanwhile prepare a blond roux with the butter and flour and make into a velouté with the cooking liquor. Cook out for approximately 20 minutes.

8 Correct the seasoning and consistency, and pass through a fine strainer on to the meat, which has been placed in a clean pan.

8 Reheat, mix in the cream and serve, finished with chopped parsley.

9 To enrich this dish a liaison of yolks and cream is sometimes added at the last moment to the boiling sauce, which must not be allowed to reboil, otherwise the eggs will scramble and the sauce will curdle.

 HEALTHY EATING TIP

- Trim as much fat as possible from the lamb before cooking.

- Use the minimum amount of salt.

- Reduce the fat content by using low-fat yoghurt in place of the cream when reheating.

- Serve with mashed potato with spring onion and colourful vegetables.

Chef's tip
Be very careful when adding the liaison of yolks and cream; make sure the sauce does not come back to the boil or it will curdle.

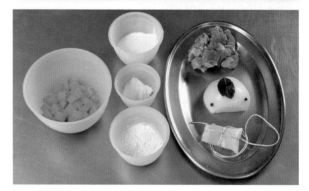
Ingredients for blanquette of lamb

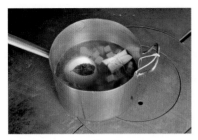
Cook the meat on the stove

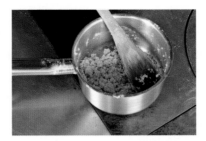
Make a roux

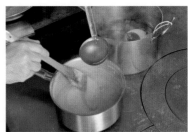
Make a velouté by combining the roux with the liquid

* Using butter and 2 tbsp low-fat yoghurt

25 Lamb fillets with beans and tomatoes

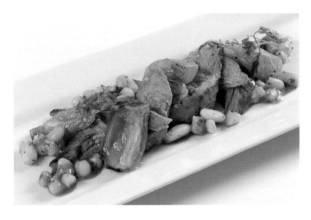

	4 portions	10 portions
olive oil	approx. 50 ml	approx. 125 ml
onions, finely chopped	50 g	125 g
garlic, crushed and chopped	2	5
dried cannellini beans, soaked	500 g	1¼ kg
lamb stock	1 litre	2½ litres
bay leaves	2	5
salt, pepper		
cherry tomatoes	750 g	1 kg
lamb fillets	900 g	2¼ kg

1 Heat the olive oil in a suitable pan, and gently fry the onion and garlic. Rinse the beans, drain and add to the pan.

2 Add the stock and bay leaves. Bring to the boil. Simmer for approximately 1 hour until the beans are tender. Season.

3 Cook the cherry tomatoes in a hot oven at 190°C with a drizzle of oil.

4 Rub a little olive oil into the lamb fillets. Leave for approximately 20 minutes at room temperature.

5 Season the lamb and shallow-fry. Serve with the tomatoes and the beans nearly arranged on a plate.

Chef's tip
Lamb fillets only need a little cooking. Cook them at the last minute so that they will look and taste as good as possible.

26 Valentine of lamb

1 Prepare a short saddle with all the bones, kidneys and internal fat removed.

2 Split into two loins.

3 Trim off excess fat and sinew.

4 Cut across the muscle grain into thick boneless chops.

5 Slice three parts through the lean meat and open to give a double-sized cut surface (butterfly cut).

Valentines are cooked in the same way as noisettes and rosettes. They may also be grilled or braised. Best end may be used in place of the loin.

HEALTHY EATING TIP

- Grilling or braising is a healthier way of cooking.

- Add starchy carbohydrate and vegetables to proportionally reduce the amount of fat.

- Trim off as much fat as possible before cooking.

27 Braised lamb shanks with ratatouille

cal	kcal	fat	sat fat	carb	sugar	protein	fibre
2020 KJ	483 kcal	27.3 g	9.6 g	23.7 g	10.5 g	37.1 g	8.6 g

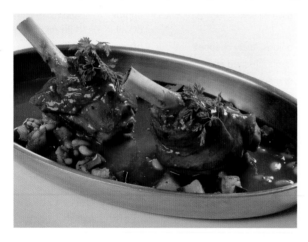

	4 portions	10 portions
lamb shanks	4	10
olive oil	3 tbsp	7 tbsp
red onions, finely chopped	50 g	125 g
garlic cloves, crushed, finely chopped	2	5
aubergine large, diced 1 cm (½ inch) dice	1	2
courgettes diced 1 cm (½ in) dice	3	7
plum tomatoes (canned)	400 g	1 kg
lamb stock	250 ml	625 ml
flageolet beans (canned), rinsed and drained	400 g	1 kg
fresh oregano, chopped	1 tbsp	2½ tbsp
fresh rosemary, chopped	1 tbsp	2½ tbsp
clear honey	1 tbsp	2½ tbsp
salt, pepper		

1 Season the lamb shanks. Heat the oil in a suitable braising pan, fry the shanks on all sides until golden brown. Remove from pan and set aside.

2 Add the chopped onion and garlic, sweat until soft.

3 Add the diced aubergine and courgettes, cook for 5 minutes.

4 Stir in the chopped plum tomatoes and stock.

5 Place the lamb shank back with the vegetables. Bring to the boil, reduce heat, cover and braise in the oven for 1 hour.

6 Remove the lamb. Stir in the flageolet beans, add the herbs and honey. Simmer, check all the vegetables are soft.

7 Replace the lamb and allow the shanks to steep in the vegetables.

8 Correct the seasoning and consistency.

9 Serve with mashed potatoes or couscous.

HEALTHY EATING TIP

- Fry the shanks in a little olive oil and drain off any excess fat.

- Skim any fat from the cooked sauce before adding the beans.

- Serve with a large portion of potatoes or couscous and colourful seasonal vegetables.

- Add the minimum amount of salt.

Chef's tip
Browning the lamb before it is braised will give the sauce a good colour and flavour.

Using edible portion of meat (90 g), with broad beans used to replace flageolet beans

---

28 Roast saddle of lamb with rosemary mash

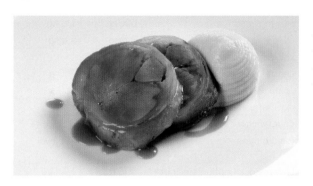

	4 portions	10 portions
saddle of lamb, boned		
milk	250 ml	625 ml
rosemary	2 sprigs	5 sprigs
potato, mashed	1.3 kg	3.2 kg

1 Bone the saddle of lamb and roast in the normal way.

2 Bring the milk to the boil with the rosemary. Remove from the heat, cover and leave to infuse for 10–15 minutes.

3 To make the rosemary mash, prepare a potato purée using the milk infused with rosemary.

---

29 Mixed grill

cal	kcal	fat	sat fat	carb	sugar	protein	fibre
2050 KJ	488 kcal	40.8 g	19.3 g	0.0 g	0.0 g	30.4 g	0.0 g

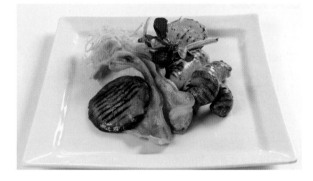

	4 portions	10 portions
sausages	4	10
cutlets	4	10
kidneys	4	10
tomatoes	4	10
mushrooms	4	10
rashers streaky bacon	4	10
deep-fried potato, to serve		
watercress, to serve		
parsley butter, to serve		

1 Grill in the order listed above.

2 Dress neatly on an oval flat dish or plates.

3 Garnish with deep-fried potato, watercress and a slice of compound butter on each kidney or offered separately.

These are the usually accepted items for a mixed grill, but it will be found that there are many variations to this list (e.g. steaks, liver, a Welsh rarebit and fried egg).

Chef's tip
The items must be cooked in the order listed above, so that they are all fully and evenly cooked at the end.

 HEALTHY EATING TIP

- Add only a small amount of compound butter and serve with plenty of potatoes and vegetables.

* 1 portion (2 cutlets). With deep-fried potatoes, parsley and watercress, 1 portion provides: 3050 kJ/726 kcal Energy; 59.2 g Fat; 26.6 g Sat Fat; 20.2 g Carb; 2.5 g Sugar; 29.5 g Protein; 4.9 g Fibre

30 Brown lamb or mutton stew (*navarin d'agneau*)

cal	kcal	fat	sat fat	carb	sugar	protein	fibre
1320 KJ	314 kcal	18.7 g	6.2 g	9.4 g	3.2 g	27.9 g	1.3 g *

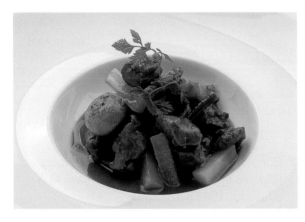

	4 portions	10 portions
stewing lamb	500 g	1 ½ kg
oil	2 tbsp	5 tbsp
salt, pepper		
carrot	100 g	250 g
onion	100 g	250 g
clove of garlic (if desired)	1	3
flour (white or wholemeal)	25 g	60 g
tomato purée	1 level tbsp	2¼ level tbsp
brown stock (mutton stock or water)	500 g	1¼ litre
bouquet garni		
parsley, chopped, to serve		

1 Trim the meat and cut into even pieces.

2 Partly fry off the seasoned meat in the oil, then add the carrot, onion and garlic, and continue frying.

3 Drain off the surplus fat, add the flour and mix.

4 Singe in the oven or brown on top of the stove for a few minutes, or add previously browned flour.

5 Add the tomato purée and stir with a kitchen spoon.

6 Add the stock and season.

7 Add the bouquet garni, bring to the boil, skim and cover with a lid.

8 Simmer gently until cooked (preferably in the oven) for approx. 1–2 hours.

9 When cooked, place the meat in a clean pan.

10 Correct the sauce and pass it on to the meat.

11 Serve sprinkled with chopped parsley.

Making brown lamb stew
http://bit.ly/y9YRJl

Chef's tip
Make sure the oil is hot before placing the meat in the pan to brown quickly all over.

Do not allow the meat to boil in the oil, because this will spoil the flavour and texture.

Try something different

A variation includes a garnish of vegetables (glazed carrots and turnips, glazed button onions, potatoes, peas and diamonds of French beans), which may be cooked separately or in the stew).

* Using sunflower oil

31 Hot pot of lamb or mutton

cal	kcal	fat	sat fat	carb	sugar	protein	fibre
1505 KJ	360 kcal	17.0 g	6.4 g	22.0 g	1.8 g	29.0 g	2.5 g

	4 portions	10 portions
stewing lamb	500 g	1¼ kg
salt, pepper		
onions, shredded	100 g	250 g
potatoes	400 g	1¼ kg
brown stock	1 litre	2½ litres
oil (optional)	25 g	60 g
parsley, chopped		

1 Trim the meat and cut into even pieces.

2 Place in a deep earthenware dish. Season with salt and pepper.

3 Lightly sauté the onions in the oil, if desired. Mix the onion and approx. three-quarters of the potatoes (thinly sliced) together.

4 Season and place on top of the meat; cover three parts with stock.

5 Neatly arrange an overlapping layer of the remaining potatoes on top, sliced about 2 mm thick.

6 Thoroughly clean the edges of the dish and place to cook in a hot oven at 230–250°C until lightly coloured.

7 Reduce the heat and simmer gently until cooked, approximately 1½–2 hours.

8 Press the potatoes down occasionally during cooking.

9 Serve with the potatoes brushed with butter or margarine and sprinkle with the chopped parsley.

Neck chops or neck fillet make a succulent dish.

Chef's tip
When the dish is ready, the top layer of potatoes should be golden brown.

Try something different

Variations include:

- use leek in place of onion
- add 200 g lambs' kidneys
- quickly fry off the meat and sweat the onions before putting in the pot
- add 100–200 g sliced mushrooms
- add a small tin of baked beans, or a layer of thickly sliced tomatoes before adding the potatoes
- use sausages in place of lamb.

* Using sunflower oil

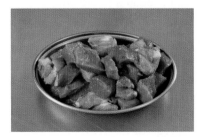
Chop the lamb into even-sized pieces

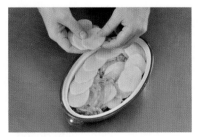
Layer the potatoes over the lamb

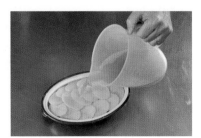
Pour over the stock

32   Shepherd's pie (cottage pie)

cal	kcal	fat	sat fat	carb	sugar	protein	fibre
1744 KJ	415 kcal	25.3 g	9.1 g	22.1 g	2.5 g	26.3 g	1.6 g *

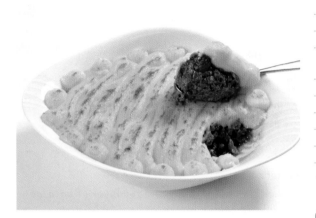

	4 portions	10 portions
onions, chopped	100 g	250 g
oil	35 g	100 g
lamb or mutton (minced), cooked	400 g	1¼ kg
salt, pepper		
Worcester sauce	2–3 drops	5 drops
potato, cooked	400 g	1¼ kg
butter or margarine	25 g	60 g
milk or eggwash		
jus-lié or demi-glace	125–250 ml	300–600 ml

1 Cook the onion in the fat or oil without colouring.

2 Add the cooked meat from which all fat and gristle has been removed.

3 Season and add Worcester sauce (sufficient to bind).

4 Bring to the boil; simmer for 10–15 minutes.

5 Place in an earthenware or pie dish.

6 Prepare the potatoes – mix with the butter or margarine, then mash and pipe, or arrange neatly on top.

7 Brush with the milk or eggwash.

8 Colour lightly under salamander or in a hot oven.

9 Serve accompanied with a sauceboat of jus-lié.

This dish prepared with cooked beef is known as cottage pie.

Chef's tips

Pipe the potato carefully so that the meat is completely covered.

When using reheated meats, care must be taken to heat thoroughly and quickly.

HEALTHY EATING TIP

- Use an oil rich in unsaturates (olive or sunflower) to lightly oil the pan.

- Drain off any excess fat after the lamb has been fried.

- Try replacing some of the meat with baked beans or lentils, and add tomatoes and/or mushrooms to the dish.

- When served with a large portion of green vegetables, a healthy balance is created.

Try something different

Variations include:

- add 100–200 g sliced mushrooms

- add a layer of thickly sliced tomatoes, then sprinkle with rosemary

- mix a tin of baked beans in with the meat

- sprinkle with grated cheese and brown

- vary the flavour of the mince by adding herbs or spices

- the potato topping can also be varied by mixing in grated cheese, chopped spring onions or herbs, or by using duchess potato mixture

- serve lightly sprinkled with garam masala and with grilled pitta bread.

Using sunflower oil, with hard margarine in topping

33 Samosas

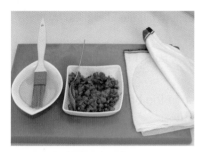

Prepare the pastry, filling and eggwash

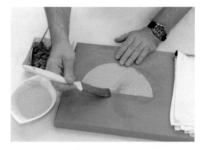

Form the pastry into a semicircle and eggwash the straight edge

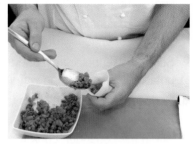

Shape the pastry into a cone

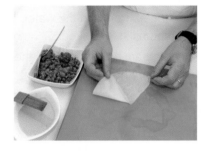

Fill the cone

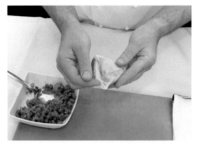

Seal the top

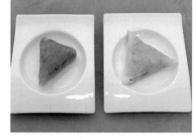

Samosas before and after frying

Samosa pastry	40–60 pasties	100–150 pasties
short pastry made from ghee fat and fairly strong flour as the dough (should be fairly elastic)	400 g	1 kg

1 Take a small piece of dough, roll into a ball 2 cm in diameter. Keep the rest of the dough covered with either a wet cloth, clingfilm or plastic, otherwise a skin will form on the dough.

2 Roll the ball into a circle about 9 cm round on a lightly floured surface. Cut the circle in half.

3 Moisten the straight edge with eggwash or water.

4 Shape the semicircle into a cone. Fill the cone with approximately 1½ tsp of filling, moisten the top edges with beaten egg white, flour paste or eggwash and press together well.

5 The samosas may be made in advance, covered with clingfilm or plastic, and refrigerated before being deep-fried.

6 Deep-fry at 180°C until golden brown; remove from fryer and drain well.

7 Serve on a suitable dish. Savoury samosas can be garnished with coriander leaves and served with chutney.

Filling 1: potato

	4 portions	10 portions
potatoes, peeled	200 g	500 g
vegetable oil	1½ tsp	3¾ tsp
black mustard seeds	½ tsp	1¼ tsp
onions, finely chopped	50 g	125 g
fresh ginger, finely chopped	12 g	30 g
fennel seeds	1 tsp	2½ tsp
cumin seeds	¼ tsp	1 tsp
turmeric	¼ tsp	1 tsp
frozen peas	75 g	187 g
salt, to taste		
water	2½ tsp	6¼ tsp
fresh coriander, finely chopped	1 tsp	2½ tsp
garam masala	½ tsp	2½ tsp
pinch of cayenne pepper		

1 Cut the potatoes into ½ cm dice; cook in water until only just cooked.

2 Heat the oil in a suitable pan, add the mustard seeds and cook until they pop.

3 Add the onions and ginger. Fry for 7–8 minutes, stirring continuously until golden brown.

4 Stir in the fennel, cumin and turmeric, add the potatoes, peas, salt and water.

5 Reduce to a low heat, cover the pan and cook for 5 minutes.

6 Stir in the coriander; cook for a further 5 minutes.

7 Remove from the heat, stir in the garam masala and the cayenne seasoning.

8 Remove from the pan, place into a suitable bowl to cool before using.

 HEALTHY EATING TIP

- Use the minimum amount of salt.

- Use a small amount of unsaturated oil to fry the mustard seeds and the onion.

- Skim any fat from the finished dish.

Filling 2: lamb

	4 portions	10 portions
saffron	½ tsp	1¼ tsp
boiling water	2½ tsp	6¼ tsp
vegetable oil	3 tsp	7½ tsp
fresh ginger, finely chopped	12 g	30 g
cloves garlic, crushed and chopped	2	5
onions, finely chopped	50 g	125 g
salt, to taste		
lean lamb, minced	400 g	1 kg
pinch of cayenne pepper		
garam masala	1 tsp	2½ tsp

HEALTHY EATING TIP

- No added salt is necessary.

- Use a small amount of unsaturated oil to fry the onions and lamb.

- Drain off the excess fat before adding the water.

1 Infuse the saffron in the boiling water; allow to stand for 10 minutes.

2 Heat the vegetable oil in a suitable pan. Add the ginger, garlic, onions and salt, stirring continuously. Fry for 7–8 minutes, until the onions are soft and golden brown.

3 Stir in the lamb, add the saffron with the water. Cook, stirring the lamb until it is cooked.

4 Add the cayenne and garam masala, reduce the heat and allow to cook gently for a further 10 minutes.

5 The mixture should be fairly tight with very little moisture.

6 Transfer to a bowl and allow to cool before using.

34 Fricassée of veal *(fricassée de veau)*

cal	kcal	fat	sat fat	carb	sugar	protein	fibre
992 KJ	236 kcal	13.6 g	7.5 g	5.3 g	0.4 g	23.3 g	0.2 g	*

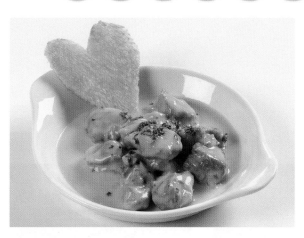

	4 portions	10 portions
boned stewing veal (shoulder or breast)	400 g	1¼ kg
margarine, butter or oil	35 g	100 g
flour	25 g	60 g
white veal stock	500 ml	1¼ litres
salt, pepper		
egg yolk	1	2–3
cream (dairy or vegetable)	2–3 tbsp	5–7 tbsp
squeeze of lemon juice		
parsley, chopped, to finish		
heart-shaped croutons, to finish		

1 Trim the meat. Cut into even 25 g pieces.

2 Sweat the meat gently in the butter without colour in a sauté pan.

3 Mix in the flour and cook out without colour.

4 Allow to cool.

5 Gradually add boiling stock just to cover the meat, stir until smooth.

6 Season, bring to the boil, skim.

7 Cover and simmer gently on the stove until tender (approx. 1½–2 hours).

8 Pick out the meat into a clean pan. Correct the sauce.

9 Pass on to the meat and reboil. Mix the yolk and cream in a basin.

10 Add a little of the boiling sauce, mix in and pour back on to the meat, shaking the pan until thoroughly mixed; do not reboil. Add the lemon juice.

11 Serve, finished with chopped parsley and heart-shaped croutons fried in butter or oil.

HEALTHY EATING TIP

- Add the minimum amount of salt.

- Serve with oven-baked croutons brushed with olive oil or sippets.

- A large serving of starchy carbohydrates and vegetables will help to proportionally reduce the fat content.

Try something different

A variation is to add mushrooms and button onions. Proceed as for this recipe but, after 1 hour's cooking, pick out the meat, strain the sauce back on to the meat and add 8 small button onions. Simmer for 15 minutes, add 8 small white button mushrooms, washed and peeled if necessary, then complete the cooking. Finish and serve as in this recipe. This is known as *fricassée de veau à l'ancienne*.

* *Using butter*

Chef's tips

After adding the flour, cook carefully so that it does not colour.

Add the liaison of yolks and cream carefully. Do not allow the sauce to boil after this, because it will curdle.

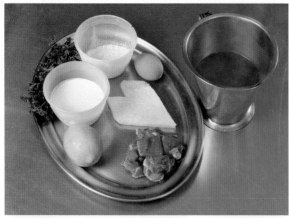

Ingredients for fricassée of veal

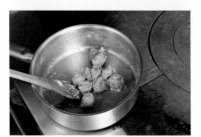

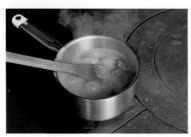

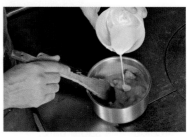

Cook the meat and flour   Add the stock and continue to cook   Add the liaison of egg yolk and cream

---

35 White stew or blanquette of veal *(blanquette de veau)*

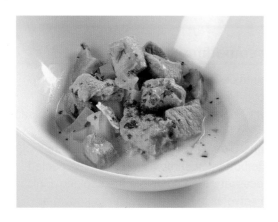

Proceed as for white lamb stew (recipe 24), using 400 g of prepared stewing veal.

36 Roast veal four-bone rib

cal	kcal	fat	sat fat	carb	sugar	protein	fibre	salt
394 KJ	118 kcal	3.1 g	1.0 g	1.0 g	0.3 g	21.6 g	0.1 g	0.8 g

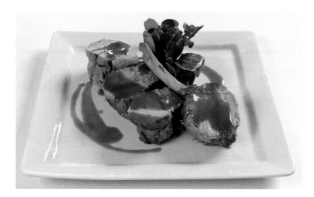

	6–8 portions
veal	4-bone rib (approx. 800 g)
salt, pepper	
Dijon mustard	2 tsp
garlic cloves, cut into slivers	2
cold water	
fresh thyme	2 sprigs

1 Place the joint in a roasting tray and season. Score the joint, rub the mustard into the joint and insert garlic into the incisions.

2 Pour sufficient cold water into the tray to cover the base. Add the thyme to the water and place in the oven at 200°C for 10–15 minutes. Then cover with foil and reduce the temperature to 190°C. Cook for a further 20 minutes per 450 g.

3 Add more water as necessary to keep liquid in the bottom of the pan, and baste occasionally.

4 After cooking allow the joint to rest in a warm place for 15–20 minutes before carving.

5 Use the pan juices to make the gravy or sauce, or serve with a suprême sauce with mushrooms.

ASSESSMENT

37 Veal stuffing

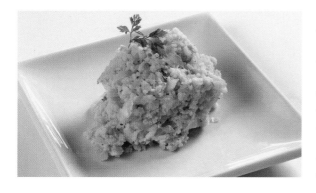

	4 portions	10 portions
breadcrumbs (white or wholemeal)	100 g	250 g
onion, cooked in oil, butter or margarine without colour	50 g	125 g
pinch of chopped parsley		
suet, chopped	50 g	125 g
good pinch of powdered thyme or rosemary		
lemon, grated zest and juice of	½	1
salt, pepper		

1 Combine all the ingredients.

2 This mixture may be used for stuffing joints or may be cooked separately in buttered paper or in a basin in the steamer for approximately 1 hour.

Try something different

The stuffing for veal joints may be varied by using:

● orange in place of lemon

● the addition of duxelle

● leeks in place of onion

- various herbs
- adding a little spice (e.g. ginger, nutmeg, allspice).

HEALTHY EATING TIP

- Use the minimum amount of salt; rely on the herbs and lemon for flavour.
- Use a little unsaturated oil to cook the onion.

38 Grilled veal cutlet *(côte de veau grille)*

cal	kcal	fat	sat fat	carb	sugar	protein	fibre
990 KJ	236 kcal	9.7 g	2.6 g	0.0 g	0.0 g	36.9 g	0.0 g	*

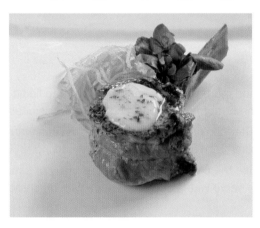

1 Lightly season the prepared chop with salt and mill pepper.
2 Brush with oil. Place on previously heated grill bars.
3 Cook on both sides for 8–10 minutes in all.
4 Brush occasionally to prevent the meat from drying.

5 Serve with watercress, a deep-fried potato and a suitable sauce or butter, such as béarnaise or compound butter, or on a bed of plain or flavoured mashed potato (see page 224).

Sprigs of rosemary may be added to the chop before or halfway through cooking.

HEALTHY EATING TIP

- Use the minimum amount of salt to season the meat.
- Serve with a small amount of sauce or butter and a large portion of mixed vegetables.

* Using sunflower oil

39 Braised shin of veal (osso buco)

cal	kcal	fat	sat fat	carb	sugar	protein	fibre *
1748 KJ	416 kcal	28.6 g	7.8 g	9.3 g	4.1 g	28.5 g	1.9 g

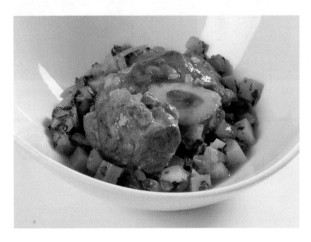

	4 portions	10 portions
meaty knuckle of veal	1½ kg	3¾ kg
salt, pepper		
flour	25 g	60 g
butter or margarine	50 g	125 g
oil	60 ml	150 ml
onion	50 g	125 g
small clove garlic	1	2–3
carrot	50 g	125 g
leek	25 g	60 g
celery	25 g	60 g
dry white wine	60 ml	150 ml
white stock	60 ml	150 ml
tomato purée	25 g	60 g
bouquet garni		
tomatoes, concassée	200 g	500 g
parsley and basil, chopped		
lemon or orange, grated zest and juice of	½	1

1 Prepare the veal knuckle by cutting and sawing through the bone in 5 cm thick pieces.

2 Season the veal pieces with salt and pepper, and pass through flour on both sides.

3 Melt the butter and oil in a sauté pan.

4 Add the veal slices and cook on both sides, colouring slightly.

5 Add the finely chopped onion and garlic, cover with a lid and allow to sweat gently for 2–3 minutes.

6 Add the carrot, leek and celery cut in brunoise, cover with a lid and allow to sweat for 3–4 minutes. Pour off the fat.

7 Deglaze with the white wine and stock. Add the tomato purée.

8 Add the bouquet garni, replace the lid and allow the dish to simmer gently, preferably in an oven, for 1 hour.

9 Add the tomato concassée, correct the seasoning.

10 Replace the lid, return to the oven and allow to continue simmering until the meat is so tender that it can be pulled away from the bone easily with a fork.

11 Remove the bouquet garni, add the lemon juice, correct the seasoning and serve sprinkled with a mixture of chopped fresh basil, parsley, and grated orange and lemon zest (known as gremolata).

A risotto with saffron may be served separately. *Osso buco* is an Italian regional dish that has many variations.

Chef's tip
At step 4, only colour the veal lightly.

🍎 HEALTHY EATING TIP

- Use the minimum amount of salt to season the meat and in the finished sauce.

- Lightly oil the pan with an unsaturated oil and drain off any excess after the frying is complete.

- Serve with a large portion of risotto.

* Using hard margarine and sunflower oil

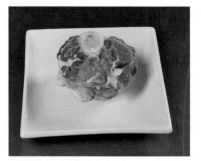

Raw shin of veal

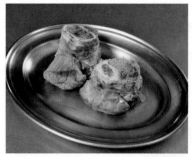

Colour the meat

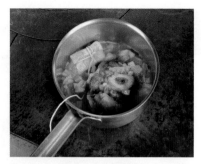

Combine all the ingredients for braising

40 Hot veal and ham pie

cal	kcal	fat	sat fat	carb	sugar	protein	fibre
1394 KJ	332 kcal	20.7 g	8.1 g	8.9 g	0.8 g	27.9 g	0.7 g

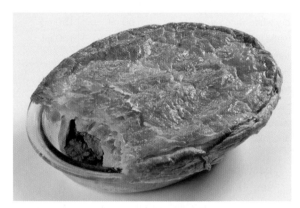

	4 portions	10 portions
bacon rashers	100 g	250 g
stewing veal without bone	400 g	1¼ kg
hardboiled egg, chopped or quartered	1	2
parsley, chopped	1 tsp	2 tsp
onion, chopped	50 g	125 g
salt, pepper		
stock (white)	250 ml	625 ml
rough puff or puff paste (see page 502)	100 g	250 g

1 Bat out the bacon thinly and use it to line the bottom and sides of a ½ litre pie dish, reserving two or three pieces for the top.

2 Trim the veal, cut it into small pieces and mix with the egg, parsley and onion. Season and place in the pie dish.

3 Just cover with stock. Add the rest of the bacon.

4 Roll out the pastry, eggwash the rim of the pie dish and line with a strip of pastry 1 cm wide. Press this down firmly and eggwash.

5 Without stretching the pastry, cover the pie and seal firmly.

6 Trim off any excess pastry with a sharp knife, notch the edge neatly, eggwash and decorate.

7 Allow to rest in the refrigerator or a cool place.

8 Place on a baking sheet in a hot oven at 200°C for 10–15 minutes until the paste has set and is lightly coloured.

9 Remove the pie from oven, cover with foil and return to the oven, reducing the heat to 190°C for 15 minutes, to 160°C for a further 15 minutes, then to 140°C.

10 Complete the cooking at this temperature ensuring that the liquid is gently simmering. Cook the pie for approx. 1–1½ hours, or less if the pieces of meat are small (e.g. 50 minutes – 1 hour if using 1 cm pieces).

Variations include rabbit, pork, chicken or guinea fowl in place of veal.

 HEALTHY EATING TIP

- Little or no salt is needed – there is plenty in the bacon.

- Serve with plenty of starchy carbohydrate and vegetables to proportionally reduce the fat.

41 Escalope of veal

cal	kcal	fat	sat fat	carb	sugar	protein	fibre
2079 KJ	495 kcal	39.8 g	11.4 g	10.3 g	0.5 g	24.7 g	1.0 g

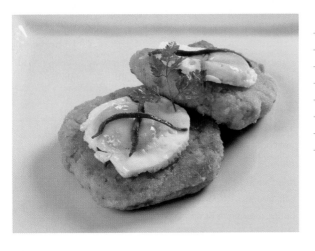

	4 portions	10 portions
nut or cushion of veal	400 g	1¼ kg
seasoned flour	25 g	60 g
egg	1	2
breadcrumbs	50 g	125 g
oil for frying	50 g	125 g
butter	50 g	125 g
beurre noisette (optional)	50 g	125 g
jus-lié	60 ml	150 ml

1 Trim and remove all sinew from the veal.

2 Cut into four even slices and bat out thinly using a little water.

3 Flour, egg and crumb. Shake off surplus crumbs. Mark with a palette knife.

4 Place the escalopes into shallow hot fat and cook quickly for a few minutes on each side.

5 Dress on a serving dish or plate.

6 An optional finish is to pour over 50 g *beurre noisette* (nut brown butter), and finish with a cordon of jus-lié.

> **Chef's tip**
> *The escalopes need to be batted out thinly. Excess breadcrumbs must be shaken off before the escalopes are placed into the hot fat.*

🍎 HEALTHY EATING TIP

- Use an unsaturated oil to fry the veal.
- Make sure the fat is hot so that less will be absorbed into the crumb.
- Drain the cooked escalope on kitchen paper.
- Use the minimum amount of salt.
- Serve with plenty of starchy carbohydrate and vegetables.

Try something different

Variations include the following.

- **Escalope of veal Viennoise:** as for this recipe, but garnish the dish with chopped yolk and white of egg and chopped parsley; on top of each escalope place a slice of peeled lemon decorated with chopped egg yolk, egg white and parsley, an anchovy fillet and a stoned olive; finish with a little lemon juice and nut brown butter.

- **Veal escalope Holstein:** prepare and cook the escalopes as for this recipe; add an egg fried in butter or oil, and place two neat fillets of anchovy criss-crossed on each egg; serve.

- **Escalope of veal with spaghetti and tomato sauce:** prepare escalopes as for this recipe, then garnish with spaghetti with tomato sauce (page 430), allowing 10 g spaghetti per portion.

* Fried in sunflower oil, using butter to finish

42 Veal escalopes with Parma ham and mozzarella cheese *(involtini di vitello)*

cal	kcal	fat	sat fat	carb	sugar	protein	fibre
1642 KJ	394 kcal	26.1 g	15.5 g	0.1 g	0.1 g	39.8 g	0.0 g

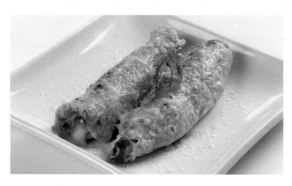

	4 portions	10 portions
small, thin veal escalopes	400 g (8 in total)	1¼ kg (20 in total)
flour		
Parma ham, thinly sliced	100 g	250 g
mozzarella cheese, thinly sliced	200 g	500 g
fresh leaves of sage	8	20
or		
dried sage	1 tsp	2½ tsp
salt, pepper		
butter, margarine or oil	50 g	125 g
Parmesan cheese, grated		

1 Sprinkle each slice of veal lightly with flour and flatten.

2 Place a slice of Parma ham on each escalope.

3 Add several slices of mozzarella cheese to each.

4 Add a sage leaf or a light sprinkling of dried sage.

5 Season, roll up each escalope, and secure with a toothpick or cocktail stick.

6 Melt the butter in a sauté pan, add the escalopes and brown on all sides.

7 Transfer the escalopes and butter to a suitably sized ovenproof dish.

8 Sprinkle generously with grated Parmesan cheese and bake in a moderately hot oven at 190°C for 10 minutes.

9 Clean the edges of the dish and serve.

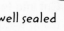

Chef's tip

Make sure the ham and cheese are well sealed within the escalope before cooking.

HEALTHY EATING TIP

- Use a small amount of oil to fry the escalopes, and drain the cooked escalopes on kitchen paper.

- No added salt is necessary as there is plenty of salt in the cheese.

- Serve with plenty of vegetables.

43 | # Roast leg of pork

| cal 1357 KJ | kcal 323 kcal | fat 22.4 g | sat fat 8.9 g | carb 0.0 g | sugar 0.0 g | protein 30.4 g | fibre 0.0 g | * |

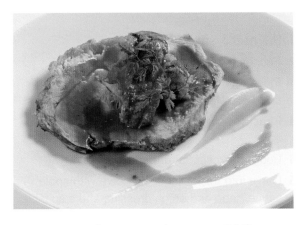

1 Prepare leg for roasting (see page 308).

2 Moisten with water, oil, cider, wine or butter and lard then sprinkle with salt, rubbing it well into the cracks of the skin. This will make the crackling crisp.

3 Place on a trivet in a roasting tin with a little oil or dripping on top.

4 Start to cook in a hot oven at 230–250°C, basting frequently.

5 ⚠ Gradually reduce the heat to 180–185°C, allowing approximately 25 minutes per ½ kg plus another 25 minutes. Pork must always be well cooked. If using a probe, the minimum temperature should be 72°C for 2 minutes.

6 When cooked, remove from the pan and prepare a roast gravy from the sediment.

7 Remove the crackling and cut into even pieces for serving.

8 Serve the joint garnished with picked watercress and accompanied by roast gravy, sage and onion dressing and apple sauce (page 192). If to be carved, proceed as for roast lamb (page 304).

Note:

Other joints can also be used for roasting (e.g. loin, shoulder and spare rib).

For the roast gravy

1 After removing the cooked joint from the roasting tray, place the tray on the stove over a gentle heat to allow the sediment to settle.

2 Carefully strain off the fat, leaving the sediment in the tray.

3 Return to the stove and brown carefully. Deglaze with brown stock.

4 Allow to simmer for a few minutes.

5 Correct the seasoning and colour, then strain and skin.

For the sage and onion dressing

	4 portions	10 portions
onion, chopped	50 g	125 g
pork dripping	50 g	125 g
white breadcrumbs	100 g	250 g
pinch chopped parsley		
good pinch powdered sage		
salt, pepper		

1 Cook the onion in the dripping without colour.

2 Combine all the ingredients. Dressing is usually served separately.

🍎 **HEALTHY EATING TIP**

● Use a small amount of unsaturated oil to cook the onion.

● Add the minimum amount of salt.

Modern practice is to refer to this as a dressing if served separately to the meat, but as stuffing if used to stuff the meat.

* 113 g portion

44 Slow roast pork belly

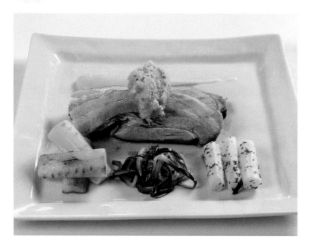

	4 portions	10 portions
pork belly	1.2 kg	3 kg

1 Pre-heat oven to 145°C.
2 Season the pork with salt and pepper.
3 Place on a rack in a large roasting tray, skin side up.
4 Roast for 4½–5 hours, then remove from the tray.
5 Pour off excess fat and make a gravy.
6 Carve into thick slices and serve with apple sauce, sage and onion dressing and a suitable potato and vegetable.

45 Spare ribs of pork in barbecue sauce

cal	kcal	fat	sat fat	carb	sugar	protein	fibre	salt
6151 KJ	1465 kcal	12.6 g	37.3 g	20.3 g	17.1 g	63.5 g	0.3 g	1.45 g

*

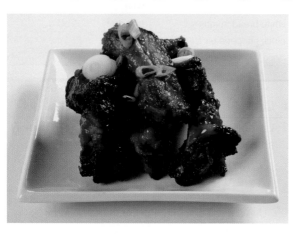

	4 portions	10 portions
onion, finely chopped	100 g	250 g
clove of garlic, chopped	1	2
oil	60 ml	150 ml
vinegar	60 ml	150 ml
tomato purée	150 g	375 g
honey	60 ml	150 ml
brown stock	250 ml	625 ml
Worcester sauce	4 tbsp	10 tbsp
dry mustard	1 tsp	2 tsp
pinch thyme		
salt		
spare ribs of pork	2 kg	5 kg

1 Sweat the onion and garlic in the oil without colour.
2 Mix in the vinegar, tomato purée, honey, stock, Worcester sauce, mustard and thyme, and season with salt.
3 Allow the barbecue sauce to simmer for 10–15 minutes.
4 Place the prepared spare ribs fat side up on a trivet in a roasting tin.
5 Brush the spare ribs liberally with the barbecue sauce.
6 Place in a moderately hot oven: 180–200°C.
7 Cook for ¾–1 hour.
8 Baste generously with the barbecue sauce every 10–15 minutes.
9 The cooked spare ribs should be brown and crisp.

10 Cut the spare ribs into individual portions and serve.

Chef's tip

Apply plenty of barbecue sauce before and during cooking, to give the ribs a good flavour.

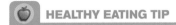 **HEALTHY EATING TIP**

- Sweat the onion and garlic in a little unsaturated oil.
- No added salt is necessary as the Worcester sauce is salty.

* Using sunflower oil

---

46 **Pork loin chops with pesto and mozzarella**

cal	kcal	fat	sat fat	carb	sugar	protein	fibre
3531 KJ	844 kcal	66.3 g	25.6 g	0.5 g	0.4 g	61.2 g	0.0 g

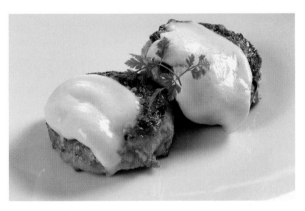

	4 portions	10 portions
salt, pepper		
loin chops	4	10
olive oil (if frying)	2 tbsp	5 tbsp
pesto	4 tsp	10 tsp
mozzarella	4 slices	10 slices

1 Season, then shallow-fry or grill the chops until almost cooked.

2 Spread the pesto on top of each chop and top each with a slice of mozzarella.

3 Finish under the grill for approximately 1 minute until the cheese is golden and just cooked through.

4 Serve with a suitable pasta, e.g. butttered noodles and a green vegetable or tossed salad.

Chef's tip
When ready, the cheese should be a golden brown colour.

*Using a 225 g portion of pork and 60 g of mozzarella

47 Raised pork pie/hot water paste

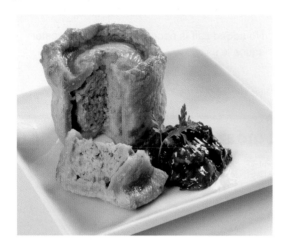

Raised pork pie

	4 portions	10 portions
shoulder of pork, without bone	300 g	1 kg
bacon	100 g	250 g
allspice (or mixed spice) and chopped sage	½ tsp	1½ tsp
salt, pepper		
bread soaked in milk	50 g	125 g
stock or water	2 tbsp	5 tbsp
In addition		
eggwash		
stock, hot	125 ml	375 ml
gelatine	5 g	12.5 g
picked watercress and salad to serve		

Hot water paste

	4 portions	10 portions
strong plain flour	250 g	500 g
salt		
lard or margarine (alternatively use 100 g lard and 25 g butter or margarine)	125 g	300 g
water	125 ml	300 ml

1 Sift the flour and salt into a basin. Make a well in the centre.
2 Boil the fat with the water and pour immediately into the flour.
3 Mix with a kitchen spoon until cool.
4 Mix to a smooth paste and use while still warm.

The cooking times in this recipe are for a 4-portion pie. For individual pies, at step 9, bake for approx. 30 minutes.

1 Cut the pork and bacon into small even pieces and combine with the rest of the main ingredients.
2 Keep one-quarter of the paste warm and covered.
3 Roll out the remaining three-quarters and carefully line a well-greased raised pie mould or mould the paste around a mould for a hand-raised pie (as shown here).
4 Add the filling and press down firmly.
5 Roll out the remaining pastry for the lid, and eggwash the edges of the pie.
6 Add the lid, seal firmly, neaten the edges, cut off any surplus paste; decorate if desired.
7 Make a hole 1 cm in diameter in the centre of the pie; brush all over with eggwash.
8 Bake in a hot oven (230–250°C) for approximately 20 minutes.
9 ⚠ Reduce the heat to moderate (150–200°C) and cook for 1½–2 hours in all. Use a temperature probe to check that the meat is cooked: the temperature should be 72°C.
10 If the pie colours too quickly, cover with greaseproof paper or foil. Remove from the oven and carefully remove tin. Eggwash the pie all over and return to the oven for a few minutes.

11 Remove from the oven and fill with approximately 125 ml of good hot stock in which 5 g of gelatine has been dissolved.

12 Serve when cold, garnished with picked watercress and chutney, and offer a suitable salad.

 HEALTHY EATING TIP

- The paste, pork and bacon result in a high-fat dish. Serve with plenty of potato, rice or pasta and a large salad to proportionally reduce the fat.

- Little or no added salt is needed – there is plenty in the bacon.

---

48 Pork escalopes

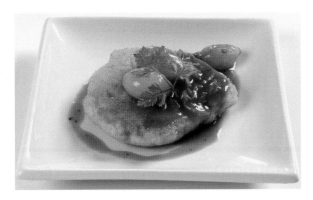

Pork escalopes are usually cut from the prime cuts of meat in the leg or loin, and can be dealt with in the same way as a leg of veal. They may be cut into 75–100 g slices, flattened with a meat bat, and used plain or crumbed and served with vegetables or a pasta (noodles) with a suitable sauce (e.g. Madeira, or as for veal escalopes (recipes 40 and 41).

Chef's tip
Bat out the escalopes thinly.

---

49 Sweet and sour pork

cal	kcal	fat	sat fat	carb	sugar	protein	fibre	
3067 KJ	730 kcal	43.9 g	9.2 g	69.7 g	54.7 g	13.4 g	1.6 g	*

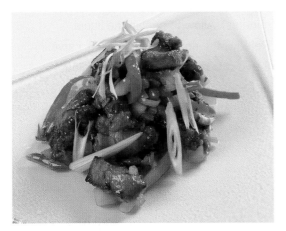

	4 portions	10 portions
loin of pork, boned	250 g	600 g
sugar	12 g	30 g
dry sherry	70 ml	180 ml
soy sauce	70 ml	180 ml
cornflour	50 g	125 g
vegetable oil, for frying	70 ml	180 ml
oil	2 tbsp	5 tbsp
clove garlic	1	2
fresh root ginger	50 g	125 g
onion, chopped	75 g	180 g
green pepper, in 1 cm dice	1	2½
chillies, chopped	2	5
sweet and sour sauce (page 183)	210 ml	500 ml
pineapple rings (fresh or canned)	2	5
spring onions	2	5

1 Cut the boned loin of pork into 2 cm pieces.

2 Marinate the pork for 30 minutes in the sugar, sherry and soy sauce.

3 Pass the pork through cornflour, pressing the cornflour in well.

4 Deep-fry the pork pieces in oil at 190°C until golden brown, then drain. Add the tablespoons of oil to a sauté pan.

5 Add the garlic and ginger, and fry until fragrant.

6 Add the onion, pepper and chillies, sauté for a few minutes.

7 Stir in the sweet and sour sauce (page 183), bring to the boil.

8 Add the pineapple cut into small chunks, thicken slightly with diluted cornflour. Simmer for 2 minutes.

9 Deep-fry the pork again until crisp. Drain, mix into the vegetables and sauce or serve separately.

10 Serve garnished with rings of spring onions or button onions.

Chef's tip

It is important to allow the pork enough time to marinate.

HEALTHY EATING TIP

- Use hot sunflower oil to fry the pork and a small amount of an unsaturated oil to fry the vegetables.

- No added salt is needed, as the soy sauce is high in sodium.

- Serve with plenty of rice or noodles, and additional vegetables.

Using sunflower oil

---

50 Boiled bacon (hock, collar or gammon)

cal	kcal	fat	sat fat	carb	sugar	protein	fibre
1543 KJ	367 kcal	30.5 g	12.2 g	0.0 g	0.0 g	23.1 g	0.0 g

*

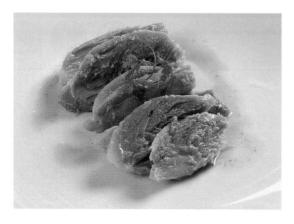

1 Soak the bacon in cold water for 24 hours before cooking. Change the water (see note, page 289).

2 Bring to the boil, skim and simmer gently (approx. 25 minutes per ½ kg, plus another 25 minutes). Allow to cool in the liquid.

3 Remove the rind and brown skin; carve.

4 Serve with a little of the cooking liquor.

Boiled bacon may be served with pease pudding and a suitable sauce such as parsley (page 186).

Using 113 g per portion

51 Griddled gammon with apricot salsa

cal	kcal	fat	sat fat	carb	sugar	protein	fibre
1112 KJ	266 kcal	14.2 g	4.2 g	8.1 g	7.4 g	26.9 g	1.0 g

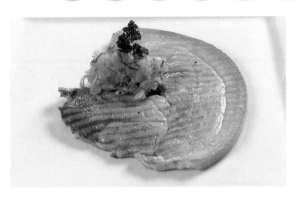

	4 portions	10 portions
gammon steaks	4 × 150 g	10 × 150 g
oil		
Apricot salsa		
fresh apricots or dried, reconstituted, stoned and chopped	200 g	500 g
lime, grated rind and juice	1	3
fresh root ginger, grated	2 tsp	5 tsp
clear honey	2 tsp	5 tsp
olive oil	1 tbsp	2½ tsp
sage, chopped, fresh	1 tbsp	2½ tbsp
spring onions, chopped	4	10
salt, pepper		

1 Heat the griddle pan, lightly oil it then cook the gammon steaks.
2 Make the salsa: mix together in a processor the apricots, lime rind and juice, ginger, honey, olive oil and sage.
3 Add the finely chopped spring onions, correct the seasoning then mix well.

The texture should be the consistency of thick cream but coarse. A little extra olive oil or some apricot juice may be required.

HEALTHY EATING TIP

- Use more juice and less oil in the salsa to reduce the fat.
- Gammon is a salty meat, so no extra salt is needed.
- Serve with a large portion of potatoes and vegetables or salad.

52 Potted meats

cal	kcal	fat	sat fat	carb	sugar	protein	fibre	
1160 KJ	280 kcal	23.8 g	14.5 g	0.2 g	0.2 g	16.4 g	0.0 g	*

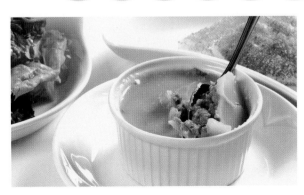

cooked meat, e.g. beef, salt	
beef, tongue, venison,	
chicken or a combination	200 g
salt, pepper and mace	
clarified butter	100 g

1 Using an electric blender or chopper, reduce the meat, seasoning and 85 g of the butter to a paste.
2 Pack firmly into an earthenware or china pot and refrigerate until firm.
3 Cover with 1 cm of clarified butter and refrigerate.
4 Serve with a small tossed green salad and hot toast.

Chef's tip
Carefully purée the meat to give the desired texture.

* 1 of 4 portions

HEALTHY EATING TIP

- Keep added salt to a minimum.
- Serve with plenty of salad vegetables and butter or toast (optional butter or spread).

53 Oxtail with Guinness

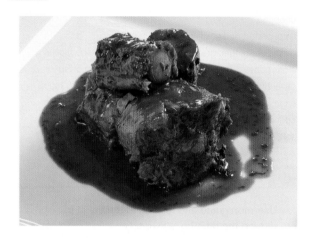

	4 portions	10 portions
oxtail	1.2 kg	4 kg
flour, to coat		
olive oil	3 tbsp	7 tbsp
celery, cut into batons	4 sticks	10 sticks
onions, finely chopped	2	5
carrots, thinly sliced	2	5
Guinness	440 ml	1 litre
tinned tomatoes	750 g	1875 g
bay leaves	2	5
garlic cloves	6	15
salt, pepper		

1 Place the oxtail pieces through the flour.
2 Heat the oil in a suitable pan. Fry the oxtail on both sides until golden brown. Remove.
3 Heat the remaining oil in the pan. Cook the celery, onion and carrots until they begin to soften.
4 Pour on the Guinness and bring to the boil.
5 In a clean pan, layer the oxtail with the vegetable and beer mixture, tomatoes (chopped), bay leaves and garlic. Season. Top up with water or brown stock to cover the oxtail.

6 Bring to the boil. Place in an oven at 140°C and cook for 3–3½ hours.
7 When cooked, serve with potato and celeriac mash and roasted root vegetables.

Chef's tip
Cut the oxtail into neat portions before shallow frying to brown them.

54 Grilled lambs' kidneys *(rognons grillés)*

cal	kcal	fat	sat fat	carb	sugar	protein	fibre
614 KJ	147 kcal	10.3 g	5.9 g	0.1 g	0.1 g	13.7 g	0.0 g

1 Season the prepared skewered kidneys.

2 Brush with melted butter, margarine or oil.

3 Place on preheated greased grill bars or on a greased baking tray.

4 Grill fairly quickly on both sides (approx. 5–10 minutes depending on size).

5 Serve with parsley butter, picked watercress and straw potatoes.

Chef's tip

Cook kidneys to order so that they are fresh and tasty.

HEALTHY EATING TIP

- Use the minimum amount of salt.
- Serve with plenty of starchy carbohydrate and vegetables.

55 Braised lambs' hearts *(coeurs d'agneau braisés)*

cal	kcal	fat	sat fat	carb	sugar	protein	fibre
1489 KJ	354 kcal	19.0 g	5.6 g	5.0 g	4.3 g	41.2 g	1.7 g

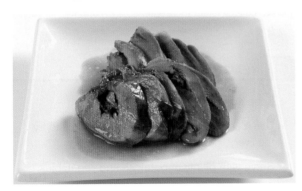

	4 portions	10 portions
lambs' hearts	4	10
salt, pepper		
fat or oil	25 g	60 g
onions	100 g	250 g
carrots	100 g	250 g
brown stock	500 ml	1¼ litre
bouquet garni		
tomato purée	10 g	25 g
demi-glace or jus-lié	250 ml	625 ml

1 Remove tubes and excess fat from the hearts.

2 Season and colour quickly on all sides in hot fat to seal the pores.

3 Place into a small braising pan (any pan with a tight-fitting lid that may be placed in the oven) or in a casserole.

4 Place the hearts on the lightly fried sliced vegetables.

5 Add the stock, which should come two-thirds of the way up the meat; season lightly.

6 Add the bouquet garni and tomato purée and, if available, add a few mushroom trimmings.

7 Bring to the boil, skim, cover with a lid and cook in a moderate oven at 150–200°C.

8 After 1½ hours add the demi-glace or jus-lie, reboil, skim and strain.

9 Continue cooking until tender.

10 Remove the hearts and correct the seasoning, colour and consistency of the sauce.

11 Pass the sauce on to the sliced hearts and serve.

Chef's tip

Shallow frying the hearts in hot oil before braising gives the finished dish its attractive golden brown colour.

Try something different

The hearts can be prepared and cooked as above and, prior to cooking, the tube cavities can be filled with a firm stuffing (e.g. recipe 17).

* Using sunflower oil

 HEALTHY EATING TIP

- Lightly oil the pan using an unsaturated oil (olive or sunflower).

- Drain off any excess fat and skim all fat from the finished dish.

- Keep added salt to a minimum.

---

56 Fried lambs' liver and bacon (foie d'agneau au lard)

cal	kcal	fat	sat fat	carb	sugar	protein	fibre
1039 KJ	250 kcal	20.1 g	3.8 g	0.1 g	0.1 g	17.2 g	0.0 g

*

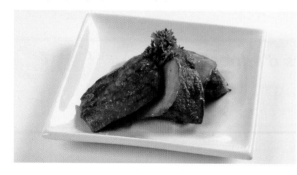

	4 portions	10 portions
liver	300 g	1 kg
butter, margarine or oil, for frying	50 g	125 g
streaky bacon	50 g (approx. 4 rashers)	125 g (approx. 10 rashers)
jus-lié, reduced lamb stock or red wine jus	125 ml	300 ml

1 Skin the liver and remove the gristle. Cut into thin slices on the slant.

2 Pass the slices of liver through seasoned flour. Shake off the excess flour.

3 Fry quickly on both sides in hot fat. (Liver is often served still pink in the centre but it is safer to cook it to a higher core temperature.)

4 Remove the rind and bone from the bacon and grill on both sides.

5 Serve the liver and bacon with a cordon and a sauceboat of jus or reduced stock.

HEALTHY EATING TIP

- Keep added salt to a minimum.

- Use a small amount of an unsaturated oil to fry the liver.

- Serve with plenty of potatoes and vegetables.

* Using oil, jus-lié and reduced stock

57 Kidney sauté (rognons sautés)

cal	kcal	fat	sat fat	carb	sugar	protein	fibre	*
1680 KJ	400 kcal	28.3 g	4.3 g	15.5 g	3.7 g	21.8 g	1.8 g	

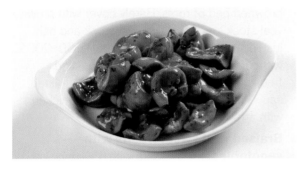

	4 portions	10 portions
sheep's kidneys	8	20
butter, margarine or oil	50 g	125 g
demi-glace, lamb jus or jus-lié	250 ml	625 ml

1 Skin and halve the kidneys. Remove the sinews.

2 Cut each half into 3 or 5 pieces and season.

3 Fry quickly in a frying pan using the butter, margarine or oil for approximately 4–5 minutes.

4 Place in a colander to drain, then discard the drained liquid.

5 Deglaze pan with demi-glace or jus, correct the seasoning and add the kidneys.

6 Do not reboil before serving as kidneys will toughen.

Try something different

After draining the kidneys, the pan may be deglazed with white wine, sherry or port. As an alternative, a sauce suprême (see page 186) may be used in place of demi-glace.

 HEALTHY EATING TIP

- Lightly oil the pan using an unsaturated oil (olive or sunflower).

- Drain off any excess fat.

- Add the minimum amount of salt to the demi-glace.

- Serve with plenty of starchy carbohydrates and vegetables.

An alternative recipe is **kidney sauté Turbigo**. Cook as for kidney sauté, then add 100 g small button mushrooms cooked in a little butter, margarine or oil, and 8 small 2 cm long grilled or fried chipolatas. Serve with the kidneys in an entrée dish, garnished with heart-shaped croutons (double these amounts for 10 portions).

* Using sunflower oil

58 Braised veal sweetbreads (white) *(ris de veau braisé – à blanc)*

cal	kcal	fat	sat fat	carb	sugar	protein	fibre	*
1103 KJ	263 kcal	20.7 g	4.4 g	1.7 g	0.0 g	17.6 g	0.0 g	

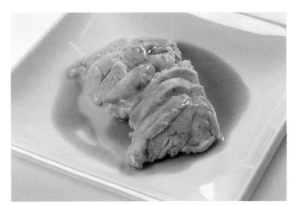

	4 portions	10 portions
heart-shaped sweetbreads	8	20
salt, pepper		
onion	100 g	250 g
carrot	100 g	250 g
oil, margarine or butter	50 g	125 g
bouquet garni		
veal stock	250 ml	625 ml

1 Wash, blanch, refresh and trim the sweetbreads (see page 286).

2 Season and place in a casserole or sauté pan on a bed of roots smeared with the oil, margarine or butter.

3 Add the bouquet garni and stock.

4 Cover with buttered greaseproof paper and a lid.

5 Cook in a moderate oven at 150–200°C for approximately 45 minutes.

6 Remove the lid and baste occasionally with cooking liquor to glaze.

7 Serve with some of the cooking liquor, thickened with diluted arrowroot if necessary, and passed on to the sweetbreads.

> Sweetbreads are glands, and two types are used for cooking. The thymus glands (throat) are usually long in shape and are of inferior quality. The pancreatic glands (stomach) are heart-shaped and of superior quality.

Try something different

Variations include the following.

- **Braised veal sweetbreads (brown):** prepare as in this recipe, but place on a lightly browned bed of roots. Barely cover with brown veal stock, or half-brown veal stock and half jus-lié. Cook in a moderate oven at 150–200°C without a lid (for approx. 1 hour), basting frequently. Cover with the corrected, strained sauce to serve. (If veal stock is used, thicken with arrowroot.)

- **Braised veal sweetbreads with vegetables:** braise white with a julienne of vegetables in place of the bed of roots, the julienne served in the sauce.

* Using hard margarine and sunflower oil

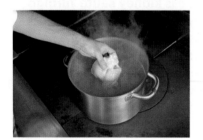
Blanch the sweetbreads

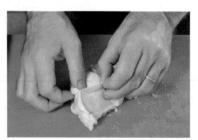
Peel the sweetbreads

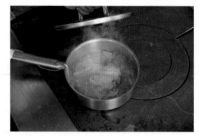
Add the stock and braise

59 Sweetbread escalope *(escalope de ris de veau)*

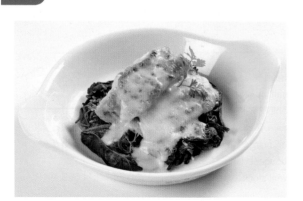

1 Braise the sweetbreads white, press slightly between two trays and allow to cool.

2 Cut into slices ½–1 cm thick, dust with flour and shallow-fry.

3 Serve with suitable garnish and sauce (e.g. on a bed of leaf spinach; coat with mornay sauce and glaze).

Chef's tip

Pressing the sweetbread escalope between two trays gives it a good shape.

60 Grilled veal sweetbreads

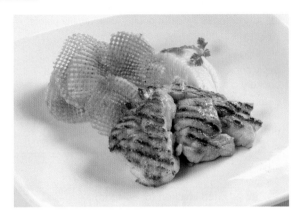

1 Blanch, braise, cool and press the sweetbreads.
2 Cut in halves crosswise, pass through melted butter and grill gently on both sides.
3 Serve with a sauce and garnish as indicated.

> In some recipes, the sweetbreads may be passed through butter and crumbs before being grilled, and garnished with noisette potatoes, buttered carrots, purée of peas and béarnaise sauce.

61 Lambs' kidneys bouchées

	12 bouchées
puff pastry (see page 502)	200 g
lambs' kidneys	8
vegetable oil	50 ml
butter	50 g
sherry vinegar	50 ml
parsley, chopped	1 tsp

1 Roll out the pastry approximately ½ cm thick. Cut out with a round, fluted 5 cm cutter.
2 Place the rounds on a greased, dampened baking sheet; eggwash. Dip a plain 4 cm diameter cutter into hot fat or oil and make an incision 3 mm deep in the centre of each. Allow to rest in a cool place.
3 Bake at 220°C for about 20 minutes.

4 Remove from the oven and allow to cool. Remove the caps or lids carefully and remove all the raw pastry from inside the cases.
5 Remove the fat from the kidneys and skin them. Cut them into small pieces.
6 Heat the oil in a shallow pan, add the kidneys and sauté for 1–2 minutes. Add the butter and baste the kidneys.
7 Add the sherry vinegar and chopped parsley. (A little jus-lié may also be added.) Baste the kidneys in the liquor.
8 Fill each bouchée with the cooked kidneys. Serve immediately.

A filled bouchée may be offered as a canapé or an amuse-bouche. Alternative fillings include sautéd chicken liver prepared in a similar way.

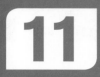
Number	Recipe title	Page number
Chicken		
2	Chicken à la king (*emincé de volaille à la king*)	347
3	Chicken in red wine (*coq au vin*)	348
13	Chicken Kiev (traditional)	356
1	Chicken sauté chasseur (*poulet sauté chasseur*)	346
4	Chicken spatchcock (*poulet grillé à la crapaudine*)	349
11	Chicken tikka	354
5	Crumbed breast of chicken with asparagus (*suprême de volaille aux pointes d'asperges*)	350
	Fricassée de volaille à l'ancienne	351
6	Fricassée of chicken (*fricassée de volaille*)	350
7	Fried chicken (deep-fried)	351
8	Grilled chicken (*poulet grillé*)	352
9	Roast chicken with dressing (*poulet rôti à l'anglaise*)	352
12	Tandoori chicken	355
10	Terrine of chicken and vegetables	353
Other poultry		
17	Confit duck leg with red cabbage and green beans	358
18	Duckling with orange sauce (*caneton bigarade*)	359
19	Roast duck or duckling (*canard/caneton rôti*)	361
14	Roast turkey (*dinde rôti*)	356
16	Suprêmes of guineafowl with a pepper and basil coulis	358
15	Turkey escalopes	357

In this chapter, you will learn how to:

1. prepare and cook poultry, including:

- using tools and equipment correctly, in a safe and hygienic way
- demonstrating preparation skills, portion control, cooking and finishing skills
- producing sauces, dressings, garnishes and accompaniments

2. you should have the knowledge to:

- identify different types of poultry, their quality points, weights and commonly used cuts
- store poultry safely at the correct temperatures
- apply cooking principles and suitable methods of cookery
- determine when poultry is cooked and the required safe temperature has been reached, and check the finished dish.

Poultry

The word 'poultry' means all domestic fowl (birds) bred for food. It includes chickens, turkeys, ducks, geese and pigeons. Chicken is the type most commonly used in cooking, and in this first section chicken is the poultry that will be used for examples; turkeys, geese and ducks are discussed in more detail later in the chapter.

Originally chickens were classified according to size and cooking method by specific names, as shown in Table 11.1.

Table 11.1 Traditional classification of fowl

	Weight (kg)	Number of portions
single baby chicken (poussin)	3/10–½	1
double baby chicken (poussin)	½–3/4	2
small roasting chicken	3/4–1	3–4
medium roasting chicken	1–2	4–6
large roasting or boiling chicken	2–3	6–8
capon	3–4½	8–12
old boiling fowl	2½–4	

There is approximately 15–20 per cent bone in poultry.

Types of chicken

There are different types of chicken available. Different chickens are good for different things.

- **Spring chickens** (poussins) are 4–6 weeks old and are used for roasting or grilling.
- **Broiler chickens** are 3–4 months old and are used for roasting, grilling and casseroles.
- **Medium roasting chickens** are fully grown, tender prime birds used for roasting, grilling, sautéing, casseroles, suprêmes and pies.
- **Large roasting chickens** are used for roasting, boiling and casseroles.
- **Capons** are large, specially bred cock birds used for roasting.
- **Old hen birds** are used for stocks and soups.

Food value

The flesh of poultry is more easily digested than that of butchers' meat. It contains protein, so it is useful for building and repairing body tissues and providing heat and energy. The fat content is low and contains a high percentage of unsaturated fat.

Storage

Chilled birds should be stored between 3°C and 5°C. Oven-ready birds are eviscerated (gutted) and should be stored in a refrigerator. Frozen birds must be kept in a deep freeze until required, but must be completely thawed, preferably in a refrigerator, before being cooked. This procedure is essential to reduce the risk of food poisoning: chickens are potential carriers of salmonella, and if birds are cooked from frozen there is a risk that the degree of heat required to kill off salmonella may not reach the centre of the bird.

When using frozen poultry, check that:

- the packaging is undamaged
- there are no signs of freezer burns, which are indicated by white patches on the skin.

Frozen birds should removed from the freezer and put into a refrigerator to defrost.

Quality points

Good-quality chickens should have the following features:

- The breast should be plump and firm.
- The wishbone (breastbone) should be easy to bend between your fingers and thumb.
- The skin should be white and unbroken. Broiler chickens have a faint bluish tint.
- Corn-fed chickens are yellow. Free range chickens have more colour, a firmer texture and more flavour.
- Bresse chickens are specially bred in France and are highly regarded.
- Old birds have coarse scales, large spurs on the legs and long hairs on the skin.

Trussing

Roasting

- Clean the legs by dipping in boiling water for a few seconds, then remove the scales with a cloth.
- Cut off the outside claws, leaving the centre ones; trim these to half their length.
- To make carving easier, remove the wishbone.
- Place the bird on its back.
- Hold the legs back firmly.
- Insert a trussing needle through the bird, midway between the leg joints.

- Turn on to its side.
- Pierce the winglet, the skin of the neck, the skin of the carcass and the other winglet.
- Tie the ends of the string securely.
- Secure the legs by inserting the needle through the carcass and over the legs; take care not to pierce the breast.

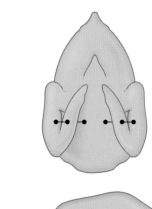

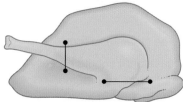

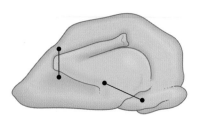

Trussing a chicken for roasting and boiling

Boiling and pot roasting

- Proceed as for roasting.
- Cut the leg sinew just below the joint.
- Bend back the legs so that they lie parallel to the breast, and secure them when trussing; *or* insert the legs through incisions made in the skin at the rear end of the bird, and secure when trussing.

Cutting for sauté, fricassée, pies, etc.

Using a large, sharp knife:

- Remove the feet at the first joint.
- Remove the legs from the carcass.
- Cut each leg in two at the joint.
- Remove the wishbone.
- Remove the winglets (small bones attached to the wings) and trim.
- Remove the wings carefully, leaving two equal portions on the breast.
- Remove the breast and cut in two.
- Trim the carcass and cut into three pieces.

Cuts of chicken

The pieces of cut chicken are (the numbers refer to the next diagram):

1 wing
2 breast
3 thigh ⎫
4 drumstick ⎬ leg
5 winglet
6 carcass

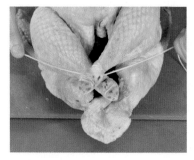

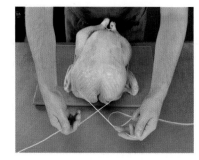

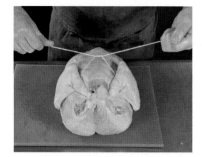

Poultry may be trussed without using a needle

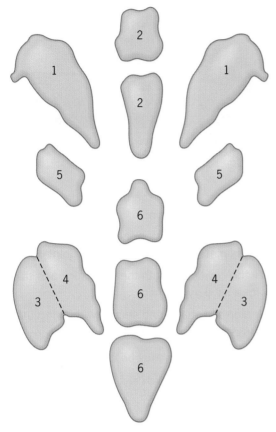

Cuts of chicken

Preparation for grilling (spatchcock)

- Remove the wishbone.
- Cut off the feet at the first joint.
- Place the bird on its back.
- Insert a large knife through the neck end and out of the vent (the gap at the other end, just under the parson's nose).
- Cut through the backbone and open out the bird.
- Remove the back and rib bones.

Preparation for suprêmes

A suprême is the wing and half the breast of a chicken with the trimmed wing bone attached; one chicken yields two suprêmes.

1 Use a chicken weighing 1¼–1½ kg.
2 Cut off both the legs.
3 Remove the skin from the breasts.
4 Remove the wishbone.
5 Scrape the wing bone bare where it meets the breast.
6 Cut off the winglets near the joints, leaving 1½–2 cm of bare bone attached to the breasts.

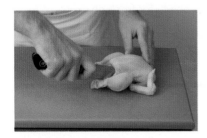

Preparing chicken for sauté: remove the winglets

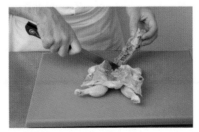

Remove the legs and divide them into thigh and drumstick

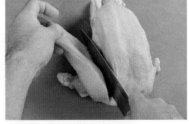

Remove each breast and cut it into two pieces

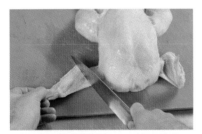

To spatchcock a chicken for grilling, first insert the knife into the neck end and cut through the back

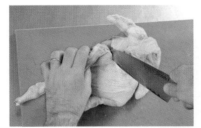

Turn the chicken over, open up the cut and remove the backbone

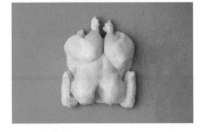

Chicken spatchcock with the rib bones removed, ready for cooking

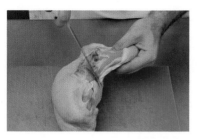

To prepare chicken suprêmes, cut off both legs and then the winglets

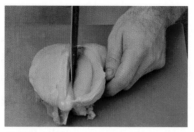

Cut the breasts close to the breastbone and follow the bone down to the wing joint

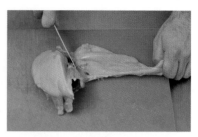

Cut through the joint. Pull the suprêmes off, using a knife to assist

7 Cut the breasts close to the breastbone and follow the bone down to the wing joint.

8 Cut through the joint.

9 Lay the chicken on its side and pull off the suprêmes, using the knife to help.

10 Lift the fillets (the small, tender part that is slightly separate from the rest of the breast) from the suprêmes and remove the sinew from both.

11 Make an incision lengthways, along the thick side of the suprêmes (do not cut all the way through); open this and place the fillets inside.

12 Close, lightly flatten with a bat moistened with water, and trim if necessary.

Preparation for ballotines

A ballotine is a boned, stuffed leg of bird.

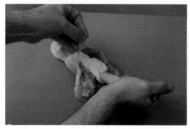

Stuffing a chicken leg for a ballotine

● Using a small, sharp knife, remove the thigh bone.

● Scrape the flesh off the bone of the drumstick towards the claw joint.

● Cut off the drumstick bone, leaving approximately 2–3 cm at the claw joint end.

● Fill the cavities in both the drumstick and thigh with a savoury stuffing.

● Neaten the shape and secure with string using a trussing needle.

Ballotines of chicken may be cooked and served using any of the recipes for sautéed chicken presented in this chapter.

Cutting cooked chicken (roasted or boiled)

● Remove the legs and cut in two (drumstick and thigh).

● Remove the wings.

● Separate the breast from the carcass and divide in two.

● Serve a drumstick with a wing and a thigh with a breast.

✎ ACTIVITY

1 Give another name for supême of chicken.

2 List the quality points for fresh chicken.

3 Name the food poisoning bacteria associated with fresh chicken.

Turkey

Turkeys can vary in weight from 3½ to 20 kg. They are trussed in the same way as a chicken.

The wishbone should always be removed before trussing, to make carving easier. The sinews should be drawn out of the legs. Allow 200 g per portion raw weight.

When cooking a large turkey, the legs may be removed, boned, rolled, tied and roasted separately from the remainder of the bird. This will reduce the cooking time, and help the legs and breast to cook more evenly (see recipe 14).

Stuffings may be rolled in foil, steamed or baked and thickly sliced. If a firmer stuffing is required, mix in one or two raw eggs before cooking.

Quality points

Good-quality turkeys should have the following features:

- Large full breast with undamaged skin and no signs of stickiness.
- Legs smooth with supple feet and a short spur. As birds age the legs turn scaly and the feet harden.

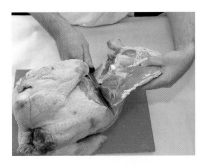
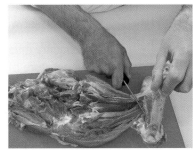
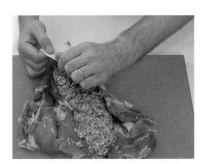
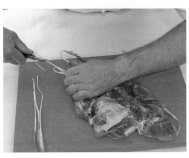
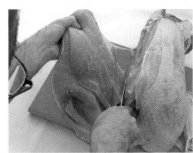
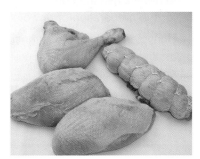

Boning, stuffing, rolling and tying turkey in six steps

Duck, duckling, goose, gosling

Approximate sizes are as follows:

- **duck**: 3–4 kg
- **goose**: 6 kg
- **duckling**: 1½–2 kg
- **gosling**: 3 kg

Quality points

Good-quality birds should have the following features:

- Plump breasts.
- Webbed feet should tear easily.
- The lower back should bend easily.
- Feet and bill should be yellow.

Roasting

Preparation is the same as for chicken (page 341 and recipe 9). The only difference is that these birds have a gizzard, which should not be split but should be trimmed off with a knife.

Roast birds can be served whole and carved at the table, or can be carved up before they are served, in which case:

- Remove the legs and cut into two (drumstick and thigh).

- Remove the wings and divide the breast into two.

- Serve a drumstick with a wing and a thigh piece with a piece of breast.

Food safety

For information on maintaining a safe and secure working environment, a professional and hygienic appearance, clean food production areas, equipment and utensils, and food hygiene, please refer to Chapters 2 and 3. Additional health and safety points to reduce the risk of cross-contamination are as follows.

- When preparing uncooked poultry, and then cooked food, or changing from one type of meat or poultry to another, equipment, working areas and utensils must be thoroughly cleaned, or changed.

- If colour-coded boards are used, it is essential to always use the correct colour-coded boards for the preparation of raw or cooked poultry.

- Unhygienic equipment, utensils and preparation areas increase the risk of cross-contamination and danger to health.

- Store uncooked poultry on trays to prevent dripping, in a separate refrigerator at a temperature of 3–5°C, preferably at the lower temperature. If separate refrigerators are not available then store in a separate area within the refrigerator.

- Wash all work surfaces with a bactericidal detergent to kill bacteria. This is particularly important when handling poultry.

All poultry must be cooked until it reaches a core temperature of 75°C, even if this is not stated in the recipe.

Test yourself

1 List the quality points for a good quality chicken.
2 Describe a spatchcock chicken.
3 How many edible pieces does a chicken cut for sauté yield?
4 What is the safe internal temperature required for cooked poultry?
5 Describe chicken à la king.

ASSESSMENT

1 Chicken sauté chasseur (poulet sauté chasseur)

cal	kcal	fat	sat fat	carb	sugar	protein	fibre
2430 KJ	579 kcal	45.8 g	20.7 g	2.1 g	1.6 g	37.6 g	1.5 g

	4 portions	10 portions
butter, margarine or oil	50 g	125 g
salt, pepper		
chicken, 1¼–1½ kg, cut for sauté	1	2½
shallots, chopped	10 g	25 g
button mushrooms	100 g	250 g
dry white wine	3 tbsp	8 tbsp
jus-lié, demi-glace or reduced brown stock	250 ml	625 ml
tomatoes concassée	200 g	500 g
parsley and tarragon, chopped		

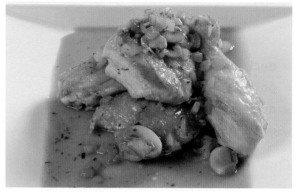

1 Place the butter, margarine or oil in a sauté pan on a fairly hot stove.

2 Season the pieces of chicken and place in the pan in the following order: drumsticks, thighs, carcass, wings, winglets and breast.

3 Cook to a golden brown on both sides.

4 Cover with a lid and cook on the stove or in the oven until tender. Dress neatly in a suitable dish.

5   Add the shallots to the sauté pan, cover with a lid, cook on a gentle heat for 1–2 minutes without colour.

6   Add the washed, sliced mushrooms and cover with a lid; cook gently for 3–4 minutes without colour. Drain off the fat.

7   Add the white wine and reduce by half. Add the jus-lié, demi-glace or reduced brown stock.

8   Add the tomatoes concassée; simmer for 5 minutes.

9   Correct the seasoning and pour over the chicken.

10 Sprinkle with chopped parsley and tarragon; serve.

Ballotines of chicken chasseur can be prepared as above or lightly braised (as shown).

Chef's tips

The leg meat takes longer to cook than the breast meat, which is why the drumsticks and thighs should be added first.

Add the soft herbs and tomatoes just before serving.

*Using butter

Cutting chicken for sauté
http://bit.ly/xBU6qv

---

2   Chicken à la king (eminçé de volaille à la king)

cal	kcal	fat	sat fat	carb	sugar	protein	fibre
1226 KJ	292 kcal	16.7 g	7.8 g	3.2 g	0.8 g	30.4 g	0.9 g

	4 portions	10 portions
button mushrooms	100 g	250 g
butter, margarine or oil	25 g	60 g
red pimento, skinned	50 g	125 g
cooked boiled chicken	400 g	1¼ kg
sherry	30 ml	75 ml
chicken velouté	125 ml	150 ml
cream or non-dairy cream	30 ml	75 ml

1   Wash, peel and slice the mushrooms.

2   Cook them without colour in the butter or margarine.

3   If using raw pimento, discard the seeds, cut the pimento into dice and cook with the mushrooms.

4   Cut the chicken into small, neat slices.

5   Add the chicken to the mushrooms and pimento.

6   Drain off the fat. Add the sherry.

7   Add the velouté and bring to the boil.

8   Finish with the cream and correct the seasoning.

9   Place in a serving dish and decorate with small strips of cooked pimento.

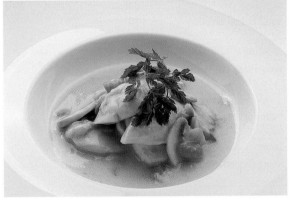

1 or 2 egg yolks may be used to form a liaison with the cream, mixed into the boiling mixture at the last possible moment and immediately removed from the heat. Chicken à la king may be served in a border of golden brown duchess potato, or a pilaff of rice (see page 421) may be offered as an accompaniment. It is suitable for a hot buffet dish.

Chef's tip

Use a velouté with a good chicken flavour, to create the best sauce.

- Use the minimum amount of salt.

- Remove the skin from the cooked chicken.

- Try reducing or omitting the cream used to finish the sauce.

- Serve with plenty of rice and vegetables or salad.

* Using butter or hard margarine

3 Chicken in red wine *(coq au vin)*

cal	kcal	fat	sat fat	carb	sugar	protein	fibre
4794 KJ	1141 kcal	95.7 g	32.9 g	16.6 g	2.3 g	49.0 g	1.7 g

	4 portions	10 portions
roasting chicken, 1½ kg	1	2–3
lardons	50 g	125 g
small chipolatas	4	10
button mushrooms	50 g	125 g
butter or margarine	50 g	125 g
sunflower oil	3 tbsp	7 tbsp
small button onions	12	30
red wine	125 ml	300 ml
brown stock *or* red wine	500 ml	900 ml
butter or margarine	25 g	60 g
flour	25 g	60 g
heart-shaped croutons	4	10
parsley, chopped		

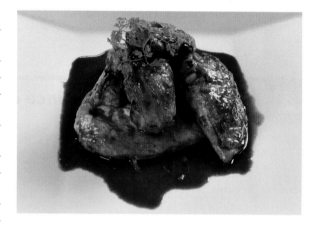

1 Cut the chicken as for sauté (page 343). Blanch the lardons.

2 If the chipolatas are large divide into two.

3 Wash and cut the mushrooms into quarters.

4 Sauté the lardons, mushrooms and chipolatas in a mixture of butter/margarine and oil. Remove when cooked.

5 Lightly season the pieces of chicken and place in the pan in the correct order (see recipe 1) with button onions. Sauté until almost cooked. Drain off the fat.

6 Just cover with red wine and brown stock; cover with a lid and finish cooking.

7 Remove the chicken and onions, place into a clean pan.

8 Lightly thicken the liquor with a *beurre manié* from the 25 g (or 60 g) butter/margarine and 25 g (or 60 g) flour.

9 Pass the sauce over the chicken and onions, add the mushrooms, chipolatas and lardons. Correct the seasoning and reheat.

10 Serve garnished with heart-shaped croutons with the points dipped in chopped parsley.

Chef's tip

Add the beurre manié slowly, mixing well, to create a thick, smooth sauce.

HEALTHY EATING TIP

- Use a well-seasoned pan to dry-fry the lardons and chipolatas, then add the mushrooms.

- Use the minimum amount of added salt.

- Drain all the fat from the cooked chicken.

- Garnish with ovenbaked croutons.

- Serve with plenty of starchy carbohydrate and vegetables.

* Using sunflower oil and hard margarine

4 · Chicken spatchcock *(poulet grillé à la crapaudine)*

cal	kcal	fat	sat fat	carb	sugar	protein	fibre
1560 KJ	372 kcal	24.1 g	8.0 g	0.0 g	0.0 g	38.9 g	0.0 g

	4 portions	10 portions
chicken, 1¼–1½ kg	1	2½

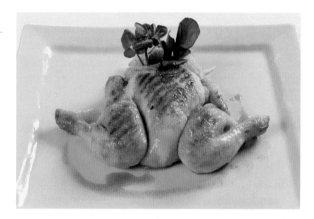

1 Cut horizontally from below the point of the breast over the top of the legs down to the wing joints, without removing the breasts. Fold back the breasts.

2 Snap and reverse the backbone into the opposite direction so that the point of the breast now extends forward.

3 Flatten slightly. Remove any small bones.

4 Skewer the wings and legs in position.

5 Season with salt and mill pepper.

6 Brush with oil or melted butter.

7 Place on preheated grill bars or on a flat tray under a salamander.

8 Brush frequently with melted fat or oil during cooking and allow approximately 15–20 minutes on each side.

9 Test if cooked by piercing the drumstick with a needle or skewer – there should be no sign of blood.

10 Serve garnished with picked watercress and offer a suitable sauce separately (e.g. devilled sauce or a compound butter).

🍎 HEALTHY EATING TIP

- Use a minimum amount of salt to season the chicken.

- The fat content can be reduced if the skin is removed from the chicken.

- Use a small amount of an unsaturated oil to brush the chicken.

- Serve with a large portion of potatoes and vegetables.

5 Crumbed breast of chicken with asparagus (*suprême de volaille aux pointes d'asperges*)

cal	kcal	fat	sat fat	carb	sugar	protein	fibre
1831 KJ	439 kcal	26.4 g	8.9 g	15.7 g	1.5 g	35.5 g	1.3 g

	4 portions	10 portions
suprêmes of chicken (page 344)	4 × 125 g	10 × 125 g
egg	1	2
breadcrumbs (white or wholemeal)	50 g	125 g
oil	50 g	125 g
butter or margarine	50 g	125 g
butter	50 g	125 g
jus-lié	60 ml	150 ml
asparagus	200 g	500 g

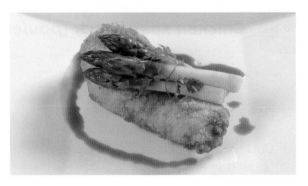

1 Pané the chicken suprêmes (this means passing it through flour, beaten egg and then breadcrumbs). Shake off all surplus crumbs.
2 Neaten and mark on one side with a palette knife.
3 Heat the oil and fat in a sauté pan.
4 Gently fry the suprêmes to a golden brown on both sides (6–8 minutes).
5 Dress the suprêmes on a flat dish and keep warm.
6 Mask the suprêmes with the remaining butter cooked to the nut brown stage.
7 Surround the suprêmes with a cordon of jus-lié.
8 Garnish each suprême with a neat bundle of asparagus points (previously cooked, refreshed and reheated with a little butter).

 HEALTHY EATING TIP

- Use a minimum amount of salt.
- Remove the skin from the suprêmes and fry in a little unsaturated vegetable oil. Drain on kitchen paper.
- Try omitting the additional cooked butter.
- Serve with plenty of boiled new potatoes and vegetables.

ASSESSMENT

6 Fricassée of chicken (*fricassée de volaille*)

cal	kcal	fat	sat fat	carb	sugar	protein	fibre
2699 KJ	643 kcal	51.3 g	23.3 g	7.4 g	0.6 g	38.2 g	0.4 g

	4 portions	10 portions
chicken, 1¼–1½ kg	1	2–3
salt, pepper		
butter, margarine or oil	50 g	125 g
flour	35 g	100 g
chicken stock	½ litre	1¼ litres
egg yolks	1–2	5
cream or non-dairy cream	4 tbsp	10 tbsp
parsley, chopped		

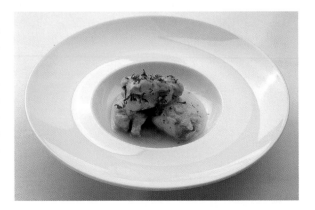

1 Cut the chicken as for sauté (page 343); season with salt and pepper.

2 Place the butter in a sauté pan. Heat gently.

3 Add the pieces of chicken. Cover with a lid.

4 Cook gently on both sides without colouring. Mix in the flour.

5 Cook out carefully without colouring. Gradually mix in the stock.

6 Bring to the boil and skim. Allow to simmer gently until cooked.

7 Mix the yolks and cream in a basin (liaison).

8 Pick out the chicken into a clean pan.

9 Pour a little boiling sauce on to the yolks and cream and mix well.

10 Pour all back into the sauce, combine thoroughly but do not reboil.

11 Correct the seasoning and pass through a fine strainer.

12 Pour over the chicken, reheat without boiling.

13 Serve sprinkled with chopped parsley.

14 Garnish with heart-shaped croutons, fried in butter, if desired.

Try something different

Fricassée de volaille à l'ancienne, a fricassée of chicken with button onions and mushrooms can be made in a similar way, with the addition of 50–100 g button onions and 50–100 g button mushrooms. They are peeled and the mushrooms left whole, turned or quartered depending on size and quality. The onions are added to the chicken as soon as it comes to the boil and the mushrooms 15 minutes later. Heart-shaped croutons may be used to garnish. This is a classic dish.

Chef's tips

Sauté the chicken lightly.
Add the liaison of yolks and cream carefully. Do not allow the sauce to come back to the boil once the liaison has been added, or it will curdle.

 HEALTHY EATING TIP

- Keep added salt to a minimum throughout the cooking.

- Use a little unsaturated oil to cook the chicken, and drain off all excess fat after cooking.

- Try oven-baking the croutons brushed with olive oil.

- The sauce is high in fat, so serve with plenty of starchy carbohydrate and vegetables.

* Using butter

---

7 | ## Fried chicken (deep-fried)

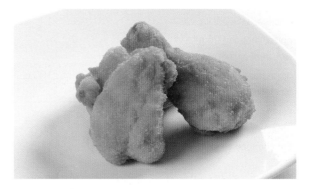

cal	kcal	fat	sat fat	carb	sugar	protein	fibre
1754 KJ	421 kcal	28.6 g	6.1 g	14.5 g	0.4 g	27.2 g	0.5 g

1 Cut the chicken as for sauté and: coat with either flour, egg and crumbs (pané, as shown here); or pass through a light batter (page 386) to which herbs can be added.

2 For suprêmes, make an incision, stuff with a compound butter, flour, egg and crumb, and deep-fry as in Chicken Kiev (recipe 13).

 HEALTHY EATING TIP

- The fat content can be reduced if the skin is removed from the chicken.

8 Grilled chicken *(poulet grillé)*

cal	kcal	fat	sat fat	carb	sugar	protein	fibre
975 KJ	234 kcal	15.7 g	4.3 g	0.0 g	0.0 g	23.3 g	0.0 g

*

1 Season the chicken with salt and mill pepper, and prepare as for grilling (see page 343).

2 Brush with oil or melted butter or margarine, and place on preheated greased grill bars or on a barbecue or a flat baking tray under a salamander.

3 Brush frequently with melted fat during cooking; allow approximately 15–20 minutes each side.

4 Test if cooked by piercing the drumstick with a skewer or trussing needle; there should be no sign of blood issuing from the leg.

5 Serve garnished with picked watercress and offer a suitable sauce separately.

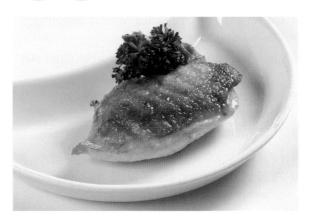

Grilled chicken is frequently served garnished with streaky bacon, tomatoes and mushrooms. The chicken may be marinated for 2–3 hours before grilling, in a mixture of oil, lemon juice, spices, herbs, freshly grated ginger, finely chopped garlic, salt and pepper. Chicken or turkey portions can also be grilled and marinated beforehand if wished (breasts or boned-out lightly battered thighs of chicken).

HEALTHY EATING TIP

- Use a minimum amount of salt and an unsaturated oil.
- Garnish with grilled tomatoes and mushrooms.
- Serve with Delmonico potatoes and green vegetables.

* Based on chicken with bone, wing and leg quarters

9 Roast chicken with dressing *(poulet rôti à l'anglaise)*

cal	kcal	fat	sat fat	carb	sugar	protein	fibre
1363 KJ	327 kcal	20.4 g	3.7 g	6.7 g	0.7 g	29.5 g	0.3 g

*

chicken, 1¼–1½ kg	1
onion, chopped 25 g	
salt, pepper	
oil, butter or margarine	100 g
pinch chopped parsley	
pinch powdered thyme	
breadcrumbs (white or wholemeal)	50 g
the chopped chicken liver (raw) (optional)	

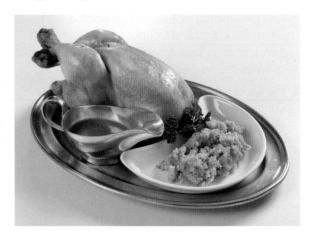

1 Lightly season the chicken inside and out with salt.

2 Place on its side in a roasting tin.

3 Cover with 50 g of oil, butter or margarine.

4 Place in a hot oven for approximately 20–25 minutes, then turn on to the other leg.

5 Cook for approximately a further 20–25 minutes. Baste frequently.

6 To test whether the chicken is fully cooked, pierce it with a fork between the drumstick and thigh, and hold it over a plate. The juice issuing from the chicken should not show any sign of blood. If using a temperature probe, insert in the thickest part of the leg; it should read 77°C. Place the cooked chicken breast side down to retain all the cooking juices.

7 To make the dressing, gently cook the onion in 50 g of oil, butter or margarine without colour.

8 Add the seasoning, herbs and breadcrumbs.

9 Mix in the liver.

10 Correct the seasoning and bake or steam the dressing separately, for approximately 20 minutes.

> *Arrange the chicken to cook sitting on one leg, then the other leg and then with the breast upright, so that the whole bird cooks evenly.*

HEALTHY EATING TIP

- Use a little unsaturated oil to cook the onion.
- Keep the added salt to a minimum.
- Serve with plenty of potatoes and vegetables.

* Based on average edible portion of roasted meat (100 g)

---

10   Terrine of chicken and vegetables

cal	kcal	fat	sat fat	carb	sugar	protein	fibre
930 KJ	226 kcal	17.3 g	9.4 g	2.0 g	1.8 g	15.5 g	0.9 g

	8–10 portions
carrots, turnips and swedes, peeled and cut into 7 mm dice	50 g of each
broccoli, small florets	50 g
baby corn, cut into 7 mm rounds	50 g
French beans, cut into 7 mm lengths	50 g
chicken (white meat only), minced	400 g
egg whites	2
double cream	200 ml
salt, mill pepper	

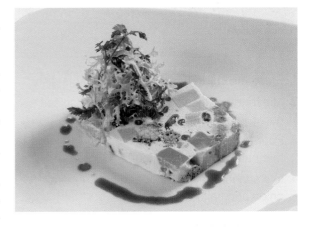

1 Blanch all the vegetables individually in boiling salted water, ensuring that they remain firm. Refresh in cold water, and drain well.

2 Blend the chicken and egg whites in a food processor until smooth. Turn out into a large mixing bowl and gradually beat in the double cream.

3 Season with salt and mill pepper, and fold in the vegetables.

4 Line a lightly greased 1-litre terrine with clingfilm.

5 Spoon the farce into the mould and overlap the clingfilm.

6 Cover with foil, put the lid on and cook in a bain-marie in a moderate oven for about 45 minutes.

7 When cooked, remove the lid and leave to cool overnight.

11 Chicken tikka

cal	kcal	fat	sat fat	carb	sugar	protein	fibre
1780 KJ	427 kcal	27.1 g	5.2 g	5.5 g	5.1 g	41.3 g	0.6 g

	4 portions	10 portions
chicken, cut for sauté	1 × 1½ kg	2½ × 1½ kg
natural yoghurt	125 ml	250 ml
grated ginger	1 tsp	2½ tsp
ground coriander	1 tsp	2½ tsp
ground cumin	1 tsp	2½ tsp
chilli powder	1 tsp	2½ tsp
clove garlic, crushed and chopped	1	2–3
lemon, juice of	½	1
tomato purée	50 g	125 g
onion, finely chopped	50 g	125 g
oil	60 ml	150 ml
lemon, wedges of	4	10
seasoning		

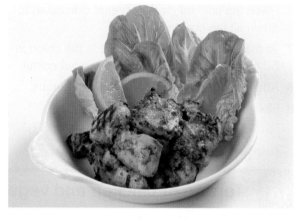

1 Place the chicken pieces into a suitable dish.

2 Mix together the yoghurt, seasoning, spices, garlic, lemon juice and tomato purée.

3 Pour this over the chicken, mix well and leave to marinate for at least 3 hours.

4 In a suitable shallow tray, add the chopped onion and half the oil.

5 Lay the chicken pieces on top and grill under the salamander, turning the pieces over once or gently cook in a moderate oven at 180°C for 20–30 minutes.

6 Baste with the remaining oil.

7 Serve on a bed of lettuce garnished with wedges of lemon.

Chef's tip

Baste the chicken during grilling so that it does not become too dry.

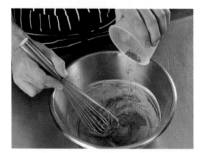

Mix together the spices

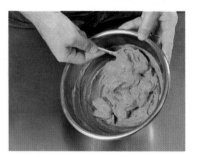

Mix the chicken pieces into the marinade

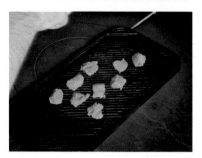

Griddle the chicken in a shallow tray

HEALTHY EATING TIP

- Skin the chicken and keep the added salt to a minimum.

- Use half the amount of unsaturated oil.

- Serve with rice and a vegetable dish.

* Estimated edible meat used

12 Tandoori chicken

cal	kcal	fat	sat fat	carb	sugar	protein	fibre
1436 KJ	342 kcal	14.1 g	4.6 g	10.1 g	8.6 g	44.6 g	0.3 g

*

	4 portions
chicken, cut as for sauté (page 343)	1¼–1½ kg
salt	1 tsp
lemon, juice of	1
plain yoghurt	300 ml
small onion, chopped	1
clove garlic, peeled	1
ginger, piece of, peeled and quartered	5 cm
fresh hot green chilli, sliced	½
garam masala	2 tsp
ground cumin	1 tsp
few drops each red and yellow colouring	

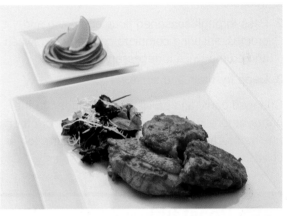

Chef's tip
If cooking in a tandoori oven, make sure the chicken is secure on the skewer, so that it cannot slip off during cooking.

1 Cut slits bone-deep in the chicken pieces.

2 Sprinkle the salt and lemon juice on both sides of the pieces, lightly rubbing into the slits; leave for 20 minutes.

3 Combine the remaining ingredients in a blender or food processor.

4 Brush the chicken pieces on both sides, ensuring the marinade goes into the slits. Cover and refrigerate for 6–24 hours.

5 Preheat the oven to the maximum temperature.

6 Shake off as much of the marinade as possible from the chicken pieces; place on skewers and bake for 15–20 minutes or until cooked.

7 Serve with red onion rings and lime or lemon wedges.

 HEALTHY EATING TIP

- Skin the chicken and reduce the salt by half.

- Serve with rice and vegetables.

* Estimated edible meat used; vegetable oil used

13 Chicken Kiev (traditional)

	4 portions	10 portions
suprêmes of chicken	4 x 150 g	10 x 150 g
butter	100 g	250 g
seasoned flour	25 g	65 g
eggs	2	5
breadcrumbs	100 g	250 g

1 Make an incision along the thick sides of the suprêmes. Insert 25 g cold butter into each. Season.

2 Pass through seasoned flour, egg wash and crumbs, ensuring complete coverage. Eggwash and crumb twice if necessary.

3 Deep fry, drain and serve.

Chopped garlic and parsley can be added to the butter before insertion to add a variation, or other fine herbs can be used – for example, tarragon or chives.

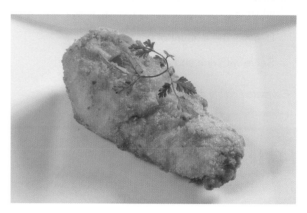

Chef's tip

The butter must be pushed well into the suprême, and the incision must be sealed, or the butter will leak out during cooking.

14 Roast turkey (*dinde rôti*)

cal	kcal	fat	sat fat	carb	sugar	protein	fibre
836 KJ	200 kcal	11.75 g	4.0 g	0.0 g	0.0 g	29.0 g	0.0 g

	4 portions	10 portions
Chestnut stuffing		
chestnuts	200 g	500 g
sausage meat	600 g	1 ½ kg
chopped onion	50 g	125 g
Parsley and thyme stuffing		
chopped onion	50 g	125 g
oil, butter or margarine	100 g	250 g
salt, pepper		
breadcrumbs (white or wholemeal)	100 g	250 g
pinch powdered thyme		
pinch chopped parsley		
turkey liver (raw), chopped		
turkey	5 kg	12 kg
fat bacon	100 g	250 g

brown stock	375 ml	1 litre
bread sauce, to serve		

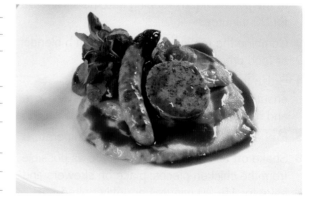

1 Slit the chestnuts on both sides using a small knife.

2   Boil the chestnuts in water for 5–10 minutes.

3   Drain and remove the outer and inner skins while warm.

4   Cook the chestnuts in a little stock for 5 minutes.

5   When cold, dice and mix into the sausage meat and cooked onion.

6   For the parsley and thyme stuffing, cook the onion in oil, butter or margarine without colour.

7   Remove from the heat, and add the seasoning, crumbs and herbs.

8   Mix in the raw chopped liver (optional) from the bird.

9   Truss the bird firmly (removing the wishbone first).

10 Season with salt and pepper.

11 Cover the breast with fat bacon.

12 Place the bird in a roasting tray on its side and coat with 200 g dripping or oil.

13 Roast in a moderate oven at 180–185°C.

14 Allow to cook on both legs; complete the cooking with the breast upright for the last 30 minutes.

15 Baste frequently and allow 15–20 minutes per ½ kg. If using a temperature probe, insert in the thickest part of the leg for a reading of 77°C.

16 Bake the two stuffings separately in greased trays until well cooked.

17 Prepare the gravy from the sediment and the brown stock. Correct the seasoning and remove the fat.

18 Remove the string and serve with the stuffings, roast gravy, bread sauce and/or hot cranberry sauce.

19 The turkey may be garnished with chipolata sausages and bacon rolls.

Chef's tips

Arrange the turkey to cook sitting on one leg, then the other leg and then with the breast upright, so that the whole bird cooks evenly. When the turkey is cooked, to facilitate carving, remove and de-bone the legs. For ease of carving, before cooking turkeys may be completely boned and the tough sinew removed from each leg. The breasts and the legs can both be stuffed, rolled and tied prior to roasting. (For safety reasons, it is not a good idea to stuff a whole bird for roasting.)

* No accompaniments, 200 g raw with skin and bone. With stuffing, roast gravy and bread sauce, 1 portion (200 g raw, with skin and bone) provides: 1589 kJ/380 kcal Energy; 24.0 g Fat; 8.4 g Sat Fat; 8.6 g Carb; 1.6 g Sugar; 34.0 g Protein; 0.9 g Fibre

15 Turkey escalopes

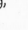

1   100 g slices cut from boned out turkey breast can be: lightly floured and gently cooked on both sides in butter, oil or margarine with a minimum of colour; or floured, egged and crumbed, and shallow-fried.

2   Serve with a suitable sauce and/or garnish (e.g. pan-fried turkey escalope cooked with oyster mushrooms and finished with white wine and cream).

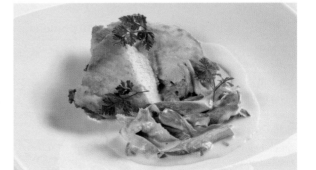

Chef's tip

The oil or fat must be hot enough before the escalopes are placed in the pan. If it is too cool, the breadcrumbs will absorb the fat and the dish will be greasy.

---

16 Suprêmes of guineafowl with a pepper and basil coulis

cal	kcal	fat	sat fat	carb	sugar	protein	fibre	
904 KJ	216 kcal	4.7 g	1.3 g	7.8 g	7.3 g	35.8 g	0.5 g	*

	4 portions	10 portions
red peppers	3	7
olive oil	150 ml	375 ml
fresh basil, chopped	2 tbsp	5 tbsp
salt, pepper		
guineafowl suprêmes (approx. 150 g each)	4	10

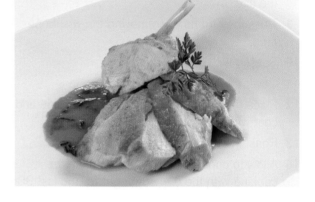

1 Skin the peppers by brushing with oil and gently scorching in the oven or under the grill. Alternatively, use a blowtorch with great care. Once scorched, peel the skin from the peppers, cut in half and deseed.

2 Place the skinned and deseeded peppers in a food processor, blend with the olive oil and pass through a strainer.

3 Add the chopped basil and season.

4 Season the guineafowl and either shallow-fry or grill.

5 Pour the coulis on to individual plates. Place the guineafowl on top and serve immediately.

Using chicken instead of guineafowl

---

17 Confit duck leg with red cabbage and green beans

	4 portions	10 portions
confit oil*	1 litre	2½ litres
garlic cloves	4	10
bay leaf	1	3
sprig of thyme	1	2
duck legs	4 × 200 g	10 × 200 g
butter	50 g	125 g
green beans, cooked and trimmed	300 g	750 g
braised red cabbage	250 g	625 g
seasoning		

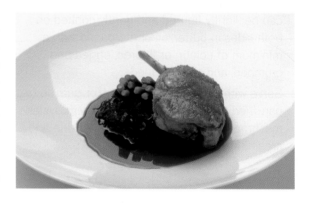

* Confit oil is 50/50 olive oil and vegetable oil, infused with herbs, garlic, whole spice or any specific flavour you wish to impart into the oil; then, through slow cooking in the oil, the foodstuff picks up the flavour.

1 Gently heat the confit oil, add the garlic, bay leaf and thyme.

2 Put the duck legs in the oil and place on a medium to low heat, ensuring the legs are covered.

3 Cook gently for 4–4½ hours (if using goose, 5–6½ hours may be needed).

4 To test if the legs are cooked, squeeze the flesh on the thigh bone and it should just fall away.

5 When cooked, remove the legs carefully and place on a draining tray.

6 When drained, put the confit leg on a baking tray and place in a pre-heated oven at 210°C; remove when the skin is golden brown (approx.

9–10 minutes), taking care as the meat is delicate.

7 Heat the butter in a medium sauté pan and reheat the green beans.

8 Place the braised cabbage in a small pan and reheat slowly.

9 Place the duck leg in a serving dish or plate along with the red cabbage and green beans.

> Confit duck legs can be prepared up to three or four days in advance. Remove them carefully from the fat they are stored in, clean off any excess fat and place directly into the oven. This is a great time-saver in a busy service.

Chef's tip
Control the temperature carefully as the duck legs cook, to obtain the right texture and flavour.

---

18 Duckling with orange sauce (*caneton bigarade*)

cal	kcal	fat	sat fat	carb	sugar	protein	fibre
3125 KJ	744 kcal	60.1 g	17.1 g	11.8 g	9.3 g	39.9 g	0.1 g

*

	4 portions	10 portions
duckling, 2 kg	1	2–3
butter	50 g	125 g
carrots	50 g	125 g
onions	50 g	125 g
celery	25 g	60 g
bay leaf	1	2–3
small sprig thyme	1	2–3
salt, pepper		
brown stock	250 ml	625 ml
arrowroot	10 g	25 g
oranges	2	5
lemon	1	2
vinegar	2 tbsp	5 tbsp
sugar	25 g	60 g

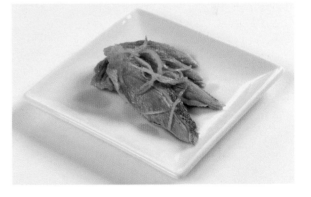

1 Clean and truss the duck. Use a fifth of the butter to grease a deep pan. Add the mirepoix (vegetables and herbs).

2 Season the duck. Place the duck on the mirepoix.

3 Coat the duck with the remaining butter.

4 Cover the pan with a tight-fitting lid.

5 Place the pan in the oven at 200–230°C.

6 Baste occasionally; cook for approximately 1 hour.

7 Remove the lid and continue cooking the duck, basting frequently until tender (about a further 30 minutes).

8 Remove the duck, cut out the string and keep the duck in a warm place. Drain off all the fat from the pan.

9 Deglaze with the stock, bring to the boil and allow to simmer for a few minutes.

10 Thicken by adding the arrowroot diluted in a little cold water.

11 Reboil, correct the seasoning, degrease and pass through a fine strainer.

12 Thinly remove the zest from half the oranges and the lemon(s), and cut into fine julienne.

13 Blanch the julienne of zest for 3–4 minutes, then refresh.

14 Place the vinegar and sugar in a small sauteuse and cook to a light caramel stage.

15 Add the juice of the oranges and lemon(s).

16 Add the sauce and bring to the boil.

17 Correct the seasoning and pass through a fine strainer.

18 Add the julienne to the sauce; keep warm.

19 Remove the legs from the duck, bone out and cut into thin slices.

20 Carve the duck breasts into thin slices and dress neatly.

21 Coat with the sauce and serve.

An alternative method of service is to cut the duck into eight pieces, which may then be either left on the bone or the bones removed.

Chef's tip

Baste the duck during cooking; the butter will give it flavour.

HEALTHY EATING TIP

- Use the minimum amount of salt to season the duck and the final sauce.

- Take care to remove all the fat from the roasting tray before deglazing with the stock.

- Reduce the fat by removing the skin from the duck, and 'balance' this fatty dish with a large portion of boiled potatoes and vegetables.

*Using butter

19 Roast duck or duckling *(canard ou caneton rôti)*

cal	kcal	fat	sat fat	carb	sugar	protein	fibre
3083 KJ	734 kcal	60.5 g	16.9 g	8.2 g	7.8 g	40.0 g	1.4 g

*

	4 portions	10 portions
duck	1	2–3
salt		
oil		
brown stock	¼ litre	600 ml
salt, pepper		
bunch watercress	1	2
apple sauce (page 217)	125 ml	300 ml

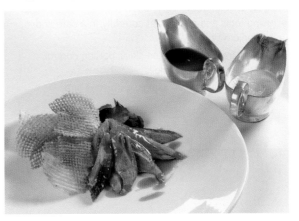

1 Lightly season the duck inside and out with salt.

2 Truss and brush lightly with oil.

3 Place on its side in a roasting tin, with a few drops of water.

4 Place in a hot oven for 20–25 minutes.

5 Turn on to the other side.

6 Cook for a further 20–25 minutes. Baste frequently.

7 To test if cooked, pierce with a fork between the drumstick and thigh and hold over a plate. The juice issuing from the duck should not show any signs of blood. If using a probe, the temperature should be 62°C. If the duck is required pink, the temperature should be 57°C.

8 Prepare the roast gravy with the stock and the sediment in the roasting tray. Correct the seasoning, remove the surface fat.

9 Serve garnished with picked watercress.

10 Accompany with a sauceboat of hot apple sauce, a sauceboat of gravy, and game chips. Also serve a sauceboat of sage and onion dressing as described on page 327.

Preparing a duck
http://bit.ly/z2rBxZ

* With apple sauce and watercress

Chef's tips

Arrange the duck to cook sitting on one leg, then the other leg and then with the breast upright, so that the whole bird cooks evenly.

The temperatures in this recipe reflect industry standards for cooking duck. An environmental health officer may advise higher temperatures of 75–80°C. You must use these higher temperatures if cooking for someone in a high-risk group (see Chapter 2).

12 Prepare and cook fish and shellfish

In this chapter, you will learn how to:

1. prepare and cook fish and shellfish, including:

- using tools and equipment correctly, in a safe and hygienic way
- demonstrating preparation skills, portion control, cooking and finishing skills
- producing sauces, dressings, garnishes and accompaniments

2. you should have the knowledge to:

- identify different types of fish and shellfish, their quality points, weights and commonly used cuts
- store fish and shellfish safely
- describe the preservation methods used for fish and shellfish
- apply cooking principles and suitable methods of cookery
- determine when fish and shellfish are cooked and check the finished dish.

Number	Recipe title	Page number
Fish		
19	Baked cod with a herb crust	393
5	Fillets of fish Véronique (*filets de poisson Véronique*)	383
6	Fillets of fish with white wine sauce (*filets de poisson vin blanc*)	384
	Fish *belle meunière*	383
	Fish *bonne-femme*	384
	Fish Bretonne	383
	Fish *bréval*	384
	Fish Doria	383
	Fish Grenobloise	383
25	Fish kebabs	397
26	Fish kedgeree (*cadgery de poisson*)	398
4	Fish meunière	382
27	Fish pie	398
1	Fried egg and breadcrumbed fish	381
9	Fried fish in batter	386
2	Fried sole (*sole frite*)	381

3	Goujons of fish	381
15	Griddled monkfish with leeks and Parmesan	390
8	Grilled fish fillets (sole, plaice, haddock)	385
16	Grilled round fish	390
22	Grilled salmon, pea soup and quails' eggs	395
17	Grilled swordfish and somen noodle salad with cilantro vinaigrette	391
30	Haddock and smoked salmon terrine	400
12	Nage of red mullet with baby leeks	388
11	Pan-fried fillets of sea bass with rosemary mash and mushrooms	387
21	Poached salmon	394
13	Poached smoked haddock	389
20	Red mullet ceviche with organic leaves	393
18	Roast fillet of sea bass with vanilla and fennel	392
23	Sardines with tapenade	396
7	Skate with black butter (*raie au beurre noir*)	385
28	Smoked mackerel mousse	399

29	Soused herring or mackerel	400
14	Steamed fish with garlic, spring onions and ginger	389
10	Whitebait (*blanchailles*)	386
24	Whole trout baked in salt	396
Shellfish		
35	Crab cakes with rocket salad and lemon dressing	405
37	Lobster thermidor (*homard thermidor*)	407
36	Mussels gratin with white wine sauce	406
33	Oyster tempura	403

32	Oysters in their own shells	402
34	Poached langoustines with aioli dip	404
38	Scallop ceviche with organic leaves	408
31	Scallops with caramelised cauliflower	401
Other seafood		
39	*Kalamarakia yemista* (stuffed squid)	409
41	Seafood in puff pastry (*bouchées de fruits de mer*)	410
40	Seafood stir-fry	411

Fish

Origins

Fish are vertebrates (animals with a backbone) and are split into two main groups: flat and round. From this they can be split again, into subgroups or secondary groups such as pelagic (oil-rich fish that swim mid-water, such as mackerel and herring) and demersal (white fish that live at or near the bottom of the sea, such as cod, haddock, whiting and plaice).

Marine and freshwater fish were a crucial part of man's diet long before prehistoric societies learnt how to cultivate vegetables and domesticate livestock. Fish provided essential proteins and vitamins; they were easy to catch and eat, and predominantly eaten raw.

There are more than 20,000 species of fish in the seas of the world, yet we use only a fraction of the resources available. Undoubtedly certain types are neither edible nor ethical – however, the European market has a dozen types of fish that make up a large percentage of our consumption. The Japanese and, closer to home, the Portuguese are the exceptions to the rule when it comes to using a high proportion of fish species.

Ethical: In keeping with generally accepted rules of right and wrong. Using certain types of fish might be considered wrong or not ethical (unethical) if, for example, there was a danger that it could kill off the species, or very greatly reduce its numbers.

Because of health considerations many people choose to eat fish in preference to meat, and

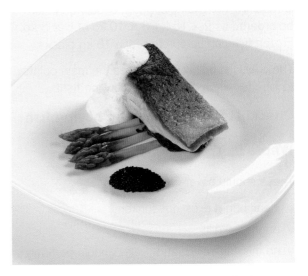

Fish dishes, like the crispy seared salmon shown here, are very popular (recipe available on Dynamic Learning)

consequently consumption of fish is steadily increasing. This popularity has resulted in a far greater selection becoming available and, due to swift and efficient transport, well over 200 types of fish are on sale throughout the year. However, it has also led to overfishing, causing a steep decline in the stocks of some species. Because of this, it is now necessary to have fish farms (such as those for trout and salmon, turbot, bass and cod) to supplement natural sources.

Although fish is plentiful in the UK because we are surrounded by water, the overfishing and pollution are affecting supplies of certain fish. Most catches are made off Iceland or Scotland, in the North Sea, Irish Sea and the English Channel. Salmon are caught in certain English and Scottish rivers, and are also extensively farmed. Frozen fish is imported from Scandinavia, Canada, Japan and other countries worldwide; Canada and Japan both export frozen salmon to Britain.

Choosing and buying fish

As already mentioned, fish can be oily or white:

- **Oily fish** are round in shape (e.g. herring, mackerel, salmon, tuna, sardines).
- **White fish** are round (e.g. cod, whiting, hake) or flat (e.g. plaice, sole, turbot).

Fresh fish is bought by the kilogram, by the number of fillets or whole fish of the weight that is required. For example, 30 kg of salmon could be ordered as 2 × 15 kg, 3 × 10 kg or 6 × 5 kg. Frozen fish can be purchased in 15 kg blocks.

The checklist below summarises the main points to look for when choosing and buying fish.

Checklist for choosing and buying fish

Whole fish

These should have:

- clear, bright eyes, not sunken
- bright red gills
- no missing scales and scales should be firmly attached to the skin

- moist skin (fresh fish feels slightly slippery)
- shiny skin with bright natural colouring
- a stiff tail firm flesh
- a fresh sea smell and no trace of ammonia.

Fillets

These should be:

- neat and trim with firm flesh
- firm and closely packed together, not ragged or gaping
- a translucent white colour if they are from a white fish, with no discoloration.

Smoked fish

These should have:

- a bright, glossy surface
- firm flesh (sticky or soggy flesh means the fish may have been poor quality or undersmoked)
- a pleasant, smoky smell.

Frozen fish

This should:

- be frozen hard with no signs of thawing
- be in packaging that is not damaged
- show no evidence of freezer burn (i.e. dull, white, dry patches).

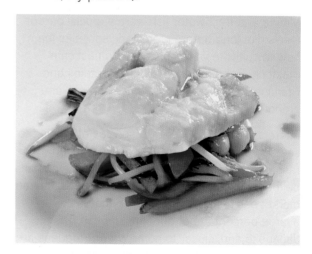

When cod is cooked, it takes on an opaque white colour, as in this baked dish (recipe available on Dynamic Learning)

Cooking

Fish is very economical to prepare as it cooks quickly and so can save fuel. When cooked, fish loses its translucent look and in most cases takes on an opaque white colour. It will also flake easily and should be considered as a delicate product after preparation.

Fish easily becomes dry and loses its flavour if overcooked, so it is important to consider methods of cookery carefully. Overcooked and dry fish will be far less enjoyable to eat than fish that is cooked well.

Storage

Spoilage is mainly caused by the actions of enzymes and bacteria. There are enzymes in the gut of the living fish that help convert its food to tissue and energy. When the fish dies, these enzymes carry on working and help the bacteria in the digestive system to penetrate the belly wall and start breaking down the flesh itself. Bacteria also exist on the skin and in the fish intestine. While the fish is alive, the normal defence mechanisms of the body prevent the bacteria from invading the flesh. Once the fish dies, however, the bacteria invade the flesh and start to break it down – the higher the temperature the faster the deterioration. Although these bacteria are harmless to humans, they reduce the eating quality of the fish and quickly make it smell bad. In order to avoid a deterioration in the quality of the fish it should be stored correctly.

Fish, once caught, has a shelf life of 10 to 12 days if kept properly in a refrigerator at a temperature of between 0°C and 5°C. If the fish is delivered whole with the innards still in the fish, then it should be gutted and the cavity washed well before it is stored.

Fresh fish should be used as soon as possible, but it can be stored overnight. Rinse, pat dry, cover with clingfilm and store towards the bottom of the refrigerator.

Ready-to-eat cooked fish, such as 'hot' smoked mackerel, prawns and crab, should be stored on shelves above other raw foodstuffs to avoid cross-contamination.

Food value

Fish is as useful a source of animal protein as meat. The oily fish (sardines, mackerel, herring, salmon, sardines) contain fat-soluble vitamins (A and D) in their flesh and omega-3 fatty acids (these are unsaturated fatty acids that are essential for good health). It is recommended that we eat more oily fish.

The flesh of white fish does not contain any fat. Vitamins A and D are only present in the liver (e.g. cod liver or halibut liver oil).

The small bones in sardines, whitebait and tinned salmon provide the human body with calcium and phosphorus.

Owing to its fat content, oily fish is not so digestible as white fish and is not suitable to use in cooking for people who are ill.

Preservation

Freezing

Fish is either frozen at sea or as soon as possible after reaching port. It should be thawed out before being cooked. Plaice, halibut, turbot, haddock, sole, cod, trout, salmon, herring, whiting, scampi, smoked haddock and kippers are available frozen.

Frozen fish should be checked for:

- no evidence of freezer burn
- undamaged packaging
- minimum fluid loss during thawing
- flesh that is still firm after thawing.

Frozen fish should be stored at −18°C to −20°C and thawed out overnight in a refrigerator. It should *not* be thawed out in water as this spoils the taste and texture of the fish, and valuable water-soluble nutrients are lost. Fish should not be re-frozen as this will impair its taste and texture.

Fish should be frozen as quickly as possible. The longer it takes to freeze, the larger and more angular the ice crystals become, and they invariably sever the protein strands, allowing the liquid contained in them to flow out once it has been defrosted, leaving you with an inferior product. If, however, you freeze the fish quickly, the ice crystals that form are small (remember: quick = small), so cause less damage. There will always be some loss of liquid, but if the fish is frozen quickly the loss will be less dramatic.

Canning

Oily fish are usually canned. Sardines, salmon, anchovies, pilchards, tuna, herring and herring roe (unfertilised eggs) are canned either in their own juice (as with salmon), or in oil or tomato sauce.

Salting

- In the UK, the salting of fish is usually accompanied by a smoking process (see below).
- Cured herrings are packed in salt.
- Caviar – the roe (unfertilised eggs) of the sturgeon – is slightly salted then sieved, tinned and refrigerated. Imitation caviar is also obtainable.

Pickling and smoking

Herrings pickled in vinegar are filleted, rolled and skewered, and known as rollmops.

Fish that is to be smoked may be gutted or left whole. It is then soaked in a strong salt solution (brine) and in some cases a dye is added to improve colour. After this, it is drained, hung on racks in a kiln and exposed to smoke for five or six hours.

Cold smoking takes place at no more than 33°C, to avoid cooking the flesh. Therefore, all cold-smoked fish is raw and is usually cooked before being eaten, except smoked salmon.

Hot-smoked fish is cured between 70°C and 80°C in order to cook the flesh at the same time, so does not require further cooking.

Note

There is a high salt content in salted, pickled and smoked fish. There is no need to add extra salt.

Smoked fish should be wrapped up well and kept separate from other fish to prevent the smell and dye penetrating other foods.

Cooking methods

The following are the main methods used for cooking fish.

En sous vide

This is a well-matched method of cookery for fish, as it helps to reduce the moisture loss and also isolates the fish, preventing it from absorbing outside flavours or liquids, thus offering a truer taste. The dish *escabeche* (cured fish) benefits very well from this method as it helps with the marinating process and distributes the liquor evenly around the fish.

Frying

Frying is probably the most popular method of cooking fish. Described below are the three main types of frying.

Shallow frying (recipes 2, 4 and 11)

The fish should be seasoned and lightly coated with flour or crumb before frying, in order to protect it and seal in the flavour. Use a mixture of oil and butter when frying, and turn the fish only once during cooking, to avoid it breaking up.

This method is suitable for small whole fish, cuts or fillets that are cooked in oil or fat in a frying pan. The fish are usually coated with flour but semolina, matzo meal, oatmeal or breadcrumbs may also be used. If the frying medium is to be butter, it must be clarified, otherwise there is a risk that the fish may burn. Oil is the best medium, to which a little butter may be added for flavour.

Deep frying (recipes 1, 3, 9 and 10)

Deep frying fish
http://bit.ly/wSSk0e

This method is suitable for small whole white fish, cuts and fillets. Any white fish are suitable for deep frying in batter, including cod, haddock, skate and rock salmon (a term used for catfish, coley, dog-fish and so on when cleaned and skinned). Depending on size, the fish may be left whole, or may be portioned or filleted.

The fish should be seasoned and coated before frying, usually with a batter or an egg and breadcrumb mixture. This forms a surface that prevents penetration of the cooking fat or oil into the fish. Coatings can be either:

- flour, egg and breadcrumbs
- milk and flour
- batter.

Use a suitable container and heat the oil to 190°C. Test the temperature before cooking the fish. Drain the fish on absorbent paper after cooking.

For further information, refer to the text on deep-frying in Chapter 7.

Stir-frying (recipe 40)

This is a very fast and popular method of cooking. Use a wok or deep frying pan and a high cooking temperature. Food should be cut into thin strips and prepared before cooking begins. This method is very well suited to cooking firm-fleshed fish.

It is suitable for fish fillets cut into finger-sized pieces which are quickly fried in hot oil. Finely cut ginger and vegetables (e.g. garlic, shallots, broccoli sprigs, mushrooms and beanshoots) may be added. Soy sauce is often used as a seasoning.

Grilling (recipes 8, 15–17, 22 and 23)

Grilling, or griddling, is cooking under radiant heat, and is a fast and convenient method suitable for fillets or small whole fish. When grilling whole fish, cut through the thickest part of the fish to allow even cooking. Lightly oil and season fish or fillets and, to avoid breaking, do not turn more than once.

Poaching (recipes 5, 6, 13 and 21)

Poaching is sometimes referred to as boiling, and is suitable for:

- whole fish (e.g. salmon, trout, bass) and
- certain cuts on the bone (e.g. salmon, turbot, brill, halibut, cod, skate).

In either case, the prepared fish should be completely immersed in the cooking liquid, which can be either water, water and milk, fish stock (for white fish), or a court bouillon (water, vinegar, onion, carrot, thyme, bay leaf, parsley stalks and peppercorns) for oily fish. Most kinds of fish can be cooked in this way and should be poached gently for 5–8 minutes, depending on the thickness of the fish. Whole fish are covered with a cold liquid and brought to the boil then simmered *gently*. Cut fish are usually placed in a *gently* simmering liquid to cook. The resulting liquid is ideal for use in sauces and soups (unless it is from smoked fish).

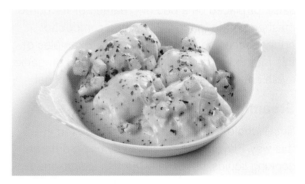

Poached fish served with a sauce (fillet of fish Dugléré – recipe available on Dynamic Learning)

When poaching smoked fish, place in cold, unsalted water and bring to a steady simmer. This liquid will be salty and may not be suitable for reuse.

Roasting (recipe 18)

Roasting is a term commonly used nowadays and, particularly when describing a method of cookery on a menu, it is used quite loosely. It is not impossible to roast fish, but a fishbone trivet should be used, primarily to prevent the fish frying in the oil or cooking medium, and also to impart more flavour to the fish while cooking.

This method of cookery, when used with fish, should be quick and used only with thick cuts of fish such as cod, salmon, turbot, sea bass and monkfish. Depending on size, the fish may be roasted whole (e.g. sea bass). However, fish is more usually portioned, with the skin left on, and lightly seared in hot oil, skin side down in a pan, then roasted in a hot oven (230°C) skin side up. Finely sliced vegetables and sprigs of herbs can be added to the roasting tray and, when the fish is cooked and removed, the tray can be deglazed with a suitable wine (usually a dry white) and fish stock to form the basis of an accompanying sauce.

If the fish is skinned after it has been seared, it can be coated in a light crust of breadcrumbs mixed with a good oil, butter or margarine, lemon juice, fresh chopped herbs (e.g. parsley, tarragon, chervil, rosemary), a duxelle-based mixture or a light coating of creamed horseradish.

The fish portions may be served with a sauce or salsa, or placed on a bed of creamed or flavoured mashed potato (page 224) with a compound butter sauce and quarters of lemon. Examples of this method of cooking include roast cod on garlic mash and roast sea bass flavoured with fennel.

Steaming (recipe 14)

Small whole fish or fillets are good cooked in this way. Flavour can be added by using different cooking liquids, but usually the fish is seasoned. Place it in a steamer, cover it tightly and cook over simmering water for 10–15 minutes, depending on the thickness of the fish or the fillets. If a steamer is not available, fish can be steamed between two plates above a pan of boiling water.

Fish is prepared as for poaching. Any fish that can be poached or boiled may also be cooked by steaming. This method has a number of advantages.

- It is an easy method of cooking.
- Because it is quick, it conserves flavour, colour and nutrients.
- It is suitable for large-scale cookery.

The liquor from the steamed fish should be strained off, reduced and incorporated into the sauce. Preparation can also include adding finely cut ingredients (e.g. ginger, spring onions, garlic, mushrooms and soft herbs), lemon juice and dry white wine, either to the fish on the steamer dish before cooking or when the fish is served.

Baking (recipes 19 and 24)

Many fish (whole, portioned or filleted) may be oven-baked. To retain their natural moisture it is necessary to protect the fish from direct heat. There are various ways of preparing fish for baking:

- whole fish (scaled, gutted and washed)
- whole fish stuffed, e.g. a duxelle-based mixture, breadcrumbs, herbs
- wrapped in pastry (puff or filo)
- completely covered with a thick coating of dampened sea salt
- portions of fish (e.g. cod, hake, haddock).

Then proceed as follows.

- Depending on the size and shape of the fish, 100–150 g thick portions can be cut, leaving the skin on (this helps to retain the natural moisture of the fish).
- Place the prepared portions in a greased ovenproof dish, brush with oil and bake slowly, skin side up, basting frequently.
- Add herbs (e.g. parsley, rosemary, thyme) and finely sliced vegetables (e.g. mushrooms, onions, shallots).
- The fish can then be simply served, e.g. on a bed of creamy or flavoured mashed potato (page 224) with a suitable sauce, such as compound butter (page 202) or a salsa (page 194).

Health, safety and hygiene

For information on maintaining a safe and secure working environment, a professional and hygienic appearance, clean food production areas, equipment and utensils, and food hygiene, please refer to Chapters 2 and 3. Additional food safety points relating to fish preparation and cookery are as follows.

- Store fresh fish in containers with ice (changed daily) in a refrigerator at a temperature of 1–2°C.
- To avoid the risk of cross-contamination, fish should be stored in a separate refrigerator away from other foods; cooked and raw fish must be kept separate.
- Frozen fish should be stored in a deep-freezer at −18°C. When required, frozen fish should be defrosted in a refrigerator. If the frozen food is

removed from the freezer and left uncovered in the kitchen, there is a danger of contamination.

- Smoked fish should be kept in a refrigerator.
- Use the correct colour-coded boards for preparing raw fish, and different ones for cooked fish. Keep the boards clean using fresh disposable wiping cloths.
- Use equipment reserved for raw fish. If this is not possible, wash and sanitise equipment before and immediately after each use.
- Unhygienic equipment, utensils and preparation areas increase the risk of cross-contamination and danger to health.
- Fish offal and bones present a high risk of contamination and must not be mixed or stored with raw prepared fish.
- Wash equipment, knives and hands regularly using a bactericide detergent, or sanitising agent, to kill germs.
- Dispose of all wiping cloths immediately after use. Reused cloths may cause contamination.

Basic fish preparation

Unless otherwise stated, as a guide allow 100 g fish off the bone and 150 g on the bone for a portion.

- All fish should be washed under running cold water before and after preparation.
- Whole fish are trimmed to remove the scales, fins and head using fish scissors and a knife. If the head is to be left on (as in the case of a salmon for the cold buffet), the gills and the eyes are removed.

Gutting and scaling

If the fish has to be gutted, the following procedure should be used.

- Cut from the vent (hole) to two-thirds along the fish.
- Draw out the intestines with the fingers or, in the case of a large fish, use the hook handle of a utensil such as a ladle.
- Ensure that the blood lying along the main bone is removed, then wash and drain thoroughly.

- If the fish is to be stuffed then it may be gutted by removing the innards through the gill slits, thus leaving the stomach skin intact, forming a pouch in which to put the stuffing. When this method is used, care must be taken to ensure that the inside of the fish is clear of all traces of blood.

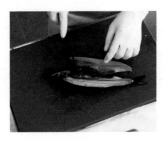

Gutting a red mullet

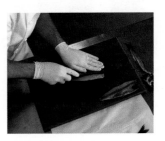

Cleaning the blood line after gutting

Skinning and filleting
Filleting round fish

- Remove the head and clean thoroughly.
- Remove the first fillet by cutting along the backbone from head to tail.
- Keeping the knife close to the bone, remove the fillet.
- Reverse the fish and remove the second fillet in the same way, this time cutting from tail to head.

Filleting a round fish
http://bit.ly/wNRqo6

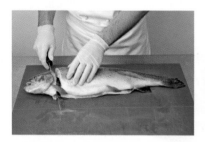

(1) To fillet a trout, first cut off the head

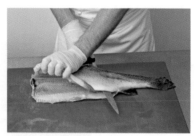

(2) Cut down the back

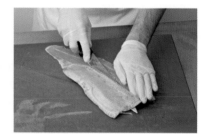

(3) Cut into the flesh to remove the ribcage

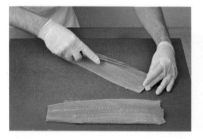

(4) Trim the fillets

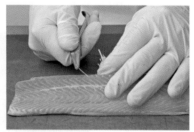

(5) Pin bone each fillet

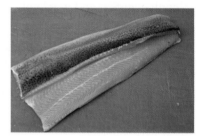

Fillets ready for use

Filleting flat fish, with the exception of Dover sole

- Using a filleting knife, make an incision from the head to tail down the line of the backbone.
- Remove each fillet, holding the knife almost parallel to the work surface and keeping the knife close to the bone.

Skinning flat fish fillets, with the exception of Dover sole

- Hold the fillet firmly at the tail end.
- Cut the flesh as close to the tail as possible, as far as the skin.
- Keep the knife parallel to the work surface, grip the skin firmly and move the knife from side to side to remove the skin.

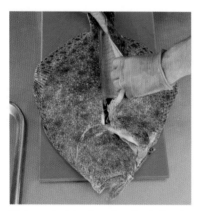

Make an incision from head to tail and remove the first fillet

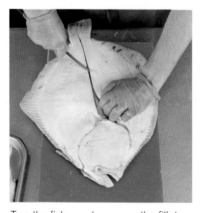

Turn the fish over to remove the fillets from the underside

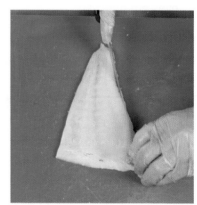

Trim the fillets

Preparation of whole Dover sole

- Hold the tail firmly, then cut and scrape the skin until you have lifted enough to grip.
- Pull the skin away from the tail to the head.

- Both black and white skins may be removed in this way.
- Trim the tail and side fins with fish scissors, remove the eyes, and clean and wash the fish thoroughly.

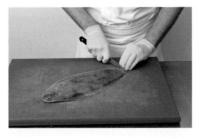

To remove the skin from a whole Dover sole, first score the skin just above the tail

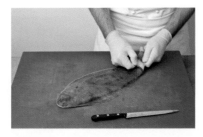

Lift the edge of the skin

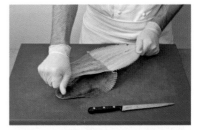

Pull back the skin, holding the fish firmly

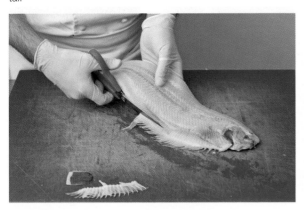

Trim the fish before use

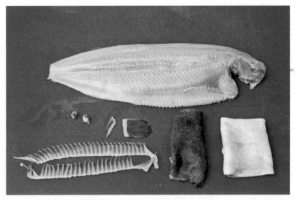

Whole Dover sole, ready for use, with all the parts that have been removed

Preparation of turbot

- Remove the head with a large chopping knife.
- Cut off the side bones.
- Commencing at the tail end, chop down the centre of the backbone, dividing the fish into two halves.
- Divide each half into steak portions (tronçons) as required.

Commencing: Starting or beginning.

Cutting a fillet of salmon into suprêmes
http://bit.ly/wt3MOt

> **Note**
>
> Allow approximately 300 g per portion on the bone. A 3½ kg fish will yield approximately 10 portions.

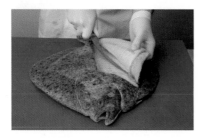

Filleting turbot

Cuts of fish

Steaks:

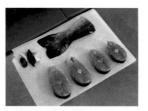

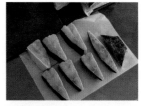

- These are thick slices of fish on or off the bone.
- Steaks of round fish (salmon, cod) may be called darnes.
- Steaks of flat fish on the bone (turbot, halibut) may be called tronçons.

Darne of salmon   Tronçons of white fish

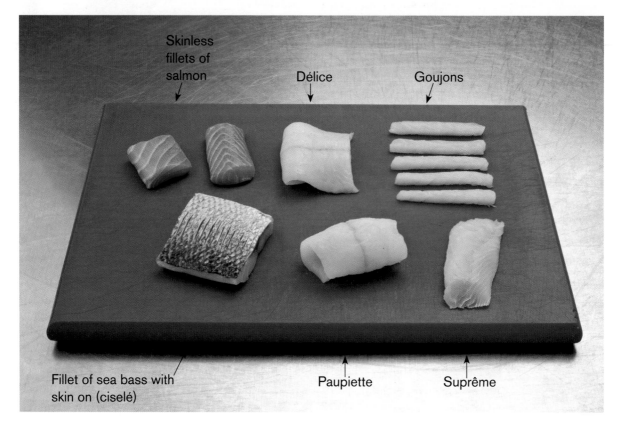

Cuts of fish

Fillets are cuts that do not contain any bones. A round fish yields two fillets, a flat fish four fillets.

Suprêmes are prime cuts without bone or skin (pieces cut from fillets of salmon, turbot, brill, etc.).

Goujons are made up of filleted fish cut into strips approximately 8 × 0.5 cm.

Cutting a fillet of fish into goujons
http://bit.ly/yoWESI

Paupiettes are fillets of fish (e.g. sole, plaice, whiting) spread with a stuffing and rolled.

Plaited fish is also known as *en tresse* – for example, sole fillets cut into three even pieces lengthwise to within 1 cm of the top, and neatly plaited.

Fish types

Table 12.1 gives examples of the 200-plus fish types that are available.

Table 12.1 Examples of fish types available, and suitable cooking methods (O = oily, W = white)

		Baking	Boiling	Deep frying	Grilling	Poaching	Roasting	Shallow (pan) frying	Steaming	Stir-frying
Barracuda	O				✓			✓		
Cod	W	✓	✓	✓	✓	✓	✓	✓	✓	
Coley	W		✓	✓	✓			✓		
Dorade (red sea bream)	O	✓			✓			✓		✓
Dover Sole	W			✓	✓	✓		✓		
Emperor bream	O	✓			✓			✓		
Grouper	W				✓		✓	✓		
Haddock	W	✓		✓	✓	✓		✓		
Hake	W	✓			✓	✓		✓		
Halibut	W	✓			✓	✓	✓	✓	✓	✓
Herring	O				✓			✓		
Huss	W			✓	✓	✓		✓		
John Dory	W	✓				✓		✓		
Lemon sole	W	✓		✓	✓	✓		✓		
Mackerel	O	✓			✓	✓				
Marlin	O	✓			✓	✓		✓		
Monkfish	W	✓					✓	✓		✓

Plaice	W	✓		✓	✓			✓			
Red mullet	O	✓			✓		✓	✓			
Red snapper	O	✓			✓	✓		✓			
Salmon	O	✓	✓		✓	✓	✓	✓	✓		✓
Sardines	O				✓			✓			
Sea bass	W	✓			✓	✓		✓	✓		
Shark	W	✓			✓	✓	✓	✓	✓		✓
Skate wings	W		✓	✓		✓		✓			
Swordfish	W	✓			✓			✓			✓
Trout	O	✓			✓			✓			
Tuna	O				✓	✓		✓			✓
Turbot	W	✓	✓	✓	✓	✓	✓	✓			✓
Whitebait	O			✓							

Seasonality and availability of fish

Seasonality

The quality of fish can vary due to local climatic and environmental conditions. Generally, all fish spawn over a period of four to six weeks. During spawning, they use up a lot of their reserves of fat and protein in the production of eggs. This has the effect of making their flesh watery and soft. Fish in this condition are termed 'spent fish'. This takes anything between one and two months, depending on local environmental conditions.

Availability

See Table 12.2. Naturally, prevailing weather conditions have an enormous bearing on fishing activities. The full range of species may not always be available during stormy weather, for instance.

Spawn: When fish release or deposit their eggs (which are also called 'spawn').

Cooking fish

 To maintain the quality and food safety of fish and shellfish dishes it is advisable to check the internal temperature using a probe. It is recommended that all fish and shellfish should be cooked to an internal temperature of 62°C.

Note

Environmental Health Officers may require higher temperatures.

ACTIVITY

1 Name three examples of flat fish.

2 Name three examples of round fish.

3 List the quality points to be considered when purchasing fresh fish.

4 How should raw fresh fish be stored?

5 How much fish should be used for one portion?

Table 12.2 Seasonality of fish

	JAN	FEB	MAR	APR	MAY	JUN	JUL	AUG	SEP	OCT	NOV	DEC
Bream					*	*	*					
Brill			*	*	*							
Cod			*	*								
Eel												
Mullet (grey)			*	*								
Gurnard												
Haddock												
Hake			*	*	*							
Halibut				*	*							
Herring												
John Dory												
Mackerel												
Monkfish												
Plaice			*	*								
Red mullet												
Salmon (farmed)												
Salmon (wild)												
Sardines												
Sea bass				*	*							
Sea trout								*	*	*	*	
Skate												
Squid												
Sole (Dover)	*											
Sole (lemon)												
Trout												
Tuna												
Turbot				*	*	*						
Whiting												

Key:

Available	At best

* Spawning and roeing – this can deprive the flesh of nutrients and will decrease the yield.

Shellfish

Origins

Shellfish, such as lobsters and crabs, are all invertebrates (i.e. they do not possess an internal skeleton) and are split into two main groups: **molluscs** have either an external hinged double shell (e.g. scallops, mussels) or a single spiral shell (e.g. winkles, whelks), or have soft bodies with an internal shell (e.g. squid, octopus); **crustaceans** have tough outer shells that act like armour, and also have flexible joints to allow quick movement (e.g. crab, lobster).

Choosing and buying

Shellfish are prized for their tender, fine-textured flesh, which can be prepared in a variety of ways, but are prone to rapid spoilage. The reason for this is that they contain quantities of certain proteins, amino acids, which encourage bacterial growth.

To ensure freshness and best flavour it is preferable to choose live specimens and cook them yourself. This is often possible with the expansion of globalisation and air freight creating a healthy trade in live shellfish.

Bear in mind the following points when choosing shellfish:

- Shells should not be cracked or broken.
- The shells of mussels and oysters should be tightly shut; open shells that do not close when tapped sharply should be discarded.
- Lobsters, crabs and prawns should have a good colour and be heavy for their size.
- Lobsters and crabs should have all their limbs.

Cooking

The flesh of fish and shellfish is different from meat: the connective tissue is very fragile, the muscle fibres shorter and the fat content relatively low. Generally, care should be taken when cooking and shellfish should be cooked as

Table 12.3 Seasonality of shellfish

	JAN	FEB	MAR	APR	MAY	JUN	JUL	AUG	SEP	OCT	NOV	DEC
Crab (brown cock)	▓	▓	▓	▓								
Crab (spider)	▓	▓	▓	▓	▓	▓	▓	▓	▓	▓		
Crab (brown hen)	▓	▓						▓	▓	▓	▓	▓
Clams	▓	▓	▓	▓							▓	▓
Cockles	▓	▓	▓	▓	▓	▓	▓	▓	▓	▓	▓	▓
Crayfish (signal)					▓	▓	▓	▓	▓			
Lobster							▓	▓	▓	▓	▓	▓
Langoustines			▓	▓	▓							
Mussels	▓	▓	▓						▓	▓	▓	▓
Oysters (rock)	▓	▓	▓	▓					▓	▓	▓	▓
Oysters (native)	▓	▓							▓	▓	▓	▓
Prawns								▓	▓	▓	▓	
Scallops						▓	▓	▓	▓	▓	▓	▓

Key:

Available	At best

little as possible, to the point that the protein in the muscle groups just coagulates. Beyond this point the flesh tends to dry out, making it tougher and drier. Shellfish are known for their dramatic colour change, from blue/grey to a vibrant orange colour. This is because they contain red and yellow pigments called carotenoids, bound to molecules of protein. The protein bonds obscure the yellow/red pigment and, once heat is applied, the bonds are broken and the vibrant pigmentation is revealed.

Storage

All shellfish will start to spoil as soon as they have been removed from their natural environment, therefore, the longer shellfish are stored the more they will deteriorate due to the bacteria present (see the guidelines on choosing and buying, above). Best practice is to cook immediately and store in the same way as cooked fish. Shellfish can be blanched quickly to remove the shell and membrane (especially in lobsters), but they will still need to be stored as a raw product as they will require further cooking.

Bear in mind the following quality, purchasing and storage points:

- Whenever possible, all shellfish should be purchased live so as to ensure freshness.
- Shellfish should be kept in suitable containers, covered with damp seaweed or damp cloths, and stored in a cold room or refrigerator.
- Shellfish should be cooked as soon as possible after purchasing.

Shrimps and prawns

These are often bought cooked, either in the shells or peeled. Smell is the best guide to freshness. Shrimps and prawns can be used for garnishes, decorating fish dishes, cocktails, sauces, salads, hors d'oeuvres, omelettes, and snack and savoury dishes. They can also be used for a variety of hot dishes: stir-fries, risotto, curries, etc. Potted shrimps are also a popular dish. Freshly cooked prawns in their shells may also be served cold, accompanied by a mayonnaise-based sauce, such as garlic mayonnaise. **King prawns**

are a larger variety, which can also be used in any of the ways listed.

Raw and cooked shrimps and prawns are prepared by removing the head, carapace (upper shell), legs, tail section and the dark intestinal vein running down the back.

Scampi, crayfish, Dublin Bay prawns

Scampi, saltwater crayfish and Dublin Bay prawns are also known as Norway lobster or langoustine and are sold fresh, frozen, raw or cooked. Their tails are prepared like shrimps and they are used in a variety of ways: salads, rice dishes, stir-fries, deep-fried, poached and served with a number of different sauces. They are also used as garnishes to hot and cold fish dishes.

Freshwater crayfish are also known as *écrevisse*. These are small freshwater crustaceans with claws, found in lakes and lowland streams. They are prepared and cooked like shrimps and prawns, and used in many dishes, including soup. They are often used whole to garnish hot and cold fish dishes.

Lobster

Purchasing points

- Purchase alive, with both claws attached, to ensure freshness.
- Lobsters should be heavy in proportion to their size.
- The coral (the roe) of the hen (female) lobster is necessary to give the required colour for certain soups, sauces and lobster dishes.
- Hen lobsters are distinguished from cock lobsters by their broader tails.

Cooking lobster

- Wash then plunge them into a pan of boiling salted water containing 60 ml of vinegar to 1 litre of water.
- Cover with a lid, re-boil, then allow to simmer for 15–20 minutes according to size.
- Overcooking can cause the tail flesh to toughen and the claw meat to become hard and fibrous.

- Allow to cool in the cooking liquid when possible.

Cleaning cooked lobster

- Remove the claws and the pincers from the claws.
- Crack the claws and joints and remove the meat.
- Cut the lobster in half by inserting the point of a large knife 2 cm above the tail on the natural central line.
- Cut through the tail firmly.
- Turn the lobster around and cut through the upper shell (carapace).
- Remove the halves of the sac (which contains grit). This is situated at the top, near the head.
- Using a small knife, remove the intestinal tract from the tail and wash if necessary.

Uses

Lobsters are served cold in cocktails, lobster mayonnaise, hors d'oeuvres, salads, sandwiches and in halves on cold buffets. They are used hot in soups, sauces, rice dishes, stir-fry dishes and in numerous ways served in the half shell with various sauces. They are also used to garnish fish dishes.

Crawfish

These are sometimes referred to as 'spiny lobsters', but unlike lobsters they have no claws and their meat is solely in the tail. Crawfish vary considerably in size from 1 to 3 kg; they are cooked in the same way as lobsters, and the tail

meat can be used in any of the lobster recipes. Because of their impressive appearance, crawfish dressed whole are sometimes used on special cold buffets. They are very expensive and are also available frozen.

Crab

Purchasing points

- Buy alive to ensure freshness.
- Ensure that both claws are attached.
- Crabs should be heavy in relation to size.

Cooking

- Place the crabs in boiling salted water with a little vinegar added.
- Re-boil, then simmer for 15–30 minutes according to size. These times apply to crabs weighing from ½–2½ kg.
- Allow the crabs to cool in the cooking liquor.

Uses

Crab meat can be used cold for hors d'oeuvres, cocktails, salads, sandwiches and dressed crab. Used hot, it can be covered with a suitable sauce and served with rice, in bouchées or pancakes, or made into crab fish cakes.

Cockles

Cockles are enclosed in small, attractive, cream-coloured shells. As they live in sand it is essential to purge them by washing well under running cold water and leaving them in cold salted water

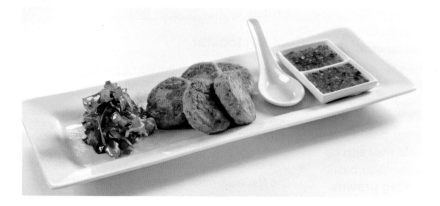

Crab cakes (recipe available on Dynamic Learning)

(changed frequently) until no traces of sand remain.

Cockles can be cooked either by steaming, boiling in unsalted water, on a preheated griddle, or as for any mussel recipe. They should be cooked only until the shells open.

They can be used in soups, sauces, salads, stir-fries and rice dishes, and as garnish for fish dishes.

Mussels

Mussels are extensively cultivated on wooden hurdles in the sea, producing tender, delicately flavoured plump flesh. They are produced in Britain and imported from France, Holland and Belgium. French mussels are small; Dutch and Belgian mussels are plumper. The quality tends to vary from season to season.

Purchasing points

- The shells must be tightly closed, indicating that the mussels are alive.
- They should be of a good size.
- There should not be an excessive number of barnacles attached.
- They should smell fresh.

Storage

Mussels should be kept in containers, covered with damp seaweed or cloths, and stored in a cold room or refrigerator.

Uses

Mussels can be used for soups, sauces and salads, and cooked in a wide variety of hot dishes.

Cooking

- Scrape the shells to remove any barnacles, etc. Wash well and drain in a colander.
- In a thick-bottomed pan with a tight-fitting lid, place 25 g chopped shallot or onion for each litre of mussels.
- Add the mussels, cover with a lid and cook on a fierce heat for 4–5 minutes until the shells open completely.

- Remove the mussels from the shells, checking carefully for sand, weed, etc.
- Retain the carefully strained liquid for the sauce.

Scallops

There are a number of varieties of scallop:

- great scallops are up to 15 cm in size
- bay scallops are up to 8 cm
- queen scallops, also known as queenies, are small, cockle-sized scallops.

Scallops are found on the seabed and are therefore dirty, so it is advisable to purchase them ready cleaned. If scallops are bought in their shells, the shells should be tightly shut, which indicates they are alive and fresh. The roe (orange in colour) should be bright and moist. Scallops in their shells should be covered with damp seaweed or cloths and kept in a cold room or refrigerator. To remove from the shells, place the shells on top of the stove or in an oven for a few seconds, when they will open and the flesh can then be removed with a knife. Scallops should then be well washed. Remove the trail, leaving only the white scallop.

Cooking

Scallops should be only lightly cooked.

- Poach gently for 2–3 minutes in dry white wine with a little onion, carrot, thyme, bay leaf and parsley. Serve with a suitable sauce (e.g. white wine, mornay).
- Lightly fry on both sides for a few seconds in butter or oil in a very hot pan (if the scallops are very thick they can be cut in half sideways) and serve with a suitable garnish (sliced wild or cultivated mushrooms, or a fine brunoise of vegetables and tomato) and a liquid that need not be thickened (white wine and fish stock, or cream- or butter-mounted sauce). Fried scallops can also be served hot on a plate of salad leaves.
- Deep-fry, either coated in egg and crumbs or passed through a light batter, and served with segments of lemon and a suitable sauce (e.g. tartare).
- Wrap in thin streaky bacon and place on skewers for grilling or barbecuing.

Whelks

The common whelk is familiar around the coast of Britain. It is actually a gastropod, which means it has a large, strong, flat foot to move around on. Whelks are also equipped with a thick siphon, which is used for breathing and feeling around for food.

Whelks can often be bought in jars, packed in vinegar and water.

Basic cooking:

- Place the whelks in a saucepan and add water to cover them by 1 cm. Add a sprig of thyme and a bay leaf.
- Bring to a boil and cook at a bare simmer.
- Whelks require only a very short cooking time, otherwise the flesh has a tendency to become tough.

British winkles

The main types of British winkle, which can be readily identified on rocky shores, are:

- small periwinkle – approximately 4 mm
- rough periwinkle – at least four different subspecies, with the largest reaching 30 mm
- flat periwinkle.

To remove the winkles easily from their shells they need to be cooked.

Basic cooking:

- Place the winkles in a saucepan and cover with water. Add salt and a bay leaf.
- Turn on the heat, wait for the first sign of boiling and allow 2 to 3 minutes longer – no more.
- Take out one winkle to test if cooked; if it isn't cooked enough it will resist, still clinging firmly to its shell.
- When the winkles are cooked, run them quickly under cold water, otherwise they will toughen.
- Serve them simply in melted butter.

Oysters

Oysters are bivalve (two-shell) molluscs found near the bottom of the sea in coastal areas. The upper shell (valve) is flattish and attached by an elastic ligament hinge to the lower, bowl-shaped shell. Oysters are high in protein and low in fat; they are rich in zinc and contain many other nutrients such as calcium, iron, copper, iodine, magnesium and selenium.

Size, shape and colour vary considerably. Native oysters are pricier and generally thought of as superior. Pacific or rock oysters tend to have a frillier shell and are smaller, with milder meat.

Oysters may be cooked, but are usually served raw, freshly opened on ice with lemon.

Purchasing points

The shells should be clean, bright, tightly closed and unbroken.

Storage

Oysters should be stored at a low temperature and should smell briny fresh. Unopened live oysters can be kept in the fridge covered with wet cloths for two to three days; discard any that open. Do not store in an airtight container or under fresh water as this will cause them to die. Shucked oysters (ones that have been removed from their shells) can be kept refrigerated in a sealed container for four to five days.

 ACTIVITY

1 Explain the difference between molluscs and crustaceans.

2 How should mussels be opened?

3 Name two ways of preparing/cooking oysters.

4 List the hygiene precautions that have to be taken when preparing and cooking shellfish.

Test yourself • • • • • • • • • • • • • •

1 State the difference between oily and white fish.

2 Describe the difference between a tronçon and a suprême.

3 At what temperatures should fresh fish and frozen fish be stored?

4 Describe how you would skin a Dover sole.

5 State the quality points to look for when purchasing lobsters.

• •

1   Fried egg and breadcrumbed fish

1. For fish fillets, pass through flour, beaten egg and fresh white breadcrumbs. (Pat the surfaces well to avoid loose crumbs falling into the fat, burning and spoiling both the fat and the fish.)
2. Deep-fry at 175°C, until the fish turns a golden-brown. Remove and drain well.
3. Serve with either lemon quarters or tartare sauce.

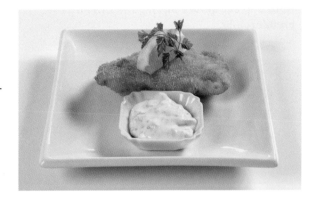

2   Fried sole *(sole frite)*

For fish courses use 200–250 g sole per portion; for main course 300–400 g sole per portion.

1. Remove the black and white skin. Remove the side fins.
2. Remove the head. Clean well.
3. Wash well and drain. Pané and deep-fry at 175°C.
4. Serve on a dish paper with picked or fried parsley and a quarter of lemon on a flat dish, and with a suitable sauce, such as tartare or anchovy.

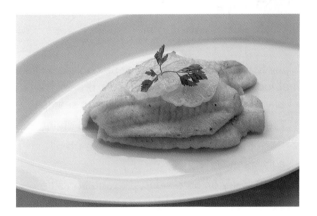

3   Goujons of fish

1. Cut fish fillets (e.g. sole, plaice, salmon) into strips approx. 8 × ½ cm. Wash and dry well.
2. Pass through flour, beaten egg and fresh white breadcrumbs. Pat the surfaces well so that there are no loose crumbs which could fall into the fat and burn.
3. Deep-fry at 175°C, then drain well.
4. Serve with lemon quarters and a suitable sauce (e.g. tartare).

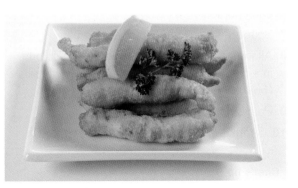

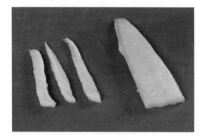

Cut the fish fillet into goujons

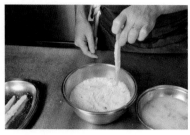

Pané the fish in breadcrumbs

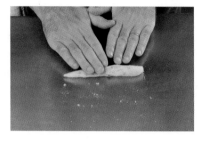

Roll the goujons to make sure the coating sticks

4 Fish meunière

cal	kcal	fat	sat fat	carb	sugar	protein	fibre
1314 KJ	313 kcal	24.1 g	10.3 g	3.1 g	0.0 g	21.2 g	0.1 g

Many fish, whole or filleted, may be cooked by this method, for example, sole, sea bass, bream, fillets of plaice, trout, brill, cod, turbot, herring, scampi.

1 Prepare and clean the fish, wash and drain.
2 Pass through seasoned flour, shake off all surplus.
3 Shallow-fry on both sides, presentation side first, in hot clarified butter, margarine or oil.
4 Dress neatly on an oval flat dish or plate/plates.
5 Peel a lemon, removing the peel, white pith and pips.
6 Cut the lemon into slices and place one on each portion.
7 Squeeze some lemon juice on the fish.
8 Allow 10–25 g butter per portion and colour in a clean frying pan to the nut-brown stage (*beurre noisette*).
9 Pour over the fish.
10 Sprinkle with chopped parsley and serve.

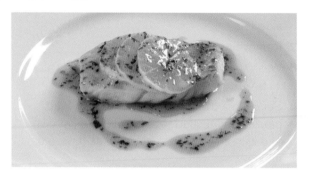

Making fish meunière
http://bit.ly/xzAnYO

Try something different

Variations include the following.

- **Fish meunière with almonds:** as for fish meunière, adding 10 g of almonds cut in short julienne or coarsely chopped into the meunière butter just before it begins to turn brown. This method is usually applied to trout.

- **Fish belle meunière:** as for fish meunière, with the addition of a grilled mushroom, a slice of peeled tomato and a soft herring roe (passed through flour and shallow-fried), all neatly dressed on each portion of fish.

- **Fish Doria:** as for fish meunière, with a sprinkling of small turned pieces of cucumber carefully cooked in 25 g of butter in a small covered pan, or blanched in boiling salted water.

- **Fish Grenobloise:** as for fish meunière, the peeled lemon being cut into segments, neatly dressed on the fish, with a few capers sprinkled over.

- **Fish Bretonne:** as for fish meunière, with a few picked shrimps and cooked sliced mushrooms sprinkled over the fish.

ASSESSMENT

5   Fillets of fish Véronique *(filets de poisson Véronique)*

cal	kcal	fat	sat fat	carb	sugar	protein	fibre
1077 KJ	256 kcal	19.3 g	10.7 g	6.9 g	2.1 g	11.8 g	0.4 g

	4 portions	10 portions
fillets of white fish	400–600 g	1–1.5 kg
butter, for dish and greaseproof paper		
shallots, finely chopped	10 g	25 g
fish stock	60 ml	150 ml
dry white wine	60 ml	150 ml
lemon, juice of	¼	½
fish velouté	250 ml	625 ml
egg yolk or spoonful of sabayon	1	2½
butter	50 g	125 g
cream, lightly whipped	2 tbsp	5 tbsp
white grapes, blanched, skinned and pipped	50 g	125 g

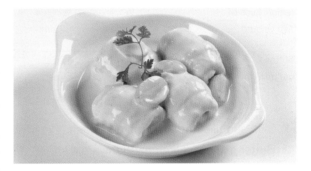

1 Skin and fillet the fish, trim and wash.

2 Butter and season an earthenware dish.

3 Sprinkle with the sweated chopped shallots and add the fillets of fish.

4 Season, add the fish stock, wine and lemon juice.

5 Cover with buttered greaseproof paper.

6 Poach in a moderate oven at 150–200°C for 7–10 minutes.

7 Drain the fish well and retain the cooking liquor. Dress the fish neatly on a flat dish or clean earthenware dish.

8 Bring the cooking liquor to the boil with the velouté and egg yolk or sabayon.

9 Correct the seasoning and consistency, and pass through double muslin or a fine strainer.

10 Mix in the butter then, finally, add the cream.

11 Coat the fillets with the sauce. Glaze under the salamander.

12 Arrange the grapes neatly on the dish.

Chef's tip

Chill the grapes well before use, so that they provide a real contrast of flavour.

   HEALTHY EATING TIP

- Keep the added salt to a minimum. Reduce the amount of butter and cream added to finish the sauce. Less sauce could be added plus a large portion of potatoes and vegetables.

6 Fillets of fish with white wine sauce (filets de poisson vin blanc)

cal	kcal	fat	sat fat	carb	sugar	protein	fibre
1421 KJ	342 kcal	24.0 g	12.8 g	5.8 g	0.9 g	25.9 g	0.2 g

	4 portions	10 portions
fillets of white fish	400–600 g	1–1.5 kg
butter, for dish and greaseproof paper		
shallots, finely chopped and sweated	10 g	25 g
fish stock	60 ml	150 ml
dry white wine	60 ml	150 ml
lemon, juice of	¼	½
fish velouté	250 ml	625 ml
butter	50 g	125 g
cream, lightly whipped	2 tbsp	5 tbsp

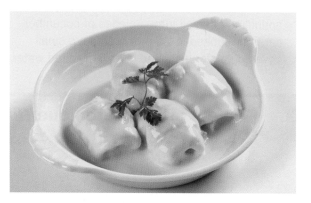

Chef's tip

In this recipe, the shallots should be sweated before use; however, if they are very finely chopped, they could be added raw.

1 Skin and fillet the fish, trim and wash.

2 Butter and season an earthenware dish.

3 Sprinkle with the sweated chopped shallots and add the fillets of sole.

4 Season, add the fish stock, wine and lemon juice.

5 Cover with buttered greaseproof paper.

6 Poach in a moderate oven at 150–200°C for 7–10 minutes.

7 Drain the fish well; dress neatly on a flat dish or clean earthenware dish.

8 Bring the cooking liquor to the boil with the velouté.

9 Correct the seasoning and consistency, and pass through double muslin or a fine strainer.

10 Mix in the butter then, finally, add the cream.

11 Coat the fillets with the sauce. Garnish with *fleurons* (puff paste crescents).

Filleting a flat fish
http://bit.ly/wJKnim

Try something different

Add to the fish before cooking:

- **fish *bonne-femme*** – 100 g thinly sliced white button mushrooms and chopped parsley
- **fish *bréval*** – as for *bonne-femme* plus 100 g diced, peeled and deseeded tomatoes.

7 ## Skate with black butter *(raie au beurre noir)*

cal	kcal	fat	sat fat	carb	sugar	protein	fibre
725 KJ	174 kcal	10.8 g	6.5 g	0.1 g	0.1 g	19.0 g	0.0 g

	4 portions	10 portions
skate wings	400–600 g	1¼ kg
court bouillon (see recipe 34)		
butter	50 g	125 g
vinegar	1 tsp	2½ tsp
parsley, chopped		
capers	10 g	25 g

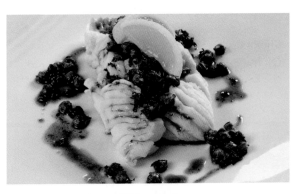

1 Cut the skate into 4 (or 10) even pieces.
2 Simmer in a court bouillon until cooked (approximately 10 minutes).
3 Drain well, place on a serving dish or plates.
4 Heat the butter in a frying pan until well browned, almost black; add the vinegar, pour over the fish, sprinkle with chopped parsley and a few capers and serve.

Try something different

Proceed as for steps 1–3, then drain well and serve on a bed of plain or herb-flavoured mashed potato, accompanied by a compound butter sauce (page 202) or a salsa (page 194).

 HEALTHY EATING TIP

- Pour less black butter over the cooked fish.
- Serve with a large portion of potatoes and vegetables.

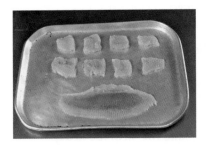

Raw skate

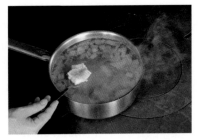

Poach the fish

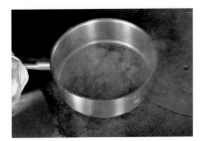

Heat the butter

8 ## Grilled fish fillets (sole, plaice, haddock)

1 Remove the black skin from sole and plaice. Wash the fillets and dry them well.
2 Pass through flour, shake off surplus and brush with oil.
3 Place on hot grill bars, a griddle or a greased baking sheet if grilling under a salamander. Brush occasionally with oil.

4 Turn the fish carefully and grill on both sides. Do not overcook.

5 Serve with lemon quarters and a suitable sauce (e.g. compound butter or salsa).

> **Chef's tip**
> Oil the grill bars well, so that the fish does not stick.

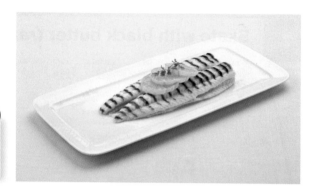

9 Fried fish in batter

To make the batter

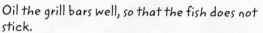

	4 portions	10 portions
flour	200 g	500 g
salt		
yeast	10 g	25 g
water or milk	250 ml	625 ml

1 Sift the flour and salt into a basin.

2 Dissolve the yeast in a little of the water.

3 Make a well in the flour. Add the yeast and the liquid.

4 Gradually incorporate the flour and beat to a smooth mixture.

5 Allow to rest for at least 1 hour before using.

To prepare the fish

1 Pass the prepared, washed and well-dried fish through flour, shake off the surplus and pass through the batter.

2 Place carefully away from you into the hot

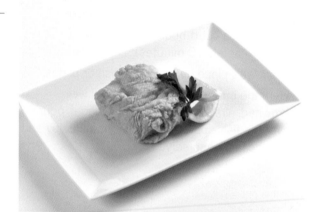

deep-fryer at 175°C until the fish turns a golden-brown. Remove and drain well.

3 Serve with either lemon quarters or tartare sauce.

> **Chef's tip**
> Remove any excess batter before frying; too much batter will make the meal too heavy.

10 Whitebait *(blanchailles)*

 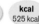   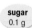

cal	kcal	fat	sat fat	carb	sugar	protein	fibre
2174 KJ	525 kcal	47.5 g	0.0 g	5.3 g	0.1 g	19.5 g	0.2 g

Allow 100 g per portion.

1 Pick over the whitebait, wash carefully and drain well.

2 Pass through milk and seasoned flour.

3 Shake off surplus flour in a wide-mesh sieve and place fish into a frying-basket.

4 Plunge into very hot fat, just smoking (195°C).

5 Cook until brown and crisp (approximately 1 minute).

6 Drain well.

7 Season lightly with salt and cayenne pepper.

8 Serve garnished with fried or picked parsley and quarters of lemon.

Chef's tip

It is important to shake off any excess flour before frying; too much flour will cause the fish to stick together.

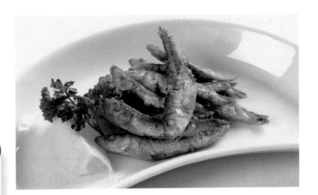

11 Pan-fried fillets of sea bass with rosemary mash and mushrooms

cal	kcal	fat	sat fat	carb	sugar	protein	fibre
1183 KJ	282 kcal	11.6 g	3.6 g	17.3 g	0.6 g	28.2 g	1.3 g

	4 portions	10 portions
vegetable oil	10 ml	25 ml
salt, pepper		
sea bass portions, skin on	4 × 100 g	10 × 100 g
wild mushrooms, sliced	200 g	600 g
extra virgin olive oil	10 ml	25 ml
rosemary, chopped	pinch	1 tsp
mashed potato (see page 224)	400 g	1 kg

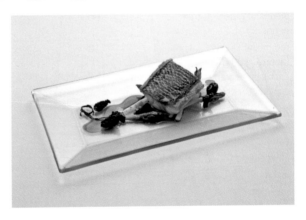

1 Heat the vegetable oil in a non-stick pan, season and then fry the lemon sole, skin side first, until it has a golden colour and is crispy.

2 Turn the fish over and gently seal without colouring.

3 Remove from the pan (skin side up) and keep warm.

4 Quickly and lightly fry the mushrooms in extra virgin olive oil.

5 Mix the rosemary into the mashed potato.

6 Arrange the potato in the centre of hot plates.

7 Place the fish on top, skin side down.

8 Garnish with the mushrooms and olive oil and serve.

HEALTHY EATING TIP

- Using an unsaturated oil (sunflower or olive), lightly oil the non-stick pan to fry the sole.
- Use a little olive oil to fry the mushrooms.
- Keep added salt to a minimum.
- Serve with plenty of seasonal vegetables and new potatoes.

Try something different

- A sauce of light veal or chicken jus flavoured with fennel can be served around the plates.

- If the rosemary is in fresh sprigs it can be used to garnish the dish instead of being put into the potato.

- Girolle or button mushrooms can be used in place of wild mushrooms.

- Sautéed leeks, small stewed baby leeks or points of cooked asparagus can be used to garnish the dish and add colour.

* Using lemon sole in place of sea bass, and button mushrooms.

---

12 **Nage of red mullet with baby leeks**

	4 portions	10 portions
mussels, cooked and out of shell	16	40
lemons, juice of	2	5
baby spinach	200 g	500 g
baby leeks	12	30
spears of baby asparagus	12	30
pieces of green beans	24	60
red mullet fillets (approx. 120 g each), pinned and scaled	4	10
Nage		
large onion	1	3
carrots, peeled	2	5
celery sticks	2	5
leeks	2	5
garlic cloves	1	3
half white and half pink peppercorns	12	30
star anise	1	3
white wine	375 ml	950 ml
Noilly Prat	375 ml	950 ml
chervil	10 g	25 g
parsley	10 g	25 g
tarragon	10 g	25 g
chives, chopped	1 tbsp	3 tbsp

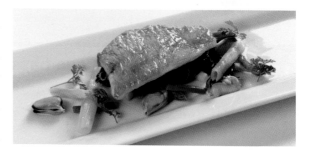

1. In a large pan place the onions, carrots, celery and leeks, which have been cut into 2 cm pieces.

2. Just cover the vegetables with water. Bring to the boil. Simmer for 4–5 minutes. Remove from the heat and add the rest of the ingredients.

3. Cover with clingfilm and allow to cool to room temperature. Place into a plastic container and store in the fridge overnight to develop flavour.

4. Pass through a fine sieve. The resulting nage can be bottled for later use.

5. To finish, place 500 ml of the vegetable nage in a pan, add the mussels, a squeeze of lemon, spinach, baby leeks, asparagus and green beans.

6. Bring to the boil, check the seasoning and retain.

7. Heat a non-stick pan with a little vegetable oil. Season the mullet fillets and cook for one minute on each side (thickness dependent), starting with the skin side down.

8. Divide the vegetable garnish between the bowls. Place the red mullet on top of the vegetable garnish and, returning the pan the mullet was cooked in to the stove, pour in the nage.

9. When the nage has returned to the boil, spoon over the fish and garnish. Serve immediately.

> This dish is open to many substitutions of fish and shellfish but one key point to remember is that the nage should not be allowed to overpower the main ingredients.

13 Poached smoked haddock

	4 portions	10 portions
smoked haddock fillets	400–600 g	1.2 kg
milk and water		

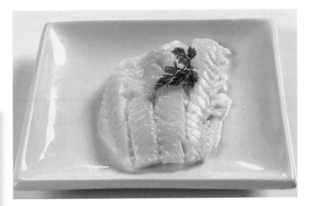

This is a popular breakfast dish and is also served as a lunch and a snack dish. For example:

- when cooked, garnish with slices of peeled tomato or tomato concassée, lightly coat with cream, flash under the salamander and serve
- top with a poached egg
- when cooked, lightly coat with Welsh rarebit mixture (see Appendix), brown under the salamander and garnish with peeled slices of tomato or tomato concassée.

1 Cut fillets into even portions, place into a shallow pan and cover with half milk and water.

2 Simmer gently for a few minutes until cooked.

3 Drain well and serve.

14 Steamed fish with garlic, spring onions and ginger

cal 468 KJ	kcal 112 kcal	fat 3.5 g	sat fat 0.7 g	carb 1.2 g	sugar 0.4 g	protein 18.7 g	fibre 0.1 g	*

   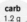

	4 portions	10 portions
white fish fillets, e.g. cod, sole	400 g	1.5 kg
salt		
ginger, freshly chopped	1 tbsp	2½ tbsp
spring onions, finely chopped	2 tbsp	5 tbsp
light soy sauce	1 tbsp	2½ tbsp
garlic cloves, peeled and thinly sliced		
oil	1 tbsp	2½ tbsp

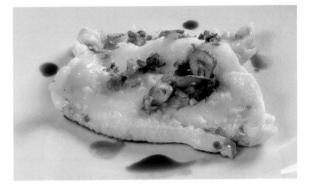

1 Wash and dry the fish well; rub *lightly* with salt on both sides.

2 Put the fish onto plates, scatter the ginger evenly on top.

3 Put the plates into the steamer, cover tightly and steam gently until just cooked (5–15 minutes, according to the thickness of the fish).

4 Remove the plates, sprinkle on the spring onions and soy sauce.

5 Brown the garlic slices in the hot oil and pour over the dish.

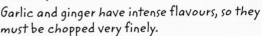

Chef's tip

Garlic and ginger have intense flavours, so they must be chopped very finely.

Try something different

This is a Chinese recipe that can be adapted in many ways – for example, replace the spring onions and garlic and use thinly sliced mushrooms, diced tomato (skinned and deseeded), *finely* chopped shallots, lemon juice, white wine, chopped parsley, dill or chervil.

HEALTHY EATING TIP

- Steaming is a healthy way of cooking.
- Serve with a large portion of rice or noodles and stir-fried vegetables.

* Using 2 cloves of garlic

---

15 Griddled monkfish with leeks and Parmesan

cal	kcal	fat	sat fat	carb	sugar	protein	fibre
1009 KJ	239 kcal	8.3 g	5.0 g	1.0 g	0.8 g	40.3 g	0.6 g

	4 portions	10 portions
oil		
leeks, finely sliced	100 g	250 g
Parmesan, grated	100 g	250 g
salt, pepper		
prepared monkfish fillets	750 g	1.8 kg
egg white, lightly beaten	2	5
lemons	1	3
mixed salad leaves, to serve		

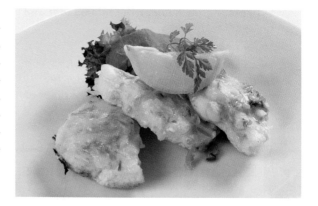

1 Heat the griddle pan and oil lightly.
2 Cut the leeks into fine julienne with the Parmesan, then season.
3 Cut the monkfish into 1.5 cm thick slices. Dry, dip in the beaten egg white, then in the leek and Parmesan.
4 Place the monkfish on the griddle to cook (approximately 3–4 minutes).
5 Garnish with lemon wedges and mixed leaves.

HEALTHY EATING TIP

- There is no need to add salt – there is plenty in the cheese.
- Serve with a large portion of potatoes and vegetables or salad.

---

16 Grilled round fish (herring, mackerel, bass, mullet)

1 Descale fish where necessary, using the back of a knife.
2 Remove heads, clean out intestines, trim off all fins and tails using fish scissors. Leave herring roes in the fish.
3 Wash and dry well.
4 Make three light incisions 2 mm deep on either

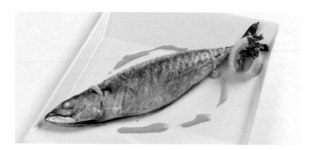

side of the fish. This is known as 'scoring' and helps the heat to penetrate the fish.

5 Pass through flour, shake off surplus and brush with oil.

6 Place on hot grill bars, a griddle or a greased baking sheet if grilling under a salamander. Brush occasionally with oil.

7 Turn the fish carefully and grill on both sides. Do not overcook.

8 Serve with lemon quarters and a suitable sauce (e.g. compound butter or salsa).

> Herrings are traditionally served with a mustard sauce.
> Mackerel may be butterfly filleted and grilled.

---

17 Grilled swordfish and somen noodle salad with cilantro vinaigrette

cal	kcal	fat	sat fat	carb	sugar	protein	fibre
2599 KJ	623 kcal	42.6 g	6.1 g	40.3 g	2.7 g	21.2 g	2.5 g

	4 portions	10 portions
swordfish fillets	4 × 75 g	10 × 75 g
buckwheat somen noodles	200 g	500 g
romaine lettuce	¼	½
celery, finely diced	50 g	125 g
chopped onion (red)	50 g	125 g
Vinaigrette		
olive oil	70 ml	170 ml
sesame oil	35 ml	85 ml
canola oil	35 ml	85 ml
rice wine	2 tbsp	4½ tbsp
lemon, juice of	½	1
lime, juice of	1	2
fresh ginger, chopped	2 tbsp	5 tbsp
garlic, chopped	1 clove	3 cloves
cilantro leaves	1 tbsp	2½ tbsp
sesame seeds (black)	2 tbsp	5 tbsp
seasoning		

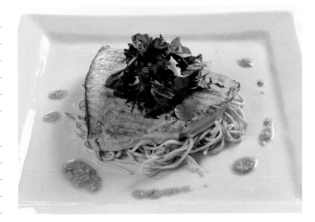

1 Prepare the vinaigrette by placing all the ingredients in a liquidiser, purée until smooth. Season to taste.

2 Season the swordfish fillets, brush with the vinaigrette. Grill for 2 to 3 minutes on each side until cooked. Allow to cool.

3 Cook the noodles in boiling water, refresh and drain. Allow to cool.

4 Shred the lettuce finely, mix with the diced celery and finely chopped red onion. Season with the vinaigrette.

5 Serve by arranging the noodles in the centre of each plate.

6 Place the swordfish fillets on the noodles, season with vinaigrette.

7 Garnish with romaine lettuce. Freshly ground black pepper may be used to finish the dish.

HEALTHY EATING TIP

- Keep added salt to a minimum.
- Adding less vinaigrette to the finished dish can reduce the fat content.

* Using vegetable oil for canola; coriander for cilantro; wheat pasta for buckwheat pasta

18   Roast fillet of sea bass with vanilla and fennel

	4 portions	10 portions
sea bass fillets (approx. 160 g each, cut from a 2–3 kg fish) skin on, scaled and pin-boned	4	10
seasoning		
vegetable oil	50 ml	125 ml
Fennel		
bulbs of baby fennel	8	20
vegetable oil	50 ml	125 ml
fish stock	500 ml	1¼ litres
clove of garlic	1	3
Vanilla sauce		
shallots, peeled and sliced	1	3
fish stock	500 ml	1¼ litres
white wine	200 ml	500 ml
vanilla pods	2	5
butter	50 g	125 g
chives, chopped	1 tsp	3 tsp
tomato concassée	100 g	250 g

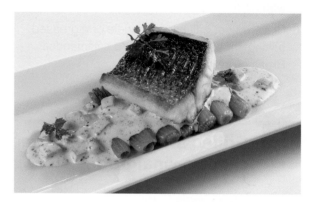

For the fennel

1 Trim the fennel bulbs well, ensuring they are free from blemishes and root.
2 Heat the oil in a pan, place in the fennel and slightly brown.
3 Add the stock and garlic, bring to the boil and cook until tender.

For the sauce

1 Heat a small amount of vegetable oil in a pan.
2 Place in the shallot and cook without colour, add the stock, white wine and split vanilla, and reduce by two-thirds.

3 Pass through a chinois and reserve for serving.
4 Add the butter and chopped chives.

To finish

1 Pre-heat the oven to 180°C.
2 Heat the oil in a non-stick pan and place the seasoned sea bass fillets in skin side down.
3 Cook for 2 minutes on the stove and then place in the oven for 3 minutes (depending on thickness) still with the skin side down.
4 Meanwhile, reheat the fennel and add the tomato concassée to the sauce.
5 Remove the sea bass from the oven and turn in the pan, finishing the flesh side for 30 seconds to 1 minute.
6 Lay the fennel in the centre of the plate and place the sea bass on top.
7 Finish the dish with the sauce over the bass and around, serve immediately.

A marriage of flavour: vanilla, bass and fennel are made for each other. This fish can also be steamed.

19   Baked cod with a herb crust

cal	kcal	fat	sat fat	carb	sugar	protein	fibre
1882 KJ	452 kcal	30.8 g	18.7 g	12.7 g	0.8 g	31.7 g	0.4 g

*

	4 portions	10 portions
cod fillets, 100–150 g each	4	10
herb mustard		
fresh breadcrumbs	100 g	250 g
butter, margarine or oil	100 g	250 g
Cheddar cheese, grated	100 g	250 g
parsley, chopped	1 tsp	1 tbsp
salt, pepper		

1. Place the prepared, washed and dried fish on a greased baking tray or ovenproof dish.
2. Combine the ingredients for the herb crust (the mustard, breadcrumbs, butter or oil, cheese, parsley and seasoning) and press evenly over the fish.
3. Bake in the oven at 180°C for approx. 15–20 minutes until cooked and the crust is a light golden-brown.
4. Serve either with lemon quarters or a suitable salsa (page 194) or sauce, e.g. tomato or egg.

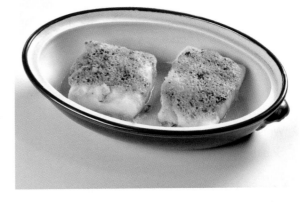

HEALTHY EATING TIP

- Use a little sunflower oil when making the herb crust.
- Cheese is salty – no added salt is needed.
- Serve with a large portion of tomato or cucumber salsa and new potatoes.

* Using mustard powder (1 tsp) for herb mustard

Chef's tip
Add a little bit of beaten egg to the breadcrumb mixture; this will help bind the mixture together.

20   Red mullet ceviche with organic leaves

4 portions	10 portions	
2	5	shallots, finely diced
1 tbsp	3 tbsp	olive oil
50 ml	125 ml	white wine vinegar
1 litre	2½ litres	fish stock
1	3	lemons, juice of
2 tbsp	5 tbsp	cucumber, diced
4	10	red mullet fillets (approx. 120 g each), pinned and scaled

300 g	750 g	organic salad leaf (5 varieties)
50 ml	125 ml	vinaigrette
50 g	125 g	caviar (optional)
Saffron dressing		
10 ml	25 ml	water
		saffron
50 ml	125 ml	vegetable oil
10 ml	25 ml	vinegar

1 Bring the shallots, olive oil, white wine vinegar and fish stock to the boil. Add the lemon and cucumber, and allow to cool at room temperature.

2 Place the red mullet in a container and cover with the liquid. Top with clingfilm to ensure all the air is kept out, capitalising on maximum curing. This will need to remain in the fridge for a minimum of 6 hours.

To make the dressing

1 Add water and a pinch of saffron to a pan and bring to the boil.

2 Whisk in the vegetable oil and vinegar.

3 Season.

> A cured dish always tastes of the true ingredients. Using red mullet, as here, the flavours are bold and earthy, and paired with the saffron it makes a perfect summer starter.

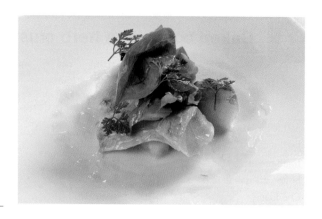

To finish

1 Mix the dressed leaves lightly in vinaigrette.

2 Place the red mullet carefully on a plate with a little of the curing liquor, shallots and cucumber.

3 Top with the organic salad and finish with the saffron dressing and caviar (if using).

21 Poached salmon

1 Place the prepared and washed darnes of salmon in a simmering court bouillon for approximately 5 minutes.

2 Drain well and carefully remove centre bone and outer skin. (The bone is easy to remove.) Ensure that the fish is cleaned of any cooked blood.

3 Serve with a suitable sauce (e.g. hollandaise) or melted herb butter, and thinly sliced cucumber.

> Depending on the size of the salmon, either a whole or half a darne would be served as a portion.

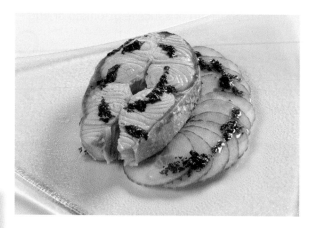

22 Grilled salmon, pea soup and quails' eggs

	4 portions	10 portions
Soup		
vegetable oil	50 ml	125 ml
shallots, peeled and sliced	2	5
garlic cloves, crushed	1	3
raw potato, chopped	200 g	500 g
peas	600 g	1½ kg
milk	500 ml	1½ litres
stem of mint	1	3
Salmon		
salmon fillet	4 x 150 g	10 x 150 g
plain flour	25 g	60 g
olive oil	4 tbsp	9 tbsp
To finish		
spinach, washed	200 g	500 g
peas, cooked and crushed	600 g	1½ kg
butter	50 g	125 g
seasoning		
quails' eggs, lightly poached	8	20
first press olive oil		
fresh herbs		

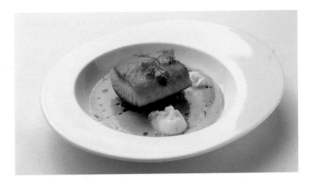

For the salmon

1 Heat a lower-heat grill ensuring the bars are clean.

2 Lightly oil the bars and then dust the salmon fillet in the flour.

3 Carefully place the salmon fillet on the grill and score.

4 Once sealed rotate the fish 45 degrees and mark, creating a diamond shape.

5 After 2–3 minutes turn the salmon over taking care not to break the flesh.

6 After 2 minutes cooking on the other side check if cooked by gently pushing your index finger into the centre – the fish should still have a little structure.

To make the soup

1 Heat the oil and add the shallots and garlic, cook without colour for 2 minutes.

2 Then add the potato and cook for a further 2 minutes.

3 Add the peas and milk, bring to the boil and remove from the heat.

4 Add the mint sprig and allow to infuse for 3-4 minutes. Remove and then blitz the soup in a processor.

5 Pass through a strainer and retain.

To finish

1 Wilt the spinach in a hot pan, add the peas and butter and season.

2 Place the poached eggs in the soup and quickly re-heat.

3 Place a mound of spinach and peas in the centre of a bowl with the salmon on top and 2 quails' eggs per bowl.

4 Finish the dish with a drizzle of fine olive oil and fresh herbs.

This is a suitable summer dish, light and very seasonal. As an alternative, replace the salmon with salt cod.

23 Sardines with tapenade

	4 portions	10 portions
sardines	8–12	20–30
For the tapenade		
kalamata olives	20	50
capers	1 tbsp	2½ tbsp
lemon juice	1 tsp	2½ tsp
olive oil	2 tsp	5 tsp
anchovy paste (optional)	½ tsp	1¼ tsp
freshly ground black pepper		

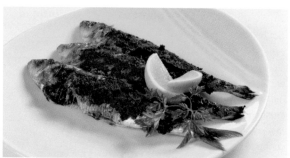

1 Finely chop the olives and capers. Add the lemon juice, olive oil, anchovy paste and black pepper. Mix well.

2 Allow 2–3 sardines per portion. Clean them, and grill them on both sides, either on an open flame grill or under the salamander.

3 When cooked, smear the tapenade on top. The tapenade can be heated slightly before spreading.

A little chopped basil and a crushed chopped clove of garlic may also be added to the tapenade.

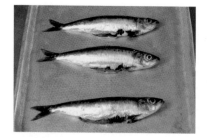

Raw sardines

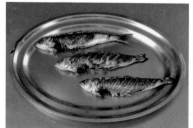

Grilled sardines

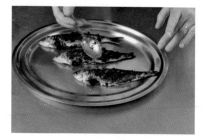

Smear the sardines with tapenade

24 Whole trout baked in salt

egg whites	6
coarse sea salt	600 g
trout, gutted, cleaned and washed	1

1 Preheat the oven to 185°C.

2 Whisk the egg whites slightly to make them more liquid.

3 Mix the egg whites in to the salt.

4 Place a bed of the salt mixture, as long as the trout and 1 cm thick, in the bottom of a dish that is suitable for service at the table.

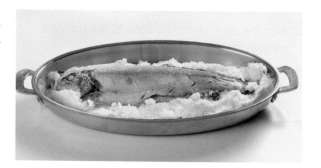

5 Place the trout on top of the salt.

6 Cover the trout completely with the remaining salt mixture, ensuring a seal. Make sure that the dish is clean, because any stray salt may burn.

7 Cook for 35 minutes in a preheated fan-assisted oven.

8 Remove from the oven. Inconspicuously pierce the trout with a metal skewer to ensure that it is cooked through to the centre.

9 Serve at the table by cracking open the top crust. Carefully remove the salt and skin from the top of the fish. Lift the fillet off the bone.

Serve with butter sauce and green salad.

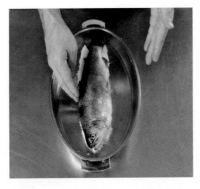

Place the trout in the pan on a bed of salt

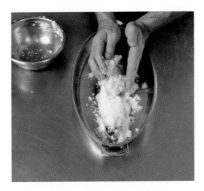

Add a crust of salt on top of the fish

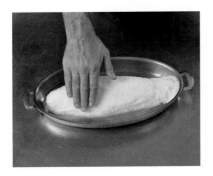

Make sure the crust is tidy, with no stray salt, before baking

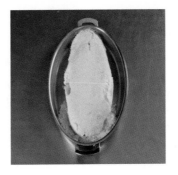

Baked trout, before the crust is broken

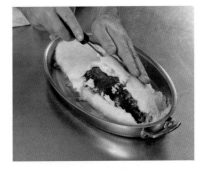

Break the salt crust and carefully remove it and the skin

25 Fish kebabs

Fish kebabs or brochettes are best made using a firm fish (e.g. salmon, tuna, marlin, turbot). The fish (free from skin and bone) is cut into cubes and can be (a) simply seasoned with salt and pepper or (b) lightly rolled in herbs (e.g. cumin seeds and mustard) or (c) placed in a simple marinade (e.g. olive oil, lemon juice and chopped parsley) for 30 minutes. Other ingredients to be threaded on the skewers can be halves of small, par-boiled new potatoes, cherry tomatoes and mushrooms. The

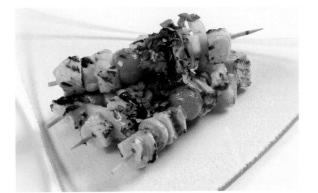

kebabs are lightly brushed with oil and cooked on a fierce grill or barbecue.

Scallops are also suitable for kebabs (see page 308).

Scallops are also suitable for kebabs (see page 308).

Chef's tip
Brushing the kebabs with oil stops them from sticking to the grill.

26 Fish kedgeree *(cadgery de poisson)*

cal	kcal	fat	sat fat	carb	sugar	protein	fibre	*
1974 KJ	472 kcal	28.2 g	15.3 g	29.3 g	4.7 g	25.7 g	1.2 g	

	4 portions	10 portions
fish (usually smoked haddock or fresh salmon)	400 g	1 kg
rice pilaff (see page 442)	200 g	500 g
eggs, hard-boiled	2	5
butter	50 g	125 g
salt, pepper		
curry sauce, to serve	250 ml	625 ml

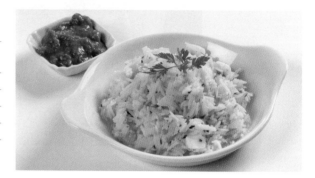

1 Poach the fish. Remove all skin and bone. Flake.

2 Cook the rice pilaff. Cut the eggs into dice.

3 Combine the eggs, fish and rice, and heat in the butter. Correct the seasoning.

4 Serve hot with a sauceboat of curry sauce.

This dish is traditionally served for breakfast, lunch or supper. The fish used should be named on the menu (e.g. salmon kedgeree).

 **HEALTHY EATING TIP**

- Reduce the amount of butter used to heat the rice, fish and eggs.

- Garnish with grilled tomatoes and serve with bread or toast.

Using smoked haddock

27 Fish pie

cal	kcal	fat	sat fat	carb	sugar	protein	fibre
879 KJ	209 kcal	12.0 g	5.3 g	11.9 g	3.2 g	14.1 g	0.9 g

	4 portions	10 portions
béchamel sauce (thin) (see page 184)	250 ml	625 ml
cooked fish (free from skin and bone)	200 g	500 g
mushrooms, cooked and diced	50 g	125 g
egg, hard-boiled and chopped	1	3
parsley, chopped		
salt, pepper		
mashed or duchess potatoes	200 g	500 g
eggwash or milk, to finish		

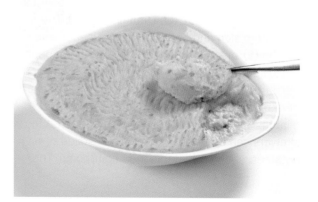

1 Bring the béchamel to the boil.

2 Add the fish, mushrooms, egg and parsley. Correct the seasoning.

3 Place in a buttered pie dish.

4 Place or pipe the potato on top. Brush with eggwash or milk.

5 Brown in a hot oven or under the salamander and serve.

Try something different

- Add prawns or shrimps.

- Add herbs such as dill, tarragon or fennel.

- Poach raw fish in white wine, strain off the cooking liquor, add double cream instead of béchamel and reduce to a light consistency.

🍎 HEALTHY EATING TIP

- Keep the added salt to a minimum.

- This is a healthy main course dish, particularly when served with plenty of vegetables.

---

28 Smoked mackerel mousse

cal	kcal	fat	sat fat	carb	sugar	protein	fibre
1192 KJ	289 kcal	27.5 g	10.7 g	0.4 g	0.4 g	9.8 g	0.0 g *

	4 portions	10 portions
smoked mackerel, free from bone and skin	200 g	500 g
optional seasoning: pepper, chopped parsley, fennel or chervil, 1 tbsp tomato ketchup, two ripe tomatoes free from skin and pips		
double cream (or non-dairy cream)	90 ml	250 ml

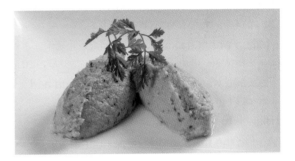

1 Ensure that the mackerel is completely free from skin and bones.

2 Liquidise with the required seasoning.

3 Three-quarter whip the cream.

4 Remove mackerel from liquidiser and fold into the cream. Correct the seasoning.

5 Serve in individual dishes accompanied with hot toast.

> This recipe can be used with smoked trout or smoked salmon trimmings. It can also be used for fresh salmon, in which case 50 g of cucumber can be incorporated with the selected seasoning.

🍎 HEALTHY EATING TIP

- Serve with plenty of salad vegetables and bread or toast (optional butter or spread).

- Use the minimum amount of salt.

* Using double cream

29 Soused herring or mackerel

cal	kcal	fat	sat fat	carb	sugar	protein	fibre
2419 KJ	576 kcal	44.5 g	9.4 g	3.0 g	3.0 g	41.0 g	1.1 g *

	4 portions	10 portions
herrings or mackerel	2	5
salt, pepper		
button onions	25 g	60 g
carrots, peeled and fluted	25 g	60 g
bay leaf	½	1½
peppercorns	6	12
thyme	1 sprig	2 sprigs
vinegar	60 ml	150 ml

1 Clean, scale and fillet the fish.
2 Wash the fillets well and season with salt and pepper.
3 Roll up with the skin outside. Place in an earthenware dish.
4 Peel and wash the onion. Cut the onion and carrots into neat, thin rings.
5 Blanch for 2–3 minutes.
6 Add to the fish with the remainder of the ingredients.
7 Cover with greaseproof paper and cook in a moderate oven for 15–20 minutes.

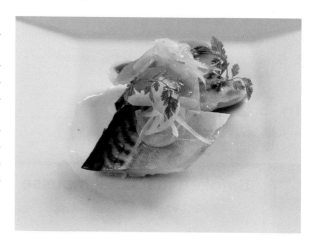

8 Allow to cool, place in a dish with the onion and carrot.
9 Garnish with picked parsley, dill or chives.

HEALTHY EATING TIP

- Serve with plenty of salad vegetables and bread or toast (optional butter or spread).
- Keep the added salt to a minimum.

* For 4 portions

30 Haddock and smoked salmon terrine

cal	kcal	fat	sat fat	carb	sugar	protein	fibre
563 KJ	133 kcal	3.4 g	0.7 g	0.1 g	0.1 g	25.7 g	0.1 g

	4 portions	10 portions
smoked salmon	140 g	350 g
haddock, halibut or Arctic bass fillets, skinned	320 g	800 g
salt, pepper		
eggs, lightly beaten	1	2
crème fraiche	40 ml	105 ml
capers	3 tbsp	7 tbsp
green or pink peppercorns	1 tbsp	2 tbsp

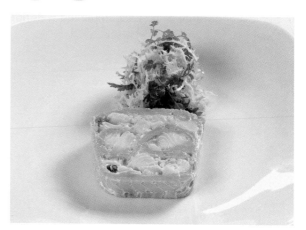

1 Grease a 1 litre loaf tin with oil; alternatively, line with clingflim.

2 Line the tin with thin slices of smoked salmon. Let the ends overhang the mould. Reserve the remaining salmon until needed.

3 Cut two long slices of haddock the length of the tin and set aside.

4 Cut the rest of the haddock into small pieces. Season all the haddock with salt and pepper.

5 In a suitable basin, combine the eggs, crème fraiche, capers, and green or pink peppercorns. Add the pieces of haddock.

6 Spoon the mixture into the mould until one-third full. Smooth with a spatula.

7 Wrap the long haddock fillets in the reserved smoked salmon. Lay them on top of the layer of the fish mixture in the terrine.

8 Fill with the remainder of the haddock and crème fraiche mixture.

9 Smooth the surface and fold over the overhanging pieces of smoked salmon.

10 Cover with tin foil, secure well.

11 Cook in a water bath (bain-marie) of boiling water. Place in the oven at 200°C for approximately 45 minutes, until set.

12 Remove from oven and bain-marie. Allow to cool. Do not remove foil cover.

13 Place heavy weights on top and leave in refrigerator for 24 hours.

14 When ready to serve, remove the weights and foil. Remove from mould.

15 Cut into thick slices, serve on suitable plates with a dill mayonnaise and garnished with salad leaves and fresh dill.

Chef's tip
Line the tin carefully so that the finished terrine will look attractive.

 HEALTHY EATING TIP

- Season with the minimum amount of salt.
- Offer the customer the mayonnaise separately.
- Serve with a warm bread or rolls (butter optional).

---

31 Scallops with caramelised cauliflower

	4 portions	10 portions
raisins	100 g	250 g
capers	100 g	250 g
water	180 ml	450 ml
sherry vinegar	1 tbsp	2 tbsp
grated nutmeg		
salt and cayenne pepper		
butter	30 g	75 g
head of cauliflower, sliced into ½ cm-thick pieces	½	1
large hand-dived scallops (roe removed)	12	30

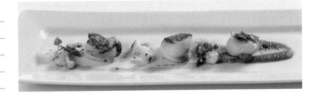

1 In a small saucepan, cook the raisins and capers in the water until the raisins are plump, about 5 minutes.

2 Pour mixture into blender and add the vinegar, nutmeg, salt and pepper, blend just until smooth.

3 Set sauce aside.

4 In a sauté pan, heat butter and cook the cauliflower until golden on both sides. To prevent cauliflower from burning, if necessary, add about 1 tablespoon of water to pan during cooking. Set cauliflower aside.

5 In a separate pan, sauté the scallops in a little butter, about 1½ minutes on each side. To serve, place 3 scallops on each plate, top with cauliflower and finish with the caper-raisin emulsion.

When using scallops, always use hand-dived scallops as first choice, as dredged scallops are sometimes unethically sourced. You will pay a bit more for the hand-dived variety but the difference is certainly worth it.

Chef's tip

Be careful not to overcook the scallops, as they will become tough.

32 Oysters in their own shells

Serves 4

24 rock or native oysters

1 lemon

To accompany

brown bread and butter

Tabasco or chilli sauce

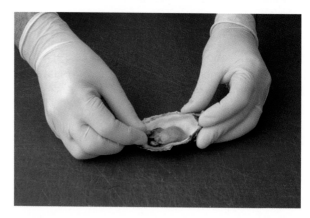

1 Select only those oysters that are tightly shut and have a fresh smell (category A is best, which means the waters they have grown in are clean).

2 To open an oyster, only the point of the oyster knife is used. Hold the oyster with a thick oven cloth to protect your hand.

3 With the oyster in the palm of your hand, push the point of the knife about 1 cm deep into the 'hinge' between the 'lid' and the body of the oyster.

4 Once the lid has been penetrated, push down. The lid should pop open. Lift up the top shell, cutting the muscle attached to it.

5 Remove any splintered shell from the flesh and solid shell.

6 Return each oyster to its shell and serve on a bed of crushed ice with chilli sauce, brown bread and lemon.

Make sure the oysters have been grown in or fished from clean waters, and take note of the famous rule only to use them when there is an 'r' in the month, although rock oysters are available throughout the year.

33 Oyster tempura

The recipe for tempura batter is on page 250.

1 Open the fresh oysters.
2 Place each oyster on a tray on absorbent kitchen paper.
3 Lightly sprinkle with finely chopped herbs, parsley, basil and chives.
4 Pass each oyster through seasoned flour.
5 Dip in tempura batter and fry in hot deep oil at 180°C until golden brown.
6 Remove from the oil and drain well.

Serve as a garnish or as a hot hors d'oeuvre with a suitable dip, such as tomato chilli and lemon and garlic mayonnaise.

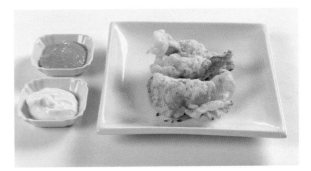

Chef's tip
Make sure the oil is at the right temperature. Cook the oysters quickly until crisp and golden brown.

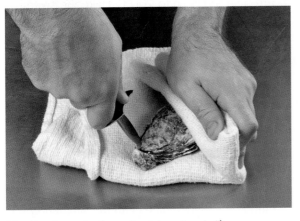

Shucking the oyster (removing it from the shell)

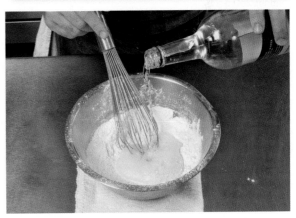

Add sparkling water to flour to make the batter

34   Poached langoustines with aioli dip

	4 portions	10 portions
raw langoustine tails, large (or king or tiger prawns)	36	90
Court bouillon		
carrots	2	5
fennel bulbs	1	3
garlic cloves	2	5
water	1400 ml	3½ litres
white wine	290 ml	725 ml
a few fresh parsley and chervil stalks		
white peppercorns, crushed	3	7
Aioli		
sweet potato (about 250 g each), orange flesh	1	2½
mayonnaise	3 tbsp	7½ tbsp
pinches saffron strands, soaked in a little water	2	5
eggs, boiled and yolks removed and reserved	3	7
crushed garlic	½ tsp	1½ tsp
a little olive oil		
salt and pepper		
lemon, juice of	½	1

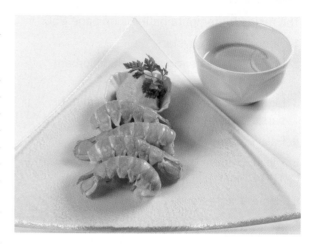

Langoustines are normally bought 'dipped'. This means they have already been blanched; they are not alive.

To make the bouillon

1 Place vegetables in pan and cover with water.
2 Gently bring to the boil and simmer for 5–10 minutes.
3 Add the white wine, parsley, chervil stalks and crushed peppercorns.
4 Cook for a further 10 minutes then leave to stand until cool.
5 Strain out the vegetables and chill the liquid.

To make the aioli

1 Pre-heat the oven to 200°C. Bake the sweet potato for about 35–45 minutes or until tender. Peel off the skin and gently crush the flesh.
2 Place sweet potato flesh in a liquidiser, add the mayonnaise, saffron, egg yolks and garlic and blend.
3 Add olive oil to moisten, season and finish with a squeeze of lemon juice.
4 Remove entrails from langoustines by taking the middle segment or tail shell between thumb and forefinger, then twist it and pull.
5 Plunge the langoustines into the simmering court bouillon for 30–40 seconds. Remove and leave to cool naturally. Serve with the aioli.

> **Chef's tips**
> Allow the bouillon to simmer gently and bring out the flavours.
> Be careful not to overcook the langoustines, as they will become tough.

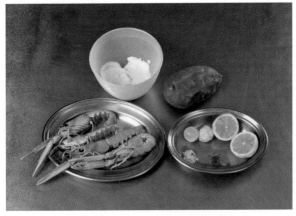

Ingredients for poached langoustines with aioli dip

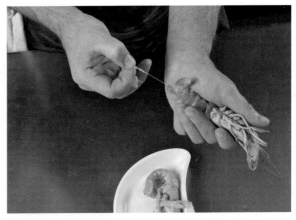

Pull out the cord from each langoustine before cooking

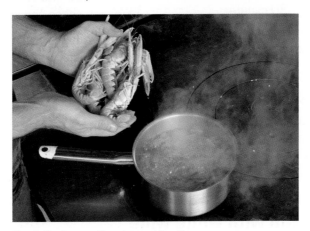

Poach the langoustines in court bouillon

35   Crab cakes with rocket salad and lemon dressing

4 portions	10 portions	
Crab cakes		
25 g	60 g	shallots, finely chopped
4	10	spring onions, finely chopped
75 ml	185 ml	fish/shellfish glaze
400 g	1 kg	crab meat
75 g	185 g	mayonnaise
1	3	lemons, juice of
2	5	plum tomatoes skinned, cut into concassée
1 tsp	3 tsp	wholegrain mustard
		seasoning

200 g	500 g	fresh white breadcrumbs
2	5	eggs, beaten with 100 ml of milk
		flour for rolling
Salad and dressing		
170 ml	425 ml	vegetable oil
25 ml	60 ml	white wine vinegar
1	3	lemons, juice of
		seasoning
250 g	625 g	washed and picked rocket
100 g	250 g	shaved Reggiano Parmesan

To make the crab cakes

1 Mix the shallots, spring onion and the fish glaze with the hand-picked crab meat.

2 Add the mayonnaise, lemon juice, tomato concassée and mustard, check and adjust the seasoning.

3 Allow to rest for 30 minutes in the refrigerator.

4 Scale into 80–90 g balls and shape into discs 1½ cm high, place in the freezer for 30 minutes to harden.

5 When firm to the touch, coat in breadcrumbs using the flour, egg and breadcrumbs.

6 Allow to rest for a further 30 minutes.

7 Heat a little oil in a non-stick pan, carefully place the cakes in and cook on each side until golden brown.

To make the salad and dressing

1 Combine the oil, vinegar and lemon juice together, check the seasoning.

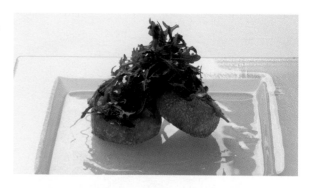

2 Place the rocket and Parmesan in a large bowl and add a little dressing, just to coat.

3 Place this in the centre of each plate, top with the crab cakes and serve.

Any excess crab meat can be used up in this recipe – a quick, classic dish. The crab can be exchanged for salmon or most fresh fish trimmings.

> **Chef's tip**
> Make sure that the crab mixture is divided into equal-sized cakes.

36 Mussels gratin with white wine

	4 portions	10 portions
shallots, chopped	50 g	125 g
parsley, chopped	1 tbsp	2 tbsp
white wine	60 ml	150 ml
strong fish stock	200 ml	500 ml
mussels	2 kg	5 kg
butter	25 g	60 ml
flour	25 g	60 ml
seasoning		
Gruyere cheese, grated		
fresh breadcrumbs		

1 Take a thick-bottomed pan and add the shallots, parsley, wine, fish stock and the cleaned mussels.

2 Cover with a tight-fitting lid and cook over a high heat until the shells open.

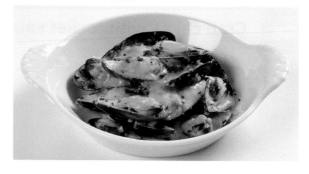

3 Drain off all the cooking liquor in a colander set over a clean bowl to retain the cooking juices.

4 Carefully check the mussels and discard any that have not opened.

5 Place in a dish and cover to keep warm.

6 Make a beurre manié from the flour and butter; pour over the cooking liquor, ensuring it is free from sand and stirring continuously to avoid lumps.

7 Correct the seasoning and garnish with more chopped parsley. Pour over the mussels.

8 Mix equal quantities of grated Gruyère and fresh breadcrumbs, sprinkle over the dish and gratinate until golden brown under the salamander; alternatively, bake in a moderate to high oven until golden brown on the top.

Chef's tip

Before starting to cook, check all the mussels and discard any that are already open: they are not fresh enough to use.

---

37 Lobster thermidor (homard thermidor)

cal	kcal	fat	sat fat	carb	sugar	protein	fibre
1973 KJ	475 kcal	35.8 g	19.5 g	10.8 g	1.1 g	28.1 g	0.4 g *

	4 portions	10 portions
lobsters, cooked	2	5
butter	25 g	60 g
shallots, finely chopped	12 g	30 g
dry white wine	60 ml	150 ml
English mustard, diluted	½ tsp	1 tsp
parsley, chopped		
mornay sauce (see page 210)	¼ litre	5/8 litre
Parmesan cheese, grated	25 g	60 g
picked parsley, to garnish		

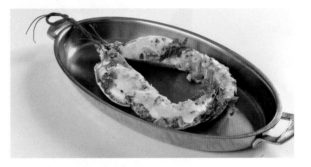

1 Remove the lobsters' claws and legs.

2 Carefully cut the lobsters in halves lengthwise. Remove the meat.

3 Discard the sac and remove the trail from the tail.

4 Wash the halves of shell and drain on a baking sheet.

5 Cut the lobster meat into thick escalopes.

6 Melt the butter in a sauteuse, add the chopped shallots and cook until tender, without colour.

7 Add the white wine to the shallots and allow to reduce to a quarter of its original volume.

8 Mix in the mustard and chopped parsley.

9 Add the lobster slices, season lightly with salt, mix carefully and allow to heat slowly for 2–3 minutes. If this part of the process is overdone the lobster will become tough and chewy.

10 Meanwhile, spoon a little of the warm mornay sauce into the bottom of each lobster half-shell.

11 Neatly add the warmed lobster pieces and the juice in which they were reheated. If there is an excess of liquid it should be reduced and incorporated into the mornay sauce.

12 Coat the half lobsters with the remaining mornay sauce, sprinkle with the Parmesan and place under a salamander until golden-brown. Serve garnished with picked parsley.

🍎 HEALTHY EATING TIP

- Use a small amount of unsaturated oil (olive or sunflower) to cook the lobster.

- Use little or no salt as the cheese will provide the necessary seasoning.

* Using mornay sauce as per Chapter 8

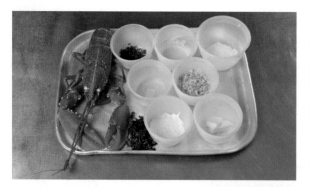

Ingredients for lobster thermidor

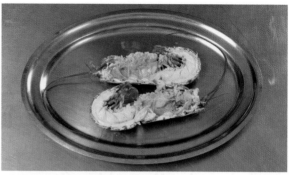

Open lobster halves

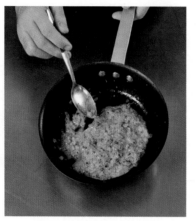

Prepare the shallot mixture

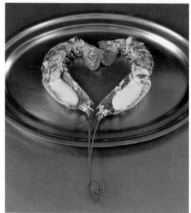

Fill the lobster halves and coat with sauce

38 Scallop ceviche with organic leaves

This recipe should be made one day prior to serving.

	4 portions	10 portions
large scallops (roe removed)	12	30
limes, juice of	2	5
oranges, juice of	1	3
lemons, grated rind	1	3
limes grated rind	1	3
orange	1	1
salt and freshly cracked pepper to taste		
orange liqueur	2 tbsp	5 tbsp
vinaigrette	50 ml	125 ml
organic leaves (5 varieties)	500 g	1¼ kg

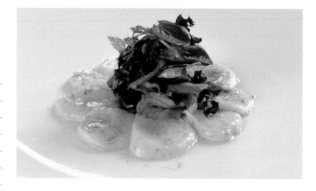

1 Slice the raw scallops thinly (laterally into 3) and lay on a clean non-reactive tray.

2 Mix all the other ingredients (except the organic leaves) and pour evenly over the scallops.

3 Leave covered in the refrigerator overnight. (The acid in the citrus juice will cure the scallops.)

4 To serve, arrange the scallops in a circle form (9 slices), dress the leaves and arrange in the centre of the scallops.

5 Drizzle any excess cure/dressing around the scallops and serve.

> Only the freshest scallops can be used for this recipe as the slightest taint of age will dominate and spoil the dish.
>
> ⚠ Some food safety experts discourage the consumption of uncooked shellfish.

---

39   Kalamarakia yemista (stuffed squid)

cal	kcal	fat	sat fat	carb	sugar	protein	fibre
1984 KJ	474 kcal	26.2 g	3.0 g	42.2 g	20.5 g	19.9 g	1.9 g

*

	4 portions	10 portions
medium-sized squid	4	10
onion, finely chopped	50 g	125 g
clove garlic, crushed and chopped	1	2–3
oil	60 ml	150 ml
wholegrain rice	100 g	250 g
fish stock	250 ml	725 ml
pine kernels	50 g	125 g
raisins	100 g	250 g
parsley, chopped		
salt, pepper		
dry white wine	125 ml	250 ml
tomatoes, skinned, deseeded, diced	200 g	500 g

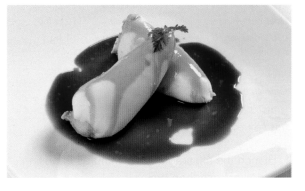

1 Prepare the squid: pull the body and head apart, remove the transparent pen from the bag and any soft remaining part. Rinse under cold water. Pull off the thin purple membrane on the outside.

2 Remove the tentacles and cut into pieces. Remove the ink sac. Reserve the ink to finish the sauce.

3 Sweat the onion and garlic in the oil.

4 Add the rice and moisten with half the fish stock. Stir and add the chopped tentacles, pine kernels, raisins and chopped parsley. Season. Stir well and allow to simmer for 5–8 minutes so that the rice is partly cooked.

5 Stuff the squid loosely with this mixture. Seal the end by covering with aluminium foil.

6 Lay the squid in a sauté pan with the remaining fish stock, white wine and tomatoes.

7 Cover with a lid and cook in a moderate oven at 180°C for 30–40 minutes, turning the squid gently during cooking. Cook very gently or the squid will burst.

8 When cooked, remove the squid and place in a suitable serving dish.

9 Reboil the cooking liquor and reduce by one-third. Strain the ink into the sauce, boil and reduce for 5 minutes. Check the seasoning.

10 Mask the squid with the sauce and finish with chopped parsley to serve.

🍎 HEALTHY EATING TIP

- Season with the minimum amount of salt.
- Use an unsaturated oil (olive or sunflower) and reduce the quantity used.
- Serve with a large mixed salad.

* Using approx. 400 g raw squid

40 Seafood stir-fry

cal	kcal	fat	sat fat	carb	sugar	protein	fibre
724 KJ	172 kcal	4.9 g	0.8 g	9.1 g	4.9 g	23.2 g	2.1 g

		4 portions	10 portions
small asparagus spears		100 g	250 g
sunflower or groundnut oil		1 tbsp	2½ tbsp
fresh ginger, grated		1 tsp	2½ tsp
leeks, cut into julienne		100 g	250 g
carrots, cut into julienne		100 g	250 g
baby sweetcorn		100 g	250 g
light soy sauce		2 tbsp	5 tbsp
oyster sauce		1 tbsp	2½ tbsp
clear honey		1 tsp	2½ tsp
cooked assorted shellfish	prawns	400 g	1 kg
	mussels		
	scallops		
Garnish			
large cooked prawns		4	10
fresh chives		25 g	62 g

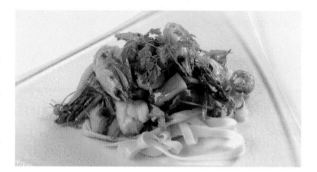

1 Blanch the asparagus for 2 minutes in boiling water, refresh then drain.

2 Heat the oil in a wok, add the ginger, leek, carrots and sweetcorn, stir-fry for 3 minutes without colour.

3 Add the soy and oyster sauce and honey. Stir.

4 Stir in the cooked shellfish and continue to stir-fry for 2–3 minutes until the vegetables are just tender and the shellfish is thoroughly heated through.

5 Add the blanched asparagus and stir-fry for another 1 minute.

6 Serve with fresh cooked noodles garnished with large fresh prawns and chopped chives.

Chef's tip

If you blanch the vegetables before stir-frying them, they will keep their colour and flavour, and can be fried more quickly.

HEALTHY EATING TIP

- No added salt is needed – soy sauce is high in sodium.

- Increasing the ratio of vegetables to seafood will improve the 'balance' of this dish.

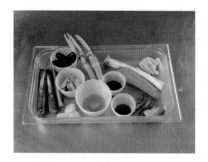

Ingredients for seafood stir-fry

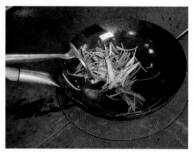

Fry the ginger and vegetables

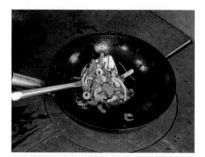

Combine all the ingredients and continue to stir-fry

41 Seafood in puff pastry (bouchées de fruits de mer)

cal	kcal	fat	sat fat	carb	sugar	protein	fibre	salt
1327 KJ	316 kcal	17.6 g	3.1 g	28.9 g	1.1 g	12.2 g	1.2 g	1.2 g *

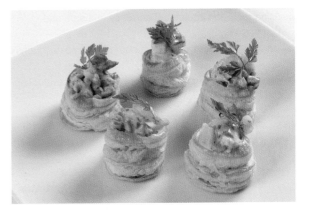

	4 portions	10 portions
button mushrooms	50 g	125 g
butter	25 g	60 g
lemon, juice of	¼	½
cooked lobster, prawns, shrimps, mussels, scallops	200 g	500 g
white wine sauce (see page 182)	125 ml	300 ml
chopped parsley		
salt, pepper		
puff pastry *bouchée* cases	4	10
picked parsley, to garnish		

1 Peel and wash the mushrooms, cut into neat dice.
2 Cook in butter with the lemon juice.
3 Add the cooked shellfish (mussels, prawns, shrimps left whole, the scallops and lobster cut into dice).
4 Cover the pan with a lid and heat through slowly for 3-4 minutes.
5 Add the white wine sauce and chopped parsley, and correct the seasoning.
6 Meanwhile warm the *bouchées* in the oven or hot plate.
7 Fill the bouchées with the mixture and place the lids on top.
8 Serve garnished with picked parsley.

Vol-au-vents can be prepared and cooked in the same way as *bouchées*.

Chef's tip
Try sweating the mushrooms in butter and white wine to bring out the flavour.

HEALTHY EATING TIP

- The white wine sauce is seasoned, so added salt is not required.
- Serve with a salad garnish.

* Fried in peanut oil

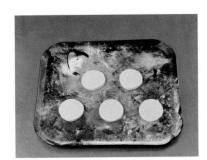
Raw puff pastry *bouchées*, before baking

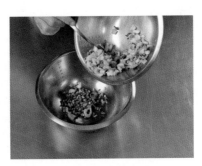
Combine the shellfish with the mushrooms

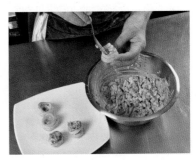
Fill the pastry cases

13 Prepare and cook rice, pasta, grains and egg dishes

In this chapter, you will learn how to:

1. prepare and cook rice, pasta, grains and eggs:

- using tools and equipment correctly, in a safe and hygienic way
- using the correct type and amount of rice, pasta, grains or eggs
- preparing, cooking, assembling, finishing and evaluating the dish

2. you should have the knowledge to:

- identify types of rice, pasta, grains and eggs, and their uses
- apply cooking principles and suitable methods of cookery, and identify adjustments needed
- identify sauces and accompaniments
- hold, cool and store dishes safely.

Number	Recipe title	Page number
Rice		
1	Braised or pilaff rice (*riz pilaff – Indian pilau*)	421
5	Paella (savoury rice with chicken, fish, vegetables and spices)	423
3	Plain boiled rice	422
7	Risotto of Jerusalem artichoke and truffle	425
6	Risotto with Parmesan (*risotto con Parmigiano*)	424
2	Steamed rice	422
4	Stir-fried rice	422
Pasta		
11	Cannelloni	429
17	Fresh egg pasta dough	433
8	Lasagne	426
14	Macaroni cheese	432
15	Noodles with butter	432
9	Pumpkin tortellini with brown butter balsamic vinaigrette	427
10	Ravioli	428
13	Spaghetti bolognaise (*spaghetti alla bolognese*)	431
12	Spaghetti with tomato sauce (*spaghetti alla pomodoro*)	430
18	Stuffings for pasta	434
16	Tagliatelle carbonara	433
	Wholewheat pasta dough	434

Number	Recipe title	Page number
Grains		
20	Couscous with chorizo sausage and chicken	436
19	Crisp polenta and roasted Mediterranean vegetables	435
Gnocchi		
21	Gnocchi parisienne (choux paste)	437
22	Gnocchi romaine (semolina)	438
Eggs		
30	Egg white omelette	443
	Eggs florentine	441
33	Eggs in cocotte (basic recipe) (*oeufs en cocotte*)	444
34	Eggs *sur le plat*	445
	Eggs Washington	441
28	French-fried eggs (deep-fried eggs)	442
27	Fried eggs (*oeufs frits*)	441
24	Hard-boiled eggs with cheese and tomato sauce (*oeufs aurore*)	439
	Mushroom omelette	443
29	Omelettes (basic recipe) (*omelette nature*)	442
26	Poached eggs with cheese sauce (*oeufs pochés mornay*)	440
32	Scotch eggs	444
23	Scrambled eggs (basic recipe) (*oeufs brouillés*)	439
25	Soft-boiled eggs (*oeufs mollets*)	440
31	Spanish omelette	443

Rice

Rice, a type of grain, is one of the world's most important crops. There are three basic kinds in culinary terms: long, medium and short grain. **Long-grain** is traditionally used in savoury dishes and **short-grain** in dessert cooking, although this varies across the globe. Wholegrain rice has a nuttier taste and contains more fibre and nutrients, but takes longer to cook (use one part grain to two parts water for 35–40 minutes). Arborio rice is a medium- to long-grain rice and is used in risottos because it can absorb a good deal of cooking liquid without becoming too soft. Rice flour is available but, because it is gluten free, it can't be used to make a yeasted loaf. Rice flakes (brown and white) can be added to muesli or made into a milk pudding or porridge.

Varieties

A hot, wet atmosphere is required for the cultivation of rice, and it is grown chiefly in India, the Far East, South America, Italy and the southern states of the USA. Rice is the main food crop for about half the world's population. In order to grow, it needs more water than any other cereal crop. There are around 250 different varieties of rice. The main ones are described below.

- **Long-grain:** a narrow, pointed grain that has had the full bran and most of the germ removed so that it is less fibrous than brown rice. Because of its firm structure, which helps to keep the grains separate when cooked, it is suitable for plain boiling and savoury dishes such as kedgeree and curry.

- **Brown grain:** any rice that has had the outer covering removed, but retains its bran and, as a result, is more nutritious and contains more fibre. It takes longer to cook than long-grain rice. The nutty flavour of brown rice lends itself to some recipes, but does not substitute well in traditional dishes such as paella, risotto or puddings. Any other rice recipes can be used (see recipes 1 to 4), but allow extra cooking time to soften the grain.

- **Short-grain:** a short, rounded grain with a soft texture, suitable for sweet dishes and risotto. *Arborio* is an Italian short-grain rice.

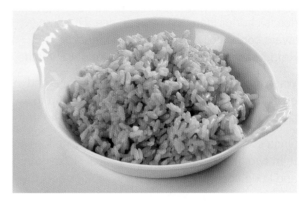

Brown rice

Many other types of rice are now available, which can add different colours and textures to dishes. Some of these are described below.

- **Basmati:** a narrow long-grain rice with a distinctive flavour, suitable for serving with Indian dishes. Basmati rice needs to be soaked before being cooked to remove excess starch.

- **Wholegrain rice:** the whole unprocessed grain of the rice.

- **Wild rice:** is not, in fact, a rice, but the seed of an aquatic grass. Difficulty in harvesting makes it expensive, but the colour (a purplish black) and its subtle nutty flavour make it a good base for a special dish or rice salad, and it can be economically mixed with other rices (but may need pre-cooking as it takes 45–50 minutes to cook, using one part grain to three parts water).

- **Red rice:** an unmilled short-grain rice from the Camargue in France, with a brownish-red colour and a nutty flavour. It is slightly sticky when cooked, and particularly good in salads.

- **Precooked instant rice:** par-boiled, ready cooked and boil-in-the-bag rice are similar.

- **Ground rice:** used for milk puddings (see page 476). *Rice flour* can be used for thickening cream soups. *Rice paper* is used for macaroons and nougat.

Aquatic: Relating to water. Wild rice is the seed of an 'aquatic grass' – one that grows in water.

Rice is a very useful and versatile carbohydrate. When added to dishes it helps to proportionally reduce the fat content.

Storage

Uncooked rice can be stored on the shelf in a tightly sealed container. The shelf life of brown rice is shorter than that of white rice. The bran layers contain oil that can become rancid. Refrigeration is recommended for longer shelf life.

Washing rice is not necessary; just measure and cook. Cooked rice can be refrigerated for up to seven days or stored in the freezer for six months.

Once cooked, keep hot (above 65°C for no longer than two hours) or cool quickly (within 90 minutes) and keep cool (below 5°C). If this is not done, the spores of *Bacillus cereus* (a bacterium found in the soil) may revert to bacteria and multiply.

ACTIVITY

1 How should cooked rice be stored?

2 Name two types of long-grain rice.

3 What is wild rice?

4 How is pilaff rice cooked?

5 What is the basic difference between pilaff and risotto?

6 Which type of bacillus bacteria is associated with rice?

Pasta

Pasta is the name for a type of food consisting of dough made from durum wheat and water, thought to be originally from Italy. The dough is stretched and flattened into various shapes and either used fresh or dried.

Food value

Durum wheat has a 15 per cent protein content, which makes it a good alternative to rice and potatoes for vegetarians. Pasta also contains carbohydrates in the form of starch, which gives the body energy.

Storage

Dry pasta can be stored almost indefinitely if kept in a tightly sealed package or a covered container in a cool, dry place.

If cooked pasta is not to be used immediately, drain and rinse thoroughly with cold water. If it is left to sit in water, it will continue to absorb water and become mushy. When the pasta is cool, drain and toss lightly with salad oil to prevent it

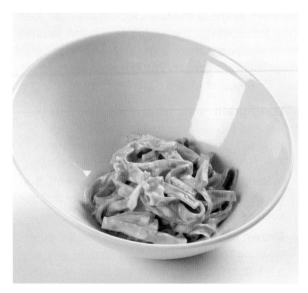

Green fettucine pasta with ham and creamy cheese (recipe available on Dynamic Learning)

from sticking and drying out. Cover tightly and refrigerate or freeze. Refrigerate the pasta and sauce separately or the pasta will become soggy. To reheat, put pasta in a colander and immerse in rapidly boiling water just long enough to heat through. Do not allow it to continue to cook. Pasta may also be reheated in a microwave.

Preparation

Cooking fresh and dried pasta
http://bit.ly/wTU9K2

Bring plenty of water (at least 3.8 litres for every 585 g of dry pasta) to a rolling boil. Add about 1 tbsp of salt per 4 litres of water, if desired. Add the pasta in small quantities to maintain the rolling boil. Stir frequently to prevent sticking. Do not cover the pan. Follow package directions for cooking time. Do not overcook. Pasta should be 'al dente' (meaning 'to the tooth' – tender, yet firm). It should be slightly resistant to the bite, but cooked through. Drain to stop the cooking action. Do not rinse unless the recipe says to do so. For salads, drain and rinse pasta with cold water.

About dried pasta

There is an almost infinite number of types of pasta asciutta. Almost 90 per cent of the pasta eaten in Italy is dried. A rule of thumb for portion weights is 80–100 g per portion as a starter course and, if larger portions are required, increase accordingly; traditionally pasta is eaten predominantly as a starter.

Most types of dried pasta will cook perfectly well in under 10 minutes. The cooking times on British packaging are often too long. Spaghetti that has been stored for too long and is over-dry may take longer and you might not want to eat the result.

Allow 500 ml to 1 litre of water per person – the more the better. The reason for this is that the water should always be at a rolling boil. The more water in proportion to pasta the quicker it will return to the boil after the pasta is added. This means fast cooking and better-textured pasta.

Some recipe books suggest that you add a little oil to the water when cooking pasta. This has no benefit when cooking dried pasta; it was a

method of storage in restaurants when the pasta (predominantly spaghetti) was pre-cooked and a little oil was added to the reheating water to prevent it sticking together.

> **Infinite:** Endless; so many that it cannot be measured.

Types of pasta and sauces

There are basically four types of pasta, each of which may be plain, or flavoured with spinach or tomato:

1 dried durum wheat pasta

2 egg pasta

3 semolina pasta

4 wholewheat pasta.

These come in myriad shapes and sizes, the most common in the UK include spaghetti, fettuccini (long, narrow ribbons), penne (short tubes cut diagonally), farfalle (bow tie or butterfly shaped), and fusilli (short spirals). Stuffed pasta includes cannelloni (tubes), ravioli and tortellini (see below). Sheets of pasta are used for lasagne.

Examples of sauces to go with pasta include:

- tomato sauce
- cream, butter or béchamel-based sauces
- rich meat sauce
- olive oil and garlic
- soft white or blue cheese
- pesto (see page 197).

Tortellini and its history

Tortellini literally means 'navel of Venus' (the Roman goddess of love) and derives from its shape. As legend would have it, Venus and Jupiter were planning to get together one night. When Venus checked into an inn, the chef found out. He went to her room, peeped through the keyhole and saw Venus lying there, half-naked in bed on her back. When the chef saw her navel, he was inspired to rush to the kitchen to create a stuffed pasta that looked like it, and thus arose the legend of the famous tortellina (tortellini is plural). About the size of a 10 pence piece, this is a round, wrinkled pasta, usually filled with cheese and other variant ingredients like meat.

Pasta cooking with cheese

Examples of cheeses used in pasta cooking include those described below.

Parmesan

The most popular hard cheese used with pasta, ideal for grating. The flavour is best when it is freshly grated. If it is bought ready grated, or if it is grated and stored, the flavour deteriorates.

Pecorino

A strong ewes' milk cheese, sometimes studded with peppercorns. Used for strongly flavoured dishes, it can be grated or thinly sliced.

Ricotta

Creamy-white in colour, made from the discarded whey of other cheeses, ricotta is widely used in fillings for pasta such as cannelloni and ravioli, and for sauces.

Mozzarella

Traditionally made from the milk of the water buffalo, mozzarella is pure white and creamy, with a mild but distinctive flavour, and usually round or pear-shaped. It will keep for only a few days in a container half-filled with milk and water.

Gorgonzola or Dolcelatte

These are both distinctive blue cheeses that can be used in sauces.

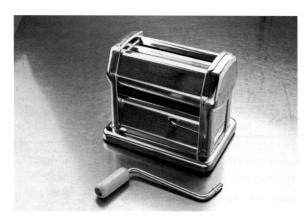

Pasta machine

Ingredients for pasta dishes

The following are some examples of ingredients that can be used in pasta dishes. The list is almost endless, but can include:

smoked salmon	prawns
shrimps	mussels
scallops	tongue
lobster	chicken livers
tuna fish	smoked ham
crab	mustard and cress
anchovies	parsley
cockles	rosemary
avocado	basil
mushrooms	tarragon
tomatoes	fennel
onions	chives
courgettes	spring onions
peas	marjoram
spinach	pine nuts
chillies	walnuts
peppers	stoned olives
broad beans	capers
broccoli	cooked, dried beans
sliced sausage	eggs
salami	grated lemon zest
ham	saffron
bacon	grated nutmeg
beef	sultanas
chicken	balsamic vinegar
duck	

Summary: cooking pasta

- Allow 50 g dry weight as a first course, 100 g as a main course.
- Always cook pasta in plenty of gently boiling salted water.
- Stir to the boil.
- Do not overcook.
- When cooking fresh pasta, add a little oil to the water to prevent the pieces sticking together.
- If not to be used immediately, refresh and reheat carefully in hot salted water when required. Drain well in a colander.
- With most pasta, freshly grated cheese (Parmesan) should be served separately.

✎ ACTIVITY

1 Which type of flour is used for pasta dough?

2 Name four different pasta shapes.

3 What does 'al dente' mean?

4 How should cooked pasta be stored?

5 What is the difference between the techniques for making ravioli and cannelloni?

Grains

Grain is the term used for any cultivated cereal used as food. There are many different varieties.

Barley

Barley grows in a wider variety of climatic conditions than any other cereal. Usually found in the shops as whole or pot barley (or polished pearl barley) you can also buy barley flakes or kernels. It can be cooked on its own (one part grain to three parts water for 45–60 minutes) as an alternative to rice, pasta or potatoes, or added to stews. Malt extract is made from sprouted barley grains.

Barley must have its fibrous hull (outer shell) removed before it is eaten (hulled barley). Hulled barley still has its bran and germ and is considered a whole grain, making it a popular health food. Pearl barley is hulled barley that has been processed further to remove the bran.

Buckwheat

When roasted, the seeds of buckwheat are dark reddish-brown. It can be cooked (one part grain to two parts water for 6 minutes, leave to stand for 6 minutes) and served like rice, or it can be added to stews and casseroles. Buckwheat flour can be added to cakes, muffins and pancakes, where it gives a distinctive flavour. Soba noodles, made from buckwheat, are an essential ingredient in Japanese cooking. Buckwheat is gluten free.

Corn/maize

Fresh corn – available in the form of **sweetcorn** and **corn on the cob** – is eaten as a vegetable.

The dried grain is most often eaten as cornflakes or popcorn. Tortillas are made from maize meal, as are quite a lot of snack foods. The flour made from corn (cornmeal or maize meal) is used to make Italian **polenta**, and can be added to soup, pancakes and muffins. When cooking polenta (one part grain to three parts water, for 15–20 minutes), stir carefully to avoid lumps. Use it like mashed potato: it is quite bland, so try stirring in tasty ingredients like Gorgonzola, Parmesan and fresh herbs, or press it when cold, cut into slices, brush with garlicky olive oil, and grill. You can also get readymade polenta. Don't confuse cornmeal with refined corn starch/flour, used for thickening. Corn is gluten free.

Millet

The millets are a group of small-seeded cereal crops or grains widely grown around the world for food and fodder. The main millet varieties are:

- pearl millet
- foxtail millet
- proso millet, also known as common millet, broom corn millet, hog millet or white millet
- finger millet.

As none of the millets is closely related to wheat, they can be eaten by those with coeliac disease or other forms of allergies/intolerances to wheat. Coeliac patients can replace certain cereal grains in their diets with millets in various forms, including breakfast cereals. Millet can also often be used in place of buckwheat, rice or quinoa.

Coeliac disease: A disease in which a person is unable to digest the protein gluten (found in wheat, and other cereals). Gluten causes the person's immune system to attack its own tissues, specifically the lining of the small intestine. Symptoms include diarrhoea, bloating, abdominal pain, weight loss and malnutrition.

In western India, millet flour (called 'bajari' in Marathi) has been commonly used with 'jowar' (sorghum) flour for hundreds of years to make the local staple flat bread, 'bhakri'.

The protein content in millet is very close to that of wheat; both provide about 11 per cent protein by weight. Millets are rich in B vitamins (especially niacin, B6 and folacin), calcium, iron, potassium, magnesium and zinc. Millets contain no gluten, so they cannot rise for bread. However, when combined with wheat or xanthan gum (for those who have coeliac disease), they can be used to make raised bread. Alone, they are suited to flatbread.

Millet can be used as an alternative to rice, but the tiny grains need to be cracked before they will absorb water easily. Before boiling, sauté with a little vegetable oil for 2–3 minutes until some crack, then add water carefully (one part grain to three parts water). Bring to the boil and simmer for 15–20 minutes until fluffy. Millet flakes can be made into porridge or added to muesli. Millet flour is available, sometimes made into pasta.

Oats

There are various grades of oatmeal, rolled oats or jumbo oat flakes. All forms can be used to make porridge, combined with groundnuts to make a nut roast, or added to stews. Oatmeal is low in gluten so can't be used to make a loaf, but can be mixed with wheat flour to add flavour and texture to bread, muffins and pancakes. Oatmeal contains some oils and can become rancid, so keep an eye on the best-before date.

Oatmeal is created by grinding oats into coarse powder; various grades are available depending on thoroughness of grinding (including coarse, pinhead and fine). The main uses of oats are:

- as an ingredient in baking
- in the manufacture of bannocks or oatcakes
- as a stuffing for poultry
- as a coating for some cheeses
- as an ingredient of black pudding
- for making traditional porridge (or 'porage').

Rye

Rye is one of the few cereals (along with wheat and barley) that has enough gluten to make a yeasted loaf. However, with less gluten than wheat, rye flour makes a denser, richer-flavoured bread. It is more usual to mix rye flour with wheat flour. Rye grains should be cooked using one part grain to three parts water for 45–60 minutes. Kibbled (cracked) rye is often added to granary-type loaves. Rye grains can be added to stews, and rye flakes are good in muesli.

Spelt

Originating in the Middle East, spelt is closely related to common wheat and has been popular for decades in eastern Europe. It has an intense nutty, wheaty flavour. The flour is excellent for breadmaking and spelt pasta is becoming more widely available.

Wheat

This is the most familiar cereal in Britain today, used for bread, cakes, biscuits, pastry, breakfast cereals and pasta. Wheat grains can be eaten whole (cook one part grain to three parts water for 40–60 minutes) and have a satisfying, chewy texture. Cracked or kibbled wheat is the dried whole grains cut by steel blades. **Bulgar wheat** is parboiled before cracking, has a light texture and only needs rehydrating by soaking in boiling water or stock. **Semolina** is a grainy yellow flour ground from durum or hard wheat, and is the main ingredient of dried Italian pasta. **Couscous** is made from semolina grains that have been rolled, dampened and coated with finer wheat flour. Soak couscous in two parts of water/stock to rehydrate; traditionally, it is steamed after soaking. Strong wheat flour (with a high gluten content) is required for yeasted breadmaking. Plain flour is used for general cooking, including cakes and shortcrust pastry. Wheat flakes are used for porridge, muesli and flapjacks.

Quinoa

Quinoa is an ancient crop that fed the South American Aztec Indians for thousands of years, and has recently been cultivated in Britain. It is a seed that is high in protein, making it useful for vegetarians.

The small, round grains look similar to millet, but are pale brown in colour. The taste is mild, and the texture firm and slightly chewy. It can be cooked like millet and absorbs twice its volume in liquid. Cook for 15 minutes (one part grain to three parts water); it is ready when all the grains have turned from white to transparent, and the spiral-like germ has separated. Use in place of more common cereals or pasta, or in place of rice (risottos, pilaff) and is served in salads and some stuffings.

ACTIVITY

1 Name three different types of grain used in culinary work.

2 What is the nutritional value of grains in a menu?

3 Design a dish using a basic grain ingredient.

Eggs

Eggs are used widely in all sorts of cooking, both savoury and sweet. An important ingredient in many recipes, eggs are used for binding, enriching, colouring, emulsifying and aerating.

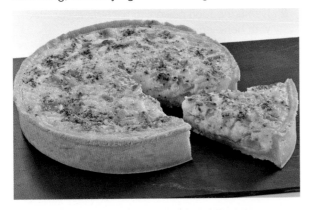

Eggs are an essential ingredient for quiche fillings

Types of egg

Hens' eggs are almost exclusively used for cookery, but eggs from turkeys, geese, ducks, guinea fowl, quail and gulls are also edible.

Quails' eggs are used in a variety of ways, for example, as a garnish to many hot and cold dishes; as a starter or main course, such as a salad of assorted leaves with hot wild mushrooms and poached quail eggs, or tartlet of quail eggs on chopped mushrooms coated with hollandaise sauce.

Sizes

Hens' eggs are graded in four sizes: small, medium, large and very large, as shown in Table 13.1.

Table 13.1 Hens' egg sizes

Very large	73 g+	Size 0
		Size 1
Large	63–73 g	Size 1
		Size 2
		Size 3
Medium	53–63 g	Size 3
		Size 4
		Size 5
Small	53 g and under	Size 5
		Size 6
		Size 7

Purchasing and quality

The size of the eggs does not affect their quality, but it does affect their price. Eggs are tested for quality, then weighed and graded. When buying eggs, the following points should be noted.

- The eggshell should be clean, well shaped, strong and slightly rough.

- When eggs are broken there should be a high proportion of thick white to thin white. If an egg is kept, the thick white gradually changes into thin white, and water passes from the white into the yolk.

- The yolk should be firm, round (not flattened) and of a good even colour. Over time, as eggs are kept, the yolk loses strength and begins to flatten, water evaporates from the egg and is replaced by air.

Food value

Eggs are useful as a main dish as they provide the energy, fat, minerals and vitamins needed for growth and repair of the body. The fat in the egg yolk is high in saturated fat. The egg white is made up of protein and water (see recipe 30, egg white omelette).

Salmonella

Hens can pass salmonella bacteria into their eggs and thus cause food poisoning. To reduce this risk, pasteurised eggs may be used where appropriate (e.g. in omelettes, scrambled eggs).

Storage

Store eggs in a cool but not too dry place – 0°C to 5°C is ideal – where the humidity of the air and the amount of carbon dioxide present are controlled. Eggs will keep for up to nine months under these conditions.

Because eggshells are porous, the eggs will absorb any strong odours, so they should not be stored near strong-smelling foods such as onions, fish and cheese.

Pasteurised eggs are washed, sanitised and then broken into sterilised containers. After combining the yolks and whites they are strained, pasteurised – heated to 63°C for 1 minute – then rapidly cooled.

Health, safety and hygiene

- Eggs should be stored in a cool place, preferably under refrigeration.

- They should be stored away from possible contaminants, such as raw meat, fish and strong-smelling foods.

- Stocks should be rotated: first in, first out.

- Hands should be washed before and after handling eggs.

- Cracked eggs should not be used.

- Preparation surfaces, utensils and containers should be cleaned regularly and always cleaned between preparation of different dishes.

- Egg dishes should be consumed as soon as possible after preparation or, if not for immediate use, refrigerated.

Versatility

Fried, scrambled, poached and boiled eggs, and omelettes are mainly served at breakfast. A variety of dishes may be served for lunch, high tea, supper and snacks. They are also used widely in baking and in desserts.

 ACTIVITY

1 How is the quality of hens' eggs determined?

2 Name the food poisoning bacteria associated with hens' eggs.

3 Name four basic egg dishes.

Test yourself • • • • • • • • • • • • • • • •

1 State the difference between wholegrain and basmati rice.

2 Describe the difference between bulgar wheat, semolina and couscous.

3 At what temperature do you poach eggs, and why add vinegar to the water?

4 Which bacteria is associated with egg contamination?

5 Describe the difference between a braised rice and a risotto.

6 State the main ingredients of a paella.

7 Describe the difference between ravioli and cannelloni.

8 State the difference between gnocchi parisienne and gnocchi romaine.

• •

1 Braised or pilaff rice *(riz pilaff* – Indian pilau)

cal	kcal	fat	sat fat	carb	sugar	protein	fibre
774 KJ	184 kcal	10.4 g	4.5 g	22.1 g	0.3 g	1.9 g	0.6 g

*

	4 portions	10 portions
butter or oil	50 g	125 g
onion, chopped	25 g	60 g
rice, long grain, white or brown	300 g	750 g
white stock (preferably chicken)	600 ml	1 litre
salt, mill pepper		
butter, to finish	50 g	125 g

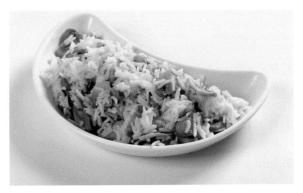

1 Place the butter or oil into a small sauteuse. Add the onion.

2 Cook gently without colouring for 2–3 minutes. Add the rice.

3 Cook gently without colouring for 2–3 minutes.

4 Add twice the amount of stock to rice.

5 Season, cover with buttered paper, bring to the boil.

6 Place in a hot oven (230–250°C) for approximately 15 minutes, until cooked.

7 Remove immediately into a cool sauteuse.

8 Carefully mix in the additional butter with a two-pronged fork.

9 Correct the seasoning and serve.

It is usual to use long-grain rice for pilaff because the grains are firm, and there is less likelihood of them breaking up and becoming mushy. During cooking, long-grain rice absorbs more liquid, loses less starch and retains its shape as it swells; short or medium grains may split at the ends and become less distinct.

Chef's tip
Cook the rice for the exact time specified in the recipe. If it cooks for longer, it will be overcooked and the grains will not separate.

Try something different

- Add wild mushrooms as shown in the photo – about 50–100 g for 4 portions.
- Pilaff may also be infused with herbs and spices such as cardamom.

HEALTHY EATING TIP

- Use an unsaturated oil (sunflower or olive). Lightly oil the pan and drain off any excess after the frying is complete.
- Keep the added salt to a minimum.

Using white rice and hard margarine. Using brown rice and hard margarine, 1 portion provides: 769 kJ/183 kcal Energy; 10.9 g Fat; 4.6 g Sat Fat; 20.7 g Carb; 0.7 g Sugar; 1.9 g Protein; 1.0 g Fibre

2 Steamed rice

cal	kcal	fat	sat fat	carb	sugar	protein	fibre
1277 KJ	305 kcal	1.4 g	0.0 g	63.7 g	0.0 g	7.1 g	0.0 g

	4 portions	12 portions
rice (dry weight)	300 g	750 g

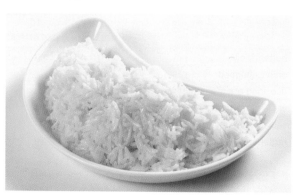

1 Place the washed rice into a saucepan and add water until the water level is 2.5 cm above the rice.

2 Bring to the boil over a fierce heat until most of the water has evaporated.

3 Turn the heat down as low as possible, cover the pan with a lid and allow the rice to complete cooking in the steam.

4 Once cooked, the rice should be allowed to stand in the covered steamer for 10 minutes.

3 Plain boiled rice

cal	kcal	fat	sat fat	carb	sugar	protein	fibre
37 KJ	90 kcal	0.1 g	0.0 g	8.2 g	20.0 g	1.9 g	0.0 g

	4 portions	12 portions
rice (dry weight)	300 g	750 g

1 Pick and wash the long-grain rice. Add to plenty of boiling salted water.

2 Stir to the boil and simmer gently until tender (approx. 12–15 minutes).

3 Pour into a sieve and rinse well under cold running water, then boiling water. Drain and leave in sieve, placed over a bowl and covered with a cloth.

4 Place on a tray in the hotplate and keep hot.

5 Serve separately in a vegetable dish.

4 Stir-fried rice

cal	kcal	fat	sat fat	carb	sugar	protein	fibre	
1423 KJ	338 kcal	10.2 g	1.9 g	30.6 g	0.6 g	32.7 g	0.6 g	*

Stir-fried rice dishes consist of a combination of cold pre-cooked rice and ingredients such as cooked meat or poultry, fish, vegetables or egg.

1 Prepare and cook meat or poultry in fine shreds; dice and lightly cook any vegetables. Add bean sprouts just before the egg.

2 Place a wok or thick-bottomed pan over fierce heat, add some oil and heat until smoking.

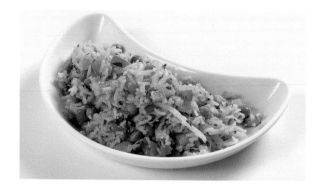

3 Add the cold rice and stir-fry for about 1 minute.

4 Add the other ingredients and continue to stir-fry over fierce heat for 4–5 minutes.

5 Add the beaten egg and continue cooking for a further 1–2 minutes.

6 Correct the seasoning and serve immediately.

 HEALTHY EATING TIP

- Use an unsaturated oil (sunflower or olive) to lightly oil the pan.

- Soy sauce adds sodium, so no added salt is needed.

Using 125 g chicken (average dark and light meat) and 25 g mung beans per portion

---

5 **Paella (savoury rice with chicken, fish, vegetables and spices)**

cal	kcal	fat	sat fat	carb	sugar	protein	fibre
3383 KJ	804 kcal	31.0 g	6.2 g	48.8 g	3.8 g	85.7 g	1.3 g

	4 portions	10 portions
cooked lobster	400 g	1 kg
squid	200 g	500 g
gambas (Mediterranean prawns), cooked	400 g	1 kg
mussels	400 g	1 kg
white stock	1 litre	2½ litres
pinch of saffron		
onion, finely chopped	50 g	125 g
clove garlic, finely chopped	1	2–3
red pepper, diced	50 g	125 g
green pepper, diced	50 g	125 g
roasting chicken, cut for sauté	1½ kg	3¾ kg
olive oil	60 ml	150 ml
short-grain rice	200 g	500 g
thyme		
bay leaf		
seasoning		
tomatoes, skinned, deseeded, diced	200 g	500 g
lemon wedges, to finish		

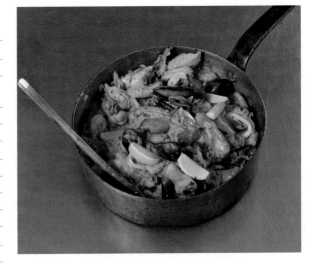

1 Prepare the lobster: cut it in half, remove the claws and legs, discard the sac and trail. Remove the meat from the claws and cut the tail into 3–4 pieces, leaving the meat in the shell.

2 Clean the squid, pull the body and head apart. Extract the transparent 'pen' from the body. Rinse well, pulling off the thin purple membrane on the outside. Remove the ink sac. Cut the body into rings and the tentacles into 1 cm lengths.

3 Prepare the gambas by shelling the body.

4 Shell the mussels and retain the cooking liquid.

5 Boil the white stock and mussel liquor together, infused with saffron. Simmer for 5–10 minutes.

6 Sweat the finely chopped onion in a suitable pan, without colour. Add the garlic and the peppers.

7 Sauté the chicken in olive oil until cooked and golden brown, then drain.

8 Add the rice to the onions and garlic and sweat for 2 minutes.

9 Add about 200 ml white stock and mussel liquor.

10 Add the thyme, bay leaf and seasoning. Bring to the boil, then cover with a lightly oiled greaseproof paper and lid. Cook for 5–8 minutes, in a moderately hot oven at 180°C.

11 Add the squid and cook for another 5 minutes.

12 Add the tomatoes, chicken and lobster pieces, mussels and gambas. Stir gently, cover with a lid and reheat the rice in the oven.

13 Correct the consistency of the rice if necessary by adding more stock, so that it looks sufficiently moist without being too wet. Correct the seasoning.

14 When all is reheated and cooked, place in a suitable serving dish, decorate with 4 (10) gambas and 4 (10) mussels halved and shelled. Finish with wedges of lemon.

> For a traditional paella, a raw lobster may be used, which should be prepared as follows. Remove the legs and claws and crack the claws. Cut the lobster in half crosswise, between the tail and the carapace. Cut the carapace in two lengthwise. Discard the sac. Cut across the tail in thick slices through the shell. Remove the trail, wash the lobster pieces and cook with the rice.

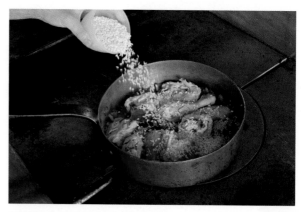

Add the rice and cook into a risotto

HEALTHY EATING TIP

- To reduce the fat, skin the chicken and use a little unsaturated oil to sweat the onions and fry the chicken.

- No added salt is necessary.

- Serve with a large green salad.

* Using edible chicken meat

ASSESSMENT

6 Risotto with Parmesan (*risotto con Parmigiano*)

cal	kcal	fat	sat fat	carb	sugar	protein	fibre	salt
2598 KJ	621 kcal	36.2 g	14.1 g	49.9 g	4.2 g	23.0 g	0.3 g	1.4 g

This is the classic risotto. With the addition of saffron and bone marrow it becomes risotto Milanese.

	4 portions	10 portions
chicken stock	1.2 litres	3 litres
butter	80 g	200 g
onion, peeled and finely chopped	½	1
Arborio rice	240 g	600 g
Parmesan, freshly grated	75 g	180 g
salt, pepper		

1 Bring the stock to a simmer, next to where you will cook the risotto. Take a wide, heavy-bottomed pan or casserole, put half the butter in over a medium heat and melt.

2 Add the onion and sweat until it softens and becomes slightly translucent.

3 Add the rice and stir with a heat-resistant spatula until it is thoroughly coated in butter (about 2 minutes). Then take a soup ladle of hot stock and pour it into the rice.

4 Continue to cook and stir until this liquid addition is completely absorbed (about 3 minutes).

5 Repeat this procedure several times until the rice has swollen and is nearly tender. The rice should not be soft but neither should it be chalky. Taste and wait: if it is undercooked, it will leave a gritty, chalky residue in your mouth.

6 Normally the rice is ready in about 20 minutes after the first addition of stock

7 Add the other half of the butter and half the Parmesan off the heat. Stir these in, season and cover. Leave to rest and swell a little more for 3 minutes. Serve immediately after this in soup plates, with more Parmesan offered separately.

 HEALTHY EATING TIP

- Use an unsaturated oil (sunflower or olive). Lightly oil the pan and drain off any excess after the frying is complete.

- Additional salt is not necessary.

- Serve with a large salad and tomato bread.

Try something different

Risotto variations include:

- **saffron or Milanese-style** – soak ¼ teaspoon saffron in a little hot stock and mix into the risotto near the end of the cooking time

- **seafood** – add any one or a mixture of cooked mussels, shrimp, prawns, etc., just before the rice is cooked; also use half fish stock, half chicken stock

- **mushrooms**.

Chef's tips
Add the stock slowly, to give the rice time to absorb the liquid.
Stir regularly during cooking.

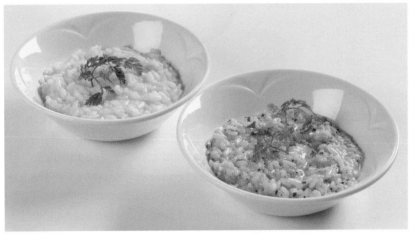

Risotto with Parmesan (left) and with Jerusalem artichoke and truffle (right)

7 Risotto of Jerusalem artichoke and truffle

	4 portions	10 portions
shallots, diced	50 g	125 g
vegetable oil	10 g	25 g
risotto rice (Carnaroli)	150 g	375 g
white wine	75 ml	180 ml
vegetable stock	1 litre	2½ litres
artichoke purée	10 g	25 g
butter	50 g	125 g
seasoning		
Parmesan Reggiano, grated		

	4 portions	10 portions
truffle oil		
chives, chopped	5 g	12 g
chervil, freshly picked		
truffle, chopped (optional)	25 g	62 g

1 Sweat the shallots in the oil, without colour, for 5 minutes.

2 Add the rice and sweat for a further minute.

3 Add the wine and cook out until completely reduced.

4 Add the stock ladle by ladle until the rice is 95 per cent cooked. (You may not need all the stock.)

5 Add the purée and butter and reduce until emulsified.

6 Season the risotto, then add the Parmesan, truffle and chives.

7 To serve, place the risotto in a bowl and garnish with some picked chervil and freshly sliced truffle (optional).

Chef's tip
Add the stock slowly, stirring well, to create a pudding-like consistency.

---

8 ## Lasagne

cal	kcal	fat	sat fat	carb	sugar	protein	fibre
2416 KJ	575 kcal	28.7 g	11.4 g	56.1 g	10.0 g	26.7 g	5.8 g

	4 portions	10 portions
lasagne	200 g	500 g
oil	1 tbsp	3 tbsp
thin strips of streaky bacon	50 g	125 g
onion, chopped	100 g	250 g
carrot, chopped	50 g	125 g
celery, chopped	50 g	125 g
minced beef	200 g	500 g
tomato purée	50 g	125 g
jus-lié or demi-glace	375 ml	1 litre
clove garlic	1	1½
salt, pepper		
marjoram	½ tsp	1½ tsp
sliced mushrooms	100 g	250 g
béchamel or mornay sauce (see pages 184 and 185)	250 ml	600 ml
Parmesan or Cheddar cheese, grated	25 g	125 g

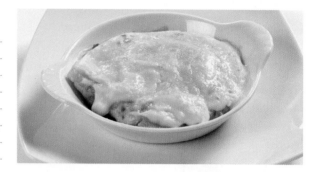

1 This recipe can be made using 200 g of ready-bought lasagne or it can be prepared fresh using 200 g flour noodle paste. Wholemeal lasagne can be made using noodle paste made with 100 g wholemeal flour and 100 g strong flour.

2 Prepare the noodle paste and roll out to 1 mm thick.

3 Cut into 6 cm squares.

4 Allow to rest in a cool place and dry slightly on a cloth dusted with flour.

5 Whether using fresh or ready-bought lasagne, cook in gently simmering salted water for approximately 10 minutes.

6 Refresh in cold water, then drain on a cloth.

7 Gently heat the oil in a thick-bottomed pan, add the bacon and cook for 2–3 minutes.

8 Add the onion, carrot and celery, cover the pan with a lid and cook for 5 minutes.

9 Add the minced beef, increase the heat and stir until lightly brown.

10 Remove from the heat and mix in the tomato purée.

11 Return to the heat, mix in the jus-lié or demi-glace, stir to boil.

12 Add the garlic, salt, pepper and marjoram, and simmer for 15 minutes. Remove the garlic.

13 Mix in the mushrooms, reboil for 2 minutes, then remove from the heat.

14 Butter an ovenproof dish and cover the bottom with a layer of the meat sauce.

15 Add a layer of lasagne and cover with meat sauce.

16 Add another layer of lasagne and cover with the remainder of the meat sauce.

17 Cover with the béchamel or mornay sauce.

18 Sprinkle with cheese, cover with a lid and place in a moderately hot oven at 190°C for approximately 20 minutes.

19 Remove the lid, cook for a further 15 minutes and serve in the cleaned ovenproof dish.

> Fillings for lasagne can be varied in many ways. Tomato sauce may be used instead of jus-lié.

Try something different

Traditionally, pasta dishes are substantial in quantity but because they are so popular they are also sometimes requested as lighter dishes. Obviously the portion size can be reduced but other variations can also be considered.

For example, freshly made pasta cut into 8–10 cm rounds or squares, rectangles or diamonds, lightly poached or steamed, well drained and placed on a light tasty mixture (e.g. a tablespoon of mousse of chicken, or fish or shellfish, well-cooked dried

spinach flavoured with toasted pine nuts and grated nutmeg, duxelle mixture) using just the one piece of pasta on top or a piece top and bottom. A light sauce should be used (e.g. a measure of well-reduced chicken stock with a little skimmed milk, blitzed to a froth just before serving, pesto sauce, a drizzle of good-quality olive oil, or a light tomato sauce. The dish can be finished with a suitable garnish (e.g. lightly fried wild or cultivated sliced mushrooms).

 HEALTHY EATING TIP

- Use an unsaturated oil (sunflower or olive). Lightly oil the pan and drain off any excess after the frying is complete. Skim the fat from the finished dish.

- Season with the minimum amount of salt.

- The fat content can be proportionally reduced by increasing the ratio of pasta to sauce and thinning the béchamel.

ASSESSMENT

9 Pumpkin tortellini with brown butter balsamic vinaigrette

cal	kcal	fat	sat fat	carb	sugar	protein	fibre
1744 KJ	417 kcal	24.6 g	9.0 g	43.2 g	4.1 g	8.2 g	3.0 g

	4 portions	10 portions
small pumpkin	1	2½
olive oil	1 tbsp	2½ tbsp
ground cinnamon	½ tsp	1¼ tsp
ground nutmeg	¼ tsp	3/4 tsp
caster sugar	1 tsp	1½ tsp
seasoning		
ravioli paste (recipe 10)		
egg	1	2
butter	50 g	125 g
shallots, finely chopped	25 g	62 g
balsamic vinegar	2 tbsp	5 tbsp
spinach leaves	100 g	250 g
sage, chopped	1 tbsp	2½ tbsp

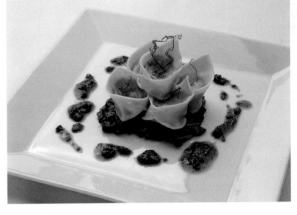

1 First prepare the pumpkin filling. Cut in half and scoop out the seeds.

2 Place in a roasting tray. Sprinkle with olive oil, cinnamon and nutmeg. Add a little water

to the pan. Roast the pumpkin at 350°C for approximately 45 minutes, until tender.

3 Remove from the oven, allow to cool, scrape out the flesh. Purée the flesh with the sugar in a food processor until smooth, then season.

4 To make the tortellini, roll out the ravioli paste into $\frac{1}{8}$ cm thick sheets. Cut the pasta sheets into 8 cm squares.

5 Place 1 teaspoon of the pumpkin filling in the centre of each square. Lightly brush two sides of the pasta with beaten egg and fold the pasta in half, creating a triangle. Join the two ends of the long side of the triangle to form the tortellini, eggwash the seam and firmly press the ends together to seal.

6 Cook the tortellini in boiling salted water for 3–4 minutes until al dente.

7 To prepare the vinaigrette, cook the butter until nut brown, remove from the heat, add the shallots and balsamic vinegar, then season.

8 Place the washed spinach leaves in a pan with one-third of the vinaigrette and quickly wilt the spinach. Season.

9 To serve, place the wilted spinach in the centre of the plates. Arrange the well-drained tortellini on the spinach. Spoon the vinaigrette around the plates. Finish with a sprinkling of fresh sage.

HEALTHY EATING TIP

- Lightly brush the pumpkin with olive oil when roasting.

- Keep the amount of added salt to a minimum throughout.

10 Ravioli

cal 1027 KJ	kcal 249 kcal	fat 9.4 g	sat fat 1.4 g	carb 38.9 g	sugar 0.8 g	protein 4.8 g	fibre 1.6 g

   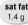 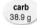 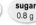

	4 portions	10 portions
flour	200 g	500 g
salt		
olive oil	35 ml	150 ml
water	105 ml	250 ml
fresh egg pasta (recipe 17) can also be used		

1 Sieve the flour and salt. Make a well. Add the liquid.

2 Knead to a smooth dough. Rest for at least 30 minutes in a cool place.

3 Roll out to a very thin oblong: 30 cm × 45 cm.

4 Cut in half and eggwash.

5 Place the stuffing in a piping bag with a large plain tube.

6 Pipe out the filling in small pieces, each about the size of a cherry, approximately 4 cm apart, on to one half of the paste.

7 Carefully cover with the other half of the paste and seal, taking care to avoid air pockets.

8 Mark each with the back of a plain cutter.

9 Cut in between each line of filling, down and across with a serrated pastry wheel.

10 Separate on a well-floured tray.

11 Poach in gently boiling salted water for approximately 10 minutes. Drain well.

12 Place in an earthenware serving dish.

13 Cover with 250 ml jus-lié, demi-glace or tomato sauce.

14 Sprinkle with 50 g grated cheese.

15 Brown under the salamander and serve.

Chef's tip

Roll out onto a board sprinkled with flour or, if possible, fine semolina. This will give the dough a good texture, as well as stopping it from sticking to the board.

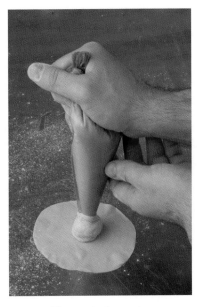

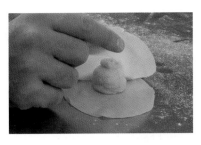

Place another piece of pasta over the top

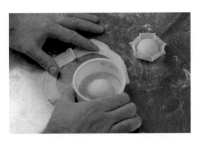

After sealing the edges, trim the ravioli into shape

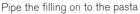
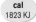

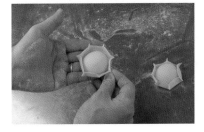

Pinch the edges up

Pipe the filling on to the pasta

11 Cannelloni

cal	kcal	fat	sat fat	carb	sugar	protein	fibre
1823 KJ	435 kcal	20.3 g	5.6 g	44.2 g	4.3 g	21.6 g	4.1 g

Use the same ingredients as for ravioli dough (recipe 10).

1 Roll out the paste as for ravioli.

2 Cut into squares approximately 6 cm × 6 cm.

3 Cook in gently boiling salted water for approximately 10 minutes. Refresh in cold water.

4 Drain well and lay out singly on the table. Pipe out the filling across each.

5 Roll up like sausage rolls. Place in a greased earthenware dish.

6 Add 250 ml demi-glace, jus-lié or tomato sauce.

7 Sprinkle with 25–50 g grated cheese.

8 Brown slowly under the salamander or in the oven, then serve.

* 1 portion with beef

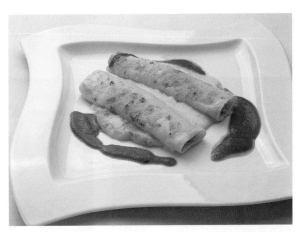

A wide variety of fillings may be used, such as those given in recipe 18.

12 Spaghetti with tomato sauce (*spaghetti alla pomodoro*)

	cal 1672 KJ	kcal 400 kcal	fat 17.2 g	sat fat 9.4 g	carb 50.0 g	sugar 10.2 g	protein 11.8 g	fibre 4.0 g

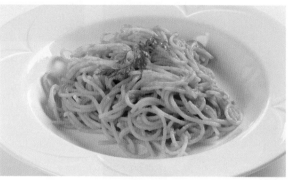

	4 portions	10 portions
spaghetti	400 g	1 kg
butter (optional) or olive oil	25 g	60 g
tomato sauce (page 181)	250 ml	625 ml
salt, mill pepper		
tomato concassée (optional)	100 g	250 g
fresh basil, to serve		
grated cheese, to serve		

1 Plunge the spaghetti into a saucepan containing boiling salted water. Allow to boil gently.

2 Stir occasionally with a wooden spoon. Cook for approximately 12–15 minutes.

3 Drain well in a colander. Return to a clean, dry pan.

4 Mix in the butter and add the tomato sauce. Correct the seasoning.

5 Add the tomato concassée and 4–5 leaves of fresh basil torn into pieces with your fingers, and serve with grated cheese.

Chef's tip
Cook pasta to an al dente texture.

HEALTHY EATING TIP

● Use very little or no salt as there is already plenty from the cheese.

● Reduce or omit the added butter and serve with a large green salad.

* Using hard margarine

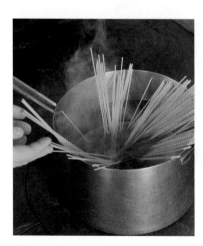

Place the spaghetti into boiling water

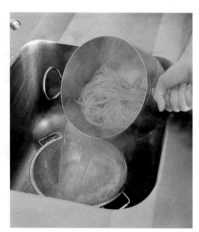

Drain the cooked pasta

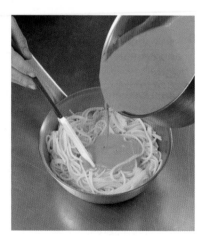

Add the sauce to the pasta

13 Spaghetti bolognaise *(spaghetti alla bolognese)*

	4 portions	10 portions
butter or oil	20 g	50 g
onion, chopped	50 g	125 g
clove garlic, chopped	1	2
lean minced beef or tail end fillet (see note), cut into 3 mm dice	400 g	1 kg
jus-lié or demi-glace	125 m	300 ml
tomato purée	1 tbsp	2½ tbsp
marjoram or oregano	1/8 tsp	¼ tsp
mushrooms, diced	100 g	250 g
salt, mill pepper		
spaghetti	400 g	1 kg

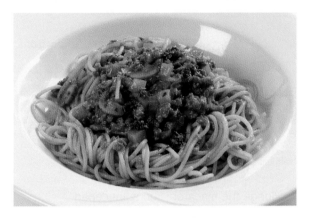

1 Place half the butter or oil in a sauteuse.

2 Add the chopped onion and garlic, and cook for 4–5 minutes without colour.

3 Add the beef and cook, colouring lightly.

4 Add the jus-lié or demi-glace, the tomato purée and the herbs.

5 Simmer until tender.

6 Add the mushrooms and simmer for 5 minutes. Correct the seasoning.

7 Meanwhile, cook the spaghetti in plenty of boiling salted water.

8 Allow to boil gently, stirring occasionally with a wooden spoon.

9 Cook for approximately 12–15 minutes. Drain well in a colander.

10 Return to a clean pan containing the rest of the butter or oil (optional).

11 Correct the seasoning.

12 Serve with the sauce in centre of the spaghetti.

13 Serve grated cheese separately.

There are many variations on bolognaise sauce, e.g. substitute lean beef with pork mince, or use a combination of both; add 50 g each of chopped carrot and celery; add 100 g chopped pancetta or bacon.

HEALTHY EATING TIP

- Use an unsaturated oil (sunflower or olive). Lightly oil the pan and drain off any excess after the frying is complete. Skim the fat from the finished dish.

- Season with the minimum amount of salt.

- Try using more pasta and extending the sauce with tomatoes.

- Serve with a large green salad.

14 Macaroni cheese

cal	kcal	fat	sat fat	carb	sugar	protein	fibre
7596 KJ	1808 kcal	116.6 g	64.2 g	136.6 g	26.6 g	60.0 g	6.8 g	*

	4 portions	10 portions
macaroni	400 g	1 kg
butter or oil, optional	25 g	60 g
grated cheese	100 g	250 g
thin béchamel (see page 184)	500 ml	1¼ litre
diluted English or continental mustard	¼ tsp	1 tsp
salt, mill pepper		

1 Plunge the macaroni into a saucepan containing plenty of boiling salted water.
2 Allow to boil gently and stir occasionally with a wooden spoon.
3 Cook for approximately 8–10 minutes and drain well in a colander.
4 Return to a clean pan containing the butter.
5 Mix with half the cheese, and add the béchamel and mustard. Season.
6 Place in an earthenware dish and sprinkle with the remainder of the cheese.
7 Brown lightly under the salamander and serve.

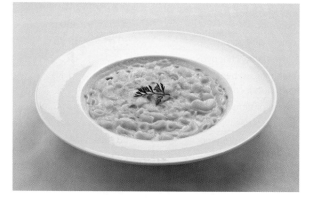

HEALTHY EATING TIP

- Half the grated cheese could be replaced with a small amount of Parmesan (more flavour and less fat).
- Use semi-skimmed milk for the béchamel. No added salt is necessary.

Try something different

Variations include the addition of cooked, sliced mushrooms, diced ham, sweetcorn, tomato, and so on. Macaroni may also be prepared and served as for any of the spaghetti dishes.

* For 4 portions

Chef's tip
Fresh pasta cooks very quickly. Dried pasta takes longer, because it needs to rehydrate: check the manufacturer's instructions. Browning the macaroni well gives it a good flavour, texture and presentation.

15 Noodles with butter

cal	kcal	fat	sat fat	carb	sugar	protein	fibre
796 KJ	191 kcal	12.3 g	7.1 g	18.0 g	0.6 g	3.1 g	0.7 g	*

	4 portions	10 portions
noodles	400 g	1 kg
salt, mill pepper		
a little grated nutmeg		
butter or sesame oil	50 g	125 g

1 Cook the noodles in plenty of gently boiling salted water.

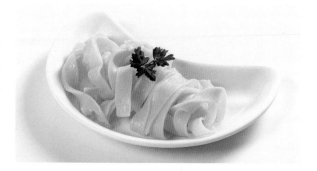

2 Drain well in a colander and return to the pan.

3 Add the seasoning and butter, and toss carefully until mixed.

4 Correct the seasoning and serve.

* *Using margarine*

Noodles may also be used as a garnish with meat and poultry dishes (e.g. braised beef).

HEALTHY EATING TIP

● Keep the added salt to a minimum.

16 Tagliatelle carbonara

	4 portions	10 portions
tagliatelle	400 g	1 kg
olive oil	1 tbsp	2½ tbsp
garlic cloves, peeled and crushed	2	5
smoked bacon, diced	200 g	500 g
eggs	4	10
double or single cream	4 tbsp	150 ml
Parmesan cheese	4 tbsp	150 ml

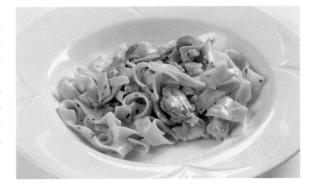

1 Cook the tagliatelle in boiling salted water until al dente. Refresh and drain.

2 Heat the oil in a suitable pan. Fry the crushed and chopped garlic. Add the diced, smoked bacon.

3 Mix together the beaten eggs, cream and Parmesan. Season with black pepper.

4 Add the tagliatelle to the garlic and bacon. Add the eggs and cream, stirring until the eggs cook in the heat. Serve immediately.

17 Fresh egg pasta dough

strong flour	400 g
salt	
eggs, beaten	4 × medium
olive oil as required	approx. 1 tbsp

1 Sieve the flour and salt, shape into a well. Pour the beaten eggs into the well.

2 Gradually incorporate the flour and only add oil to adjust to required consistency. The amount of oil will vary according to the type of flour and the size of the eggs used.

3 Pull and knead the dough until it is of a smooth, elastic consistency.

4 Cover the dough with a dampened cloth and allow to rest in a cool place for 30 minutes.

5 Roll out the dough on a well-floured surface to a thickness of ½ mm, or use a pasta rolling machine.

6 Trim the sides and cut the dough as required using a large knife.

If using a pasta rolling machine, divide the dough into three or four pieces. Pass each section through the machine, turning the rollers with the other hand. Repeat five or six times, adjusting the rollers each time to make the pasta thinner.

Fresh egg pasta requires less cooking time than dried pasta. When cooking fresh pasta, add a few drops of olive oil in the water to help prevent the pieces from sticking together. Fresh egg pasta not for immediate use must be stored in a cool, dry place. If fresh pasta is to be stored, it should be allowed to dry, then kept in a clean, dry container or bowl in a cool dry store.

> *The best way to roll out pasta dough at the correct thickness is to use a pasta machine.*

Try something different

- **Spinach:** add 75–100 g finely puréed, dry, cooked spinach to the dough.
- **Tomato:** add 2 tbsp of tomato purée to the dough. Other flavours used include beetroot, saffron and black ink from squid.
- **Wholewheat pasta:** use half wholewheat and half white flour.

Making fresh pasta
http://bit.ly/xjvhHH

Chef's tips
Do not knead the dough too much, or it will become tough.
Let it rest before rolling it out.

18 Stuffings for pasta

Here are some examples of stuffing for cannelloni, ravioli, tortellini and other pastas. Each recipe provides enough stuffing to use with 400 g pasta.

cooked minced chicken	200 g
minced ham	100 g
butter	25 g
2 yolks or 1 egg	
grated cheese	25 g
pinch of grated nutmeg	
salt and pepper, fresh white breadcrumbs	25 g

cooked dry spinach, puréed	200 g
ricotta cheese	200 g
butter	25 g
nutmeg	
salt and pepper	

cooked minced lean pork	200 g
cooked minced lean veal	200 g
butter	25 g
grated cheese	25 g
2 yolks or 1 egg	
fresh white breadcrumbs	25 g
salt and pepper	

pinch of chopped marjoram	
ricotta cheese	150 g
grated Parmesan	75 g
egg	1
nutmeg	
salt and pepper	

minced cooked meat	200 g
spinach, cooked	100 g
onion, chopped and cooked	50 g
oregano	
salt, pepper	

chopped cooked fish	200 g
chopped cooked mushrooms	100 g
chopped parsley	
anchovy paste	

Pasta that is to be stuffed must be rolled as thinly as possible. The stuffing should be pleasant in taste and plentiful in quantity. The edges of the pasta must be thoroughly sealed, otherwise the stuffing will seep out during poaching.

19 Crisp polenta and roasted Mediterranean vegetables

	4 portions	10 portions
Polenta		
water	200 ml	500 ml
butter	30 g	75 g
polenta flour	65 g	160 g
Parmesan, grated	25 g	60 g
egg yolks	1	2
crème fraiche	110 g	275 g
seasoning		
Roasted vegetables		
red peppers	2	5
yellow peppers	2	5
courgettes	2	5
red onions	2	5
vegetable oil	200 ml	500 ml
seasoning		
clove of garlic	1	3
sprigs of thyme	2	5

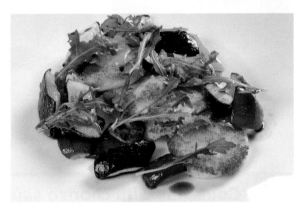

To make the polenta

1 Bring the water and the butter to the boil.

2 Season the water well and whisk in the polenta flour.

3 Continue to whisk until very thick.

4 Remove from the heat and add the Parmesan, egg yolk and crème fraiche.

5 Whisk until all incorporated; check the seasoning.

6 Set in a lined tray.

7 Once set, cut using a round cutter or cut into squares.

8 Reserve until required.

To make the roasted vegetables

1 Roughly chop the vegetables into large chunks. Ensure the seeds are removed from the peppers.

2 Toss the cut vegetables in the oil and season well.

3 Place the vegetables in an oven with the aromats for 30 minutes at 180°C.

4 Remove from the oven and drain. Reserve until required.

To serve

1 To serve the dish, shallow-fry the polenta in a non-stick pan until golden on both sides.

2 Warm the roasted vegetables and place them in the middle of the plate. Place the polenta on top.

3 Finish with rocket salad and balsamic dressing.

> **Chef's tip**
> Line the tray with clingfilm and silicone paper before pouring in the polenta – this will stop it from sticking to the tray when it sets.

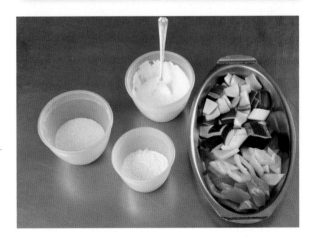

Ingredients for crisp polenta and roasted Mediterranean vegetables

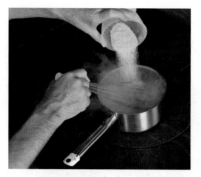

Whisk the polenta into the water

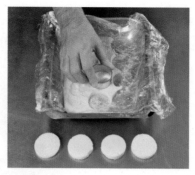

When the polenta has set, cut it into shape

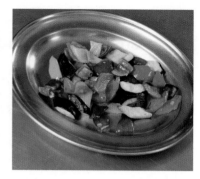

Roasted vegetables

20 Couscous with chorizo sausage and chicken

cal	kcal	fat	sat fat	carb	sugar	protein	fibre
1590 KJ	380 kcal	13.1 g	4.3 g	34.1 g	1.7 g	33.1 g	0.3 g

	4 portions	10 portions
couscous	250 g	625 g
olive oil	1 tbsp	1½ tbsp
garlic cloves, finely chopped	2	3
chorizo sausage	150 g	400 g
suprêmes of chicken, skinned	3	7
sunblush tomatoes	75 g	200 g
fresh parsley	¼ tsp	½ tsp

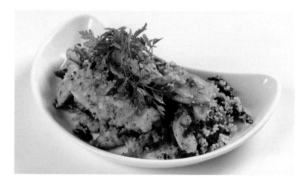

1 Prepare the couscous in a suitable bowl and gently pour over 300 ml of boiling water (750 ml for 10 portions).

2 Stir well, cover and leave to stand for 5 minutes.

3 Heat the olive oil in a suitable frying pan, add the chopped garlic, then sauté for 1 minute.

4 Add the chorizo sausage (sliced 1 cm thick) and the chicken cut into fine strips. Cook for 5–6 minutes.

5 Add the couscous, sunblush tomatoes (skinned or diced) and parsley, mix thoroughly and heat for a further 2–3 minutes.

6 Drizzle with olive oil, serve as a warm salad.

7 Garnish with mixed leaves and flat parsley.

HEALTHY EATING TIP

- Using an unsaturated oil (sunflower or olive), lightly oil the pan to sauté the garlic.

- Drain off any excess fat after cooking the sausage and chicken.

- Serve with mixed leaves.

21 Gnocchi parisienne (choux paste)

	4 portions	10 portions
water	125 ml	300 ml
margarine or butter	50 g	125 g
salt		
flour, white or wholemeal	60 g	150 g
eggs	2	5
cheese, grated	50 g	125 g
béchamel (thin) (see page 184)	250 ml	625 ml
salt, pepper, to season		

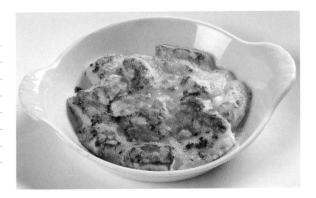

1 Boil the water, margarine or butter, and salt in a saucepan. Remove from the heat.

2 Mix in the flour with a kitchen spoon. Return to a gentle heat.

3 Stir continuously until the mixture leaves the sides of the pan.

4 Cool slightly. Gradually add the eggs, beating well. Add half the cheese.

5 Place in a piping bag with ½ cm plain tube.

6 Pipe out in 1 cm lengths into a shallow pan of gently simmering salted water. Do not allow to boil.

7 Cook for approximately 10 minutes. Drain well in a colander.

8 Combine carefully with the béchamel. Correct the seasoning.

9 Pour into an earthenware dish.

10 Sprinkle with the remainder of the cheese.

11 Brown lightly under the salamander and serve.

Gnocchi may be used to garnish goulash or navarin in place of potatoes.

Chef's tip

Mix the eggs into the paste carefully and slowly, but make sure they are well mixed in. If there is too much egg, the mixture will be slack.

HEALTHY EATING TIP

• No added salt is necessary because of the presence of the cheese.

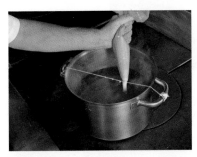

Pipe the choux paste into the simmering water; a string tied across the pan can be used to form the lengths of paste

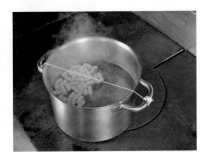

Allow the gnocchi to simmer

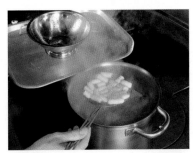

Remove the gnocchi from the water and drain them well

22 Gnocchi romaine (semolina)

cal	kcal	fat	sat fat	carb	sugar	protein	fibre	*
1066 KJ	254 kcal	12.5 g	6.9 g	27.5 g	7.0 g	9.8 g	0.8 g	

	4 portions	10 portions
milk	500 ml	1½ litre
semolina	100 g	250 g
salt, pepper		
grated nutmeg		
egg yolk	1	3
cheese, grated	25 g	60 g
butter or		
margarine	25 g	60 g
tomato sauce (see page 181)	250 ml	625 ml

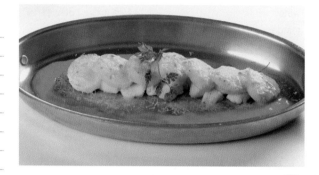

1 Boil the milk in a thick-bottomed pan.

2 Sprinkle in the semolina, stirring continuously. Stir to the boil.

3 Season and simmer until cooked (approx. 5–10 minutes). Remove from heat.

4 Mix in the egg yolk, cheese and butter.

5 Pour into a buttered tray 1 cm deep.

6 When cold, cut into rounds with a 5 cm round cutter.

7 Place the debris in a buttered earthenware dish.

8 Neatly arrange the rounds on top.

9 Sprinkle with melted butter and cheese.

10 Lightly brown in the oven or under a salamander.

11 Serve with a thread of tomato sauce round the gnocchi.

Chef's tip

Make sure the mixture has chilled until it is completely set, before cutting it into shape — it is much easier to handle once it has set.

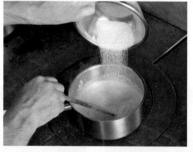

HEALTHY EATING TIP

- No added salt is necessary because of the presence of the cheese.

* Using semi-skimmed milk

Stir the semolina into the milk

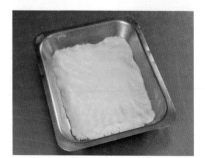

Pour the mixture into a greased tray and leave to cool

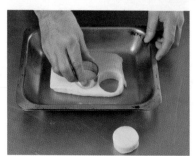

Cut the gnocchi into shape

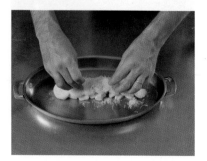

Sprinkle grated cheese over the dish

23 Scrambled eggs (basic recipe) *(oeufs brouillés)*

cal	kcal	fat	sat fat	carb	sugar	protein	fibre
1105 KJ	263 kcal	22.9 g	8.7 g	0.5 g	0.5 g	13.9 g	0.0 g

*

	4 portions	10 portions
eggs	6–8	15–20
milk (optional)	2 tbsp	5 tbsp
salt, pepper		
butter or oil	50 g	125 g

1 Break the eggs in a basin, add milk (if using), lightly season with salt and pepper and thoroughly mix with a whisk.

2 Melt half the butter in a thick-bottomed pan, add the eggs and cook over a gentle heat, stirring continuously until the eggs are lightly cooked.

3 Remove from the heat, correct the seasoning and mix in the remaining butter. (A tablespoon of cream may also be added at this point.)

4 Serve in individual egg dishes.

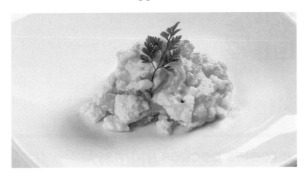

If scrambled eggs are cooked too quickly or for too long the protein will toughen, the eggs will discolour because of the iron and sulphur compounds being released, and syneresis (separation of water from the eggs) will occur. This means that they will be unpleasant to eat. The heat from the pan will continue to cook the eggs after it has been removed from the stove; therefore, the pan should be removed from the heat just before the eggs are cooked. Scrambled eggs can be served on a slice of freshly buttered toast with the crust removed.

Try something different

Scrambled eggs may be served with smoked salmon (as shown).

 HEALTHY EATING TIP

- Try to keep the butter used in cooking to a minimum and serve on unbuttered toast.

- Garnish with a grilled tomato.

* Using hard margarine

24 Hard-boiled eggs with cheese and tomato sauce *(oeufs aurore)*

	4 portions	10 portions
hard-boiled eggs	4	10
shallots, chopped	10 g	25 g
butter, margarine or oil (duxelle)	10 g	25 g
mushrooms	100 g	250 g
parsley or other fresh herbs, chopped		
salt, pepper		
béchamel sauce (see page 184)	250 ml	625 ml
tomato sauce or purée		
grated Parmesan cheese		

1 Cut the eggs in halves lengthwise.

2 Remove the yolks and pass them through a sieve.

3 Place the whites in an earthenware serving dish.

4 Prepare the duxelle by cooking the chopped shallot in the butter without colouring, add the well-washed and finely chopped mushroom or mushroom trimmings, cook for 3–4 minutes.

5 Mix the yolks with the duxelle and parsley, and correct the seasoning.

6 Spoon or pipe the mixture into the egg white halves.

7 Add a little tomato sauce or tomato purée to the béchamel sauce to give it a pinkish colour.

8 Mask the eggs with the sauce and sprinkle with grated cheese.

9 Gratinate under the salamander.

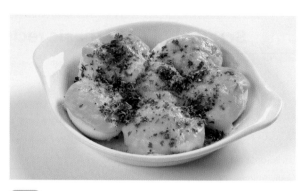

🍎 **HEALTHY EATING TIP**

● Serve with French bread or toast and a green salad.

● There is plenty of salt in the cheese, so additional salt is not necessary.

25 Soft-boiled eggs (oeufs mollets)

cal	kcal	fat	sat fat	carb	sugar	protein	fibre
1052 KJ	251 kcal	18.9 g	8.7 g	8.0 g	3.3 g	12.5 g	1.2 g	*

1 Plunge the eggs into boiling water, then reboil.

2 Simmer for 4½–5 minutes. Refresh immediately.

3 Remove the shells carefully.

4 Reheat when required for 30 seconds in hot salted water.

Boiling eggs
http://bit.ly/wgInMV

Using 1 egg per portion

26 Poached eggs with cheese sauce (oeufs pochés mornay)

cal	kcal	fat	sat fat	carb	sugar	protein	fibre
1177 KJ	280 kcal	19.1 g	8.7 g	15.2 g	3.4 g	12.8 g	0.8 g

	4 portions	10 portions
eggs	4	10
short paste tartlets	4	10
or		
half slices of buttered toast	4	10
mornay sauce (page 185)	250 ml	625 ml

1 Carefully break the eggs one by one into a pan of vinegar water (approx. 15 per cent acidulation) and make sure the water is at a gentle boil.

2 Simmer until lightly set, for approximately 3–3½ minutes.

3 Remove carefully with a perforated spoon into a bowl of ice water.

4 Trim the white if necessary.

5 Reheat, when required, by placing into hot salted water for approximately ½–1 minute.

6 Remove carefully from the water using a perforated spoon. Drain on a cloth.

7 Place tartlets or toast in an earthenware dish (the slices of toast may be halved, cut in rounds with a cutter, crust removed).

8 Add the hot, well-drained eggs.

9 Completely cover with the sauce, sprinkle with grated Parmesan cheese, brown under the salamander and serve.

Poaching eggs
http://bit.ly/zC1HWz

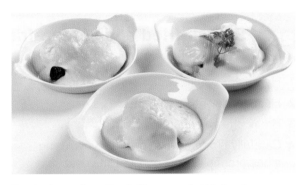

Poached eggs florentine (left), mornay (middle) and Washington (right)

Try something different

Variations include:

- *florentine* – poached eggs on a bed of leaf spinach and finished as for mornay
- *Washington* – on a bed of sweetcorn coated with suprême sauce (page 186) or cream.

27 Fried eggs *(oeufs frits)*

cal	kcal	fat	sat fat	carb	sugar	protein	fibre
536 KJ	128 kcal	31.0 g	9.8 g	0.0 g	0.0 g	7.6 g	0.0 g

1 Allow 1 or 2 eggs per portion.

2 Melt a little fat in a frying pan. Add the eggs.

3 Cook gently until lightly set. Serve on a plate or flat dish.

To prepare an excellent fried egg, it is essential to use a fresh high-quality egg, to maintain a controlled low heat and use a high-quality fat (butter or oil, such as sunflower oil).

* Fried in sunflower oil

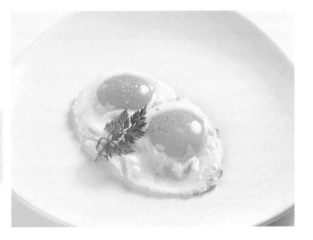

28 French-fried eggs (deep-fried eggs)

1 Half cover a shallow pan with vegetable oil.
2 Heat gently until a slight haze is seen.
3 Break a fresh egg into the oil.
4 Carefully flick the white over the yolk, using a heatproof plastic spoon, until it cooks to a golden brown colour.
5 When cooked, serve immediately.

Chef's tips
The eggs must be fried quickly. It is important to flick the white over the yolk during the cooking.

ASSESSMENT

29 Omelettes (basic recipe) *(omelette nature)*

cal	kcal	fat	sat fat	carb	sugar	protein	fibre
990 KJ	236 kcal	20.2 g	9.1 g	0.0 g	0.0 g	13.6 g	0.0 g

*

eggs, per portion	2–3
salt, pepper	
butter, margarine or oil	10 g

1 Allow 2–3 eggs per portion.
2 Break the eggs into a basin, season lightly with salt and pepper.
3 Beat well with a fork, or whisk until the yolks and whites are thoroughly combined and no streaks of white can be seen.
4 Heat the omelette pan; wipe thoroughly clean with a dry cloth.
5 Add the butter; heat until foaming but not brown.
6 Add the eggs and cook quickly, moving the mixture continuously with a fork until lightly set; remove from the heat.
7 Half fold the mixture over at right angles to the handle.
8 Tap the bottom of the pan to bring up the edge of the omelette.
9 With care, tilt the pan completely over so as to allow the omelette to fall into the centre of the dish or plate.
10 Neaten the shape if necessary and serve immediately.

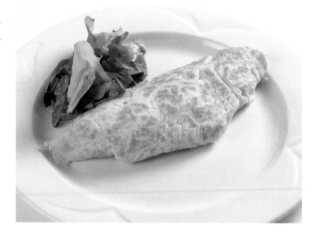

Making an omelette
http://bit.ly/zWfvHq

* *Using 2 eggs per portion.*

Try something different

Variations to omelettes can easily be made by adding the required ingredient that the guest or dish may require. For example:

- **fine herbs** (chopped parsley, chervil and chives)
- **mushroom** (cooked, sliced, wild or cultivated)
- **cheese** (25 g grated cheese added before folding)
- **tomato** (incision made down centre of cooked omelette, filled with hot tomato concassée; served with tomato sauce)
- **bacon** (grill and then julienne into small strips and fold in at the end).

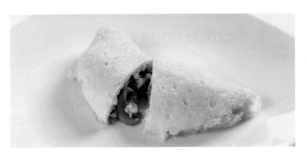

Mushroom omelette

> Omelettes are traditionally folded in a cigar shape and served baveuse (underdone and runny). Customers may prefer them to be cooked through and coloured.

30 Egg white omelette

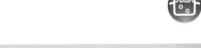

Being prepared and cooked without the egg yolks means that this is almost fat free. The whites are three-quarter whipped, lightly seasoned and then cooked as for any other omelette, folded or flat, garnished or served plain.

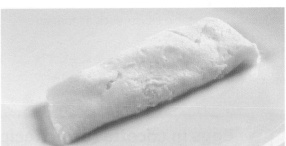

31 Spanish omelette

This omelette has tomato concassée (see page 257), cooked onions, diced red pimento and parsley added, and is cooked and served flat. Many other flat omelettes can be served with a variety of ingredients. A flat omelette is made as for a basic omelette (recipe 29) up to point 7; then sharply tap the pan on the stove to loosen the omelette and toss it over as for a pancake.

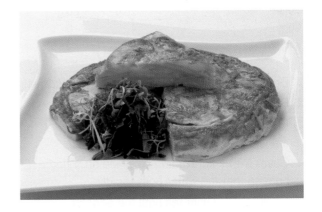

32 Scotch eggs

cal	kcal	fat	sat fat	carb	sugar	protein	fibre
2094 KJ	499 kcal	39.9 g	11.4 g	18.4 g	0.6 g	18.0 g	1.0 g

	4 portions	10 portions
hard-boiled eggs	4	10
sausage meat	300 g	1 kg
flour	25 g	60 g
beaten egg	1	3
breadcrumbs	50 g	125 g

1 Completely cover each egg with sausage meat.

2 Pass it through the flour, beaten egg and breadcrumbs. Shake off any surplus crumbs.

3 Deep-fry to a golden brown in a moderately hot fat.

4 Drain well, cut in halves and serve hot or cold.

Hot: garnish with fried or sprig parsley, and a sauceboat of suitable sauce, such as tomato (page 181).

Cold: garnish with salad in season and a sauceboat of salad dressing.

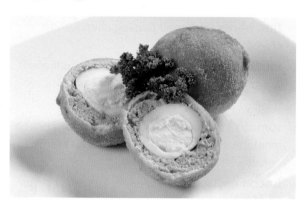

HEALTHY EATING TIP

- Make sure the fat is hot so that less fat will be absorbed into the food during cooking.

- Drain the cooked scotch eggs on kitchen paper.

33 Eggs in cocotte (basic recipe) *(oeufs en cocotte)*

cal	kcal	fat	sat fat	carb	sugar	protein	fibre
534 KJ	127 kcal	11.2 g	5.2 g	0.0 g	0.0 g	6.8 g	0.0 g

	4 portions	10 portions
butter	25 g	60 g
eggs	4	10
salt, pepper		

1 Butter the appropriate number of egg cocottes.

2 Break an egg carefully into each and season.

3 Place the cocottes in a sauté pan containing 1 cm water.

4 Cover with a tight-fitting lid, place on a fierce heat so that the water boils rapidly.

5 Cook for 2–3 minutes until the eggs are lightly set, then serve.

Try something different

Variations include:

- half a minute before the cooking is completed, add 1 tsp of cream to each egg and complete the cooking

- when cooked, add 1 tsp of jus-lié to each egg

- place diced cooked chicken, mixed with cream, in the bottom of the cocottes; break the eggs on top of the chicken and cook

- as above, using tomato concassée in place of chicken.

34   Eggs *sur le plat*

1   Take a china *sur le plat* dish. Add a teaspoon of olive oil or butter. Heat it on the side of the stove, until it is moderately hot.

2   Break in 1 or 2 eggs. Allow them to set on the stove.

3   Transfer to the oven for 2–4 minutes to finish cooking.

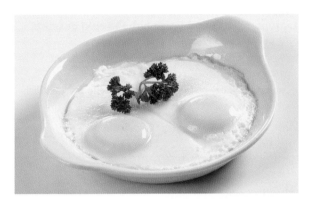

14 Produce hot and cold desserts and puddings

In this chapter, you will learn how to:

1. prepare, cook and finish hot and cold desserts and puddings, including:
- working safely and hygienically, using the correct equipment
- applying quality points and evaluating the finished dish

2. you should have the knowledge to:
- identify different hot and cold desserts and hot puddings
- understand the quality points of ingredients and how to adjust the quantity
- finish and decorate dishes, and identify sauces and accompaniments
- apply portion control
- hold and store finished dishes safely.

Number	Recipe title	Page number
Fillings and basic preparations (these are relevant throughout chapters 14–17)		
6	Almond cream (frangipane)	465
2	Boiled buttercream	462
1	Chantilly cream	462
	Crème chiboust	464
	Crème diplomat	464
3	Ganache	463
5	Italian meringue	464
4	Pastry cream (crème pâtissière)	463
Sauces		
13	Butterscotch sauce	468
12	Caramel sauce	468
10	Chocolate sauce (sauce chocolat)	467
9	Custard sauce	467
8	Fresh egg custard sauce (sauce à l'anglaise)	466
7	Fruit coulis	465
11	Stock syrup	468
Hot desserts		
32	Apple crumble tartlets	482
22	Apple fritters (beignets aux pommes)	474
30	Baked Alaska (omelette soufflée surprise)	480
19	Baked apple (pommes bonne femme)	472
14	Bramley apple spotted dick	469
23	Bread and butter pudding	474
24	Cabinet pudding (pouding cabinet)	475

Number	Recipe title	Page number
18	Chocolate fondant	471
29	Christmas pudding	479
21	Crêpes Suzette	473
	Diplomat pudding	475
17	Eve's pudding with gooseberries	471
16	Golden syrup pudding	470
27	Mango soufflé	478
20	Pancakes with apple (crêpes normande)	473
25	Rice pudding	476
28	Soufflé pudding (pouding soufflé)	478
15	Sticky toffee pudding	469
31	Tatin of apple (tarte tatin)	481
26	Vanilla soufflé (soufflé à la vanille)	476
Cold desserts		
41	Baked blueberry cheesecake	488
33	Basic fruit mousse	482
35	Bavarois: basic recipe and range of flavours	483
47	Black Forest vacherin	493
43	Burned, caramelised or browned cream (crème brûlée)	490
34	Chocolate mousse	483
44	Cream caramel (crème caramel)	491
48	Khoshaf	494
40	Lime and mascarpone cheesecake	488
37	Lime soufflé frappe	485
45	Meringue (meringue)	491
39	Poached fruits or fruit compote (compote de fruits)	487

36	Raspberry bavarois (mousse)	484
42	Trifle	489
46	Vacherin with strawberries and cream (*vacherin aux fraises*)	492
38	Vanilla panna cotta served on a fruit compote	486
Iced desserts		
52	Apple sorbet	495

50	Caramel ice cream	495
53	Chocolate sorbet	496
	Fruits of the forest sorbet	496
49	Lemon curd ice cream	494
54	Orange brandy granita	496
51	Peach ice cream	495
55	Peach Melba (*pêche Melba*)	497
56	Pear belle Hélène (*poire belle Hélène*)	497

The following information about ingredients and commodities is relevant to several units of your course: desserts and puddings; paste products; biscuits, cake and sponge products; and fermented dough products.

Ingredients used in the pastry kitchen

The principal building blocks of pastry dishes are flour, fat, sugar, raising agents, eggs and cream.

Flour

Flour is probably the most common commodity in daily use. It forms the foundation of bread, pastry and cakes and is also used in soups, sauces, batters and other foods. It is one of the most important ingredients in patisserie, if not *the* most important.

There is a great variety of high-quality flours made from cereals, nuts or legumes, such as chestnut flour, cornflour, and so on. They have been used in patisserie, baking, dessert cuisine and savoury cuisine in all countries throughout history. The king of all of them is without doubt wheat flour.

The composition of wheat flour

Wheat flour is composed of starch, gluten, sugar, fats, water and minerals.

- Starch is the main component, but gluten is also a significant element. Elastic and impermeable, it is the gluten that makes wheat flour the most common flour used in bread making.
- The quantity of sugar in wheat is very small but it plays a very important role in fermentation.
- Wheat contains a maximum of only 16 per cent water, but its presence is important.
- The mineral matter (ash), which is found mainly in the husk of the wheat grain and not in the kernel, determines the purity and quality of the flour.

From the ear to the final product, flour, wheat goes through several distinct processes. These are carried out in modern industrial plants, where wheat is subjected to the various treatments and phases necessary for the production of different types of flour. These arrive in perfect condition at our workplaces and are made into preparations like sponge cakes, yeast dough, puff pastries, biscuits, pastries and much more.

What you need to know about flour

- Flour is a particularly delicate living material, and it must be used and stored with special care. It must always be in the best condition, which is why storing large quantities is not recommended.
- It must be kept in a good environment: a clean, organised, disinfected and aerated storeroom.
- Warm and humid places must absolutely be avoided.

Impermeable: Something that liquid cannot pass through.

Aerated: To introduce air into. An 'aerated storeroom' is one that air is allowed to circulate through.

The production of flour

White flour is made up almost entirely of the part of the wheat grain known as the endosperm, which contains starch and protein. When flour is mixed with water it is converted into a sticky dough. This characteristic is due to the gluten, which becomes sticky when moistened. The relative proportion of starch and gluten varies in different wheats, and those with a low percentage of gluten (soft flour) are not suitable for bread making. For this reason, wheat is blended.

In milling, the whole grain is broken up, the parts separated, sifted, blended and ground into flour. Some of the outer coating of bran is removed, as is the wheatgerm, which contains oil and is therefore likely to become rancid and spoil the flour. For this reason wholemeal flour should not be stored for more than 14 days.

Types of flour

- White flour contains 72–85 per cent of the whole grain (the endosperm only).
- Wholemeal flour contains 100 per cent of the whole grain.
- Wheatmeal flour contains 85–95 per cent of the whole grain. Hovis flour contains 85 per cent of the whole grain.
- High-ratio or patent flour contains 40 per cent of the whole grain.
- Self-raising flour is white flour with baking powder added to it.
- Semolina is granulated hard flour prepared from the central part of the wheat grain. White or wholemeal semolina is available.

Fats

Pastry goods may be made from various types of fat, either a single named fat or a combination. Examples of fats are:

- butter
- margarine
- shortening
- lard.

Butter and other fats

Butter is the symbol of perfection in fats. It brings flowery smoothness, perfumes and aromas, and impeccable textures to our preparations. It is a point of reference for good gastronomy. Butter has a very long history, but its origin is unknown. Many books have been written about it, but we can only conclude that it was probably discovered by accident.

Butter is an emulsion – the perfect symbiosis of water and fat. It is composed of a minimum of 82 per cent fat, a maximum of 16 per cent water and 2 per cent dry extracts.

What you need to know about butter

- Butter is the most complete fat.
- It is a very delicate ingredient that can quickly spoil if a series of basic rules are not followed in its use.
- It absorbs odours very easily, so it should be kept well covered and should always be stored far from anything that produces strong odours.
- When kept at 15°C, butter is stable and retains all its properties: finesse, perfume and creaminess.
- It should not be kept too long: it is always better to work with fresh butter.
- Good butter has a stable texture, pleasing taste, fresh odour, homogenous (even) colour and, most important, it must melt perfectly in your mouth.
- It softens preparations like cookies and petit fours, and keeps products like sponge cakes soft.
- Butter enhances flavour – as in brioches, for example.
- The melting point of butter is between 30°C and 35°C, approximately.

Margarine

Margarine is often made from a blend of oils that have been hardened or hydrogenated (had hydrogen gas). Margarine may contain up to 10 per cent butterfat.

Cake margarine is again a blend of oils, hydrogenated, to which is added an emulsifying agent that helps combine water and fat. Cake margarine may contain up to 10 per cent butterfat.

Pastry margarine is used for puff pastry. It is a hard plastic or waxy fat that is suitable for layering.

Shortening

Shortening is another name for fat used in pastry making. It is made from oils and is 100 per cent fat, such as hydrogenated lard; another type of shortening is rendered pork fat.

Sugar

Sugar (or sucrose) is extracted from sugar beet or sugar cane. The juice is crystallised by a complicated manufacturing process. It is then refined and sieved into several grades, such as granulated, caster or icing sugars. Syrup and treacle are produced during the production of sugar.

Loaf or cube sugar is obtained by pressing the crystals together while they are slightly wet, drying them in blocks, and then cutting the blocks into squares.

Fondant is a cooked mixture of sugar and glucose which, when heated, is coloured and flavoured, and used for decorating cakes, buns, gâteaux and petits fours. Fondant is generally bought ready made.

Inverted sugar

When sucrose is broken down with water, in a chemical process called hydrolysis, it separates into the two types of sugar that make it: fructose and glucose. Sugar that has been treated in this way is called inverted sugar and is, after sucrose, one of the most commonly used sugars in the catering profession, thanks to its sweetening properties. Inverted sugar comes in liquid and syrup forms.

Hydrolysis: A chemical reaction in which a compound – like sugar – breaks down by reacting with water.

Liquid inverted sugar

This is a yellowish liquid with no less than 62 per cent dry matter. It contains more than 3 per cent inverted sugar, but less than 50 per cent. It is used mainly in the commercial food industry.

Inverted sugar syrup

This is a white, sticky paste and has no particular odour. It has no less than 62 per cent dry matter and more than 50 per cent inverted sugar. It is the form in which inverted sugar is most commonly used. With equal proportions of dry matter and sucrose, its sweetening capacity is 25–30 per cent greater than sucrose.

Applications of inverted sugar

- It improves the aroma of products.
- It improves the texture of doughs.
- It prevents the dehydration of frozen products.
- It reduces or stops crystallisation.
- It is essential in ice cream making – it greatly improves its quality and lowers its freezing point.

Glucose

Glucose takes on various forms:

- the characteristics of a viscous syrup, called crystal glucose
- its natural state, in fruit and honey
- a dehydrated white paste (used mainly in the commercial food industry, but also used in catering)
- 'dehydrated glucose' (atomised glucose) – a glucose syrup from which the water is evaporated; this is used in patisserie, but mainly in the commercial food industry.

Characteristics and properties of glucose syrup

- It is a transparent, viscous paste.
- It prevents the crystallisation of boiled sugars, jams and preserves.
- It delays the drying of a product.
- It adds plasticity and creaminess to ice cream and the fillings of chocolate bonbons.
- It prevents the crystallisation of ice cream.

Honey

Honey, a sweet syrup that bees make with the nectar extracted from flowers, is without doubt the oldest known sugar. A golden-brown thick paste, it is 30 per cent sweeter than sucrose.

Honey lowers the freezing point of ice cream. It can also be used like inverted sugar, but it is important to take into account that honey, unlike inverted sugar, will give flavour to the preparation. Also, it is inadequate for preparations that require long storage, since honey re-crystallises after some time.

Isomalt

Isomalt sugar is a sweetener that is still little known in the patisserie world, but it has been used for some time. It has properties distinct from those of the sweeteners already mentioned. It is produced through the hydrolysis of sugar, followed by hydrogenation (the addition of hydrogen). Produced through these industrial processes, this sugar has been used for many years in large industries, in candy and chewing gum production, and is now earning a place in gastronomy.

One of its most notable characteristics is that it can melt without the addition of water or another liquid. This is a very interesting property for making artistic decorations in caramel. Its appearance is like that of confectioners' sugar: a glossy powder. Its sweetening strength is half that of sucrose and it is much less soluble than sugar, which means that it melts less easily in the mouth.

Isomalt's main claim in gastronomy over the past few years has been as a replacement for normal sugar or sucrose when making sugar decorations, blown sugar, pulled sugar or spun sugar. Isomalt is not affected by air humidity, so sugar pieces will keep for longer.

Raising agents

A raising agent is added to a cake or bread mixture to give lightness to the product, because they produce gases, which expand when heated. The gases produced are air, carbon dioxide or water vapour. These gases are introduced before baking or are produced by substances added to the mixture before baking. When the product is cooked, the gases expand. These gases are trapped in the gluten of the wheat flour. On further heating and cooking, the product, because of the pressure of the gluten, rises and sets.

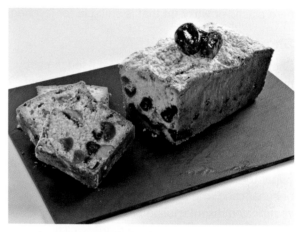

Cakes rise because of raising agents

Baking powder

Chemical raising agents cause a reaction between certain acidic and alkaline compounds, which produce carbon dioxide. The alkaline component is almost always sodium bicarbonate or sodium acid carbonate, commonly known as baking soda. It is ideal because it is cheap to produce, easily purified, non-toxic and naturally tasteless. Potassium bicarbonate is available for those on low-sodium diets, but this compound tends to absorb moisture and react prematurely, and gives off a bitter flavour.

Baking powder may be used without the addition of acid if the dough or batter is already acidic enough to react with it to produce carbon dioxide. Yoghurt and sour milk contain lactic acid, and often are used in place of water or milk in such products; sour milk can also be added along with the baking soda as a separate 'natural' component of the leavening.

Baking powder contains baking soda and an acid in the form of salt crystals that dissolve in water. Ground dry starch is also added to prevent premature reactions in humid air by absorbing moisture and to dilute the powder.

Most baking powders are 'double acting' – that is, they produce an initial set of gas bubbles when the powder is mixed into the batter and then a second set during the baking process. The first and smaller reaction is necessary to form many small gas bubbles in the batter or dough; the second is necessary to expand these bubbles to form the final light texture. This second reaction must happen late enough in the baking for the surrounding materials to have set, preventing the bubbles from escaping and the product from collapsing.

Baking powder is make from alkali (bicarbonate of soda) plus acid (cream of tartar – potassium hydrogen tartrate). Commercial baking powders differ mainly in their proportions of the acid salts. Cream of tartar is not normally used due to its high cost, so calcium phosphate and glucono-delta-lactose are now commonly used in its place. Sodium aluminium sulphate is an acid that is active only at higher oven temperatures and has an advantage over other powders, which tend to produce gas too early.

Use of water vapour

Water vapour is produced during the baking process, from the liquid content used in the mixing. Water vapour has approximately 1600 times the original volume of the water. The raising power is slower than that of a gas. This method is used in the production of choux pastry, puff pastry, rough puff, flaky and batter products.

Points to remember

- Always buy a reliable brand of baking powder.
- Store in a dry place in an airtight tin.
- Do not store for long periods of time, as the baking powder loses some of its residual carbon dioxide over time and therefore will not be as effective.
- Check the recipe carefully, making sure that the correct preparation for the type of mixture is used; otherwise, under- or over-rising may result.
- Sieve the raising agent with the flour and/or dry ingredients to give an even mix and thus an even reaction.
- Distribute moisture evenly into the mixture to ensure even action of the raising agent.

- If a large proportion of raising agent has been added to a mixture, and is not to be cooked immediately, keep it in a cool place to avoid too much reaction before baking.

What happens if too much raising agent is used?

Too much raising agent causes:

- over-risen product that may collapse, giving a sunken effect
- a coarse texture
- poor colour and flavour
- fruit sinking to the bottom of the cake
- a bitter taste.

What happens if not enough raising agent is used?

Insufficient raising agent causes:

- lack of volume
- insufficient lift
- close texture
- shrinkage.

Salt

Salt (chemical name 'sodium chloride') is one of the most important ingredients. It is well known that salt is a necessary part of the human diet, present in small or large proportions in many natural foods. Salt considerably enhances all preparations, whether they be sweet or savoury. We generally associate it with seasoning foods to improve their flavour, but it is also necessary in the making of many sweet dishes.

It is a good idea to add a pinch of salt to all sweet preparations, nougats, chocolate bonbons and cakes to intensify flavours. Salt also softens sugar and butter, activates the taste buds and enhances all aromas.

What you need to know about salt

- Salt gives us the possibility of many combinations. At times, these may seem normal (like a terrine of *foie gras* and coarse salt), others surprising (like praline with coarse salt).

- The addition of salt enhances the flavour of foods when its quantity is well adjusted; but if we add it in greater quantity than we are used to, it produces a very interesting, completely unknown result. It certainly is not adequate in all of our preparations, so we should be careful to check the results of our combinations.

- Excessive salt can cause high blood pressure, which could lead to a stroke and heart attacks, so it should be used in moderation.

Eggs

The egg is one of the principal ingredients of the gastronomy world. Its great versatility and extraordinary properties as a thickener, emulsifier and stabiliser make its presence important in various creations in patisserie: sauces, creams, sponge cakes, custards and ice creams. Although it is not often the main ingredient, it plays specific and determining roles in terms of texture, taste and aroma, among other things. The egg is fundamental in preparations such as brioches, crèmes anglaises, sponge cakes and crèmes pâtissières. The extent to which eggs are used (or not) makes an enormous difference to the quality of the product.

Hens' eggs are graded in four sizes: small, medium, large and very large. For the dessert, paste and cake recipes in this book, use medium-sized eggs (approximately 50 g).

A good custard cannot be made without eggs, as they cause the required coagulation and give it the desired consistency and finesse.

Eggs are also an important ingredient in ice cream, where their yolks act as an emulsifier, due to the lecithin they contain, which aids the emulsion of fats.

What you need to know about eggs

- Eggs act as a texture agent in, for example, patisseries and ice creams.

- They intensify the aroma of pastries like brioche.

- They enhance flavours.

- They give volume to whisked sponges and batters.

- They strengthen the structure of preparations such as sponge cakes.

- They act as a thickening agent, e.g. in crème anglaise.

- They act as an emulsifier in preparations such as mayonnaise and ice cream.

- A fresh egg should have a small, shallow air pocket inside it.

- The yolk of fresh egg should be bulbous, firm and bright.

- The fresher the egg, the more viscous the egg white.

- Eggs should be stored far from strong odours as, despite their shells, these are easily absorbed.

- In a whole 60 g egg, the yolk weighs about 20 g, the white 30 g and the shell 10 g.

- Eggs contain protein and fat.

Egg whites

- To avoid the danger of salmonella, if the egg white is not going to be cooked or will not reach a temperature of 70°C, use pasteurised egg whites. Egg white is available chilled, frozen or dried.

- Equipment must be scrupulously clean and free from any traces of fat, as this prevents the whites from whipping; fat or grease prevents the albumen strands from bonding and trapping the air bubbles.

- Take care that there are no traces of yolk in the white, as yolk contains fat.

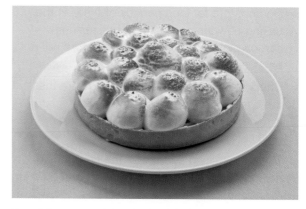

Egg whites are used to make meringues like the topping on this flan

- A little acid (cream of tartar or lemon juice) strengthens the egg white, extends the foam and produces more meringue. The acid also has the effect of stabilising the meringue.

- If the foam is over-whipped, the albumen strands, which hold the water molecules with the sugar suspended on the outside of the bubble, are overstretched. The water and sugar make contact and the sugar dissolves, making the meringue heavy and wet. This can sometimes be rescued by further whisking until it foams up, but very often you will find that you may have to discard the mixture and start again.

Beaten egg white forms a foam that is used for aerating sweets and many other desserts, including meringues (see recipe 45).

Convenience products

Convenience mixes, such as short pastry, sponge mixes and choux pastry mixes, are now becoming increasingly used in a variety of establishments. These products have improved enormously over the last few years. Using such products gives the chef the opportunity to save on time and labour; and with skill, imagination and creativity, the finished products are not impaired.

The large food manufacturer dominates the frozen puff pastry market. Not surprisingly many caterers, including some luxury establishments, have turned to using frozen puff pastry. It is now available in 30 cm squares, ready rolled, thus avoiding the possibility of uneven thickness and the waste that can occur when rolling out yourself.

Manufactured puff pastry is available in three types, defined often by their fat content. The cheapest is made with the white hydrogenated fat, which gives the product a pale colour and a waxy taste. Puff pastry made with bakery margarine has a better colour and, often, a better flavour. The best-quality puff pastry is that which is made with all butter, giving a richer texture, colour and flavour.

Pastry bought in blocks is cheaper than pre-rolled separate sheets, but has to be rolled evenly to give an even bake. The sizes of sheets do vary with manufacturers; all are interleaved with greaseproof paper.

Filo pastry is another example of a convenient pastry product; it is available in frozen sheets of various sizes. No rolling out is required; once thawed, it can be used as required and moulded if necessary.

As well as convenience pastry mixes, there is also a whole range of frozen products suitable to serve as sweets and afternoon tea pastries. These include fruit pies, flans, gâteaux and charlottes. The vast majority are ready to serve once defrosted, but very often they do require a little more decorative finish. The availability of such products gives the caterer the advantage of further labour cost reductions, while permitting the chef to concentrate on other areas of the menu.

Storage, health and safety

- Store all goods according to the Food Hygiene (Amendments) Regulations 1993/Food Safety Temperature Control Regulation 1995.

- Handle all equipment carefully to avoid cross-contamination.

- Take special care when using cream, and ensure that products containing cream are stored under refrigerated conditions.

- All piping bags must be sterilised after each use.

- Always make sure that storage containers are kept clean and returned ready for re-use. On their return they should be hygienically washed and stored.

Points to remember

- Check all weighing scales for accuracy.

- Follow the recipe carefully.

- Check all storage temperatures are correct.

- Fat is better to work with if it is 'plastic' (i.e. at room temperature). This will make it easier to cream.

- Always cream the fat and sugar well, before adding the liquid.

- Always work in a clean, tidy and organised way; clean all equipment after use.

- Always store ingredients correctly: eggs should be stored in a refrigerator, flour in a bin with a tight-fitting lid, sugar and other dry ingredients in closed storage containers.

- Ensure all cooked products are cooled before finishing.

- Understand how to use fresh cream; remember that it is easily over-whipped.

- Always plan your time carefully.

- Use silicone paper for baking in preference to greaseproof.

- Keep all small moulds clean and dry to prevent rusting.

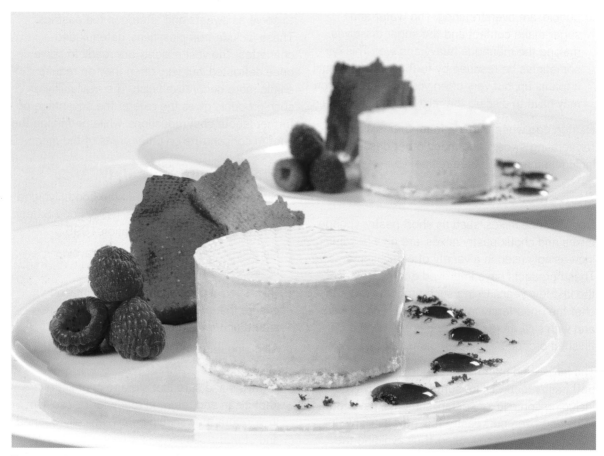

Eggs, sugar and cream are essential ingredients for many desserts, like this parfait

Healthy eating and puddings and desserts

Today desserts and puddings remain popular with the consumer, but there is now a demand for products with reduced fat and sugar content, as many people are keen to eat healthily. Chefs will continue to respond to this demand by modifying recipes to reduce the fat and sugar content; they may also use alternative ingredients, such as low-calorie sweeteners where possible and unsaturated fats. Although salt is an essential part of our diet, too much of it can be unhealthy (see page 79), and this is something else that chefs should take into consideration.

Egg custard-based desserts

Egg custard mixture provides the chef with a versatile basic set of ingredients that covers a wide range of sweets. Often the mixture is referred to as crème renversée. Some examples of sweets produced using this mixture are:

- crème caramel
- bread and butter pudding
- diplomat pudding
- cabinet pudding
- queen of puddings
- baked egg custard.

Savoury egg custard is used to make:

- quiches
- tartlets
- flans.

When a starch such as flour is added to the ingredients for an egg custard mix, this changes the characteristic of the end product.

Pastry cream (also known as confectioner's custard) is a filling used for many sweets, gâteaux, flans and tartlets, and as a basis for soufflé mixes. **Sauce anglaise** is used as a base for some ice creams. It is also used in its own right as a sauce to accompany a range of sweets.

Basic egg custard sets by coagulation of the egg protein. Egg white coagulates at approximately 60°C, egg yolk at 70°C. Whites and yolks mixed together will coagulate at 66°C. If the egg protein is overheated or overcooked, it will shrink and water will be lost from the mixture, causing undesirable bubbles in the custard. This loss of water is called syneresis.

Ingredients for egg custards

Eggs

Eggs are an essential ingredient in many desserts. Egg yolk is high in saturated fat. The yolk is a good source of protein and also contains vitamins and iron. The egg white is made up of protein (albumen) and water. The egg yolk also contains lecithin, which acts as an emulsifier in dishes such as mayonnaise – it helps to keep the ingredients mixed, so that the oils and water do not separate.

Milk

Full-cream, skimmed or semi-skimmed milk can be used for these desserts.

Milk is a basic and fundamental element of our diets throughout our lives. It is composed of water, sugar and fat (with a minimum fat content of 3.5 per cent). It is essential in an infinite number of preparations, from creams, ice creams, yeast doughs, mousses and custards to certain ganaches, cookies, tuiles and muffins. A yeast dough will change considerably in texture, taste and colour if made with milk instead of water.

Milk has a slightly sweet taste and little odour. Two distinct processes are used to conserve it:

1 **Pasteurisation** – the milk is heated to between 73°C and 85° for a few seconds, then cooled quickly to 4°C.
2 **Sterilisation (UHT)** – the milk is heated to between 140 and 150°C for 2 seconds, then cooled quickly.

Milk is homogenised to disperse the fat evenly, since the fat has a tendency to rise to the surface (see 'Cream', below).

Here are some useful facts about milk.

- Pasteurised milk has better taste and aroma than UHT milk.
- Milk is useful for developing flavour in sauces and creams, due to its lactic fermentation.
- Milk is an agent of colour, texture and aroma in doughs.
- Because of its lactic ferments, it helps in the maturation of doughs and creams.
- There are other types of milk, such as sheep's milk, that are very interesting to use in many restaurant desserts.

Milk is much more fragile than cream. In recipes, adding it in certain proportions is advisable for a much more subtle and delicate final product.

Cream

Cream is often added to egg custard desserts to enrich them and to improve the feel in the mouth (mouth-feel) of the final product. Indeed, it is used in many recipes because of its high fat content and great versatility.

Cream is the concentrated milk fat that is skimmed off the top of the milk when it has been left to sit. A film forms on the surface because of the difference in density between fat and liquid. This process is speeded up mechanically in large industries by heating and using centrifuges.

Cream should contain at least 18 per cent butter fat. Cream for whipping must contain more than 30 per cent butter fat. Commercially frozen cream is available in 2 and 10 kg slabs. Types, packaging, storage and uses of cream are listed in Table 14.1.

Table 14.1 Types of cream

Type of cream	Legal minimum fat (%)	Processing and packaging	Storage	Characteristics and uses
half cream	12	homogenised and may be pasteurised or ultra-heat treated	2–3 days	does not whip; used for pouring; suitable for low-fat diets
cream or single cream	18	homogenised and pasteurised by heating to about 79.5°C for 15 seconds then cooled to 4.5°C. Automatically filled into bottles and cartons after processing. Sealed with foil caps. Bulk quantities according to local suppliers	2–3 days in summer; 3–4 days in winter under refrigeration	a pouring cream suitable for coffee, cereals, soup or fruit. A valuable addition to cooked dishes. Makes delicious sauces. Does not whip
whipping cream	35	not homogenised, but pasteurised and packaged as above	2–3 days in summer; 3–4 days in winter under refrigeration	the ideal whipping cream. Suitable for piping, cake and dessert decoration, ice-cream, cake and pastry fillings
double cream	48	slightly homogenised, and pasteurised and packaged as above	2–3 days in summer; 3–4 days in winter under refrigeration	a rich pouring cream which will also whip. The cream will float on coffee or soup
double cream 'thick'	48	heavily homogenised, then pasteurised and packaged. Usually only available in domestic quantities	2–3 days in summer; 3–4 days in winter under refrigeration	a rich spoonable cream that will not whip
clotted cream	55	heated to 82°C and cooled for about 4½ hours. The cream crust is then skimmed off. Usually packed in cartons by hand. Bulk quantities according to local suppliers	2–3 days in summer; 3–4 days in winter under refrigeration	a very thick cream with its own special flavour and colour. Delicious with scones, fruit and fruit pies
ultra-heat treated (UHT) cream	12, 18, 35	half (12%), single (18%) or whipping cream (35%) is homogenised and heated to 132°C for one second and cooled immediately. Aseptically packed in polythene and foil-lined containers. Available in bigger packs for catering purposes	6 weeks if unopened. Needs no refrigeration. Usually date stamped	a pouring cream

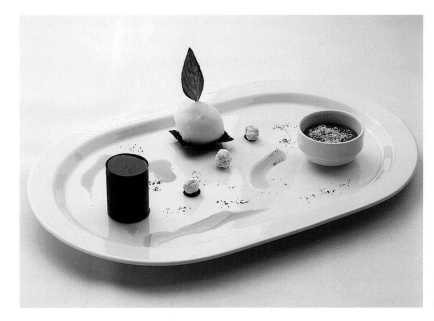

Chocolate mousse (recipe 34), lemon sorbet on a chocolate cup, and chocolate clafoutis

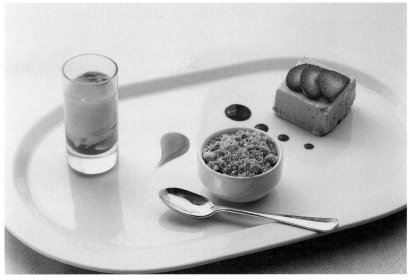

Cream caramel (recipe 44), fruit crumble and strawberry mousse (recipe 33)

Whipping and double cream may be whipped to make them lighter and to increase volume. Cream will whip more easily if it is kept at refrigeration temperature. Indeed, all cream products must be kept in the refrigerator for health and safety reasons. They should be handled with care and, as they will absorb odour, they should never be stored near onions or other strong-smelling foods.

As with milk, there are two main methods for conserving cream:

1 **Pasteurisation** – the cream is heated to between 85°C and 90°C for a few seconds and then cooled quickly; this cream retains all its flavour properties

2 **Sterilisation (UHT)** – this consists of heating the cream to between 140°C and 150°C for 2 seconds; cream treated this way loses some of its flavour properties, but it keeps for longer.

Always use pasteurised cream when possible, for example, in the restaurant when specialities are made for immediate consumption, such as 'ephemeral' patisserie (dessert cuisine), e.g. a chocolate bonbon that will be consumed immediately.

Here are some useful facts about cream.

- Cream whips with the addition of air, thanks to its fat content. This retains air bubbles formed during beating.
- Cream adds texture.
- All cream, once boiled and cooled, can be whipped again with no problem.
- Also, once it is boiled and mixed or infused with other ingredients to add flavour, it will whip again with no problem if first left to cool for 24 hours.
- To whip cream well, it must be cold (around 4°C).
- Cream can be infused with other flavours when it is hot or cold. If cold, it requires an infusion time of at least 12 hours.

Traditional custard made from custard powder

Custard powder is used to make custard sauce. It is made from vanilla-flavoured cornflour with yellow colouring added, and is a substitute for eggs. The fat content can be reduced by making it with semi-skimmed milk rather than full-fat milk.

Points to remember

Egg custard-based desserts

- Always work in a clean and tidy way, complying with food hygiene regulations.
- Prevent cross-contamination by not allowing any foreign substances to come into contact with the mixture.

- Always heat the egg yolks or eggs to 70°C, or use pasteurised egg yolks or eggs.
- Follow the recipe carefully.
- Ensure that all heating and cooling temperatures are followed.
- Always store the end product carefully at the right temperature.
- Check all weighing scales.
- Check all raw materials for correct use-by dates.
- Always wash your hands when handling fresh eggs or dairy products and other pastry ingredients.
- Never use cream to decorate a product that is still warm.
- Always remember to follow the Food Hygiene (Amendments) Regulations 1993/95.
- Check the temperature of refrigerators and freezers to ensure that they comply with the current regulations.

Fresh cream

- The piping of fresh cream is a skill; like all other skills it takes practice to become proficient. The finished item should look attractive, simple, clean and tidy, with neat piping.
- All piping bags should be sterilised after each use, as these may well be a source of contamination; alternatively use a disposable piping bag.
- Make sure that all the equipment you need for piping is hygienically cleaned before and after use to avoid cross-contamination.

Ice creams and sorbets

Ice cream

Traditional ice cream is made from a basic egg custard sauce. The sauce is cooled and mixed with fresh cream. It is then frozen by a rotating machine where the water content forms ice crystals.

Ice cream should be removed from the freezer a few minutes before serving. Long-term storage should be at between −18°C and −20°C.

The traditional method of making ice cream uses only egg yolks and sugar, and the traditional anglaise base. The more modern approach to making ice cream uses stabilisers and different sugars, plus egg whites, which prevents the high wastage of whites that might otherwise occur in the pastry section.

The Ice Cream Regulations

The Ice Cream Regulations 1959 and 1963 require ice cream to be pasteurised by heating to:

- 65°C for 30 minutes or
- 71°C for 10 minutes or
- 80°C for 15 seconds or
- 149°C for 2 seconds (sterilised).

After heat treatment, the mixture is reduced to 7.1°C within 1½ hours and kept at this temperature until the freezing process begins. Ice cream needs this treatment so as to kill harmful bacteria. Freezing without the correct heat treatment does not kill bacteria – it allows them to remain dormant. The storage temperature for ice cream should not exceed −20°C.

Any ice cream sold must comply with the following compositional standards.

- It must contain not less than 5 per cent fat and not less than 2.5 per cent milk protein (not necessary in natural proportions).
- It must conform to the Dairy Product Regulations 1995.

For further information contact the Ice Cream Alliance (see www.ice-cream.org)

The ice cream making process

1 **Weighing:** ingredients should be weighed precisely in order to ensure the best results and, what is more difficult, regularity and consistency.

2 **Pasteurisation:** this is a vital stage in making ice cream. Its primary function is to minimise bacterial contamination by heating the mixture of ingredients to 85°C, then quickly cooling it to 4°C.

3 **Homogenisation:** high pressure is applied to cause the explosion of fats, which makes ice cream more homogenous, creamier, smoother and much lighter. It is not usually done for homemade ice cream.

4 **Ripening:** this basic but optional stage refines flavour, further develops aromas and improves texture. This occurs during a rest period (4–24 hours), which gives the stabilisers and proteins time to act, improving the overall structure of the ice cream. This has the same effect on a crème anglaise, which is much better the day after it is made than it is on the same day.

5 **Churning:** here, the mixture is frozen while at the same time air is incorporated. The ice cream is removed from the machine at about 10°C.

Functions and approximate percentages of the main components of ice cream

- **Sucrose** (common sugar) not only sweetens ice cream, but also gives it body. An ice cream that contains only sucrose (not recommended) has a higher freezing point.
- The optimum sugar percentage of ice cream is between 15 and 20 per cent.
- Ice cream that contains **dextrose** (another type of sugar) has a lower freezing point, and better taste and texture.
- As much as 50 per cent of the sucrose can be substituted with other sweeteners, but the recommended amount is 25 per cent.
- **Glucose** (another type of sugar) improves smoothness and prevents the crystallisation of sucrose.
- The quantity of glucose used should be between 25 and 30 per cent of the sucrose by weight.
- **Atomised glucose** (glucose powder) is more water absorbent, so helps to reduce the formation of ice crystals.
- The quantity of dextrose used should be between 6 and 25 per cent of the substituted sucrose (by weight).
- **Inverted sugar** is a paste or liquid obtained from heating sucrose with water and an acid (e.g. lemon juice). Using inverted sugar in ice cream lowers the freezing point.
- Inverted sugar also improves the texture of ice cream and delays crystallisation.
- The quantity of inverted sugar used should be a maximum of 33 per cent of the sucrose by weight. It is very efficient at sweetening and gives the ice cream a low freezing point.

- **Honey** has more or less the same properties as inverted sugar.
- The purpose of **cream** in ice cream is to improve creaminess and taste.
- **Egg yolks** act as stabilisers for ice cream due to the lecithin they contain – they help to prevent the fats and water in the ice cream from separating.
- Egg yolks improve the texture and viscosity of ice cream.
- The purpose of stabilisers (e.g. gum Arabic, gelatine, pectin) is to prevent crystal formation by absorbing the water contained in ice cream and making a stable gel.
- The quantity of stabilisers in ice cream should be between 3 g and 5 g per kg of mix, with a maximum of 10 g.
- Stabilisers promote air absorption, making products lighter to eat and also less costly to produce, as air makes the product go further.

What you need to know about ice cream

- Hygienic conditions are essential while making ice cream – personal hygiene and high levels of cleanliness in the equipment and the kitchen environment must be maintained.
- An excess of stabilisers in ice cream will make it sticky.
- Stabilisers should always be mixed with sugar before adding, to avoid lumps.
- Stabilisers should be added at 45°C, which is when they begin to act.
- Cold stabilisers have no effect on the mixture, so the temperature must be raised to 85°C.
- Ice cream should be allowed to 'ripen' for 4–24 hours. This is a vital step that helps improve its properties.
- Ice cream should be cooled quickly to 4°C, because micro-organisms reproduce rapidly between 20°C and 55°C.

Sorbets

Sorbets belong to the ice cream family; they are a mixture of water, sucrose, atomised glucose, stabiliser, fruit juice, fruit pulp and, sometimes, liqueurs.

What you need to know about sorbet

- Sorbet is always more refreshing and easier to digest than ice cream.
- Fruit for sorbets must always be of a high quality and perfectly ripe.
- The percentage of fruit used in sorbet varies according to the type of fruit, its acidity and the quality desired.
- The percentage of sugar will depend on the type of fruit used.
- The minimum sugar content in sorbet is about 13 per cent.
- As far as ripening is concerned, the syrup should be left to rest for 4–24 hours and never mixed with the fruit because its acidity would damage the stabiliser.
- Stabiliser is added in the same way as for ice cream.
- Sorbets are not to be confused with granitas, which are semi-solid.

Stabilisers

Why do we use gelling substances?

Gelling substances, thickeners and emulsifiers are all stabilisers. They are products we use regularly, each with its own specific function; but their main purpose is to retain water to make a gel. The case of ice cream is the most obvious, in which they are used to prevent ice crystal formation. They are also used to stabilise the emulsion, increase the viscosity of the mix and give a smoother product that is more resistant to melting. There are many stabilising substances, both natural and artificial.

Edible gelatine

Edible gelatine is extracted from animals' bones (pork and veal) and, more recently, fish skin. Sold in sheets of 2 g, it is easy to precisely control the amount used and to manipulate it. Gelatine sheets should be soaked in cold water to soften, and then drained before use.

Gelatine sheets melt at 40°C and should be melted in a little of the liquid from the recipe before adding it to the base preparation.

Pectin

Pectin is another commonly used gelling substance because of its great absorption capacity. It comes from citrus peel (orange, lemon, etc.), though all fruits contain some pectin in their peel.

It is a good idea always to mix pectin with sugar before adding it to the rest of the ingredients.

Agar-agar

Agar-agar is a gelatinous marine algae found in Asia. It is sold in whole or powdered form and has a great absorption capacity. It dissolves very easily and, in addition to gelling, adds elasticity and resists heat (this is classified as a non-reversible gel).

Other stabilisers

- **Carob gum**, which comes from the seeds of the carob tree, makes sorbets creamier and improves heat resistance.
- **Guar gum** and **carrageen** are, like agar-agar, extracted from marine algae and are some of many other existing gelling substances available, but they are used less often.

Fruit-based recipes

Food value

Fruit is rich in antioxidant minerals and vitamins. Antioxidants protect cells from damage by oxygen, which may lead to heart disease and cancer. The current recommendation is to eat five portions of fruit and vegetables each day.

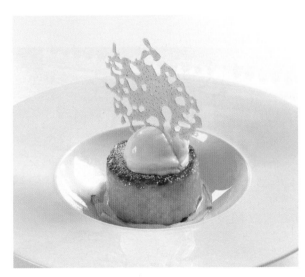

Apple Charlotte (recipe available on Dynamic Learning)

 ACTIVITY

1. How can desserts and puddings be modified to produce healthy options?
2. Name four sweets/desserts produced from milk, eggs and sugar.
3. How can egg white be strengthened during the whipping process?
4. Create your own dessert using ice cream, meringue and fresh fruit using a plate presentation.
5. Cost your dish and calculate a 70% gross profit.

Test yourself

1. State the difference between a cabinet pudding and a diplomat pudding.
2. How many eggs to ½ litre of milk for bread and butter pudding?
3. At what temperature should the oil be at for cooking apple fritters?
4. At what temperature should an individual vanilla soufflé be baked at and for how long?
5. Name three varieties of pancakes.
6. Name the classical setting agent for a fruit mousse.
7. What is a vacherin?
8. Describe a peach Melba.

1 Chantilly cream

	Makes approx. 500 ml
whipping cream	500 ml
caster sugar	100 g
vanilla arome	a few drops

1 Place all ingredients in a bowl. Whisk over ice until the mixture will form soft peaks. If using a mechanical mixer, stand and watch until the mixture is ready – do not leave it unattended.

2 Cover and place in the fridge immediately.

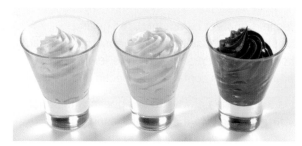

Recipes 1 to 3: chantilly cream, boiled buttercream and ganache

2 Boiled buttercream

	Makes 750 ml
medium eggs	2
icing sugar	50 g
granulated sugar or cube sugar	300 g
water	100 g
glucose	50 g
unsalted butter	400 g

1 Beat the eggs and icing sugar until at ribbon stage (sponge).

2 Boil the granulated or cube sugar with water and glucose to 118°C.

3 Gradually add the sugar at 118°C to the eggs and icing sugar at ribbon stage, whisk continuously and allow to cool to 26°C.

4 Gradually add the unsalted butter while continuing to whisk until a smooth cream is obtained.

Try something different

Buttercream may be flavoured with numerous flavours and combinations of flavours:

- chocolate and rum
- whisky and orange
- strawberry and vanilla
- lemon and lime
- apricot and passionfruit
- brandy and praline
- coffee and hazelnut.

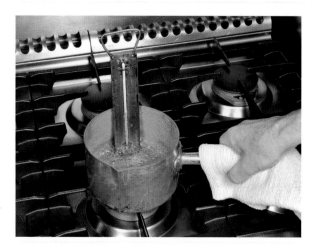

Boil the sugar with water and glucose

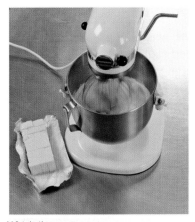

Whisk the eggs

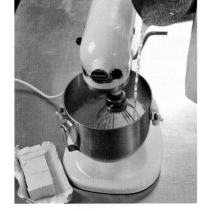

Add the sugar

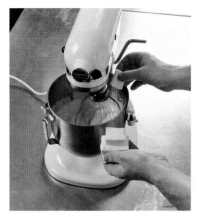

Add the butter

3 Ganache

Version 1 (makes 750 g)

double cream	300 ml
couverture, cut into small pieces	350 g
unsalted butter	85 g
spirit or liqueur	20 ml

Version 2 (makes 1 kg)

double cream	300 ml
vanilla pod	½
couverture, cut into small pieces	600 g
unsalted butter	120 g

1 Boil the cream (and the vanilla for version 2) in a heavy saucepan.

2 Pour the cream over the couverture. Whisk with a fine whisk until the chocolate has melted.

3 Whisk in the butter (and the liqueur for version 1).

4 Stir over ice until the mixture has the required consistency.

The two versions have different textures. Version 1 is ideal for truffles, version 2 for tortes or fillings.

ASSESSMENT

4 Pastry cream (*crème pâtissière*)

	Makes approx. 1 litre
milk	1 litre
vanilla pod (can be replaced with a few drops of vanilla arome)	1
eggs	4
caster sugar	200 g
strong flour	100 g
custard powder	30 g

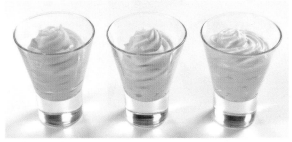

Pastry cream, crème diplomat and crème chiboust

1 Split open the vanilla pod and scrape out the seeds. Place pod and seeds in a heavy stainless steel pan, add the milk and place on the heat.

2 Whisk the eggs and sugar together.

3 Sieve the flour and custard powder onto paper and then add to the eggs. Whisk them all together to form a liaison.

4 When the milk has boiled, pour about one-third into the egg mixture and whisk in.

5 Bring the rest of the milk back to the boil, then pour in the liaison. Whisk hard until the mixture comes back to the boil again.

6 Simmer gently for 5 minutes.

7 Pour into a sterilised tray and stand on a wire rack. Stir occasionally to help the mixture cool quickly.

8 When cold, store in a plastic container in the fridge. Use within 3 days.

Try something different

- **_crème chiboust_**: when the pastry cream mixture has cooled slightly, fold in an equal quantity of Italian meringue (recipe 5)
- **_crème diplomat_**: when the pastry cream is chilled, fold in an equal quantity of whipped double cream

5 Italian meringue

	Makes 250 g
granulated or cube sugar	200 g
water	60 ml
cream of tartar	pinch
egg whites	4

1 Boil the sugar, water and cream of tartar to hard ball stage 121°C.

2 Beat the egg whites to full peak and, while stiff, beating slowly, pour on the boiling sugar. Use as required.

Making Italian meringue
http://bit.ly/AE5Ug9

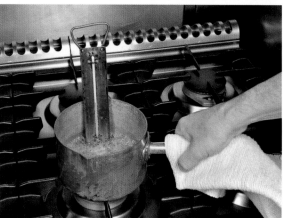

Boil the sugar

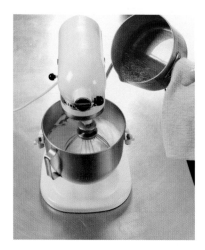

Beat the egg whites

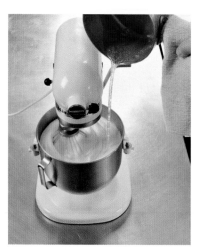

Combine the ingredients

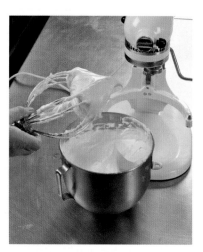

The mixture will stand up in stiff peaks when it is ready

6 Almond cream (frangipane)

	8 portions
butter	100 g
caster sugar	100 g
medium eggs	2
ground almonds	100 g
flour	10 g

1 Cream the butter and sugar.
2 Gradually beat in the eggs.
3 Mix in the almonds and flour (mix lightly).
4 Use as required.

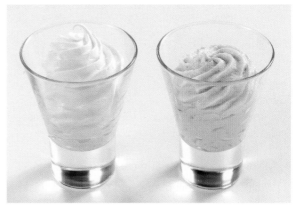

Italian meringue (recipe 5) and almond cream (recipe 6)

ASSESSMENT

7 Fruit coulis

	Makes 1500 ml
fruit purée	1 litre
caster sugar	500 g

The reason the soft ball is achieved and mixed with the purée is that this stabilises the fruit and prevents separation once the coulis has been put onto the plate.

1 Warm the purée.
2 Boil the sugar with a little water to soft-ball stage (121°C).
3 Pour the soft-ball sugar into the warm fruit purée while whisking vigorously.
4 This will then be ready to store.

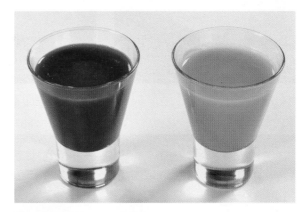

Raspberry and apricot coulis

8

Fresh egg custard sauce (sauce à l'anglaise)

cal	kcal	fat	sat fat	carb	sugar	protein	fibre
1666 KJ	397 kcal	21.7 g	9.9 g	38.0 g	38.0 g	14.7 g	0.0 g

*

	4 portions	10 portions
⚠ egg yolks, pasteurised	2	5
caster or unrefined sugar	25 g	60 g
vanilla essence or vanilla pod	2–3 drops	5–7 drops
milk, whole or skimmed	250 ml	625 ml

1 Mix the yolks, sugar and essence in a basin.
2 Whisk on the boiled milk and return to a thick-bottomed pan.
3 Place on a low heat and stir with a kitchen spoon until it coats the back of the spoon. Do not allow to boil or the eggs will scramble.
4 Put through a fine sieve into a bowl. Set on ice to arrest the cooking.

Try something different

Other flavours may be used in place of vanilla. For example:

- coffee
- curaçao
- chocolate
- Cointreau
- rum
- Tia Maria
- brandy
- whisky
- ground cinnamon
- kirsch
- orange flower water.

* Using whole milk; four portions

Making egg custard sauce
http://bit.ly/Ap8pHF

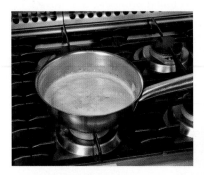

Bring the milk to the boil

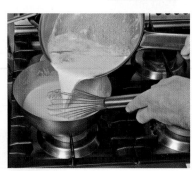

Tip the milk out, whisking it on to the eggs

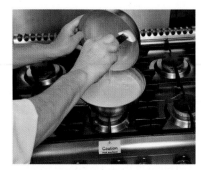

Return the mixture to the hot pan

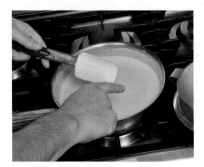

Test the consistency on the back of a spoon

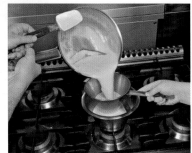

Pass the sauce

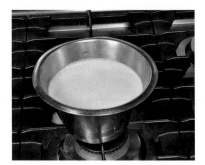

Transfer the sauce immediately to a cold pot; in the hot saucepan, it would continue to cook

9 Custard sauce

cal	kcal	fat	sat fat	carb	sugar	protein	fibre
1245 KJ	296 kcal	9.6 g	6.0 g	47.2 g	38.0 g	8.3 g	0.3 g	*

	4 portions
custard powder	10 g
milk (whole or semi-skimmed)	250 ml
caster or unrefined sugar	25 g

1 Dilute the custard powder with a little of the milk.
2 Boil the remainder of the milk.
3 Pour a little of the boiled milk on to the diluted custard powder.
4 Return to the saucepan.
5 Stir to the boil and mix in the sugar.

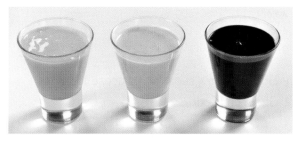

Recipes 8 to 10: custard, *sauce à l'anglais* and chocolate sauce

> See also recipe 8, for fresh egg custard sauce.

* Using whole milk

10 Chocolate sauce (*sauce chocolat*)

Method 1	
double cream	175 g
butter	40 g
milk or plain chocolate pieces	225 g

Method 2	
caster sugar	40 g
water	120 ml
dark chocolate (75% cocoa solids)	160 g
unsalted butter	25 g
single cream	80 ml

Method 1

Place butter and cream in a saucepan and gently bring to a simmer.

Add the chocolate and stir well until the chocolate has melted and the sauce is smooth.

Method 2

Dissolve the sugar in the water over a low heat.

Remove from the heat. Stir in the chocolate and butter.

When everything has melted, stir in the cream and gently bring to the boil.

11 Stock syrup

	4 portions	10 portions
water	500 ml	1¼ litres
granulated sugar	150 g	375 g
glucose	50 g	125 g

1 Boil the water, sugar and glucose together.
2 Strain and cool.

Glucose helps to prevent crystallising.

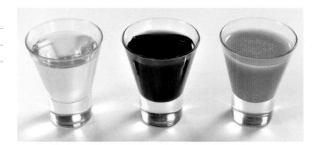

Recipes 11 to 13: stock syrup, caramel sauce and butterscotch sauce

12 Caramel sauce

	Makes 750 ml
caster sugar	100 g
water	80 ml
double cream	500 ml
egg yolks, lightly beaten (optional)	2

1 In a large saucepan, dissolve the sugar with the water over a low heat and bring to boiling point.
2 Wash down the inside of the pan with a pastry brush dipped in cold water to prevent crystals from forming.
3 Cook until the sugar turns to a deep amber colour. Immediately turn off the heat and whisk in the cream.

4 Set the pan back over a high heat and stir the sauce with the whisk. Let it bubble for 2 minutes, then turn off the heat.
5 You can now strain the sauce and use it when cooled, or, for a richer, smoother sauce, pour a little caramel onto the egg yolks, then return the mixture to the pan and heat to 80°C, taking care that it does not boil.
6 Pass the sauce through a conical strainer and keep in a cool place, stirring occasionally to prevent a skin from forming.

13 Butterscotch sauce

	4 portions	10 portions
double cream	250 ml	625 ml
butter	62 g	155 g
Demerara sugar	100 g	250 g

1 Boil the cream, then whisk in the butter and sugar, and simmer for 3 minutes.

14 Bramley apple spotted dick

	small pudding	large pudding
soft flour	350 g	700 g
baking powder	2 tsp	4 tsp
salt		
mixed spice	1 tsp	2 tsp
vegetable suet	150 g	300 g
light brown sugar	100 g	200 g
currants	150 g	300 g
Bramley apples, peeled and chopped	2	4
zest of lemons	1	3
milk	250 ml	500 ml
For the apple and vanilla compote		
sugar	300 g	
water	75 ml	
vanilla pod	1	
apples, diced	5	
sultanas	50 g	
white wine	dash	

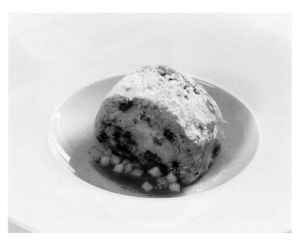

1 Sieve the flour and baking powder with a pinch of salt.

2 Stir in the rest of the pudding ingredients, adding the milk last.

3 Mix to form a sticky dough.

4 Place the mixture into greased moulds.

5 Bake in a bain-marie in the oven for 2 hours, making sure the tray is always half full of water, or cover and steam.

To make the apple and vanilla compote

1 Make a syrup from the sugar, water and vanilla.

2 Add the apples, sultanas and wine. Poach until the apple is soft.

Serve the pudding with the compote and custard.

15 Sticky toffee pudding

cal 4103 KJ	kcal 980 kcal	fat 60.4 g	sat fat 36.7 g	carb 106.7 g	sugar 78.9 g	protein 9.1 g	fibre 1.8 g

	4 portions	10 portions
Medjool dates, stoned and chopped	150 g	375 g
water	250 ml	625 ml
bicarbonate of soda	1 tsp	2½ tsp
unsalted butter	50 g	125 g
caster sugar	150 g	375 g
medium eggs	2	5
self-raising flour	150 g	375 g
vanilla essence	1 tsp	2½ tsp

1 For four portions, grease a baking tin approximately 28 × 18 cm in size (32 × 22 cm for 10 portions). (The modern version is to use individual pudding or dariole moulds.)

2 Boil the dates in the water for approximately 5 minutes until soft, then add the bicarbonate of soda.

3 Cream the butter and sugar together until light and white, gradually beat in the eggs.

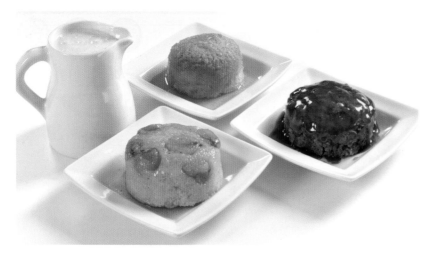

Front, Eve's pudding with gooseberries (recipe 17); back left, golden syrup pudding (recipe 16); back right, sticky toffee pudding (recipe 15)

4 Mix in the dates, flour and vanilla essence, stir well.

5 Form into the greased baking tin and bake in a pre-heated oven 180°C for approximately 30–40 minutes, until firm to the touch.

6 Carefully portion the sponge.

16 Golden syrup pudding

cal	kcal	fat	sat fat	carb	sugar	protein	fibre
1315 KJ	313 kcal	13.0 g	5.9 g	47.8 g	26.6 g	4.3 g	0.9 g

	6 portions	12 portions
flour	150 g	300 g
salt	pinch	large pinch
baking powder	10 g	20 g
or		
self-raising flour	150 g	300 g
suet, chopped	75 g	150 g
caster or unrefined sugar	50 g	100 g
lemon, zest of	1	2
egg, beaten	1	2
milk (whole or skimmed)	125 ml	250 ml
golden syrup	125 ml	250 ml

To make a treacle pudding, use a light treacle in place of the golden syrup. Vegetarian suet is available.

1 Sieve the flour, salt and baking powder (or replace the flour and baking powder with self-raising flour) into a bowl.

2 Mix the suet, sugar and zest.

3 Mix to a medium dough, with the beaten egg and milk.

4 Pour the syrup in a well-greased basin or individual moulds (1 hour cooking time). Place the pudding mixture on top.

5 Cover securely; steam for 1½ –2 hours.

6 Serve with a sauceboat of warm syrup containing the lemon juice, or with sauce anglaise or ice cream.

17 Eve's pudding with gooseberries

gooseberries, washed, topped and tailed	500 g
caster sugar	150 g plus a little for the fruit
butter	150 g
vanilla essence	
eggs, beaten	150 g
self-raising flour	240 g
milk	60 g

1 Arrange the gooseberries in the bottom of a buttered dish or individual ramekins. Sprinkle with caster sugar.

2 Cream the sugar, butter and vanilla essence together until white.

3 Gradually add the eggs to the butter mixture.

4 Sieve the flour twice, then fold it in to the eggs and butter. Adjust the consistency with milk.

5 Spread the mixture over the fruit, to a thickness of about 2 cm. This will form the sponge.

6 Bake for 30–40 minutes in a pre-heated oven at 180°C.

6 Rest for 5 minutes before removing from the dish. Brush with boiling apricot glaze. Serve with custard or *crème anglais*.

18 Chocolate fondant

cal 2830 KJ	kcal 675 kcal	fat 46.8 g	sat fat 29.6 g	carb 55.9 g	sugar 40.9 g	protein 11.0 g	fibre 0.6 g

	4 portions	10 portions
couverture chocolate	150 g	375 g
unsalted butter	125 g	312 g
eggs	3	7
yolks	2	5
caster sugar	75 g	182 g
flour	75 g	182 g
white chocolate pieces (optional)		

1 Lightly grease and flour individual dariole moulds or a ring mould.

2 Carefully melt the chocolate and butter in a suitable bowl, either in a microwave or over a pan of hot water (bain-marie).

3 In a separate bowl, whisk the eggs, egg yolks and caster sugar until aerated to ribbon stage. Pour into the chocolate and butter mix, then whisk together.

4 Add the flour, then mix until smooth.

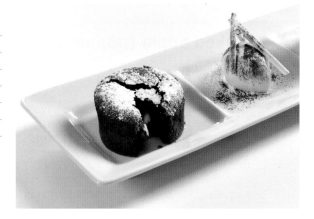

5 Pour into the moulds. Place white chocolate pieces at the centre to give a two-tone effect. Bake in the oven at 200°C for 15 minutes.

6 Remove from the oven, leave for 5 minutes before turning out onto suitable plates.

7 Serve with a suitable ice cream (e.g. vanilla, pistachio, almond or Baileys).

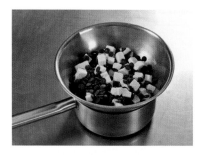

Melt the chocolate and butter in small pieces

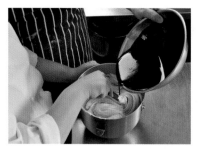

Fold the melted chocolate into the egg mixture

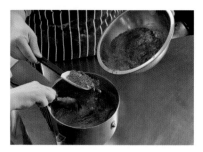

Add the dry ingredients

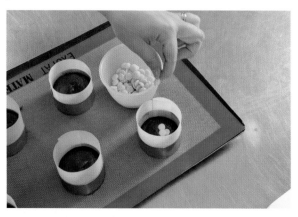

To make the centre, add white chocolate pieces on a base of the chocolate mixture

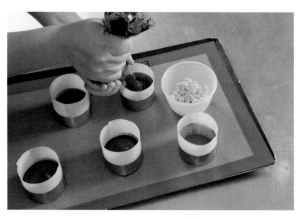

Pipe in more of the chocolate mixture until the mould is full

19 Baked apple (pommes bonne femme)

cal	kcal	fat	sat fat	carb	sugar	protein	fibre
663 KJ	156 kcal	5.1 g	2.2 g	29.7 g	29.5 g	0.4 g	2.7 g

*

	4 portions	10 portions
medium-sized cooking apples	4	10
sugar, white or unrefined	50 g	125 g
cloves	4	10
butter or margarine	20 g	50 g
water	60 ml	150 ml

1 Core the apples and make an incision 2 mm deep round the centre of each. Wash well. Peel the apples for a modern presentation.

2 Place in a roasting tray or ovenproof dish.

3 Fill the centre with sugar and add a clove to each.

4 Place 5 g butter on each. Add the water.

5 Bake in a moderate oven at 200–220°C for 15–20 minutes.

6 Turn the apples over carefully.

7 Return to the oven until cooked, about 40 minutes in all.

8 Serve with a little cooking liquor and custard, cream or ice cream.

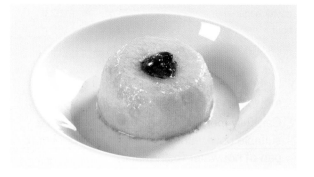

For stuffed baked apple, proceed as for baked apples, but fill the centre with washed sultanas, raisins or chopped dates, or a combination of these.

* Using hard margarine

20 Pancakes with apple *(crêpes normande)*

	4 portions	10 portions
cooked apple		
flour (white or wholemeal)	100 g	250 g
salt	pinch	large pinch
egg	1	2–3
milk (whole or skimmed)	¼ litre	625 ml
melted butter, margarine or oil	10 g	25 g
oil for frying		
caster sugar to serve		

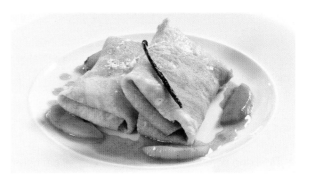

1 Place a little cooked apple in a pan, add the pancake mixture and cook on both sides.

2 Turn out, sprinkle with caster sugar and roll up.

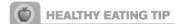 **HEALTHY EATING TIP**

- Use semi-skimmed or skimmed milk to make the batter.
- Use vegetable oil for frying.

21 Crêpes Suzette

For the crêpes	
eggs	2
salt	pinch
caster sugar	112 g
milk	575 ml
strong flour	225 g
melted butter	30 g
For the Suzette mixture	
unsalted butter	60 g
zest and juice of orange	1
caster sugar	60 g
Grand Marnier	30 ml
Cognac	30 ml
orange, peeled and divided into segments	2

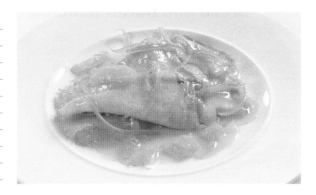

1 Make the crêpes.

2 Melt the butter. Add the sugar, zest, juice and Grand Marnier. Bring to the boil rapidly and reduce.

3 Dip each crêpe into the sauce, then fold and arrange on the plate. Keep hot.

4 Add the Cognac to the sauce and flambé.

5 Add the orange segments to the sauce and pour over the crêpes.

22 Apple fritters *(beignets aux pommes)*

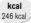

cal	kcal	fat	sat fat	carb	sugar	protein	fibre
1034 KJ	246 kcal	10.2 g	1.9 g	38.9 g	25.0 g	2.1 g	3.0 g

*

	4 portions	10 portions
cooking apples	400 g	1 kg
flour, as needed		
frying batter	150 g	375 g
apricot sauce	125 ml	300 ml

1 Peel and core the apples and cut into ½ cm rings.
2 Pass through flour, shake off the surplus.
3 Dip into the frying batter (page 386).
4 Lift out with the fingers, into fairly hot deep fat: 185°C.
5 Cook for about 5 minutes on each side.
6 Drain well on kitchen paper, dust with icing sugar and glaze under the salamander.
7 Serve with hot apricot sauce.

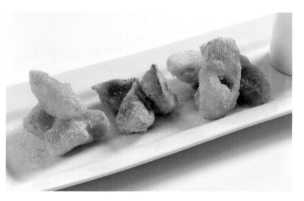

Left to right: apple, fig and banana fritters

* Fried in peanut oil

23 Bread and butter pudding

cal	kcal	fat	sat fat	carb	sugar	protein	fibre
1093 KJ	260 kcal	11.6 g	5.9 g	30.4 g	23.4 g	10.6 g	1.0 g

*

	4 portions	10 portions
sultanas	50 g	100 g
slices of white or wholemeal bread, spread with butter or margarine	2	5
eggs (medium)	3	7
sugar, caster or unrefined	50 g	125 g
vanilla essence or a vanilla pod	2–3 drops	5 drops
milk, whole or skimmed	½ litre	1¼ litres

1 Wash the sultanas and place in a pie dish or individual dishes.
2 Remove the crusts from the bread and cut each slice into four triangles; neatly arrange overlapping in the pie dish.
3 Prepare an egg custard: whisk the eggs, sugar and vanilla essence together. Warm the milk and pour it on to the eggs, whisking continuously.
4 Pass through a fine strainer on to the bread, dust lightly with sugar.
5 Stand in a roasting tray half full of water and cook slowly in a moderate oven at 160°C for 45 minutes to 1 hour.
6 Clean the edges of the pie dish and serve.

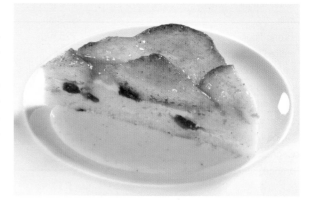

For a crisp crust finish, sprinkle with icing sugar and brown well under the salamander. Traditional bread and butter pudding is made in a pie dish and is of soft consistency. To prepare individual plated portions in the contemporary fashion requires either more egg or bread which gives a firmer consistency.

 HEALTHY EATING TIP

- Try using half wholemeal and half white bread.
- The fat content will be reduced by using semi-skimmed milk in the custard.
- Adding more dried fruit would reduce the need for so much sugar.

Try something different

- Before cooking, add freshly grated nutmeg or orange zest, or a combination of both
- Use fruit loaf, brioche or panettone
- Chocolate bread and butter pudding – add 25 g chocolate powder to the egg custard mix
- Add soft, well-drained poached (or tinned) fruit (e.g. peaches, pears) to the bottom of the dish.

* Using white bread and butter

Making bread and butter pudding
http://bit.ly/x01Z8F

---

24 Cabinet pudding (pouding cabinet)

cal	kcal	fat	sat fat	carb	sugar	protein	fibre
1427 KJ	340 kcal	15.8 g	7.2 g	40.9 g	35.5 g	11.0 g	0.7 g

	4 portions	10 portions
plain sponge cake	100 g	250 g
zest of unwaxed lemons, grated		
currants and sultanas	25 g	60 g
milk, whole or skimmed	½ litre	1¼ litres
eggs (medium)	3–4	8–10
caster or unrefined sugar	50 g	125 g
vanilla essence or a vanilla pod	2–3 drops (1 pod)	7 drops (2 pods)

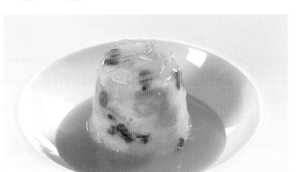

1 Cut the cake into ½ cm dice.
2 Mix with the lemon zest and fruits (which can be soaked in rum).
3 Place in a greased, sugared charlotte mould or four dariole moulds. Do not fill more than halfway.
4 Warm the milk and whisk on to the eggs, sugar and essence (or vanilla pod).
5 Strain on to the mould.
6 Place in a roasting tin, half full of water; allow to stand for 5–10 minutes.
7 Cook in a moderate oven at 150–160°C for 30–45 minutes.
8 Leave to set for a few minutes before turning out.
9 Serve a fresh egg custard (recipe 8) or hot apricot sauce separately.

Try something different

Diplomat pudding is made as for cabinet pudding, but served cold with either redcurrant, raspberry, apricot or vanilla sauce.

* Using whole milk and 3 eggs. Using whole milk and 4 eggs: 1512 kJ/360 kcal; 17.3 g Fat; 7.7 g Sat Fat; 40.9 g Carb; 35.5 g Sugar; 12.7 g Protein; 0.7 g Fibre

25 Rice pudding

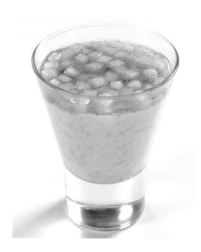

	4 portions	10 portions
rice (short or whole grain)	50 g	125 g
sugar, caster or unrefined	50 g	125 g
milk (whole or skimmed)	½ litre	1¼ litres
butter or margarine	10 g	25 g
vanilla essence	2–3 drops	6–8 drops
grated nutmeg		

1 Boil the milk in a thick-based pan.
2 Add the washed rice, stir to the boil.
3 Simmer gently, stirring frequently until the rice is cooked.
4 Mix in the sugar, flavouring and butter (at this stage an egg yolk may also be added). A vanilla pod can be used in place of essence.
5 Pour into individual dishes. Top with diced apple poached in vanilla syrup.

Candied fruit and chopped nuts may be added for variety.

 HEALTHY EATING TIP

● Use semi-skimmed milk.

26 Vanilla soufflé *(soufflé à la vanille)*

cal 757 KJ	kcal 180 kcal	fat 9.1 g	sat fat 3.5 g	carb 16.6 g	sugar 14.6 g	protein 9.1 g	fibre 0.1 g

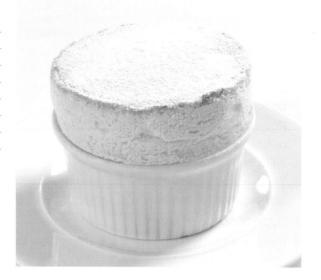

	4 portions	10 portions
butter	10 g	25 g
caster sugar, for soufflé case	50 g	125 g
milk	125 ml	300 ml
natural vanilla or pod		
medium eggs, separated	4	10
flour	10 g	25 g
caster sugar	50 g	125 g
icing sugar, to serve		

1 Lightly coat the inside of a soufflé case/dish with fresh butter.
2 Coat the butter in the soufflé case with caster sugar as needed, tap out surplus.
3 Boil the milk and vanilla in a thick-bottomed pan.

4 Mix half the egg yolks, the flour and sugar to a smooth consistency in a basin.

5 Add the boiling milk to the mixture, stir vigorously until completely mixed.

6 Return this mixture to a clean thick-bottomed pan and stir continuously with a kitchen spoon over gentle heat until the mixture thickens, then remove from heat.

7 Allow to cool slightly. Add the remaining egg yolks and mix thoroughly.

8 Stiffly whip the egg whites and *carefully* fold into the mixture, which should be just warm. (An extra egg white can be added for extra lightness.)

9 Place the mixture into the prepared case(s) and level it off with a palette knife – do not allow it to come above the level of the soufflé case.

10 Place on a baking sheet and cook in a moderately hot oven – approx. 200–230°C – until the soufflé is well risen and firm to the touch – approx. 15–20 minutes. (For individual soufflés, reduce time by 5 minutes.)

11 Remove carefully from oven, dredge with icing sugar and serve at once. A hot soufflé must not be allowed to stand or it may sink.

> A pinch of egg white powder (merri-white) can be added when whisking the whites, to strengthen them and assist in the aeration process.

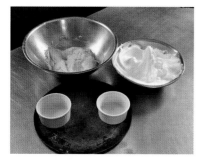

Ingredients for vanilla soufflé, with egg whites whipped

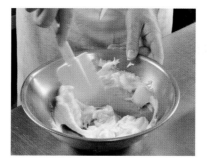

Mix half the egg whites into the flour

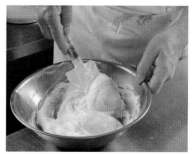

Fold the mixture

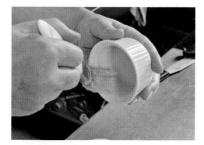

Prepare the mould

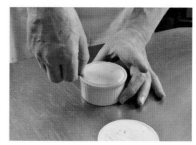

Thumb the edge

27 Mango soufflé

	4 portions
milk	100 ml
mango purée	150 ml
egg yolks	80 ml
caster sugar for liaison	60 g
cornflour for liaison	15 g
egg whites	150 ml
lemon juice	a few drops
caster sugar	30 g
cornflour	5 g
mango compote	

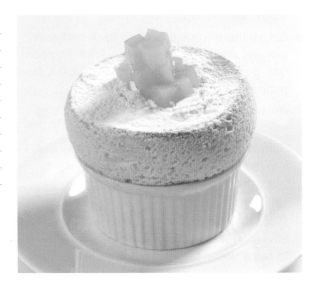

1 Bring the milk and mango purée to the boil.

2 Make the liaison by whisking the egg yolks with 60 g of caster sugar. Sieve in 15 g of cornflour and continue whisking until smooth.

3 Add one-third of the boiling liquid to the liaison.

4 Bring the rest of the liquid back to the boil. Whisk the liaison into it, then continue whisking until it returns to the boil. Simmer for 2–3 minutes. Cover and cool.

5 Whisk the egg whites, lemon juice, 30 g of sugar and 5 g of cornflour together to the

consistency of shaving foam. Fold this into the cooled mango pastry cream mixture.

6 Grease each mould and dust it with caster sugar. Place a spoonful of mango compote into the bottom of each prepared soufflé mould. Pour in the mixture.

7 Bake at 200°C for approximately 12 minutes.

ASSESSMENT

28 Soufflé pudding (pouding soufflé)

cal	kcal	fat	sat fat	carb	sugar	protein	fibre
510 KJ	122 kcal	7.6 g	3.2 g	5.9 g	4.8 g	0.2 g	0.0 g

	6 portions	10 portions
milk (whole or skimmed)	185 ml	375 ml
flour (white or wholemeal)	25 g	50 g
butter or margarine	25 g	50 g
caster or unrefined sugar	25 g	50 g
medium eggs, separated	3	6

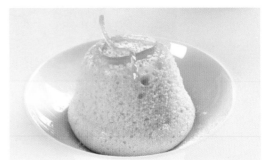

1 Boil the milk in a sauteuse.

2 Combine the flour, butter and sugar.

3 Whisk into the milk and reboil.

4 Remove from heat, add the egg yolks one at a time, whisking continuously.

5 Stiffly beat the whites and carefully fold into the mixture.

6 Three-quarters fill buttered and sugared dariole moulds.

7 Place in a roasting tin, half full of water.

8 Bring to the boil and place in a hot oven at 230–250°C for 12–15 minutes.

9 Turn out on to a flat dish and serve with a suitable hot sauce, such as custard or sabayon sauce.

> Orange or lemon soufflé pudding is made by flavouring the basic mixture with the grated zest of an orange or lemon and a little appropriate sauce. Use the juice in the accompanying sauce.

* Using white flour and hard margarine

---

29 Christmas pudding

	8–10 portions (1-litre basin)
sultanas	100 g
raisins	100 g
currants	100 g
mixed chopped candied peel	25 g
barley wine	70 ml
Guinness (stout)	70 ml
rum	2 tbsp
self-raising flour	50 g
mixed spice	1 tsp
ground nutmeg	¼ tsp
cinnamon	1 tsp
breadcrumbs (white or brown)	100 g
suet, shredded	100 g
soft dark brown sugar	200 g
ground almonds	25 g
cooking apples, peeled and chopped	75 g
orange, grated zest of	½
lemon, grated zest of	½
eggs	2

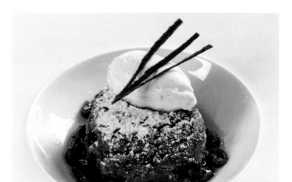

1 Place all the dried fruit and candied peel in a mixing bowl; soak overnight with the barley wine, Guinness and rum.

2 Sift the flour with the mixed spice, nutmeg and cinnamon.

3 Add breadcrumbs, suet and sugar to the flour.

4 Drain the fruit from the alcohol. Add to the flour along with the almonds, apple and grated zest.

5 In a separate basin, beat the eggs with the alcohol.

6 Add the dried fruit to the flour, mix thoroughly.

7 Pack into a lightly greased basin (1 litre). Cover with a sheet of silicone and aluminium foil. Secure well.

8 Steam for 8 hours at normal atmospheric pressure.

9 Remove from steamer and allow to cool, remove foil and silicone, replace with fresh. Secure well.

10 Allow to mature for at least 2 months. Reheat by steaming for a further 2 hours.

11 Serve with rum and brandy sauce.

30 Baked Alaska *(omelette soufflée surprise)*

cal	kcal	fat	sat fat	carb	sugar	protein	fibre
2190 KJ	521 kcal	16.4 g	7.3 g	91.3 g	81.2 g	7.7 g	0.6 g

	4 portions	10 portions
sponge cake	4 pieces	10 pieces
fruit syrup	60 ml	150 ml
vanilla ice cream or parfait	4 scoops	10 scoops
egg whites	4	10
caster sugar	200 g	500 g

1 Neatly arrange the pieces of sponge cake in the centre of a flat ovenproof dish or individual dishes.

2 Sprinkle the sponge cake with a little fruit syrup.

3 Place a flattened scoop of vanilla ice cream on each piece of sponge. Alternatively, mould a ball of parfait – this will be more stable than ice cream.

4 Surround the ice cream or parfait with sponge to conceal it (optional). Place in the freezer to prevent this from melting.

5 Meanwhile stiffly whip the egg whites and fold in the sugar.

6 Use half the meringue and completely cover the ice cream and sponge. Neaten with a palette knife.

7 Place the remainder of the meringue into a piping bag with a large tube (plain or star) and decorate over.

8 Place into a hot oven at 230–250°C and colour a golden brown or brown with a blowtorch. Serve immediately.

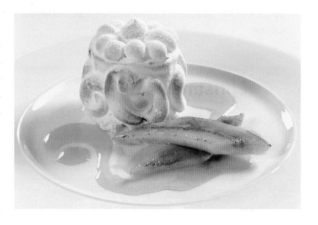

Try something different

- The fruit syrup for soaking the sponge may be flavoured with rum, sherry, brandy, whisky, Tia Maria, curaçao or any other suitable liqueur.

- **Baked Alaska with peaches:** proceed as for the basic recipe, adding a little maraschino to the fruit syrup and using raspberry ice cream instead of vanilla; cover the ice cream with four halves of peaches.

- **Baked Alaska with pears:** proceed as for the basic recipe, adding a little kirsch to the fruit syrup and adding halves of poached pears to the ice cream.

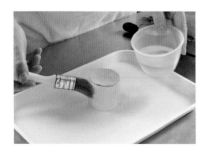

Glaze the sponge

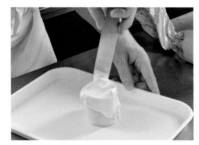

Pipe meringue to cover

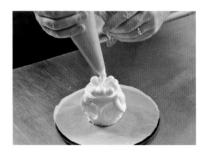

Pipe swirls of meringue to decorate

31 Tatin of apple

Makes 10 portions

100 g	caster sugar
10 g	glucose
200 ml	water
100 g	unsalted butter, diced
7	Granny Smith's apples, peeled and cored
½	lemon, juice
175 g	puff pastry (chapter 15, recipe 3)

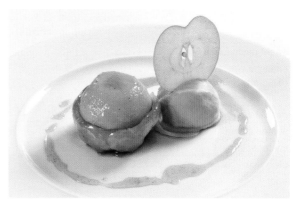

1 Cook the sugar, glucose and water in a thick-bottomed copper (bear in mind that the tatin will be cooked in this so it will need to be ovenproof) until it reaches a pale, amber colour, which is pre-caramel.

2 Remove from the heat and add the diced butter.

3 While the butter is melting, cut the apples into eighths, lightly sprinkle with lemon juice and place on top of the caramel/butter.

4 Place in the oven for 25 minutes until the apples are half-cooked and starting to caramelise.

5 Meanwhile, roll out the puff pastry, 3–4 mm thick, and slightly larger than the diameter of the pan.

6 Cover the apples with the pastry and bake for a further 15–20 minutes, until the pastry is golden.

7 Remove from the oven and leave to cool slightly before turning out.

8 Serve with vanilla ice cream, apple sorbet or crème fraîche.

Tatin of apple may also be produced individually, as shown here.

This is an apple tart that is cooked under a lid of pastry, but served with the pastry underneath the fruit. In this delicious dessert the taste of caramel is combined with the flavour of the fruit, finished with a crisp pastry base; it was created by the Tatin sisters, who ran a hotel-restaurant in Lamotte-Beuvron at the beginning of the last century. Having been made famous by the sisters the dish was first served at Maxim's in Paris, as a house speciality. It is served there to this day.

32 Apple crumble tartlets

	4 portions	10 portions
sweet paste (page 500)	175 g	435 g
eating apples, e.g. Reinette or Granny Smith, cored and thinly sliced	2	5
For the filling		
soured cream	200 ml	500 ml
caster sugar	25 g	62 g
plain flour	30 g	75 g
egg	1	3
vanilla extract		
For the crumble		
unsalted butter, melted	25 g	62 g
plain flour	30 g	75 g
walnuts, chopped	25 g	62 g
brown sugar	25 g	62 g
ground cinnamon	a good pinch	
salt		
icing sugar, to garnish		

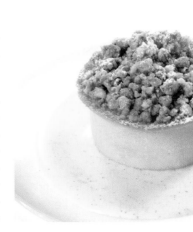

1 Line individual ramekins with sweet paste.

2 Fill each of the lined ramekins with the finely sliced apple. To make the filling, whisk the soured cream, caster sugar, flour and egg together. Pass through a fine sieve and flavour with vanilla extract.

3 Cover the apple with the filling mixture and bake at 190°C for 10 minutes.

4 To make the crumble topping, combine the walnuts, flour, brown sugar, cinnamon and a small pinch of salt. Mix with the melted butter to form a crumb.

5 Sprinkle the crumble on top of each ramekin and bake for a further 10 minutes.

6 Leave to cool slightly and then turn out onto individual plates.

7 Dust with icing sugar. Serve with warm crème anglaise. An alternative garnish would be fresh raspberries and raspberry coulis.

33 Basic fruit mousse

	9 portions (690 g)
fruit purée	225 g
egg whites, pasteurised, or Italian meringue	115 g
caster sugar	100 g
gelatine sheets (bronze)	4
semi-whipped cream	225 g
desired liquor	25 g

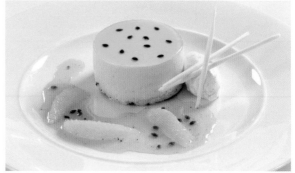

Passion fruit mousse

1 Bring the fruit purée to just under boiling point.

2 Whip the egg whites to a snow, add the sugar and combine (this offers a softer, less dense

meringue finish and homogenises into a mousse).

3 Slowly add the softened gelatine to the warmed warm purée. Cool over ice.

4 Fold in the meringue and add the other ingredients. Pour into the desired moulds.

5 To serve, unmould onto suitable plates, garnish with fresh fruit and a suitable coulis.

34 Chocolate mousse

	8 portions	16 portions
egg yolks, pasteurised	80 ml	160 ml
stock syrup at 30° Baume	125 ml	250 ml
bitter couverture	250 g	500 g
leaf gelatine (optional)	2	4
whipping cream, whipped	500 ml	1 litre

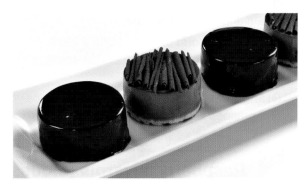

Recipes 34 and 35: chocolate mousse and chocolate bavarois

1 Boil the syrup.

2 Place the yolks into the bowl of a food mixer. Pour over the boiling syrup and whisk until thick. Remove from the machine.

3 Add all the couverture at once, and fold it in quickly until melted.

4 Drain the gelatine, melt it and fold it into the chocolate sabayon mixture.

5 Add all the whipped cream at once, and fold it in carefully.

6 Place the mixture into prepared moulds. Refrigerate or freeze immediately.

35 Bavarois: basic recipe (often referred to as a mousse)

cal	kcal	fat	sat fat	carb	sugar	protein	fibre	
970 KJ	231 kcal	18.2 g	10.9 g	11.8 g	11.8 g	5.8 g	0.0 g	*

	6–8 portions
gelatine	10 g
medium eggs, pasteurised, separated	2
caster sugar	50 g
milk, whole or skimmed	¼ litre
whipping or double cream or non-dairy cream	125 ml

1 If using leaf gelatine, soak in cold water.

2 Cream the yolks and sugar in a bowl until almost white.

3 Whisk in the milk, which has been brought to the boil; mix well.

4 Clean the milk saucepan, which should be a thick-based one, and return the mixture to it.

5 Return to a low heat and stir continuously with a wooden spoon until the mixture coats the back of the spoon. The mixture must not boil.

6 Remove from the heat; add the gelatine and stir until dissolved.

7 Pass through a fine strainer into a clean bowl, leave in a cool place, stirring occasionally until almost at setting point.

8 Fold in the lightly beaten cream.

9 Fold in the stiffly beaten whites (optional).

10 Pour the mixture into a mould or individual moulds (which may be very lightly greased with almond oil).

11 Allow to set in the refrigerator.

12 Shake and turn out on to a flat dish or plates.

Bavarois may be decorated with sweetened, flavoured whipped cream (crème Chantilly). It is advisable to use pasteurised egg yolks and whites.

HEALTHY EATING TIP

- Use semi-skimmed milk and whipping cream to reduce the overall fat content.

Try something different

- **Chocolate bavarois:** dissolve 50 g chocolate couverture in the milk. Decorate with whipped cream and grated chocolate.
- **Coffee bavarois:** proceed as for a basic bavarois, with the addition of coffee essence to taste.
- **Orange bavarois:** add grated zest and juice of 2 oranges and 1 or 2 drops orange colour to the mixture, and increase the gelatine by 2 leaves. Decorate with orange zest or a fine julienne which has been poached in stock syrup.
- **Lemon or lime bavarois:** as orange bavarois, using lemons or limes in place of oranges.
- **Vanilla bavarois:** add a vanilla pod or a few drops of vanilla essence to the milk. Decorate with vanilla-flavoured sweetened cream (crème Chantilly).

* Using whole milk and whipping cream

36 Raspberry bavarois (mousse)

cal	kcal	fat	sat fat	carb	sugar	protein	fibre
1102 KJ	265 kcal	17.7 g	10.0 g	19.0 g	19.0 g	8.5 g	0.6 g

	4 portions	10 portions
raspberries (picked, washed and sieved)	200 g	500 g
medium eggs	2	5
gelatine	10 g	25 g
milk, whole or skimmed	180 ml	500 ml
sugar, caster or unrefined	50 g	125 g
whipping or double cream or non-dairy cream	125 ml	300 ml

1 Prepare as for the basic recipe (recipe 35).
2 When the custard is almost cool, add the fruit purée.
3 Decorate with whole fruit and whipped cream.
4 Strawberries may be used instead of raspberries.

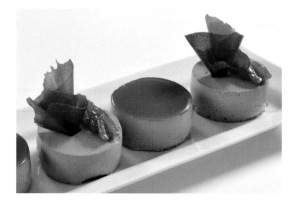

 HEALTHY EATING TIP

- Use semi-skimmed milk and whipping cream to reduce the overall fat content.

* Using whole milk and whipping cream

37 Lime soufflé frappe

	10 portions	15 portions
couverture		
sponge		
lime syrup		
For the Swiss meringue		
egg whites	190 ml	300 ml
caster sugar	230 ml	340 ml
For the sabayon		
whipping cream	600 ml	900 ml
lime zest, finely grated and blanched, and juice	8	12
egg yolks	10	15
caster sugar	170 g	250 g
leaf gelatine, soaked in iced water	9½	14
To decorate		
confit of lime segments		
moulded chocolate		

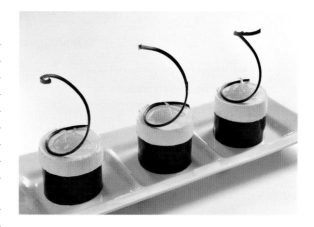

1 Use individual stainless steel ring moulds. Cut a strip of acetate, 8 cm wide, to fit inside each ring. Cut a 6 cm strip to fit inside the first, spread it with tempered couverture and place inside the first strip, in the mould.

2 Place a round of sponge in the base of each mould and moisten with lime syrup.

3 Make up the Swiss meringue.

4 Whisk the cream until it is three-quarters whipped, then chill.

5 Whisk together the egg yolks, sugar and blanched lime zest. Boil the juice and pour it over the mixture to make the sabayon. Whisk over a bain marie until it reaches 75°C, then continue whisking away from the heat until it is cold.

6 Drain and melt the gelatine. Fold it into the sabayon.

7 Fold in the Swiss meringue, and then the chilled whipped cream.

8 Fill the prepared moulds. Level the tops and chill until set.

9 To serve, carefully remove the mould, peel away the acetate, plate and decorate.

38 Vanilla panna cotta served on a fruit compote

cal	kcal	fat	sat fat	carb	sugar	protein	fibre
1565 KJ	378 kcal	34.0 g	21.1 g	16.1 g	16.1 g	2.9 g	1.5 g	*

	6 portions
milk	125 ml
double cream	375 ml
aniseeds	2
vanilla pod	½
leaf gelatine (soaked)	2 leaves
caster sugar	50 g
Fruit compote	
apricot purée	75 g
vanilla pod	½
peach	1
kiwi fruit	1
strawberries	75 g
blueberries	75 g
raspberries	50 g

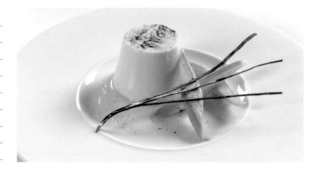

1 Prepare the fruit compote by boiling the apricot purée and infusing with vanilla pod. Remove pod, allow purée to cool.

2 Finely dice the peach and the kiwi and quarter the strawberries. Mix, then add blueberries and raspberries.

3 Bind the fruit with the apricot purée. A little stock syrup (recipe 11) may be required to keep the fruit free flowing.

4 For the panna cotta, boil the milk and cream, add aniseeds, infuse with the vanilla pod, remove after infusion.

5 Heat again and add the soaked gelatine and caster sugar. Strain through a fine strainer.

6 Place in a bowl set over ice and stir until it thickens slightly; this will allow the vanilla seeds to suspend throughout the mix instead of sinking to the bottom.

7 Fill individual dariole moulds.

8 Place the fruit compote with individual fruit plates, turn out the panna cotta, place on top of the compote, finish with a tuile biscuit.

HEALTHY EATING TIP

- This dish will contribute to the recommended five portions of fruit and vegetables per day.

* Using blackcurrants for blueberries

39 Poached fruits or fruit compote (*compote de fruits*)

	cal	kcal	fat	sat fat	carb	sugar	protein	fibre
	531 KJ	126 kcal	0.0 g	0.0 g	33.5 g	33.5 g	0.2 g	2.2 g *

	4 portions	10 portions
stock syrup (recipe 11)	¼ litre	625 ml
fruit	400 g	1 kg
sugar	100 g	250 g
lemon, juice of	½	1

Apples, pears

1 Boil the water and sugar.
2 Quarter the fruit, remove the core and peel.
3 Place in a shallow pan in sugar syrup.
4 Add a few drops of lemon juice.
5 Cover with greaseproof paper.
6 Allow to simmer slowly, preferably in the oven, cool and serve.

Soft fruits (raspberries, strawberries)

1 Pick and wash the fruit. Place in a glass bowl.
2 Pour on the hot syrup. Allow to cool and serve.

Stone fruits (plums, damsons, greengages, cherries)

1 Wash the fruit, barely cover with sugar syrup and cover with greaseproof paper or a lid.
2 Cook gently in a moderate oven until tender.

Rhubarb

1 Trim off the stalk and leaf and wash. Cut into 5 cm lengths and cook as above, adding extra sugar if necessary. A little ground ginger may also be added.

Gooseberries, blackcurrants, redcurrants

1 Top and tail the gooseberries, wash and cook as for stone fruit, adding extra sugar if necessary.
2 The currants should be carefully removed from the stalks, washed and cooked as for stone fruits.

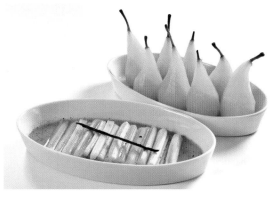

Poached rhubarb and pear

Dried fruits (prunes, apricots, apples, pears)

1 Dried fruits should be washed and soaked in cold water overnight.
2 Gently cook in the liquor with sufficient sugar to taste.

Try something different

- A piece of cinnamon stick and a few slices of lemon may be added to the prunes or pears, one or two cloves to the dried or fresh apples.
- Any compote may be flavoured with lavender and/or mint.

HEALTHY EATING TIP

- Use fruit juice to poach the fruit.
- If dried fruits are used, no added sugar is needed.

* Using pears

40 Lime and mascarpone cheesecake

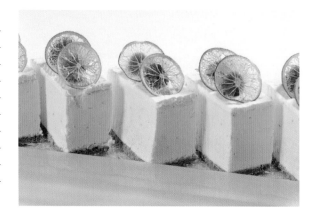

	Makes 1
packet of ginger biscuits	1
butter, melted	200 g
⚠ egg yolks, pasteurised	125 g
caster sugar	75 g
cream cheese	250 g
mascarpone	250 g
gelatine, softened in cold water	15 g
juice and grated zest of limes	2
semi-whipped cream	275 ml
white chocolate, melted	225 g

1 Blitz the biscuits in a food processor. Mix in the melted butter. Line the cake ring with this mixture and chill until required.

2 Make a sabayon by whisking the egg yolks and sugar together over a pan of simmering water.

3 Stir the cream cheese and mascarpone into the sabayon until soft.

4 Meanwhile, warm the gelatine in the lime juice, and pass through a fine chinois. Also whip the cream.

5 Pour the gelatine and melted white chocolate into the cheese mixture.

6 Remove from the food mixer and fold in the whipped cream with a spatula. Finally, whisk in the lime zest.

7 Pour over the prepared base. Chill for 4 hours.

41 Baked blueberry cheesecake

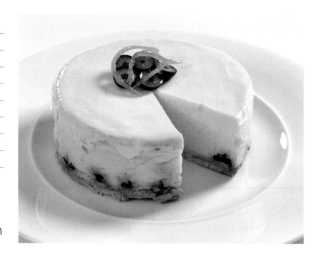

	Makes 1
digestive biscuits	150 g
butter, melted	50 g
full-fat cream cheese	350 g
caster sugar	150 g
eggs, medium	4
zest and juice of lemon	1
vanilla essence	5 ml
blueberries	125
soured cream	350 ml

1 Blitz the biscuits in a food processor. Stir in the melted butter. Press the mixture into the bottom of a lightly greased cake tin with a removable collar.

2 Whisk together the cheese, sugar, eggs, vanilla and lemon zest and juice, until smooth.

3 Stir in the blueberries, then pour over the biscuit base.

4 Bake at 160°C for approximately 30 minutes.

5 Remove from the oven and leave to cool slightly for 10–15 minutes.

6 Spread soured cream over the top and return to the oven for 10 minutes.

7 Remove and allow to cool and set. Chill.

---

42 Trifle

| cal 2280 KJ | kcal 543 kcal | fat 29.1 g | sat fat 17.1 g | carb 66.2 g | sugar 51.3 g | protein 8.2 g | fibre 1.9 g | * |

	6–8 portions
sponge (made with 3 eggs, medium)	1
jam	25 g
tinned fruit (pears, peaches, pineapple)	1
sherry (optional)	
Custard	
custard powder	35 g
milk (whole or skimmed)	375 ml
caster sugar	50 g
cream (¾ whipped) or non-dairy cream	125 ml
whipped sweetened cream or non-dairy cream	¼ litre
angelica	25 g
glacé cherries	25 g

1 Cut the sponge in half, sideways, and spread with jam.

2 Place in a glass bowl or individual dishes and soak with fruit syrup drained from the tinned fruit; a few drops of sherry may be added.

3 Cut the fruit into small pieces and add to the sponge.

4 Dilute the custard powder in a basin with some of the milk, add the sugar.

5 Boil the remainder of the milk, pour a little on the custard powder, mix well, return to the saucepan over a low heat and stir to the boil. Allow to cool, stirring occasionally to prevent a skin forming; fold in the three-quarters whipped cream.

6 Pour on to the sponge. Leave to cool.

7 Decorate with the whipped cream, angelica and cherries.

Try something different

Other flavourings or liqueurs may be used in place of sherry (e.g. whisky, rum, brandy, Tia Maria).

For raspberry or strawberry trifle use fully ripe fresh fruit in place of tinned, and decorate with fresh fruit in place of angelica and glacé cherries.

A fresh egg custard may be used with fresh egg yolks (see recipe 8).

* Using whole milk and whipping cream

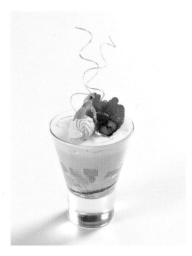

Sherry trifle

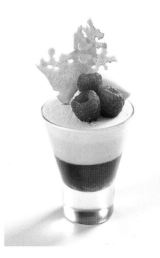

Raspberry trifle

43 Burned, caramelised or browned cream (*crème brûlée*)

cal	kcal	fat	sat fat	carb	sugar	protein	fibre
1151 KJ	278 kcal	21.9 g	12.1 g	14.8 g	14.8 g	6.2 g	0.0 g

	4 portions	10 portions
milk	125 ml	300 ml
double cream	125 ml	300 ml
natural vanilla essence or pod	3–4 drops	7–10 drops
eggs (medium)	2	5
egg yolk	1	2–3
caster sugar	25 g	60 g
demerara sugar		

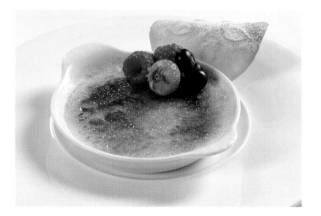

1 Warm the milk, cream and vanilla essence in a pan.

2 Mix the eggs, egg yolk and caster sugar in a basin and add the warm milk. Stir well and pass through a fine strainer.

3 Pour the cream into individual dishes and place them into a tray half-filled with warm water.

4 Place in the oven at approximately 160°C for about 30–40 minutes, until set.

5 Sprinkle the tops with demerara sugar and glaze under the salamander or by blowtorch to a golden brown.

6 Clean the dishes and serve.

Try something different

Sliced strawberries, raspberries or other fruits (e.g. peaches, apricots) may be placed in the bottom of the dish before adding the cream mixture, or placed on top after the creams are caramelised.

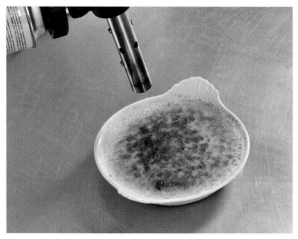

Use a blowtorch carefully to glaze the top

44 Cream caramel (*crème caramel*)

cal	kcal	fat	sat fat	carb	sugar	protein	fibre	*
868 KJ	207 kcal	7.2 g	3.3 g	30.2 g	30.2 g	7.3 g	0.0 g	

	4–6 portions	10–12 portions
Caramel		
sugar, granulated or cube	100 g	200 g
water	125 ml	250 ml
Cream		
milk, whole or skimmed	½ litre	1 litre
eggs (medium)	4	8
sugar, caster or unrefined	50 g	100 g
vanilla essence or a vanilla pod	–4 drops	6–8 drops

1 Prepare the caramel by placing three-quarters of the water in a thick-based pan, adding the sugar and allowing to boil gently, without shaking or stirring the pan.

2 When the sugar has cooked to a golden-brown caramel colour, add the remaining quarter of the water, reboil until the sugar and water mix, then pour into the bottom of dariole moulds.

3 Prepare the cream by warming the milk and whisking on to the beaten eggs, sugar and essence (or vanilla pod).

4 Strain and pour into the prepared moulds.

5 Place in a roasting tin half full of water.

6 Cook in a moderate oven at 150–160°C for 30–40 minutes.

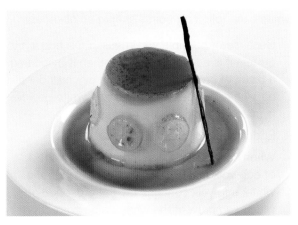

A cream caramel decorated with poached kumquats

7 When thoroughly cold, loosen the edges of the cream caramel with the fingers, shake firmly to loosen and turn out on to a flat dish or plates.

8 Pour any caramel remaining in the mould around the creams.

> Cream caramels may be served with whipped cream or a fruit sauce such as passionfruit, and accompanied by a sweet biscuit (e.g. shortbread, palmiers).
> Adding a squeeze of lemon juice to the caramel will invert the sugar, thus preventing recrystallisation.

* Using whole milk

45 Meringue (*meringue*)

cal	kcal	fat	sat fat	carb	sugar	protein	fibre	*
3491 KJ	831 kcal	0.0 g	0.0 g	210.0 g	210.0 g	10.8 g	0.0 g	

	4 portions	10 portions
⚠ egg whites, pasteurised	4	10
caster sugar	200 g	500 g

1 Whip the egg whites stiffly.

2 Sprinkle on ¼ of the sugar and carefully mix in. Mix in another ½ and then the final ¼.

3 Place in a piping bag with a large plain tube and pipe on to silicone paper on a baking sheet.

4 Bake in the slowest oven possible or in a hot plate (110°C). The aim is to dry out the meringues without any colour whatsoever.

Whipping egg whites

The reason egg whites increase in volume when whipped is because they contain so much protein

(11 per cent). The protein forms tiny filaments, which stretch on beating, incorporate air in minute bubbles then set to form a fairly stable puffed-up structure expanding to seven times its bulk. To gain maximum efficiency when whipping egg whites, the following points should be observed.

- Because of possible weakness in the egg white protein it is advisable to strengthen it by adding a pinch of cream of tartar and a pinch of dried egg white powder. If all dried egg white powder is used no additions are necessary.
- Eggs should be fresh.
- When separating yolks from whites *no* speck of egg yolk must be allowed to remain in the white; egg yolk contains fat, the presence of which can prevent the white being correctly whipped.

- The bowl and whisk must be scrupulously clean, dry and free from any grease.
- When egg whites are whipped the addition of a little sugar (15 g to 4 egg whites) will assist the efficient beating and reduce the chances of over-beating.

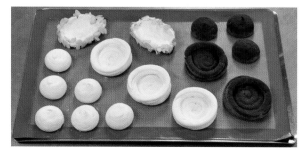

Unfilled meringues and vacherins

46 Vacherin with strawberries and cream (*vacherin aux fraises*)

cal	kcal	fat	sat fat	carb	sugar	protein	fibre	*
1436 KJ	341 kcal	12.6 g	7.9 g	56.3 g	56.3 g	3.9 g	0.6 g	

	4 portions	10 portions
egg whites	4	10
caster sugar	200 g	500 g
strawberries, picked and washed)	100–300 g	250–750 g
cream (whipped and sweetened) or non-dairy cream	125 ml	300 ml

1 Stiffly whip the egg whites. (Refer to the notes in recipe 45 for more guidance.)
2 Carefully fold in the sugar.
3 Place the mixture into a piping bag with a 1 cm plain tube.
4 Pipe on to silicone paper on a baking sheet.
5 Start from the centre and pipe round in a circular fashion to form a base 16 cm then pipe around the edge 2–3 cm high.
6 Bake in a cool oven at 100°C until the meringue case is completely dry. Do not allow to colour.
7 Allow the meringue case to cool then remove from the paper.
8 Spread a thin layer of cream on the base. Add the strawberries.
9 Decorate with the remainder of the cream.

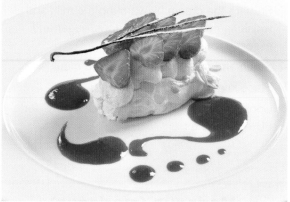

🍎 **HEALTHY EATING TIP**

- Try 'diluting' the fat in the cream with some low fat fromage frais.

A vacherin is a round meringue shell piped into a suitable shape so that the centre may be filled with sufficient fruit (such as strawberries, stoned cherries, peaches and apricots) and whipped cream to form a rich sweet. The vacherin may be prepared in one-, two- or four-portion sizes, or larger.

Try something different

- Melba sauce (recipe 55) may be used to coat the strawberries before decorating with cream.

- Raspberries can be used instead of strawberries.

* Using 280 g strawberries and whipped cream

47   Black Forest vacherin

	12 portions
egg whites	250 ml
caster sugar	500 g
lemon juice	5 ml
vanilla essence	drop
cornflour, sieved	30 g
cocoa powder, sieved	50 g
small discs of chocolate sponge	12
Kirsch syrup	100 ml
cherries (fresh, tinned or griottines)	60–72
pastry cream (see recipe 4)	200 g
Kirsch	20 ml
leaf gelatine, soaked	2
couverture, melted	200 g approx.
double cream, whipped	400 ml
chocolate shavings	
icing sugar	
cocoa powder (to dust)	

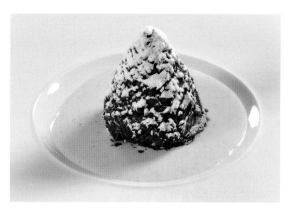

1 Whisk the egg white and one quarter of the sugar until firm. Continue to whisk while streaming in half of the sugar.

2 Add the lemon juice and vanilla. Fold in the cornflour and cocoa powder, and the remaining quarter of the sugar.

3 Pipe this vacherin mixture into 12 rounds, 80 mm in diameter. Bake at 150°C for approximately 1 hour.

4 Place a sponge disc on each vacherin. Moisten the sponge with Kirsch syrup and place 5 or 6 cherries on top.

5 Beat the pastry cream. Dissolve the gelatine in the warm Kirsch and then beat it into the pastry cream.

6 Beat in the melted couverture to taste. Fold in the cream.

7 Pipe the chocolate mixture onto the prepared bases in a spiral.

8 Cover with chocolate shavings. Dust with icing sugar first, then cocoa powder.

48 Khoshaf (dried fruit with nuts, perfumed with rose and orange water)

cal	kcal	fat	sat fat	carb	sugar	protein	fibre
1554 KJ	370 kcal	16.3 g	1.1 g	51.3 g	50.9 g	7.6 g	6.9 g

	4 portions	10 portions
dried apricots	100 g	250 g
prunes	100 g	250 g
dried figs	100 g	250 g
raisins	100 g	250 g
rose water	1 tbsp	2½ tbsp
orange blossom water	1 tbsp	2½ tbsp
blanched almonds, halved	50 g	125 g
pine kernels	50 g	125 g

1 Wash the fruit if necessary, soak overnight.

2 Drain, place fruit in a large saucepan, cover with water and bring to boil. Simmer for 10 minutes.

3 Add the rose water and the orange blossom water.

4 Place into a serving dish sprinkled with the almonds and pine kernels.

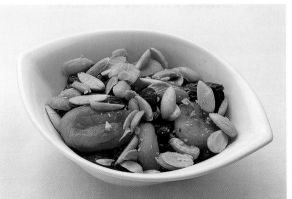

During Ramadan, Muslims fast all day and eat only after sunset. This is one of the dishes enjoyed during Ramadan. It can be served hot or cold.

49 Lemon curd ice cream

	6–8 portions
lemon curd	250 g
crème fraiche	125 g
Greek yoghurt	250 g

1 Mix all ingredients together.

2 Churn in ice cream machine.

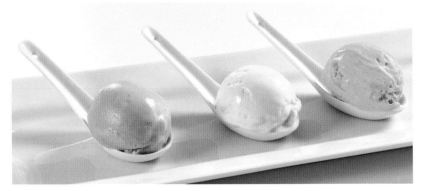

Recipes 49 to 51: caramel, lemon curd and peach ice creams

50 Caramel ice cream

For the anglaise

milk	
butter	
⚠ egg yolks, pasteurised	
sugar	
stabiliser	
For the caramel	
sugar	
unsalted butter	

1 Slowly bring the milk to the boil with the butter.
2 Whisk the egg yolks, sugar and stabiliser together to make the anglaise.

3 To make the caramel, allow the sugar to caramelise slowly over a low heat, then add the unsalted butter in small pieces.
4 Gradually add the boiling milk to the caramel.
5 Add a little of the milk and caramel mixture to the egg yolks. Pour all of this back into the rest of the milk mixture.
6 Make sure the gas is on full. Stir the mixture with a wooden spoon in a figure of eight movement, until it reaches at least 75°C.
7 Cool and allow to mature overnight.
8 Churn the following day.

51 Peach ice cream

milk	250 ml
caster sugar	175 g
orange rind	1
lemon rind	1
stabiliser (Stabilone)	100 g
single cream	250 ml
peach purée	250 ml
lemon juice	10 ml

1 Slowly bring the milk, sugar, rinds and stabiliser to the boil.
2 Remove from the heat and leave to cool slightly.
3 Add the cream and leave to cool.
4 When cold, add the peach purée and lemon juice. Leave overnight to mature.
5 Pass, then churn in the ice cream machine.
6 Place into a frozen container. Store in the freezer.

52 Apple sorbet

	8–10 portions
Granny Smith apples, washed and cored	4
juice of lemon	1
water	400 ml
sugar	200 g
glucose	50 g

1 Cut the apples into 1 cm pieces and place into lemon juice.
2 Bring the water, sugar and glucose to the boil, then allow to cool.
3 Pour the water over the apples. Blitz in a food processor.
4 Pass through a conical strainer, then churn in an ice cream machine or a Pacojet.

Try something different

Fruits of the forest sorbet: use a mixture of forest fruits instead of apples.

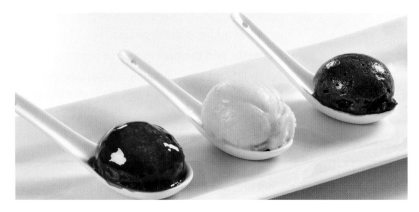

Fruits of the forest, apple and chocolate sorbets

---

53 Chocolate sorbet

water	400 ml
skimmed milk	100 ml
sugar	150 g
ice cream stabiliser	40 g
cocoa powder	30 g
dark couverture	60 g

1 Combine the water, milk, sugar, stabiliser and cocoa powder. Bring to the boil slowly. Simmer for 5 minutes.
2 Add the couverture and allow to cool.
3 Pass and churn.

---

54 Orange brandy granita

orange juice	500 ml
brandy	40 ml
stock syrup at 30° Baume	100 ml
water	175 ml

1 Mix all the ingredients together.
2 Pour into a gastronorm tray or other suitable tray and place in the freezer.
3 Fork up to produce crystals.

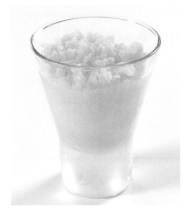

55 Peach Melba (*pêche Melba*)

	cal 607 KJ	kcal 145 kcal	fat 2.6 g	sat fat 1.3 g	carb 30.5 g	sugar 30.2 g	protein 1.6 g	fibre 1.3 g

	4 portions	10 portions
peaches	2	5
vanilla ice cream	125 ml	300 ml
Melba sauce (see below) or raspberry coulis	125 ml	300 ml

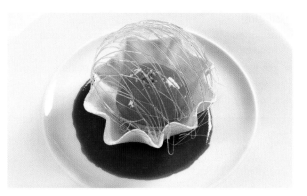

1 Poach the peaches. Allow to cool, then peel, halve and remove the stones.

2 Dress the fruit on a ball of the ice cream in an ice cream coupe, or in a tuile basket.

3 Finish with the sauce. The traditional presentation is to coat the peach in Melba sauce or coulis, and decorate with whipped cream. In this picture, the peach is garnished with crushed fresh pistachios and covered with a caramel cage; the basket is then placed carefully onto a base of coulis.

If using fresh peaches, dip them in boiling water for a few seconds, cool them by placing into cold water, then peel and halve.

1 Boil the ingredients together.

2 Cool, liquidise and strain.

To make Melba sauce

raspberry coulis	400 g
water	125 ml

Try something different

Fruit Melba can also be made using pear or banana instead of peach. Fresh pears should be peeled, halved and poached. Bananas should be peeled at the last moment.

56 Pear belle Hélène (*poire belle Hélène*)

1 Serve a cooked pear on a ball of vanilla ice cream in a coupe.

2 Decorate with whipped cream. Serve with a sauceboat of hot chocolate sauce (recipe 10).

Alternatively, present the ingredients on a plate as shown here.

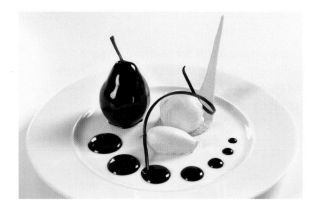

In this chapter, you will learn how to:

1. prepare, cook and finish paste products, including:

- using tools and equipment correctly, in a safe and hygienic way
- producing short, sweet, puff and choux paste products
- checking that the finished product meets requirements

2. you should have the knowledge to:

- identify different paste products, their uses and cooking methods
- understand the quality points of ingredients and how to adjust the quantity
- identify fillings, glazes, creams and icings, and finishing and decorating techniques
- store finished products safely.

Number	Recipe title	Page number
Pastes		
4	Choux paste (*pâte à choux*)	502
3	Rough puff paste	502
2	Short paste (*pâte à foncer*)	501
1	Sugar paste (*pâte à sucre*)	500
Pastry goods		
13	Baked chocolate tart (aero)	510
11	Bakewell tart	508
28	Baklava	520
15	Banana flan	511
5	Cheese and ham savoury flan (*quiche lorraine*)	504
24	Cheese straws (*paillettes au fromage*)	517
19	Chocolate éclairs (*éclairs au chocolat*)	513
	Coffee éclairs (*éclairs au café*)	513
22	Eccles cakes	515

Number	Recipe title	Page number
10	Egg custard tart	507
6	Flan	504
7	French apple flan (*flan aux pommes*)	505
17	Fruit barquettes	512
18	Fruit slice (*bande aux fruits*)	512
16	Fruit tart	512
26	Gateau pithiviers	519
12	Lemon tart (*tarte au citron*)	509
14	Mince pies	510
27	Palmiers	519
20	Paris-Brest	514
8	Pear and almond tart	506
23	Pear jalousie	516
21	Profiteroles and chocolate sauce (*profiteroles au chocolat*)	515
25	Puff pastry slice (*mille-feuilles*)	517
29	Sweet samosas	520
9	Treacle tart	507

The key ingredients for pastry work, such as flour, eggs and sugar, are described in Chapter 14 (pages 447–54). Make sure you read and understand this section.

Techniques

Adding fat to flour

Fats act as a shortening agent. The fat has the effect of shortening the gluten strands, which are easily broken when eaten, making the texture of the product more crumbly. The development of gluten in puff pastry is very important as long strands are needed to trap the expanding gases, and this is what makes the paste rise.

Ways of adding fat to flour are as follows.

- Rubbing in by hand: short pastry.
- Rubbing in by machine: short pastry.
- Creaming method by machine or by hand: sweet pastry.
- Lamination: puff pastry.
- Boiling: choux pastry.

Other techniques

Folding: for example, folding puff pastry to create its layers.

Kneading: using your hands to work dough or puff pastry in the first stage of making.

Blending: mixing all the ingredients carefully by weight.

Relaxing: keeping pastry covered with a damp cloth, clingfilm or plastic to prevent a skin forming on the surface. Relaxing allows the pastry to lose some of its resistance to rolling.

Cutting:
- Always cut with a sharp, damp knife.
- When using cutters, always flour them before use by dipping in flour. This will give a sharp, neat cut.
- When using a lattice cutter, use only on firm pastry; if the pastry is too soft, you will have difficulty lifting the lattice.

Rolling:
- Roll the pastry on a lightly floured surface; turn the pastry to prevent it sticking. Keep the

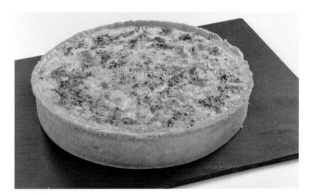

Techniques used to make this quiche include rolling and shaping the pastry

rolling pin lightly floured and free from the pastry.
- Always roll with care, treating the pastry lightly – never apply too much pressure.
- Always apply even pressure when using a rolling pin.

Shaping: producing flans, tartlets, barquettes and other such goods with pastry. Shaping also refers to crimping with the back of a small knife using the thumb technique.

Docking: this is piercing raw pastry with small holes to prevent it from rising during baking, as when cooking tartlets blind.

Glazing

A glaze is something that gives a product a smooth, shiny surface. Examples of glazes used for pastry dishes are as follows.

- A hot clear gel produced from a pectin source obtainable commercially for finishing flans and tartlets; always use while still hot. A cold gel is exactly the same except that it is used cold. The gel keeps a sheen on the goods and keeps out all oxygen, which might otherwise cause discoloration.
- Apricot glaze, produced from apricot jam, acts in the same way as gels.
- Eggwash, applied prior to baking, produces a rich glaze during the cooking process.

- Icing sugar dusted on the surface of the product caramelises in the oven or under the grill.
- Fondant gives a rich sugar glaze, which may be flavoured and/or coloured.
- Water icing gives a transparent glaze, which may also be flavoured and/or coloured.

Finishing and presentation

It is essential that all products are finished according to the recipe requirements. Finishing and presentation is often a key stage in the process, as failure at this point can affect sales. The way goods are presented is an important part of the sales technique. Each product of the same type must be of the same shape, size, colour and finish. The decoration should be attractive, delicate and in keeping with the product range. All piping should be neat, clean and tidy.

Some methods of finishing and presentation are as follows.

- **Dusting:** sprinkling icing sugar on a product using a fine sugar dredger or sieve, or muslin cloth.
- **Piping:** using fresh cream, chocolate or fondant.
- **Filling:** with fruit, cream, pastry cream, etc. Never overfill as this will often given the product a clumsy appearance.

Test yourself

1 What is the ratio of fat to flour for:
   a) short pastry
   b) puff pastry
   c) sugar pastry?
2 How is the fat added to the flour in the production of choux pastry?
3 What type of fat is required for the production of suet paste?
4 What is meant by the term 'lamination'?
5 Name the faults associated with the production of short pastry.
6 What is the filling for a classical gateau pithiviers?

1

Sugar paste (pâte à sucre)

cal	kcal	fat	sat fat	carb	sugar	protein	fibre
7864 KJ	1872 kcal	109.8 g	46.4 g	208 g	55.6 g	25.7 g	7.2 g

*

	5–8 portions	10–16 portions
medium egg	1	2–3
sugar	50 g	125 g
margarine or butter	125 g	300 g
flour (soft)	200 g	500 g
salt	pinch	large pinch

Method 1

1 Taking care not to over-soften, cream the egg and sugar.
2 Add the margarine or butter, and mix for a few seconds.
3 Gradually incorporate the sieved flour and salt. Mix lightly until smooth.
4 Allow to rest in a cool place before using.

Method 2

1 Sieve the flour and salt. Lightly rub in the margarine to achieve a sandy texture.
2 Make a well in the centre. Add the sugar and beaten egg.
3 Mix the sugar and egg until dissolved.
4 Gradually incorporate the flour and margarine, and lightly mix to a smooth paste. Allow to rest before using.

> Sugar pastry is used for flans, fruit tartlets, and so on.
> 50 per cent, 70 per cent or 100 per cent wholemeal flour may be used; the butter may be reduced from 125 to 100 g.

*5–8 portions using hard margarine

2   Short paste (pâte à foncer)

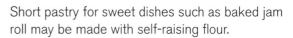

cal	kcal	fat	sat fat	carb	sugar	protein	fibre
6269 KJ	1493 kcal	92.6 g	38.0 g	155.5 g	3.1 g	18.9 g	7.2 g

*

	5–8 portions	10–16 portions
flour (soft)	200 g	500 g
salt	pinch	large pinch
lard or vegetable fat	50 g	125 g
butter or margarine	50 g	125 g
water	2–3 tbsp	5–8 tbsp

1 Sieve the flour and salt.

2 Rub in the fat to achieve a sandy texture.

3 Make a well in the centre.

4 Add sufficient water to make a fairly firm paste.

5 Handle as little and as lightly as possible.

> **Chef's tip**
>
> The amount of water used varies according to:
> * the type of flour (a very fine soft flour is more absorbent)
> * the degree of heat (e.g. prolonged contact with hot hands, and warm weather conditions).

Try something different

For wholemeal short pastry use ½ to ¾ wholemeal flour in place of white flour.

Short pastry is used in fruit pies, Cornish pasties, etc.

Making short pastry
http://bit.ly/zZFyPn

Short pastry for sweet dishes such as baked jam roll may be made with self-raising flour.

* Using lard, hard margarine (5–8 portions)

Possible reasons for faults in short pastry

* Hard:
  * too much water
  * too little fat
  * fat rubbed in insufficiently
  * too much handling and rolling
  * over-baking.

* Soft-crumbly:
  * too little water
  * too much fat.

* Blistered:
  * too little water
  * water added unevenly
  * fat not rubbed in evenly.

* Soggy:
  * too much water
  * too cool an oven
  * baked for insufficient time.

* Shrunken:
  * too much handling and rolling
  * pastry stretched whilst handling.

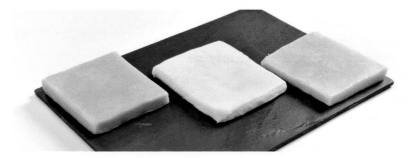

Recipes 1 to 3: short paste, rough puff paste and sweet paste

3 Rough puff paste

cal	kcal	fat	sat fat	carb	sugar	protein	fibre
7464 KJ	1777 kcal	124.3 g	53.2 g	150.8 g	3.0 g	23.2 g	0.0 g

*

	5–8 portions	10–16 portions
flour (strong)	200 g	500 g
salt		
butter or margarine	150 g	375 g
ice-cold water	125 ml	300 ml
lemon juice, ascorbic or tartaric acid	squeeze	large squeeze

1 Sieve the flour and salt (50 per cent wholemeal flour may be used).

2 Cut the fat into 10 g pieces and lightly mix them into the flour without rubbing in.

3 Make a well in the centre.

4 Add the liquid and mix to a fairly stiff dough.

5 Turn on to a floured table and roll into an oblong strip, about 30 × 10 cm, keeping the sides square.

6 Give one double turn as for puff pastry.

7 Allow to rest in a cool place, covered with cloth or plastic for 30 minutes.

8 Give three more double turns, resting between each. Allow to rest before using.

* *Using hard margarine (5–8 portions)*

Making rough puff pastry
http://bit.ly/yZjB8u

4 Choux paste (pâte à choux)

cal	kcal	fat	sat fat	carb	sugar	protein	fibre
6248 KJ	1488 kcal	106.6 g	43.3 g	99.3 g	4.1 g	38.9 g	4.5 g

*

	5–8 portions	10–16 portions
water	¼ litre	625 ml
sugar	pinch	large pinch
salt	pinch	large pinch
butter, margarine or oil	100 g	250 g
flour (strong)	125 g	300 g
eggs	4	10

1 Bring the water, sugar, salt and fat to the boil in a saucepan. Remove from heat.

2 Add the sieved flour and mix in with a wooden spoon (50 per cent, 70 per cent or 100 per cent wholemeal flour may be used).

3 Return to a moderate heat and stir continuously until the mixture leaves the sides of the pan.

4 Remove from the heat and allow to cool.

5 Gradually add the beaten eggs, beating well. Do not add all the eggs at once – check the consistency as you go. The mixture may not take all the egg. It should just flow back when moved in one direction.

Choux paste is used for éclairs, cream buns and profiteroles.

* *Using hard margarine (5–8 portions)*

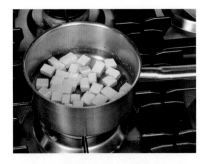

Cut the butter into cubes and then melt them in the water

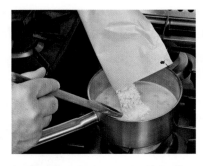

Remove from the heat and add the flour

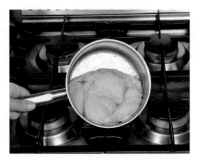

When the mixture is ready, it will start to come away from the sides

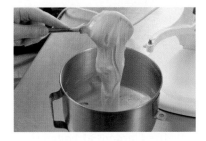

Add egg until the mixture is the right consistency: it should drop from a spoon under its own weight

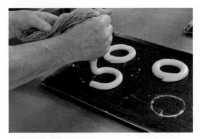

Pipe the paste into the shape required: these rings can be used for Paris-Brest (recipe 20)

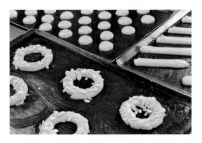

A selection of shapes in raw choux paste

Possible reasons for faults in choux paste

- Greasy and heavy:
  - basic mixture over-cooked.
- Soft, not aerated:
  - flour insufficiently cooked; eggs insufficiently beaten in the mixture; oven too cool; under-baked.

Making choux pastry
http://bit.ly/ArP7MJ

5 Cheese and ham savoury flan *(quiche lorraine)*

cal	kcal	fat	sat fat	carb	sugar	protein	fibre
2955 KJ	704 kcal	48.4 g	22.6 g	38.1 g	6.5 g	31.6 g	1.8 g

	4 portions	10 portions
rough puff, puff or short pastry	100 g	250 g
ham, chopped	50 g	125 g
cheese, grated	25 g	60 g
medium egg	1	2
milk	125 ml	300 ml
cayenne, salt		

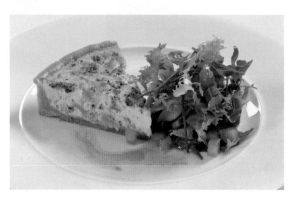

1 Lightly grease four (or ten) good-size barquette or tartlet moulds. Line thinly with pastry.

2 Prick the bottoms of the paste two or three times with a fork.

3 Cook in a hot oven at 230–250°C for 3–4 minutes or until the pastry is lightly set.

4 Remove from the oven; press the pastry down if it has tended to rise.

5 Add the chopped ham and grated cheese.

6 Mix the egg, milk, salt and cayenne thoroughly. Strain into the barquettes.

7 Return to the oven at 200–230°C and bake gently for 15–20 minutes or until nicely browned and set.

A variation is to line a 12 cm flan ring with short paste and proceed as above. The filling can be varied by using lightly fried lardons of bacon (in place of the ham), chopped cooked onions and chopped parsley.

Try something different

A variety of savoury flans can be made by using imagination and experimenting with different combinations of food (e.g. Stilton and onion; salmon and cucumber; sliced sausage and tomato).

6 Flan

1 Allow 25 g flour per portion and prepare sugar pastry as per recipe 1.

2 Grease the flan ring and baking sheet.

3 Roll out the pastry 2 cm larger than the flan ring. The pastry may be rolled between greaseproof or silicone paper.

4 Place the flan ring on the baking sheet.

5 Carefully place the pastry on the flan ring, by rolling it loosely over the rolling pin, picking up and unrolling it over the flan ring.

6 Press the pastry into shape without stretching it, being careful to exclude any air.

7 Allow a ½ cm ridge of pastry on top of the flan ring.

8 Cut off the surplus paste by rolling the rolling pin firmly across the top of the flan ring.

9 Mould the edge with thumb and forefinger. Decorate (a) with pastry tweezers or (b) with thumbs and forefingers, squeezing the pastry neatly to form a corrugated pattern.

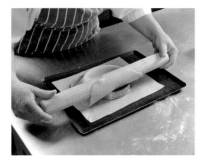

Place the pastry into the flan ring

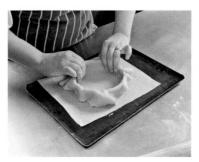

Firm the pastry into the bottom of the ring

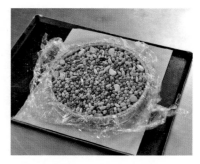

Bake blind, filled with beans, if the recipe requires

Lining a flan
http://bit.ly/xrFgiv

7 French apple flan *(flan aux pommes)*

cal	kcal	fat	sat fat	carb	sugar	protein	fibre
1428 KJ	340 kcal	13.8 g	5.8 g	53.8 g	36 g	3.5 g	2.9 g

	4 portions	10 portions
sugar paste (recipe 1)	100 g	250 g
pastry cream (chapter 14, recipe 4)	250 ml	625 ml
cooking apples	400 g	1 kg
sugar	50 g	125 g
apricot glaze	2 tbsp	6 tbsp

1 Line a flan ring with sugar paste. Pierce the bottom several times with a fork.

2 Pipe a layer of pastry cream into the bottom of the flan.

3 Peel, quarter and wash the selected apple.

4 Cut into neat thin slices and lay carefully on the pastry cream, overlapping each slice. Ensure that each slice points to the centre of the flan then no difficulty should be encountered in joining the pattern up neatly.

5 Sprinkle a little sugar on the apple slices and bake the flan at 200–220°C for 30–40 minutes.

6 When the flan is almost cooked, remove the flan ring carefully, return to the oven to complete the cooking. Mask with hot apricot glaze or flan jelly.

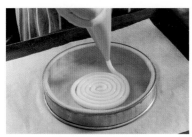

Pipe the filling neatly into the flan case

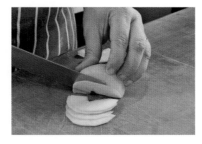

Slice the apple very thinly for decoration

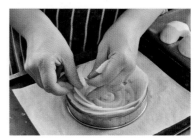

Arrange the apple slices on top of the flan

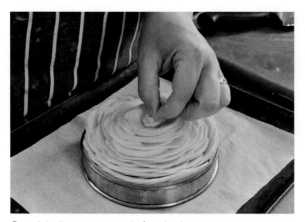

Complete the arrangement of apple slices

8 Pear and almond tart

	8 portions
sweet paste (recipe 1)	250 g
apricot jam	25 g
almond cream (chapter 14, recipe 6)	350 g
poached pears	4
apricot glaze	
flaked almonds	
icing sugar	

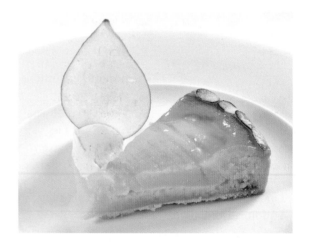

1 Line a buttered 20 cm flan ring with sweet paste. Trim and dock.

2 Using the back of a spoon, spread a little apricot jam over the base.

3 Pipe in almond cream until the flan case is two-thirds full.

4 Dry the poached pears. Cut them in half and remove the cores and string.

5 Score across the pears and arrange on top of the flan.

6 Bake in the oven at 200°C for 25–30 minutes.

7 Allow to cool, then brush with apricot glaze.

8 Sprinkle flaked almonds around the edge and dust with icing sugar.

9 Treacle tart

cal	kcal	fat	sat fat	carb	sugar	protein	fibre
1100 KJ	262 kcal	10.7 g	5.8 g	41.1 g	20.3 g	2.8 g	0.8 g

	4 portions	10 portions
Short paste		
flour	100 g	250 g
lard, margarine or vegetable fat	25 g	60 g
butter or margarine	25 g	60 g
salt	pinch	large pinch
water, to mix		
Filling		
treacle	100 g	250 g
water	1 tbsp	2½ tbsp
lemon juice	3–4 drops	8–10 drops
fresh white bread or cake crumbs	15 g	50 g

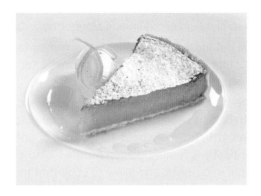

1 Make pastry as in recipe 2. Allow to rest in refrigerator.
2 Roll out to a 3 mm round.
3 Place onto a lightly greased, ovenproof plate.
4 Warm the treacle, water and lemon juice; add the crumbs.
5 Spread on the pastry and bake at 170°C for about 20 minutes.

Try something different

This tart can also be made in a shallow flan ring. Any pastry debris can be rolled and cut into ½ cm strips and used to decorate the top of the tart before baking.

Treacle tarts can also be made in individual moulds.

10 Egg custard tart

	10–12 portions
Pastry	
soft flour	500 g
salt	pinch
zest of lemon	1
butter	250 g
icing sugar	120 g
eggs	2
Egg custard filling	
egg yolks	9
caster sugar	75 g
whipping cream, gently warmed and infused with 2 sticks of cinnamon	500 ml
nutmeg, freshly grated	

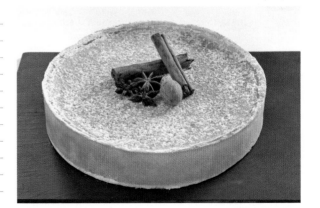

1 To make the pastry, rub together the flour, salt, lemon zest and butter until the mixture resembles breadcrumbs.

2 Add the sugar. Beat the eggs and then add them slowly, mixing until the pastry forms a ball. Wrap tightly in clingfilm and refrigerate.

3 Roll out the pastry on a lightly floured surface, to 2 mm thickness. Use it to line an 18 cm flan ring, placed on a baking sheet.

4 Line the pastry with greaseproof paper and fill with baking beans. Bake blind in a preheated oven at 175°C, for about 10 minutes or until the pastry is turning golden brown. Remove the paper and beans, and allow to cool. Turn the oven down to 130°C.

5 To make the custard filling, whisk together the egg yolks and sugar. Add the cream and mix well.

6 Pass the mixture through a fine sieve into a saucepan. Heat to blood temperature.

7 Fill the pastry case with the custard to 5 mm below the top. Place it carefully into the middle of the oven and bake for 30–40 minutes or until the custard appears to be set but not too firm.

8 Remove from the oven and cover liberally with grated nutmeg. Allow to cool to room temperature.

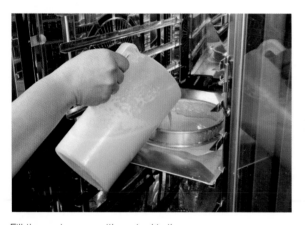

Fill the pastry case with custard in the oven

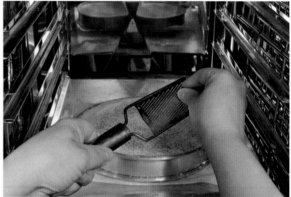

Grate nutmeg over the top

11 Bakewell tart

cal	kcal	fat	sat fat	carb	sugar	protein	fibre
2105 KJ	501 kcal	28.8 g	11.0 g	57.5 g	33.7 g	6.7 g	2.2 g

	8 portions
sugar paste (using 227 g flour) (recipe 1)	200 g
raspberry jam	50 g
eggwash	
apricot glaze	50 g
icing sugar	35 g
Frangipane (make as for chapter 14, recipe 6)	
butter or margarine	100 g
ground almonds	50 g
medium eggs	2
caster sugar	100 g
flour	50 g
almond essence	

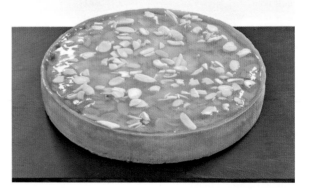

1 Line a flan ring using three-quarters of the paste, 2 mm thick.

2 Pierce the bottom with a fork.

3 Spread with jam and pipe on the frangipane.

4 Roll the remaining paste, cut into neat ½ cm strips and arrange neatly criss-crossed on the frangipane; trim off surplus paste. Brush with eggwash.

5 Bake in a moderately hot oven at 200–220°C for 30–40 minutes. Brush with hot apricot glaze.

6 When cooled brush over with very thin water icing.

* Using hard margarine

---

12 Lemon tart *(tarte au citron)*

|  cal 1978 KJ | kcal 450 kcal |  fat 28.0 g | sat fat 15.2 g |  carb 42.7 g | sugar 36.1 g |  protein 9.4 g | fibre 0.3 g |

	8 portions
sugar paste (recipe 1)	150 g
lemons	juice of 3, zest from 4
medium eggs	8
caster sugar	300 g
double cream	250 ml

1 Prepare 150 g of sugar paste, adding the zest of 1 lemon to the mix.

2 Line a 16 cm flan ring with the paste.

3 Bake blind for approximately 15 minutes.

4 Prepare the filling: mix the eggs and sugar together until smooth, add the cream, lemon juice and zest. Whisk well.

5 Seal the pastry, so that the filling will not leak out. Pour the filling into the flan case, bake for 30–40 minutes at 150°C until just set. (Take care when almost cooked as overcooking will cause the filling to rise and possibly crack.)

6 Remove from oven and allow to cool.

7 Dust with icing sugar and glaze under the grill or use a blowtorch. Portion and serve.

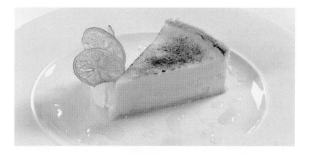

The mixture will fill one 16 × 4 cm or two 16 × 2 cm flan rings. If using two flan rings, double the amount of pastry and reduce the baking time when the filling is added.

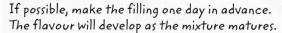

Chef's tip

If possible, make the filling one day in advance. The flavour will develop as the mixture matures.

Try something different

Limes may be used in place of lemons. If so, use the zest and juice of 5 limes or use a mixture of lemons and limes.

13   Baked chocolate tart (aero)

Makes 830 g, 1 flan cooked blind
(200 mm diameter x 35 mm height)

eggs	3
egg yolks	3
caster sugar	60 g
butter	200 g
chocolate pistoles (55% cocoa, unsweetened)	300 g

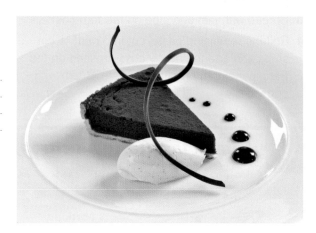

1 Whisk the eggs, yolks and sugar together.

2 Bring butter to the boil, remove and mix in chocolate pistoles until it is all melted.

3 Once sabayon is light and fluffy, fold in chocolate and butter mix very carefully, so as not to beat out the air.

4 Pour into cooked flan case (baked blind) and place in a deck oven at 150°C until the edge crusts (approx. 5 minutes). Chill.

5 Once set, remove from fridge.

6 Serve at room temperature.

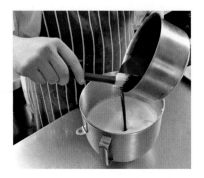

Add chocolate pistoles to the melted butter

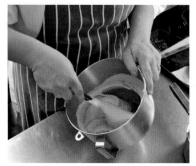

Fold in the chocolate

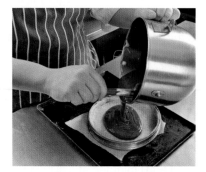

Pour the mixture into the flan case

14   Mince pies

	12 pies
sweet paste (recipe 1)	200 g
mincemeat (see below)	200 g
eggwash	
icing sugar	

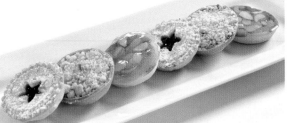

1 Roll out the pastry 3 mm thick.

2 Cut half the pastry into plain or fluted rounds 6 cm in diameter.

3 Line greased tartlet moulds with paste.

4 Fill with mincemeat.

5 Cut the remainder of the pastry into plain or fluted rounds, 8 cm in diameter.

6 Cover the mincemeat with pastry and seal the edges. Brush with eggwash.

7 Bake at 190–220°C for about 15 minutes.

8 Sprinkle with icing sugar and serve warm. Accompany with a suitable sauce (e.g. custard, brandy sauce, brandy cream).

Short or puff pastry may also be used.

To make the mincemeat

suet, chopped	100 g
mixed peel, chopped	100 g
currants	100 g
sultanas	100 g
raisins	100 g
apples, chopped	100 g
Barbados sugar	100 g
mixed spice	5 g
lemon, grated zest and juice of	1
orange, grated zest and juice of	1
rum	60 ml
brandy	60 ml

1 Mix the ingredients together.

2 Seal in jars and use as required.

15 Banana flan *(flan aux bananes)*

cal	kcal	fat	sat fat	carb	sugar	protein	fibre
1549 KJ	369 kcal	16.0 g	6.9 g	53.7 g	30.3 g	6.0 g	2.9 g

	4 portions	10 portions
sugar paste (recipe 1)	100 g	250 g
pastry cream (chapter 14, recipe 4) or thick custard	125 ml	250 g
bananas	2	5
apricot glaze	2 tbsp	5 tbsp

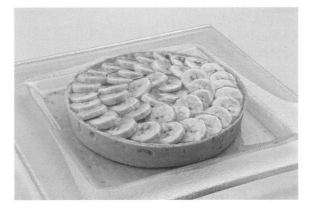

1 Line a flan ring with sugar paste. Cook blind and allow to cool.

2 Make pastry cream (chapter 14, recipe 4) or custard; pour while hot into the flan case.

3 Allow to set. Peel and slice the bananas neatly.

4 Arrange overlapping layers on the pastry cream. Coat with glaze.

16 Fruit tart

	4 portions	10 portions
sugar paste (recipe 1)	100 g	250 g
fruit	200 g	500 g
glaze	2 tbsp	5 tbsp

1 Line a flan with paste and cook it blind (see recipe 6). Allow to cool.
2 Pick and wash the small fruit, then drain well. Wash and slice the large fruit.
3 Dress neatly in the flan case. Coat with the glaze.

Use a glaze suitable for the fruit chosen; for example, with a strawberry tart, use a red glaze.

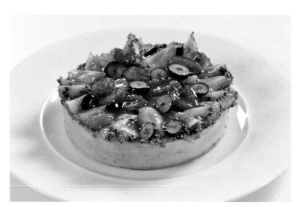

A layer of pastry cream (chapter 15, recipe 4) or thick custard may be placed in the flan case before adding the fruit.

17 Fruit barquettes

Certain fruits (e.g. strawberries, raspberries) are sometimes served in boat-shaped moulds. The preparation is the same as for tartlets. Tartlets and barquettes should be glazed and served allowing one large or two small per portion.

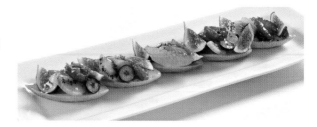

18 Fruit slice (bande aux fruits)

cal	kcal	fat	sat fat	carb	sugar	protein	fibre
767 KJ	183 kcal	7.8 g	3.4 g	28.6 g	21.3 g	1.3 g	1.6 g

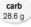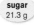

	8–10 portions
puff pastry (recipe 3)	200 g
fruit (see note)	400 g
pastry cream	250 ml approx.
sugar, to sweeten appropriate glaze	2 tbsp

1 Roll out the pastry 2 mm thick in a strip 12 cm wide.

2 Place on a greased, dampened baking sheet.
3 Moisten two edges with eggwash; lay two 1½ cm-wide strips along each edge.
4 Seal firmly and mark with the back of a knife. Prick the bottom of the slice.
5 Then, depending on the fruit used, either put the fruit (such as apple) on the slice and cook together, or cook the slice blind and afterwards

place the pastry cream and fruit (such as tinned peaches) on the pastry. Glaze and serve as for flans.

> Fruit slices may be prepared from any fruit suitable for flans/tarts.

Try something different

Alternative methods are:

- to use short or sweet pastry for the base and puff pastry for the two side strips
- to use sweet pastry in a slice mould.

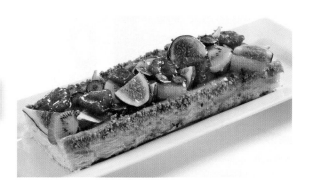

ASSESSMENT

19 Chocolate éclairs (éclairs au chocolat)

cal	kcal	fat	sat fat	carb	sugar	protein	fibre
516 KJ	123 kcal	9.5 g	5.7 g	8.8 g	7.3 g	1.1 g	0.1 g

	Makes 12
choux paste (recipe 4)	125 ml
whipped cream	¼ litre
fondant	100 g
chocolate couverture	25 g

1 Place the choux paste into a piping bag with a 1 cm plain tube.

2 Pipe into 8 cm lengths onto a lightly greased, dampened baking sheet.

3 Bake at 200–220°C for about 30 minutes.

4 Allow to cool. Make two holes using a metal piping nozzle (see photo on next page).

5 Fill with sweetened, vanilla-flavoured whipped cream, using a piping bag and small tube. The continental fashion is to fill with pastry cream.

6 Warm the fondant, add the finely cut chocolate, allow to melt slowly, adjust the consistency with a little sugar and water syrup if necessary. *Do not overheat or the fondant will lose its shine.*

7 Glaze the éclairs by dipping them in the fondant; remove the surplus with the finger. Allow to set.

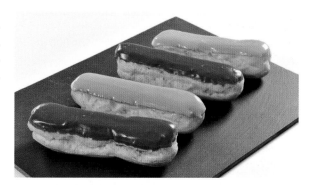

Chocolate and coffee éclairs

> Éclairs are often filled with pastry cream or crème diplomat (chapter 14, recipe 1) with a relevant flavouring, e.g. chocolate.

Try something different

Coffee éclairs (éclairs au café): add a few drops of coffee essence to the fondant instead of chocolate; coffee éclairs may also be filled with pastry cream (chapter 14, recipe 4) flavoured with coffee.

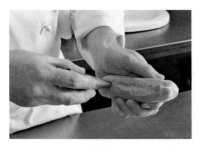

Pierce the éclair

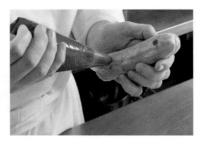

Pipe in the filling

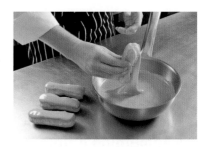

Dip the éclair in fondant; wipe the edges to give a neat finish

20   Paris-Brest

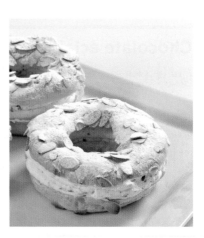

	Makes 8
choux paste	
crème diplomat or pastry cream (see chapter 14, recipes 1 and 4)	
For the praline	
flaked almonds, hazelnuts and pecans (any combination)	375 g
granulated sugar	500 g

To make the praline

1 Place the nuts on a baking sheet and toast until evenly coloured. Sprinkle with flaked almonds before baking.

2 Place the sugar in a large, heavy, stainless steel saucepan. Set the pan over a low heat and allow the sugar to caramelise. Do not over-stir, but do not allow the sugar to burn.

3 When the sugar is lightly caramelised and reaches a temperature of 170°C, remove from the heat and stir in the nuts.

4 Immediately deposit the mixture on a silpat mat. Place another mat over the top and roll as thin as possible.

5 Allow to go completely cold. Break up and store in an airtight container.

For the Paris-Brest

1 Pipe choux paste (recipe 4) into rings and bake.

2 Slice each ring in half. Fill with a mixture of crème diplomat or pastry cream (see chapter 14, recipes 1 and 4) and praline.

21 Profiteroles and chocolate sauce (*profiteroles au chocolat*)

cal	kcal	fat	sat fat	carb	sugar	protein	fibre
919 KJ	219 kcal	16.2 g	9.7 g	16.4 g	12.8 g	2.9 g	0.2 g

	8 portions
choux paste (recipe 4)	125 ml
chocolate sauce (chapter 14, recipe 10)	¼ litre
whipped, sweetened, vanilla-flavoured cream (or pastry cream)	¼ litre
icing sugar, to serve	

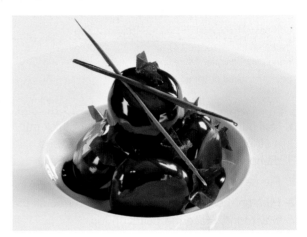

1 Line a baking sheet with greaseproof paper. Spoon the choux paste into a piping bag with a plain nozzle (approx. 1.5 cm diameter). Pipe a small blob of the paste under each corner of the paper to keep it in place.

2 Pipe walnut-sized balls of paste onto the sheet, spaced well apart. Level the peaked tops with the tip of a wet finger.

3 Bake for 18–20 minutes at 200°C, until well risen and golden brown. Remove from the oven, transfer to a wire rack and allow to cool completely.

4 Make a hole in each and fill with cream.

5 Dredge with icing sugar and serve with a sauceboat of cold chocolate sauce, or coat the profiteroles with the sauce.

22 Eccles cakes

cal	kcal	fat	sat fat	carb	sugar	protein	fibre
691 KJ	164 kcal	8.6 g	3.7 g	22.1 g	17.3 g	1.1 g	1.4 g

	12 cakes
puff or rough puff pastry (recipe 3)	200 g
egg white, to brush	
caster sugar, to coat	
Filling	
butter or margarine	50 g
raisins	50 g
demerara sugar	50 g
currants	200 g
mixed spice (optional)	pinch

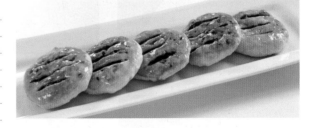

1 Roll out the pastry 2 mm thick.

2 Cut into rounds 10–12 cm diameter. Damp the edges.

3 Mix together all the ingredients for the filling and place a tbsp of the mixture in the centre of each round.

4 Fold the edges over to the centre and completely seal in the mixture.

5 Brush the top with egg white and dip into caster sugar.

6 Place on a greased baking sheet.

7 Cut two or three incisions with a knife so as to show the filling.

8 Bake at 220°C for 15–20 minutes.

23 Pear jalousie

cal	kcal	fat	sat fat	carb	sugar	protein	fibre
1178 KJ	282 kcal	17.8 g	5.1 g	27.2 g	17.5 g	3.8 g	0.8 g

	8–10 portions
puff pastry (recipe 3)	200 g
mincemeat (see recipe 14), jam or frangipane (chapter 14, recipe 6)	200 g
pears, poached or tinned	

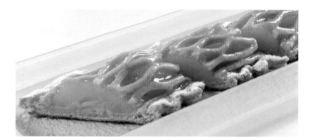

1 Roll out one-third of the pastry 3 mm thick into a strip 25 × 10 cm and place on a greased, dampened baking sheet.

2 Pierce with a docker. Moisten the edges.

3 Pipe on the frangipane, leaving 2 cm free all the way round. Place the pears on top.

4 Roll out the remaining two-thirds of the pastry to the same size.

5 Cut the dough with a trellis cutter to make a lattice.

6 Carefully open out this strip and neatly place on to the first strip.

7 Trim off any excess. Neaten and decorate the edge. Brush with eggwash.

8 Bake at 220°C for 25–30 minutes.

9 Sprinkle with icing sugar and return to a very hot oven to glaze.

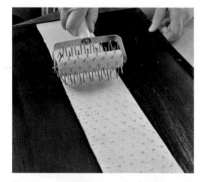

Roll the dough with a spiked roller

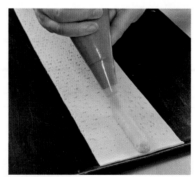

Pipe on the filling

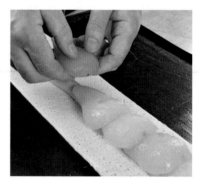

Add the fruit

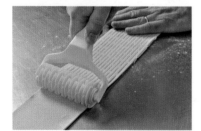

Roll the dough for the top layer with a lattice cutter

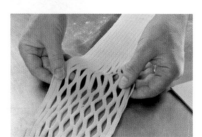

Open up the lattice

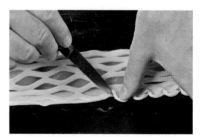

Finish and notch the edges

24 Cheese straws *(paillettes au fromage)*

cal	kcal	fat	sat fat	carb	sugar	protein	fibre
2562 KJ	610 kcal	48.1 g	24.1 g	28.7 g	0.6 g	17.4 g	1.4 g

	4 portions	10 portions
puff or rough puff paste	100 g	250 g
cheese, grated	50 g	125 g
cayenne		

1 Roll out the pastry to 60 × 15 cm.
2 Sprinkle with the cheese and cayenne.
3 Roll out to 3 mm thick.
4 Cut out four circles 4 cm in diameter.
5 Remove the centre with a smaller cutter leaving a circle ½ cm wide.
6 Cut the remaining paste into strips 8 × ½ cm.
7 Twist each once or twice.
8 Place on a lightly greased baking sheet.
9 Bake in a hot oven at 230–250°C for 10 minutes or until a golden brown.
10 To serve, place a bundle of straws into each circle.

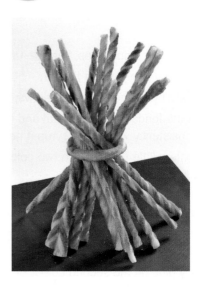

50 per cent white and 50 per cent wholemeal flour can be used for the pastry.

25 Puff pastry slice *(mille-feuilles)*

cal	kcal	fat	sat fat	carb	sugar	protein	fibre
1158 KJ	369 kcal	10.9 g	1.3 g	67.7 g	52.3 g	4.9 g	0.1 g

	6–8 slices
puff pastry (recipe 3)	200 g
pastry cream (chapter 14, recipe 4)	¼ litre
apricot jam	100 g
fondant or water icing	200 g

1 Roll out the pastry 2 mm thick into an even-sided square.
2 Roll up carefully on a rolling pin and unroll onto a greased, dampened baking sheet.
3 Using two forks or a docker, pierce as many holes as possible in the paste.
4 Cut in half with a large knife then cut each half in two to form four even-sized rectangles.

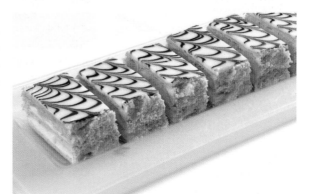

5 Bake in a hot oven at 220°C for 15–20 minutes; turn the strips over after 10 minutes. Allow to cool.

6 Keep the best strip for the top. Spread pastry cream on one strip.

7 Place another strip on top and spread with jam.

8 Place the third strip on top and spread with pastry cream.

9 Place the last strip on top, flat side up.

10 Press down firmly with a flat tray.

11 Decorate by feather-icing as follows:

12 Warm the fondant to blood heat and correct the consistency with sugar syrup if necessary.

13 Separate a little fondant into two colours and place in paper cornets.

14 Brush the top layer with apricot glaze. Pour the fondant over the mille-feuilles in an even coat.

15 Immediately pipe on one of the colours lengthwise in strips 1 cm apart.

16 Quickly pipe on the second colour between each line of the first.

17 With the back of a small knife, wiping after each stroke, mark down the slice at 2 cm intervals.

18 Quickly turn the slice around and repeat in the same direction with strokes in between the previous ones.

19 Allow to set and trim the edges neatly.

20 Cut into even portions with a sharp thin-bladed knife, dip into hot water and wipe clean after each cut.

Try something different

At steps 15 and 16, baker's chocolate or tempered couverture may be used for marbling. Whipped fresh cream may be used as an alternative to pastry cream. Also a variety of soft fruits may be incorporated in the layers, such as raspberries, strawberries, canned well-drained pears, peaches or apricots, kiwi fruit or caramelised poached apple slices. The pastry cream or whipped cream may also be flavoured with a liqueur if so desired, such as curaçao, Grand Marnier or Cointreau.

Mille-feuilles are usually made with scraps of puff pastry, rolled out very thin to make crisp layers. Full puff pastry is too active and will not form such crisp layers.

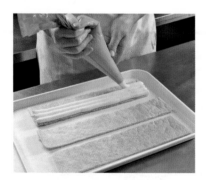
Pipe cream between layers of pastry

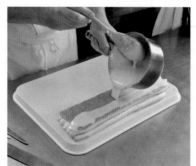
Ice the top with fondant

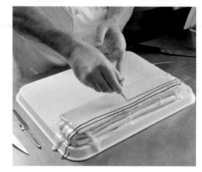
Decorate with chocolate

26 Gâteau pithiviers

cal	kcal	fat	sat fat	carb	sugar	protein	fibre
928 KJ	222 kcal	15.6 g	3.8 g	18.5 g	8.9 g	3.8 g	0.5 g

	8–10 portions	20 portions
puff pastry (recipe 3)	200 g	500 g
apricot jam	1 tbsp	3 tbsp
frangipane (chapter 14, recipe 6)	½ the recipe	1½ times the recipe

1 Roll out one-third of the pastry into a 20 cm round, 2 mm thick; moisten the edges and place on a greased, dampened baking sheet; spread the centre with jam.

2 Prepare the frangipane as per chapter 15, recipe 6, by creaming the margarine and sugar in a bowl, gradually adding the beaten eggs, and folding in the flour and almonds.

3 Spread on the frangipane, leaving a 2 cm border round the edge.

4 Roll out the remaining two-thirds of the pastry and cut into a slightly larger round.

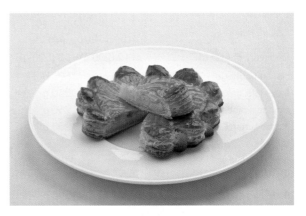

5 Place neatly on top, seal and decorate the edge.

6 Using a sharp-pointed knife, make curved cuts 2 mm deep, radiating from the centre to about 2 cm from the edge. Brush with eggwash.

7 Bake at 220°C for 25–30 minutes.

8 Glaze with icing sugar as for jalousie (recipe 23).

27 Palmiers

1 Roll out puff pastry (recipe 3), 2 mm thick, into a square.

2 Sprinkle liberally with caster sugar on both sides and roll into the pastry.

3 Fold into three from each end so as to meet in the middle; brush with eggwash and fold in two.

4 Cut into strips approximately 2 cm thick; dip one side in caster sugar.

5 Place on a greased baking sheet, sugared side down, leaving a space of at least 2 cm between each.

6 Bake in a very hot oven for about 10 minutes.

7 Turn with a palette knife, cook on the other side until brown and the sugar is caramelised.

Puff pastry trimmings are suitable for these. Palmiers may be made in all sizes. Two joined together with a little whipped cream may be served as a pastry, small ones for petits fours. They may be sandwiched together with soft fruit, whipped cream and/or ice cream and served as a sweet.

28 Baklava (filo pastry with nuts and sugar)

cal 5488 KJ	kcal 1314 kcal	fat 83.5 g	sat fat 35.8 g	carb 132.6 g	sugar 85.2 g	protein 16.6 g	fibre 6.1 g

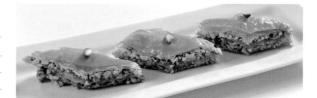

	4 portions	10 portions
filo pastry, sheets of	12 (200 g)	30 (500 g)
clarified butter or ghee	200 g	500 g
hazelnuts, flaked	100 g	250 g
almonds, nibbed	100 g	250 g
caster sugar	100 g	250 g
cinnamon	10 g	25 g
grated nutmeg		
Syrup		
unrefined sugar or caster sugar	200 g	500 g
lemons, grated zest and juice of	2	5
water	60 ml	150 ml
orange, grated zest and juice of	1	2
cinnamon stick	1	2
rose water		

1 Prepare a shallow tray slightly smaller than the sheets of filo pastry by brushing with melted clarified butter or ghee.

2 Place the sheets of filo pastry on the tray, brushing each with the fat.

3 Prepare the filling by mixing the nuts, sugar and spices together; place into the prepared tray, layered alternately with the filo pastry. Brush each layer with the clarified fat so that there are at least 2–3 layers of filling separated by filo pastry.

4 Cover completely with filo pastry and brush with the clarified fat.

5 Mark the pastry into diamonds, sprinkle with water and bake in a moderately hot oven at 190°C for approximately 40 minutes.

6 Meanwhile make the syrup: place all the ingredients, except the rose water, in a saucepan and bring to the boil. Simmer for 5 minutes, pass through a fine strainer and finish with 2–3 drops of rose water.

7 When the baklavas are baked, cut into diamonds, place on a suitable serving dish and mask with the syrup.

 HEALTHY EATING TIP

- Use oil to brush the sheets of filo pastry.

- Less sugar can be used in the filling as it should be sweet enough with the syrup used for masking.

* Using recipe of filo pastry, and ghee

29 Sweet samosas

See page 317 for the basic samosa recipe.

Filling 1: pears and ginger

de comice or conference pears	8
lemon syrup	
stem ginger, cut into brunoise	
mascarpone cheese	

1 Poach the pears in a 75% lemon syrup until they are just tender. Drain.

2 Place a small quenelle of mascarpone into each samosa, and the fruit on top.

Filling 2: apricot and almond

frangipane (see chapter 14, recipe 6)	
dried apricots, diced	

1 Pipe a little frangipane into each samosa, and top with dried apricots.

In this chapter you will learn how to:

1. prepare, cook and finish biscuit, cake and sponge products, including:

- working safely and hygienically, using the correct equipment to prepare mixtures for baking
- finishing, presenting and evaluating products

2. you should have the knowledge to:

- identify different products, their uses and cooking methods
- understand the quality points of ingredients and how to adjust the quantity
- identify fillings, glazes, creams and icings, and finishing and decorating techniques
- store finished products safely.

Number	Recipe title	Page number
Cakes and sponges		
5	Banana bread	532
2	Fresh cream and strawberry gateau	530
1	Genoese sponge (*génoise*)	529
6	Lemon drizzle cake	533
4	Rich fruit cake	531
3	Roulade sponge	531
9	Scones	535
8	Swiss roll	534
7	Victoria sandwich	533
Biscuits		
15	Brandy snaps	540
12	Cats' tongues (*langues de chat*)	538
16	Madeleines	540
13	Piped biscuits (*sablés à la poche*)	538
11	Shortbread biscuits	537
10	Sponge fingers (*biscuits à la cuillère*)	536
14	Tuiles	539

The key ingredients for biscuits, cakes and sponges, such as flour, eggs, sugar and raising agents, are described in Chapter 14 (pages 447–54). Make sure you read and understand this section.

Cake mixtures

There are three basic methods of making cake mixtures, also known as cake batters. The working temperature of cake batter should be 21°C.

Sugar batter method

For this method, the fat (cake margarine, butter or shortening) is blended in a machine with caster sugar. This is the basic or principal stage; usually the other ingredients are then added in the order shown in the diagram below.

Flour batter method

For this method the eggs and sugar are whisked to a half sponge; this is the basic or principal stage, which aims to foam the two ingredients together until half the maximum volume is achieved. Other ingredients are added as shown in the diagram on the next page.

A type of product called a humectant, which helps the product to stay moist, may be added (e.g. glycerine or honey); if so, add this at stage 2.

Blending method

This is used for high-ratio cake mixtures. It uses high-ratio flour specially produced so that it will absorb more liquid. It also uses a high-ratio fat, made from oil to which a quantity of emulsifying agent has been added, enabling the fat to take up a greater quantity of liquid.

High-ratio cakes contain more liquid and sugar, resulting in a fine stable crumb, extended shelf life, good eating and excellent freezing qualities.

The principal or basic stage is the mixing of the fat and flour to a crumbling texture. It is essential that each stage of the batter is blended into the next to produce a smooth batter, free from lumps. When using mixing machines, it is important to remember to:

- blend on a slow speed
- beat on a medium speed, using a paddle attachment.

When blending, always clear the mix from the bottom of the bowl to ensure that any first- or second-stage batter does not remain in the bowl.

Baking powder

Baking powder may be made from one part sodium bicarbonate to two parts cream of tartar. In commercial baking the powdered cream of tartar may be replaced by another acid product, such as acidulated calcium phosphate.

When used under the right conditions, with the addition of liquid and heat, it produces carbon dioxide gas. As the acid has a delayed action, only a small amount of gas is given off when the

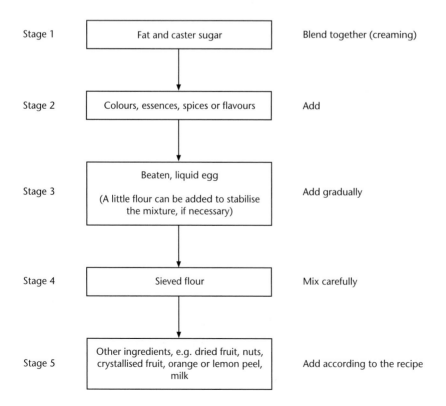

Stage 1	Fat and caster sugar	Blend together (creaming)
Stage 2	Colours, essences, spices or flavours	Add
Stage 3	Beaten, liquid egg (A little flour can be added to stabilise the mixture, if necessary)	Add gradually
Stage 4	Sieved flour	Mix carefully
Stage 5	Other ingredients, e.g. dried fruit, nuts, crystallised fruit, orange or lemon peel, milk	Add according to the recipe

The sugar batter method

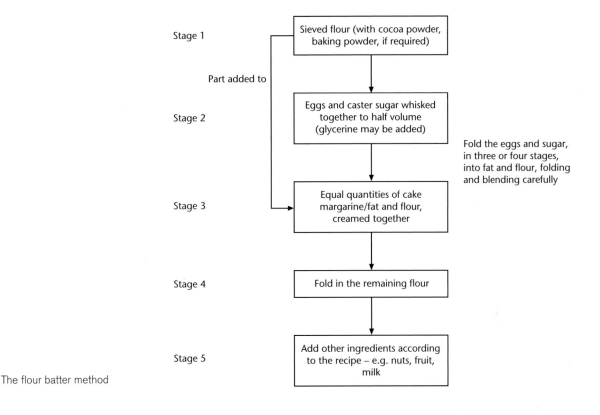

The flour batter method

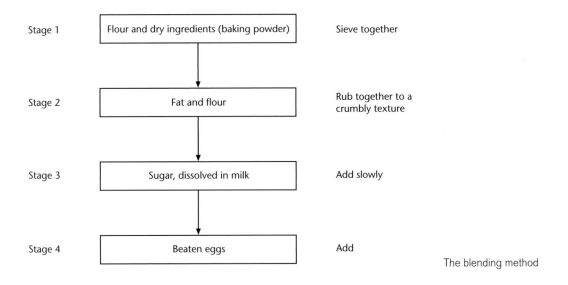

The blending method

liquid is added, and the majority is released when the mixture is heated. Therefore, when cakes are mixed they do not lose the property of the baking powder if they are not cooked right away.

Possible reasons for faults in cakes

- Uneven texture:
  - fat insufficiently rubbed in
  - too little liquid
  - too much liquid.

- Close texture:
    - too much fat
    - hands too hot when rubbing in
    - fat to flour ratio incorrect.
- Dry:
    - too little liquid
    - oven too hot.
- Bad shape:
    - too much liquid
    - oven too cool
    - too much baking powder.
- Fruit sunk:
    - fruit wet
    - too much liquid
    - oven too cool.
- Cracked:
    - too little liquid
    - too much baking powder.

Batters and whisked sponges

Batters and sponges allow us to make a large assortment of desserts and cakes. Basically, they are a mix of eggs, sugar, flour and the air incorporated when these are beaten. Certain other raw materials can be combined – for example, almonds, hazelnuts, walnuts, chocolate, butter, fruit, ginger, anise, coffee and vanilla.

Sponge mixtures are produced from a foam of eggs and sugar. The eggs may be whole eggs or separated. Examples of sponge products are gâteaux, sponge fingers and sponge cakes.

The egg white traps the air bubbles. When eggs and sugar are whisked together, they thicken until maximum volume is reached; then flour is carefully folded in by a method known as cutting in. This is the most difficult operation, as the flour must not be allowed to sink to the bottom of the bowl, otherwise it becomes lumpy and difficult to clear. However, the mixture must not be stirred as this will disturb the aeration and cause the air to escape, resulting in a much heavier sponge. If butter, margarine or oil is added, it is important that this is added at about 36°C, otherwise overheating will cause the fat or oil to act on the flour and create lumps, which are difficult, often impossible, to get rid of.

Stabilisers are often added to sponges to prevent them from collapsing. The most common are ethylmethyl cellulose and glycerol monostearate; these are added to the eggs and sugar at the beginning of the mixing.

What you need to know about sponge cakes

- You should never add flour or ground dry ingredients to a batter until the end because they impede the air absorption in the first beating stage.

> **Impede:** To restrict or prevent the progress of.

- When making sponge cakes, always sift the dry ingredients (flour, cocoa powder, ground nuts, etc.) to avoid clumping.
- Mix in the flour as quickly and delicately as possible, because a rough addition of dry ingredients acts like a weight on the primary batter and can remove part of the air already absorbed.
- Flours used in sponge cakes are low in gluten content. In certain sponge cakes, a portion of the flour can be left out and substituted with cornstarch. This yields a softer and more aerated batter.
- The eggs used in sponge cake batters should be fresh and at room temperature so that they take in air faster.
- Adding separately beaten egg whites produces a lighter and fluffier sponge cake.
- Once sponge cake batters are beaten and poured into moulds or baking trays, they should be baked as soon as possible. Otherwise, the batter loses volume.

Methods of making sponges

- **Foaming method** – whisking eggs and sugar together to ribbon stage; folding in/cutting flour.
- **Melting method** – as with foaming, but adding melted butter, margarine or oil to the mixture. The fat content enriches the sponge, improves the flavour, texture and crumb structure, and will extend shelf life.

- **Boiling method** – sponges made by this method have a stable crumb texture that is easier to handle and crumbles less when cut than the standard basic sponge containing fat (known as Genoese sponge). This method will produce a sponge that is suitable for dipping in fondant. The stages are shown in the diagram below.

- **Blending method** – this is used for high-ratio sponges, which follow the same principles as high-ratio cakes. As with cakes, high-ratio goods produce a fine, stable crumb, an even texture, excellent shelf life and good freezing qualities.

- **Creaming method** – this is the traditional method and is still used today for Victoria sandwich and light fruitcakes. The fat and sugar are creamed together, then beaten egg is added and, finally, the sieved flour is added with the other dry ingredients as desired.

- **Separate yolk and white method** – this method is used for sponge fingers (recipe 10).

Possible reasons for faults in sponges

- Close texture:
  - under-beating
  - too much flour
  - oven too cool or too hot.

- 'Holey' texture:
  - flour insufficiently folded in
  - tin unevenly filled.

- Cracked crust:
  - oven too hot.

- Sunken:
  - oven too hot
  - tin removed during cooking.

- White spots on surface:
  - insufficient beating.

Possible reasons for faults in Genoese sponges

- Close texture:
  - eggs and sugar overheated
  - eggs and sugar under-beaten
  - too much flour
  - flour insufficiently folded in
  - oven too hot.

- Sunken:
  - too much sugar
  - oven too hot
  - tin removed during cooking.

- Heavy:
  - butter too hot
  - butter insufficiently mixed in
  - flour over-mixed.

The introduction of steam or moisture

Because they become too dry while baking due to oven temperature producing a dry atmosphere, some cakes require the injection of steam. Combination ovens are ideally suited for this purpose. The steam delays the formation of the crust until the cake batter has become fully aerated and the proteins have set. Alternatively, add a tray of water to the oven while baking. If the oven is too hot the cake crust will form early and the cake batter will rise into a peak.

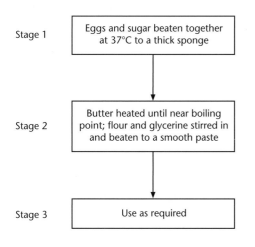

Stage 1 — Eggs and sugar beaten together at 37°C to a thick sponge

Add to stage 2 in three or four parts, beating well to produce a smooth batter

Stage 2 — Butter heated until near boiling point; flour and glycerine stirred in and beaten to a smooth paste

Stage 3 — Use as required

The boiling method

Points to remember

- Check all ingredients carefully.
- Make sure scales are accurate; weigh all ingredients carefully.
- Check ovens are at the right temperature and that the shelves are in the correct position.
- Check that all work surfaces and equipment are clean.
- Check that all other equipment required, such as cooling wires, is within easy reach.
- Always sieve flour to remove lumps and any foreign material.
- Make sure that eggs and fats are at room temperature.
- Check dried fruits carefully; wash, drain and dry if necessary.
- Always follow the recipe carefully.
- Always scrape down the sides of the mixing bowl when creaming mixtures.
- Always seek help if you are unsure, or lack understanding.
- Try to fill the oven space when baking by planning production carefully; this saves time, labour and money.
- Never guess quantities. Time and temperature are important factors; they too should not be guessed.
- The shape and size of goods will determine the cooking time and temperature: the wider the cake, the longer and more slowly it will need to cook.
- Where cakes contain a high proportion of sugar in the recipe, this will caramelise the surface quickly before the centre is cooked. Therefore cover the cake with sheets of silicone or wetted greaseproof and continue to cook.
- When cake tops are sprinkled with almonds or sugar, the baking temperature needs to be lowered slightly to prevent over-colouring of the cake crust.
- When glycerine, glucose and invert sugar, honey or treacle is added to cake mixtures, the oven temperature should be lowered as these colour at a lower temperature than sugar.
- Always work in a clean and hygienic way; remember the hygiene and safety rules, in particular the Food Safety Act.
- All cakes and sponges benefit from being allowed to cool in their tins as this makes handling easier. If sponges need to be cooled quickly, place a wire rack over the top of the tin and invert, then remove the lining paper and cool on a wire rack.

Biscuit mixtures

Biscuits and cookies may be produced by the following methods:

- rubbing in
- flour batter
- foaming
- blending
- sugar batter.

Rubbing in

This is probably the best-known method and is used in producing some of the most famous types of biscuits, such as shortbread. The method is exactly the same as that for producing short pastry.

1. Rub the fat into the flour, by hand or by machine, adding the liquid and the sugar and mixing in the flour to produce a smooth biscuit paste.
2. Do not overwork the paste otherwise it will not combine and as a consequence you will not be able to roll it out.

Foaming

This is where a foam is produced from egg whites, egg yolks or both. Sponge fingers are an example of a two-foam mixture. Meringue is an example of a single-foam mixture using egg whites. Great care must be taken not to over-mix the product.

Sugar batter method

Fat and sugar are mixed together to produce a light and fluffy cream. Beaten egg is added gradually. The dry ingredients are then carefully folded in.

Flour batter method

Half the sieved flour is creamed with the fat. The eggs and sugar are beaten together before they are added to the fat and flour mixture. Finally, the remainder of the flour is folded in, together with any other dry ingredients.

Blending method

In several biscuit recipes, the method requires the chef only to blend all the ingredients together to produce a smooth paste.

Production methods and examples

- **Rubbing in:** shortbread.
- **Foaming:** sponge fingers.
- **Sugar batter method:** cats' tongues (langues de chat), sablé biscuits.
- **Flour batter method:** cookies.
- **Blending method:** almond biscuits (using basic almond commercial mixture).

Convenience cake, biscuit and sponge mixes

There is now a vast range of prepared mixes and frozen goods available on the market. Premixes enable the caterer to calculate costs more effectively, reduce labour costs (with less demand for highly skilled labour) and limit the range of stock items to be held.

Every year, more and more convenience products are introduced onto the market by food manufacturers. The caterer should be encouraged to investigate these products, and to experiment in order to assess their quality.

Decorating and finishing for presentation

Filling

Cakes, sponges and biscuits may be filled or sandwiched together with a variety of different types of filling. Some examples are presented below.

- Creams:
    - buttercream (plain), flavoured and/or coloured
    - pastry cream, flavoured and/or coloured
    - whipped cream
    - clotted cream.
- Fruit:
    - fresh fruit purée
    - jams
    - fruit pastries
    - fruit mousses
    - preserves
    - fruit gels.
- Pastes and spreads:
    - chocolate
    - praline
    - nut
    - curds.

Spreading and coating

This is where smaller cakes and gâteaux are covered top and sides with any of the following:

- fresh whipped cream
- fondant
- chocolate
- royal icing
- buttercream
- water icing
- meringue
    - ordinary
    - Italian
    - Swiss
- commercial preparations.

Piping

Piping is a skill that takes practice. There are many different types of piping tube available. The following may be used for piping:

- royal icing
- meringue
- chocolate
- boiled sugar
- fondant
- fresh cream.

Dusting, dredging, sprinkling

These techniques are used to give the product a final design or glaze during cooking, using sugar.

- **Dusting:** a light dusting, giving an even finish.
- **Dredging:** heavier dusting with sugar.
- **Sprinkling:** a very light sprinkle of sugar.

The sugar used may be icing, caster or granulated white; demerara, Barbados or dark brown sugar. The product may be returned to the oven for glazing, or glazed under the salamander.

Other decorative media

Remember that decorating is an art form and there is a range of equipment and materials available to assist you in this work. Some examples of decorative media are as follows.

- Glacé and crystallised fruits:
  - cherries
  - lemons
  - oranges
  - pineapple
  - figs.
- Crystallised flowers:
  - rose petals
  - violets
  - mimosa
  - lilac.
- Crystallised stems:
  - angelica.
- Nuts:
  - almonds (nibbed, flaked)
  - coconut (fresh slices, desiccated)
  - hazelnuts
  - brazil nuts
  - pistachio.
- Chocolate:
  - rolls
  - vermicelli
  - flakes
  - piping chocolate
  - chips.

Biscuit pastes

Piped biscuits can be used for decoration. For example:

- cats' tongues (recipe 12)
- piped sablé paste (recipe 13)
- almond biscuits.

Test yourself

1 How much flour is required to produce a four egg Genoese sponge?
2 Describe what is meant by the 'creaming' method.
3 Describe the production of biscuit à la cuillére.
4 What is the ratio of fat to flour for shortbread biscuits?
5 Describe tuiles biscuits and what they are used for.
6 Describe the preparation and baking of the following:
   a) Madeleines
   b) Sablé à la poche.
7 List the ingredients and method for a traditional Victoria sandwich.
8 List the various shapes that can be produced from a brandy snap mixture.

1

Genoese sponge *(génoise)*

cal	kcal	fat	sat fat	carb	sugar	protein	fibre
5978 KJ	1423 kcal	65.8 g	25.6 g	182.8 g	106.6 g	36.5 g	3.6 g

*

 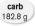

	single sponge	double sponge
medium eggs	4	10
caster sugar	100 g	250 g
flour (soft)	100 g	250 g
butter, margarine or oil	50 g	125 g

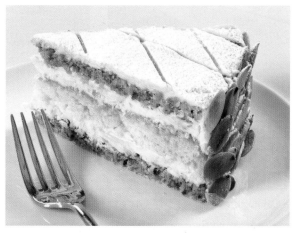

1 Whisk the eggs and sugar with a balloon whisk in a bowl over a pan of hot water.

2 Continue until the mixture is light and creamy, and has doubled in bulk.

3 Remove from the heat and whisk until cold and thick (ribbon stage). Fold in the flour very gently.

4 Fold in the melted butter very gently.

5 Place in a greased, floured Genoese mould.

6 Bake in a moderately hot oven, at 200–220°C, for about 30 minutes.

* Using hard margarine (4 portions)

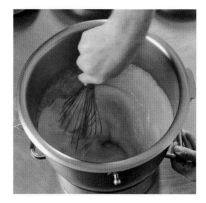

Ingredients for Genoese sponge, and boiling water ready for use

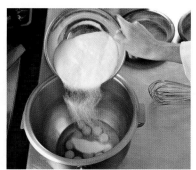

Add the sugar to the eggs

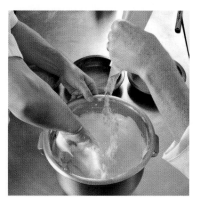

Whisk them together over boiling water

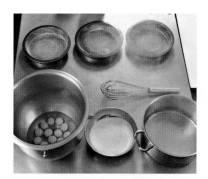

Carry on whisking as the mixture warms up

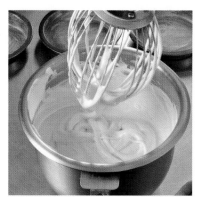

When the mixture is ready, it will form ribbons and you can draw a figure eight with it

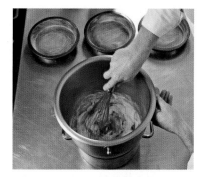

Fold in the flour

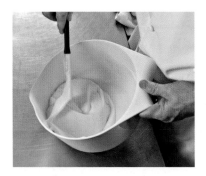

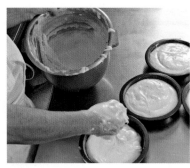

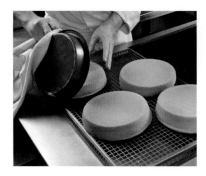

Add part of the flour mixture to the butter

Place the mixture into greased cake tins

After baking, turn the sponges out to cool on a rack

Making a Genoise
http://bit.ly/ABYLlu

2 Fresh cream and strawberry gateau

Genoese sponge made with vanilla	1
stock syrup (chapter 14, recipe 11)	100 ml
raspberry jam	50 ml
whipping or double cream	500 ml
icing sugar	75 g
strawberries, sliced	1 punnet

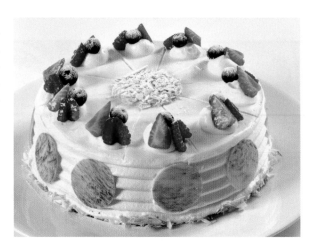

1 Carefully slice the sponge cake into three equal discs. Brush each with syrup.

2 Slowly whip the cream with the icing sugar to achieve the correct consistency.

3 Place the first piece of sponge on a cake board. Soak with syrup. Spread with a layer of jam, then a layer of cream. Scatter sliced strawberries on top.

4 Place the next piece of sponge on top. Repeat the layers of syrup, cream and strawberries. Top with additional cream.

5 Place the final piece of sponge on top.

6 Coat the top and sides with cream. Chill.

7 Comb scrape the sides of the gateau. Pipe 12 rosettes on top.

3 Roulade sponge

	24 portions
whole eggs	900 ml
egg yolks	5
caster sugar	510 g
soft flour	340 g

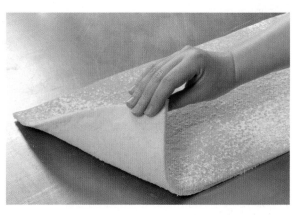

Roulade sponge should not be crisp: you should be able to bend it

1 Whisk the eggs, yolks and sugar by hand over boiling water until warm.

2 Whisk on a food mixer until the ribbon stage.

3 Sieve the flour onto paper.

4 Preheat the oven to 220°C.

5 Fold the flour into the egg mixture as quickly and lightly as possible (ask someone else to help).

6 Divide the mixture between two prepared baking sheets, as quickly as possible. Spread evenly.

7 Bake for 4–5 minutes.

8 Cool completely.

9 Cut the sheets in half. Wrap individually in clingfilm before stacking.

10 Store in the freezer, making sure they are not bent or squashed.

Try something different

To make a chocolate roulade sponge, replace the flour with a mixture of 85 g cornflour, 85 g cocoa powder and 225 g soft flour.

4 Rich fruit cake

	16 cm dia, 8 cm deep	21 cm dia, 8 cm deep	26 cm dia, 8 cm deep	31 cm dia, 8 cm deep
butter or margarine	150 g	200 g	300 g	550 g
caster or soft brown sugar	150 g	200 g	300 g	550 g
eggs	4	6	8	10
glycerine	2 tsp	3 tsp	1 tbsp	2 tbsp
soft flour	125 g	175 g	275 g	500 g
nutmeg	¾ tsp	1 tsp	1¼ tsp	2 tsp
mixed spice	¾ tsp	1 tsp	1¼ tsp	2 tsp
cinnamon	¾ tsp	1 tsp	1¼ tsp	2 tsp
ground almonds	75 g	100 g	125 g	200 g
salt	6 g	8 g	10 g	12 g
currants	150 g	200 g	300 g	550 g
sultanas	150 g	200 g	300 g	550 g
raisins	125 g	150 g	225 g	400 g
mixed peel	75 g	100 g	125 g	200 g
glacé cherries	75 g	100 g	125 g	200 g
lemon, grated rind of	½	½	1	2
oven temperature	150°C	150°C	130°C	110°C
time (approx.)	3 hours	3½ hours	4½ hours	6–7 hours

1 Cream the butter or margarine and sugar until light and fluffy.

2 Gradually beat in the eggs, creaming continuously.

3 Add the glycerine.

4 Sift the flour, nutmeg, mixed spice and cinnamon. Add the ground almonds and salt, mix well.

5 Carefully fold in the flour, nutmeg, mixed spice, cinnamon, ground almonds and salt into the eggs and sugar.

6 Fold in the dried fruit, mixed peel, glacé cherries and lemon rind.

7 Place the mixture into a prepared cake tin lined with silicone. The outside of the tin should also be well protected with paper. Bake at the required temperature for the required time.

8 To test, insert a needle into the centre of the cake; when cooked, it should come out clean and free of uncooked mixture.

9 Remove from the oven and allow to cool.

10 Wrap in tin foil and allow to mature for 2–3 weeks before coating with marzipan and icing.

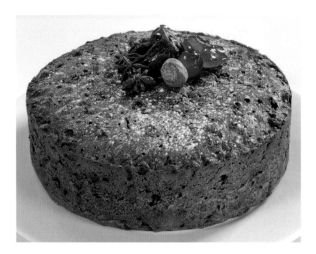

The dried fruit may be soaked in brandy for 12 hours. Allow 3 tbsp of brandy for a 16 cm diameter cake; 4 tbsp for 21 cm diameter; 5 tbsp for 26 cm diameter, etc. Alternatively, instead of soaking the fruit before baking, the brandy may be poured over the cake once it leaves the oven after baking.

5 Banana bread

	3 cakes
ripe bananas	460 g
vegetable oil	110 ml
melted butter	140 g
caster sugar	460 g
eggs	4
soft flour	460 g
baking powder	20 g
salt	2 g

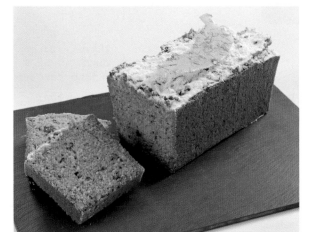

1 Beat the bananas, oil and butter together at a medium speed with the paddle attachment in a food mixer.

2 Add sugar and eggs and mix until smooth.

3 Add the dry ingredients and mix well.

4 Place mixture into 3 well greased or silicone-lined tins (7.5 cm deep × 17.5 cm long × 10 cm wide).

5 Bake at 170°C in a medium fan oven for 35 minutes and then check if cooked by inserting a skewer into the cake mixture. If the skewer comes out clean, the banana bread is done.

6 Allow to cool.

---

6 Lemon drizzle cake

butter or soft margarine	250 g
caster sugar	400 g
zest of lemons	3
soft flour	380 g
baking powder	10 g
eggs, large	4
vanilla extract	½ tsp
milk	25 ml
For the syrup	
juice of lemons	3
sugar	100 g

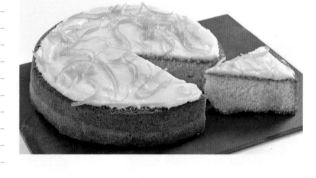

1 Cream the butter, sugar and lemon zest together until white and fluffy.

2 Sieve the flour and baking powder together.

3 Mix together the eggs and vanilla extract.

4 Mix some of the egg mixture into the creamed fat and sugar.

5 Mix in some of the flour.

6 Keep repeating, adding some eggs and then some flour, until they have all been used up.

7 Add the milk. Check that the mixture is at dropping consistency.

8 Place into a prepared tin. Bake at 165°C until cooked.

9 Make the syrup by boiling the juice and sugar together.

10 When the cake is cooked, pierce in several places with a skewer. Pour over the syrup. Leave to cool in the tin.

---

7 Victoria sandwich

cal 6866 KJ	kcal 1635 kcal	fat 94.3 g	sat fat 39.3 g	carb 184.7 g	sugar 106.6 g	protein 23.3 g	fibre 3.6 g

	single sponge	double sponge
butter or margarine	100 g	250 g
caster sugar	100 g	250 g
medium eggs	2	5
flour (soft)	100 g	250 g
baking powder	5 g	12 g

1 Cream the fat and sugar until soft and fluffy.

2 Gradually add the beaten eggs.

3 Lightly mix in the sieved flour, and baking powder.

4 Divide into two 18 cm greased sponge tins.

5 Bake at 190–200°C for 12–15 minutes.

6 Turn out on to a wire rack to cool.

7 Spread one half with jam, place the other half on top.

8 Dust with icing sugar.

* *Using hard margarine*

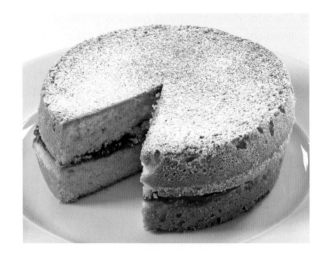

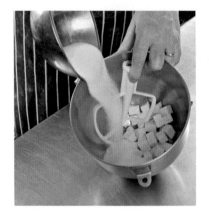

Blend the sugar and butter together

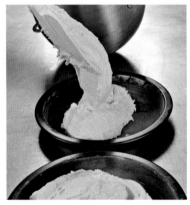

Place the mixture into greased cake tins

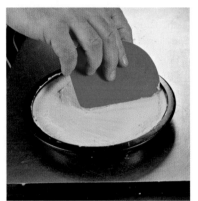

Flatten the top before baking

8 Swiss roll

cal	kcal	fat	sat fat	carb	sugar	protein	fibre
4445 KJ	1058 kcal	25.3 g	8.0 g	182.7 g	106.5 g	36.5 g	3.6 g	*

	4 portions	10 portions
Method 1		
medium eggs	4	10
caster sugar	100 g	250 g
flour (soft)	100 g	250 g
jam, as required		
Method 2		
medium eggs	250 ml	625 ml
caster sugar	175 g	425 g
flour (soft)	125 g	300 g
jam, as required		

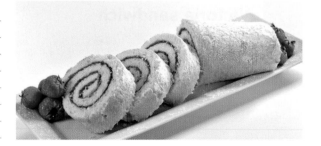

1 Whisk the eggs and sugar with a balloon whisk in a bowl over a pan of hot water, using the ingredients specified for either method 1 or 2.

2 Continue until the mixture is light, creamy and double in bulk.

3 Remove from the heat and whisk until cold and thick (ribbon stage).

4 Fold in the flour very gently.

5 Grease a Swiss roll tin and line with greased greaseproof or silicone paper.

6 Pour in the mixture and bake at 220°C for about 6 minutes.

7 Turn out on to a sheet of paper sprinkled with additional caster sugar.

8 Remove the paper from the Swiss roll, spread with warm jam.

9 Roll into a fairly tight roll, leaving the paper on the outside for a few minutes.

10 Remove the paper and allow to cool on a wire rack.

* 4 portions

---

9 ## Scones

cal	kcal	fat	sat fat	carb	sugar	protein	fibre
678 KJ	162 kcal	5.8 g	2.5 g	26.3 g	7.5 g	2.7 g	1.0 g

*

	8 scones	20 scones
self-raising flour	200 g	500 g
baking powder	5 g	12 g
salt	pinch	large pinch
butter or margarine	50 g	125 g
caster sugar	50 g	125 g
milk or water	95 ml	250 ml

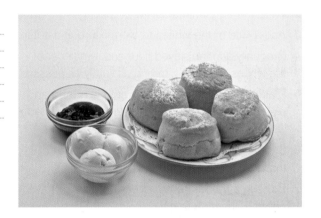

1 Sieve the flour, baking powder and salt.

2 Rub in the fat to achieve a sandy texture. Make a well in the centre.

3 Dissolve the sugar in the liquid.

4 Gradually incorporate the flour; mix lightly.

5 Roll out two rounds, 1 cm thick. Place on a greased baking sheet.

6 Cut a cross halfway through the rounds with a large knife.

7 Milkwash and bake at 200°C for 15–20 minutes.

> The comparatively small amount of fat, rapid mixing to a soft dough, quick and light handling are essentials to produce a light scone.

Try something different

● Add 50 g (125 g for 20 scones) washed and dried sultanas to the scone mixture for fruit scones; 50 per cent wholemeal flour may be used.

● Add other flavours to the mixture: try coconut or dried cranberries.

● For precisely formed scones, roll out the dough to approx. 2 cm thick and cut scones with a 4–5 cm cutter.

* Using hard margarine

10 Sponge fingers *(biscuits à la cuillère)*

cal	kcal	fat	sat fat	carb	sugar	protein	fibre
145 KJ	34 kcal	0.9 g	0.2 g	5.7 g	3.3 g	1.3 g	0.1 g

	Makes 32 fingers
medium eggs	4
caster sugar	100 g
flour (soft)	100 g
icing sugar, to sprinkle	

1 Cream the egg yolks and sugar in a bowl until creamy and almost white.

2 Whip the egg whites stiffly.

3 Add a little of the whites to the mixture and cut in.

4 Gradually add the sieved flour and remainder of the whites alternately, mixing as lightly as possible.

5 Place in a piping bag with 1 cm plain tube and pipe in 8 cm lengths on to baking sheets lined with greaseproof or silicone paper.

6 Sprinkle liberally with icing sugar. Rest for 5 minutes, repeat, then bake.

7 Bake in a moderate hot oven at 200–220°C for about 10 minutes.

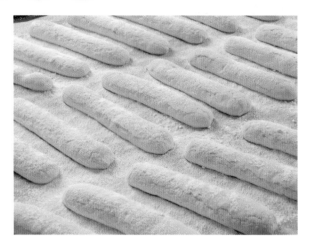

8 Remove from the oven, lift the paper on which the biscuits are piped and place upside down on the table.

9 Sprinkle liberally with water. This will assist the removal of the biscuits from the paper. (No water is needed if using silicone paper.)

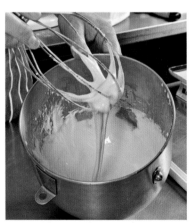

Whisk the egg yolks and sugar until creamy

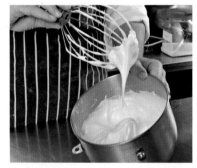

Whip the egg whites until they are stiff

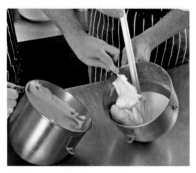

Add some egg whites to the sugar mixture

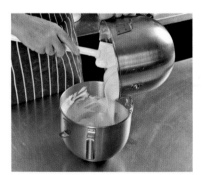

Mix lightly and pour back into the egg white container

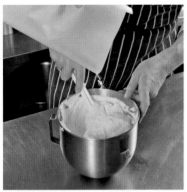
Add sieved flour

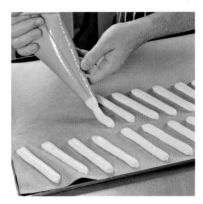
Pipe out in finger shapes

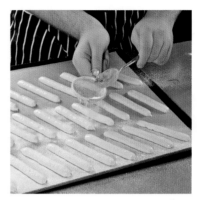
Dust with icing sugar before baking

11 Shortbread biscuits

cal	kcal	fat	sat fat	carb	sugar	protein	fibre
507 KJ	121 kcal	7.0 g	4.4 g	14.1 g	4.6 g	1.2 g	0.5 g

	12 biscuits
Method 1	
flour (soft)	150 g
salt	pinch
butter or margarine	100 g
caster sugar	50 g
Method 2	
soft flour (white or wholemeal)	100 g
rice flour	100 g
butter or margarine	100 g
caster or unrefined sugar	100 g
medium egg, beaten	1
Method 3	
butter or margarine	100 g
icing sugar	100 g
medium egg	1
flour (soft)	150 g

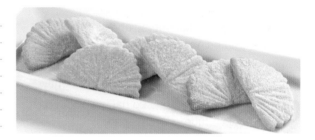

Method 1

1 Sift the flour and salt.

2 Mix in the butter or margarine and sugar with the flour.

3 Combine all the ingredients to a smooth paste.

4 Roll carefully on a floured table or board to the shape of a rectangle or round, ½ cm thick. Place on a lightly greased baking sheet.

5 Mark into the desired size and shape. Prick with a fork.

6 Bake in a moderate oven at 180–200°C for 15–20 minutes.

Method 2

1 Sieve the flour and rice flour into a basin.

2 Rub in the butter until the texture of fine breadcrumbs. Mix in the sugar.

3 Bind the mixture to a stiff paste using the beaten egg.

4 Roll out to 3 mm using caster sugar, prick well with a fork and cut into fancy shapes. Place the biscuits on a lightly greased baking sheet.

5 Bake in a moderate oven at 180–200°C for 15 minutes or until golden brown.

6 Remove with a palette knife on to a cooling rack.

Method 3

1 Cream the butter or margarine and sugar thoroughly.

2 Add the egg and mix in. Mix in the flour.

3 Pipe on to lightly greased and floured baking sheets using a large star tube.

4 Bake at 200–220°C, for approximately 15 minutes.

* Using butter

12 Cats' tongues *(langues de chat)*

	Approx. 40 biscuits
icing sugar	125 g
butter	100 g
vanilla essence	3–4 drops
egg whites	3–4
soft flour	100 g

1 Lightly cream the sugar and butter, add the vanilla essence.

2 Add the egg whites one by one, continually mixing and being careful not to allow the mixture to curdle.

3 Gently fold in the sifted flour and mix lightly.

4 Pipe on to a lightly greased baking sheet using a 3 mm plain tube, 2½ cm apart.

5 Bake at 230–250°C, for a few minutes.

6 The outside edges should be light brown and the centres yellow.

7 When cooked, remove on to a cooling rack using a palette knife.

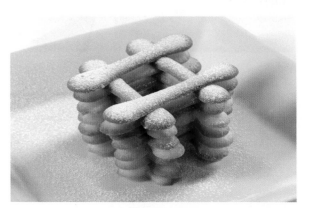

Pipe cats' tongues into their distinctive shape, thicker at the ends

13 Piped biscuits *(sablés à la poche)*

	20–30 biscuits
caster or unrefined sugar	75 g
butter or margarine	150 g
medium egg	1
vanilla essence	3–4 drops
or	
grated lemon zest	
soft flour, white or wholemeal	200 g
ground almonds	35 g

1 Cream the sugar and butter until light in colour and texture.

2 Add the egg gradually, beating continuously, add the vanilla essence or lemon zest.

3 Gently fold in the sifted flour and almonds, mix well until suitable for piping. If too stiff, add a little beaten egg.

4 Pipe on to a lightly greased and floured baking sheet using a medium-sized star tube (a variety of shapes can be used).

5 Some biscuits can be left plain, some decorated with half almonds or neatly cut pieces of angelica and glacé cherries.

6 Bake in a moderate oven at 190°C for about 10 minutes.

7 When cooked, remove on to a cooling rack using a palette knife.

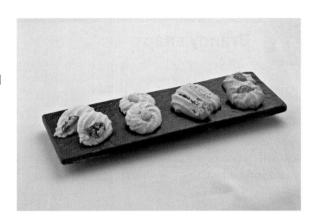

14 Tuiles

	15–20 tuiles
butter	100 g
icing sugar	100 g
flour	100 g
egg whites	2

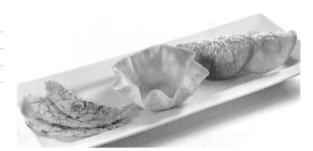

1 Mix all ingredients; allow to rest for 1 hour.

2 Spread to the required shape and size.

3 Bake at approx. 200–210°C.

4 While hot, mould the biscuits to the required shape and leave to cool.

15 Brandy snaps

	20 snaps
strong flour	225 g
ground ginger	10 g
golden syrup	225 g
butter	250 g
caster sugar	450 g

1 Combine the flour and ginger in a bowl on the scales. Make a well.

2 Pour in golden syrup until the correct weight is reached.

3 Cut the butter into small pieces. Add the butter and sugar.

4 Mix together at a slow speed.

5 Divide into four even pieces. Roll into sausage shapes, wrap each in clingfilm and chill, preferably overnight.

6 Slice each roll into rounds. Place on a baking tray, spaced well apart.

7 Flatten each round using a fork dipped in cold water, keeping a round shape.

8 Bake in a pre-heated oven at 200°C until evenly coloured and bubbly.

9 Remove from oven. Allow to cool slightly, then lift off and shape over a dariole mould.

10 Stack the snaps, no more than four together, on a stainless steel tray and store.

16 Madeleines

	45 portions (585 g)
caster sugar	125 g
eggs	3
vanilla pod, seeds from	1
flour	150 g
baking powder	1 tsp
beurre noisette	125 g

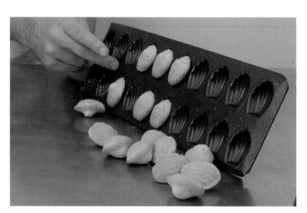

1 Whisk the sugar, eggs and vanilla seeds to a hot sabayon.

2 Fold in the flour and the baking powder.

3 Fold in the beurre noisette and chill for up to 2 hours.

4 Pipe into well buttered madeleine moulds and bake in a moderate oven.

5 Turn out and allow to cool.

17 Produce fermented dough products

In this chapter you will learn how to:

1. prepare, cook and finish fermented dough products, including:

- using tools and equipment correctly, in a safe and hygienic way
- checking that the finished product meets requirements

2. you should have the knowledge to:

- identify different products, their uses and cooking methods
- store raw dough and finished products safely
- understand the quality points of ingredients and how to adjust the quantity
- identify fillings, glazes, creams and icings, and finishing and decorating techniques.

Number	Recipe title	Page number
17	Bagels	556
9	Bath buns	551
6	Bun dough: basic recipe	549
7	Bun wash	550
15	Chapatis	554
8	Chelsea buns	550
11	Doughnuts	552
18	Focaccia	557
10	Hot cross buns	551
22	Marignans Chantilly	559
16	Naan bread	555
5	Olive bread	548
12	Parmesan rolls	552
19	Pizza	557

Number	Recipe title	Page number
13	Red onion and sage rolls	553
3	Rye bread	547
20	Savarin paste: basic recipe	558
21	Savarin with fruit (savarin aux fruits)	559
14	Seeded rolls	553
4	Soda bread	548
1	Sun-dried tomato bread	545
	Syrup for savarin, baba and marignans	559
2	Wheatmeal bread	546

The key ingredients for dough products, such as flour, eggs, sugar and raising agents, are described in Chapter 14 (pages 447–54). Make sure you read and understand this section.

Dough products

Bread and dough products basically contain wheat flour and yeast. Bread and bread products form the basis of our diet, and are staple products in our society. We eat bread at breakfast, lunch and dinner, as sandwiches, bread rolls, croissants, French sticks, etc. Bread is also used as an ingredient for many other dishes, either as slices or as breadcrumbs.

Dough consists of strong flour, water, salt and yeast, which are kneaded together to the required consistency at a suitable temperature. It is then allowed to prove (to rise and increase in size),

when the yeast produces carbon dioxide and water, which aerates the dough. When baked it produces a light digestible product with flavour and colour.

Digestible: Something that can be digested; that is possible for the body's digestive system to break down.

The basic bread dough of wheat flour, yeast and water may be enriched with fat, sugar, eggs, milk and numerous other added ingredients.

Some examples of enriched doughs or enriched breads are:

- buns
- savarins
- brioche
- croissants
- Danish pastries.

Croissants and Danish pastries are enriched doughs to which the fat is added by layering or lamination. This makes them softer to eat because the fat in the dough insulates the water molecules, keeping the moisture level higher during baking.

Salted dough is much more manageable than unsalted dough. Salt is usually added a few moments before the end of the kneading, since its function is to help expand the dough's volume.

Flour-based products provide us with variety, energy, vitamins and minerals. Wholemeal bread products also provide roughage, an essential part of a healthy diet.

Understanding fermentation

For dough to become leavened bread (bread that has risen, rather than flat bread) it must go through a fermentation process. This is brought about by the action of yeast, a living micro-organism rich in protein and vitamin B. The yeast reacts with enzymes in the dough, which convert sugar into alcohol, producing the characteristic flavour of bread. The action also produces carbon dioxide, which makes the bread rise.

Yeast requires ideal conditions for growth. These are:

- **warmth:** a good temperature for dough production is 22–30°C
- **moisture:** the liquid should be added at approximately 38°C
- **food:** this is obtained from the starch in the flour
- **time:** this is needed to allow the yeast to grow.

Dried yeast has been dehydrated and must be creamed with a little water before use. It will keep for several months in its dry state. Some types of dried yeast can be used straight from the packet.

Yeast will not survive in a high concentration of sugar or salt, and its growth will slow down in a very rich dough with a high fat and egg content.

When mixing yeast in water or milk, make sure that the liquid is at the correct temperature (38°C), and disperse the yeast in the liquid. (As a living organism cannot be dissolved, the word 'disperse' is used.)

Why does dough ferment?

The phenomenon of dough fermenting is extraordinary, but because we see it so frequently in our profession, we do not pay much attention to how it happens. It is very interesting to know why doughs ferment and what the effects are on the end product. In order to understand why yeast dough rises, we must note that the main ingredients of natural leavening are water, air and, most importantly, sugar, which is transformed into carbon dioxide and alcohol and causes the leavening. This carbon dioxide forms bubbles inside the dough and makes it rise. Fermentation is a transformation undergone by organic matter (sugars).

Points to remember

- Yeast should be removed from the refrigerator and used at room temperature.
- Check that all ingredients are weighed carefully.
- Work in a clean and tidy manner to avoid cross-contamination.
- Check all temperatures carefully.
- All wholemeal doughs absorb more water than white doughs. The volume of water absorbed by flour also varies according to the strength (protein and bran content).
- When using machines, check that they are in working order.
- Always remember the health and safety rules when using machinery.
- Divide the dough with a dough divider, hard scraper or hydraulic cutting machine.
- Check the divided dough pieces for weight.

When weighing, remember that doughs lose up to 12.5 per cent of their water during baking.

- Keep the flour, bowl and liquid warm.
- Remember to knock the dough back (re-knead it) carefully once proved, as this will expel the gas and allow the yeast to be dispersed properly, coming back into direct contact with the dough.
- Proving allows the dough to ferment; the second prove is essential for giving dough products the necessary volume and a good flavour.
- Time and temperature are crucial when cooking dough products.
- When using frozen dough products, always follow the manufacturer's instructions.
- Contamination can occur if doughs are defrosted incorrectly.

Types of dough

Enriched doughs

- **Savarin:** a rich yeast dough used for savarins, babas and marignans.
- **Brioche:** a rich yeast dough with a high fat and butter content.

Laminated doughs

- **Croissants:** made from a dough in which the fat content has been layered (laminated), as in puff pastry.
- **Danish:** also a laminated dough; Danish pastries may be filled with fruit, frangipane, apple, custard, cherries and many other ingredients.

Speciality doughs

- **Blinis:** a type of pancake.
- **Naan bread:** unleavened Indian bread, traditionally cooked in a tandoor (oven).
- **Pitta bread:** Middle Eastern and Greek bread, also unleavened.
- **Chapati:** Indian unleavened bread made from a fine ground wholemeal flour.

Storage of cooked dough products

Crusty rolls and bread are affected by changes in storage conditions; they are softened by a damp environment and humid conditions, so should be stored in a dry environment to keep them crusty.

Always store dough products in suitable containers at room temperature, and in a freezer for longer storage. Do not store in a refrigerator unless you want the bread to stale quickly for use as breadcrumbs. Staling will also occur quickly in products that contain a lot of fat and milk. Many commercial dough products contain anti-staling agents.

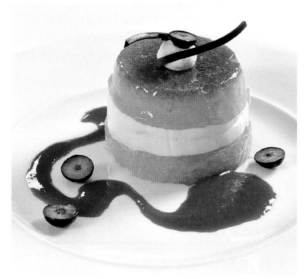

This blueberry baba is made with savarin dough (recipe available on Dynamic Learning)

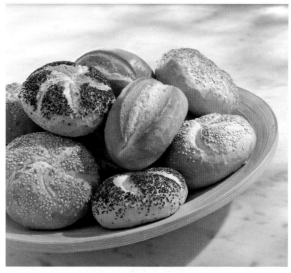

Rolls may be purchased ready for baking

Convenience dough products

There are many different types of convenience dough product on the market.

- fresh and frozen pre-proved dough products: rolls; croissants; Danish pastries; French breads
- bake-off products that are ready for baking. These can be bought either frozen or fresh, or in modified-atmosphere packaged forms (this method replaces most of the oxygen around the product to slow down spoilage). These products have to be kept refrigerated. They include garlic bread, rolls and Danish pastries.

Possible reasons for faults using yeast doughs

If your dough has a close texture this may be because:

- it was insufficiently proved
- it was insufficiently kneaded
- it contains insufficient yeast
- the oven was too hot
- too much water was added
- too little water was added.

If your dough has an uneven texture this may be because:

- it was insufficiently kneaded
- it was over-proved
- the oven was too cool.

If your dough has a coarse texture this may be because:

- it was over-proofed, uncovered
- it was insufficiently kneaded
- too much water was added
- too much salt was added

If your dough is wrinkled this may be because:

- it was over-proved.

If your dough is sour this may be because:

- the yeast was stale
- too much yeast was used.

If the crust is broken this may be because:

- the dough was under-proved at the second stage.

If there are white spots on crust this may be because:

- the dough was not covered before second proving.

Breads

It is customary today for restaurants to offer a range of different flavoured breads. Internationally there is a wide variety available; different nations and regions have their own speciality breads. Bread plays an important part in many religious festivals, especially Christian and Jewish.

Bulk fermentation

The traditional breadmaking process is known as the bulk fermentation process. This was used by many bakers before the introduction of high-speed mixing and dough conditioners, which both eliminate the need for bulk fermentation time. However, this traditional method produces a fine flavour due to the fermentation and is evident in the final product.

Bulk fermentation time (BFT) is the term used to describe the length of time that the dough is allowed to ferment in bulk. BFT is measured from the end of the mixing method to the beginning of the scaling (weighing) process. The length of BFT can be from 1 to 6 hours and is related to the level of salt and yeast in the recipe, as well as the dough temperature.

It is important during the bulk fermentation process that ideal conditions are adhered to:

- The dough must be kept covered to prevent the surface of the dough developing a skin.
- The appropriate temperature must be maintained to control the rate of fermentation.

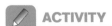 **ACTIVITY**

1 What is meant by fermentation?

2 Name two types of bread.

3 Why is temperature so important when making bread dough using yeast?

4 What is the raising agent used in soda bread?

5 What is the difference between strong and soft flour?

6 State the nutritional benefits of wholemeal flour.

Sun-dried tomato bread

	2 × 450 g loaves
sun-dried tomatoes, chopped	100 g
water	300 ml
bread flour	500 g
salt	10 g
skimmed milk powder	12½ g
shortening	12½ g
yeast (fresh)	20 g
sugar	12½ g

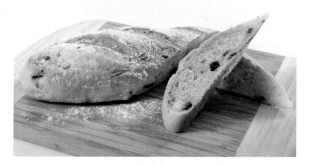

1 Soak the sun-dried tomatoes in boiling water for 30 minutes.

2 Sieve the flour, salt and skimmed milk powder.

3 Add the shortening and rub through the dry ingredients.

4 Disperse the yeast into warm water, approximately 37°C. Add and dissolve the sugar. Add to the above ingredients.

5 Mix until a smooth dough is formed. Check for any extremes in consistency and adjust as necessary until a smooth elastic dough is formed.

6 Cover the dough, keep warm and allow to prove.

7 After approximately 30–40 minutes, knock back the dough and mix in the chopped sun-dried tomatoes (well drained).

8 Mould and prove again for another 30 minutes (covered).

9 Divide the dough into two and mould round.

10 Rest for 10 minutes. Keep covered.

11 Re-mould into ball shape.

12 Place the dough pieces into 15 cm diameter hoops laid out on a baking tray. The hoops must be warm and lightly greased.

13 With the back of the hand flatten the dough pieces.

14 Prove at 38–40°C in humid conditions, preferably in a prover.

15 Bake at 225°C for 25–30 minutes.

16 After baking, remove the bread from the tins immediately and place on a cooling wire.

HEALTHY EATING TIP

- Only a little salt is necessary to 'control' the yeast. Many customers will prefer less salty bread.

2 Wheatmeal bread

	2 loaves
unsalted butter or oil	60 g
honey	3 tbsp
water, lukewarm	500 ml
fresh yeast	25 g
or	
dried yeast	18 g
salt	1 tbsp
unbleached strong white flour	125 g
stoneground wholemeal flour	625 g

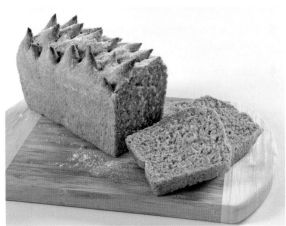

1 Melt the butter in a saucepan.
2 Mix together 1 tbsp of honey and 4 tbsp of the water in a bowl.
3 Disperse the yeast into the honey mixture.
4 In a basin, place the melted butter, remaining honey and water, the yeast mixture and salt.
5 Add the white flour and half the wholemeal flour. Mix well.
6 Add the remaining wholemeal flour gradually, mixing well between each addition.
7 The dough should pull away from the side of the bowl and form a ball. The resulting dough should be soft and slightly sticky.
8 Turn out onto a floured work surface. Sprinkle with white flour, knead well.
9 Brush a clean bowl with melted butter or oil. Place in the dough, cover with a damp cloth and allow to prove in a warm place. This will take approximately 1–1½ hours.
10 Knock back and further knead the dough. Cover again and rest for 10–15 minutes.
11 Divide the dough into two equal pieces.

12 Form each piece of dough into a cottage loaf or place in a suitable loaf tin.
13 Allow to prove in a warm place for approximately 45 minutes.
14 Place in a pre-heated oven, 220°C and bake until well browned (approx. 40–45 minutes).
15 When baked, the bread should sound hollow and the sides should feel crisp when pressed.
16 Cool on a wire rack.

Try something different

Alternatively, the bread may be divided into 50 g rolls, brushed with eggwash and baked at 200°C for approximately 10 minutes.

 HEALTHY EATING TIP

• Only a little salt is necessary to 'control' the yeast. Many customers will prefer less salty bread.

3   Rye bread

	1 medium-sized loaf
fresh yeast (or dried yeast may be used)	15 g
water	60 ml (4 tbsp)
black treacle	15 ml (1 tbsp)
vegetable oil	15 ml (1 tbsp)
caraway seeds (optional)	15 g
salt	15 g
lager	250 ml
rye flour	250 g
unbleached bread flour	175 g
polenta	
eggwash	

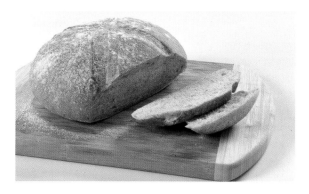

1 Disperse the yeast in the warm water (at approximately 37°C)

2 In a basin mix the black treacle, oil, two-thirds of the caraway seeds (if required) and the salt. Add the lager. Add the yeast and mix in the sieved rye flour. Mix well.

3 Gradually add the bread flour. Continue to add the flour until the dough is formed and it is soft and slightly sticky.

4 Turn the dough onto a lightly floured surface and knead well.

5 Knead the dough until it is smooth and elastic.

6 Place the kneaded dough into a suitable bowl that has been brushed with oil.

7 Cover with a damp cloth and allow the dough to prove in a warm place until it is double in size. This will take about 1½–2 hours.

8 Turn the dough onto a lightly floured work surface, knock back the dough to original size. Cover and allow to rest for approximately 5–10 minutes.

9 Shape the dough into an oval approximately 25 cm long.

10 Place onto a baking sheet lightly sprinkled with polenta.

11 Allow the dough to prove in a warm place, preferably in a prover, until double in size (approximately 45 minutes to 1 hour).

12 Lightly brush the loaf with eggwash, sprinkle with the remaining caraway seeds (if required).

13 Using a small, sharp knife, make three diagonal slashes, approximately 5 mm deep into the top of the loaf.

14 Place in a pre-heated oven 190°C (375°F) and bake for approximately 50–55 minutes.

15 When cooked, turn out. The bread should sound hollow when tapped and the sides should feel crisp.

16 Allow to cool.

 HEALTHY EATING TIP

- Only a little salt is necessary to 'control' the yeast. Many customers will prefer less salty bread.

4   Soda bread

	2 loaves
wholemeal flour	250 g
strong flour	250 g
bicarbonate of soda	1 tsp
salt	1 tsp
buttermilk	200 g
water, warm	60 ml
butter, melted	25 g

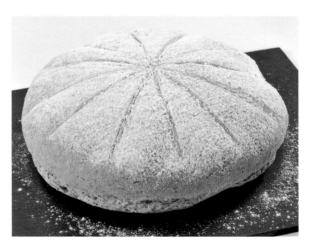

1 Sift the flours, salt and bicarbonate of soda into a bow.
2 Make a well and add the buttermilk, warm water and melted butter.
3 Work the dough for about five minutes.
4 Mould into 2 round loaves and mark the top with a cross.
5 Bake at 200°C for about 25 minutes. When the bread is ready, it should make a hollow sound when tapped.

5   Olive bread

	6 loaves
olive ferment	540 g
black olives, chopped	320 g
yeast	15 g
olive oil	150 ml
water	850 ml
no. 4 flour (strong Canadian wheat flour)	1½ kg
salt	30 g
Maldon salt	

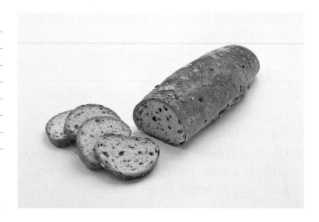

1 Place all the ingredients (three-quarters of the oil), except the flour and salt, into a large bowl. Mix the ingredients by hand.
2 Sprinkle the flour on top, then the salt, and stir to a slack dough, working in 6 turns of the bowl. Fold the edge into the centre and add a little more olive oil. Leave for 20 minutes.
3 Fold with the same method. The dough should resemble the shape of a doughnut with a dip in the centre.
4 Add a little more olive oil and leave in a warm place for 20 minutes.
5 Fold again and leave in a warm place for 20 minutes.
6 Divide the dough into approximately five 550 g balls.
7 Roll into slipper shapes divided by supported greaseproof paper.

8 Spray with water. Wrap with clingfilm and prove in the fridge overnight.

9 Remove from the fridge, unwrap and spray with water.

10 Place in a prover for approximately 30 minutes.

11 Remove, then spray again, removing greaseproof paper from the sides of the bread.

12 Divide onto oven board. Sprinkle with Maldon salt and dust with flour.

13 Cook on 230°C steaming five pulses for 4 minutes with the vent closed.

ASSESSMENT

6 Bun dough: basic recipe

cal	kcal	fat	sat fat	carb	sugar	protein	fibre
656 KJ	157 kcal	6.4 g	2.7 g	22.6 g	4.0 g	3.6 g	1.2 g

	8 buns	20 buns
flour (strong)	200 g	500 g
yeast	5 g	12 g
milk and water	60 ml (approx.)	300 ml (approx.)
medium egg	1	2–3
butter or margarine	50 g	125 g
caster sugar	25 g	60 g

1 Sieve the flour into a bowl and warm.

2 Cream the yeast in a basin with a little of the liquid.

3 Make a well in the centre of the flour.

4 Add the dispersed yeast, sprinkle with a little flour, cover with a cloth, leave in a warm place until the yeast ferments (bubbles).

5 Add the beaten egg, butter or margarine, sugar and remainder of the liquid. Knead well to form a soft, slack dough, knead until smooth and free from stickiness.

6 Keep covered and allow to prove in a warm place. Use as required.

* Using hard margarine, 1 portion (2 buns)

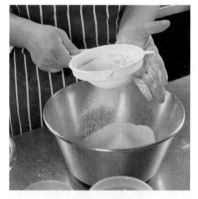
Sift the flour

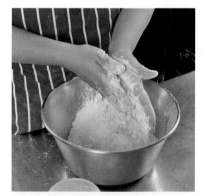
Rub in the yeast

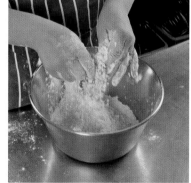
Rub in the fat

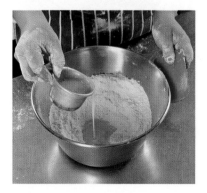
Make a well in the flour, and pour in the beaten egg

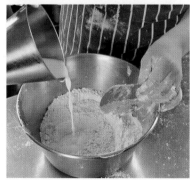
Pour in the liquid

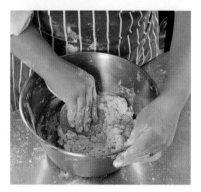
Fold the ingredients together

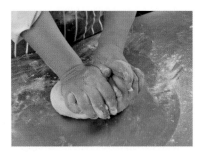

Knead the dough

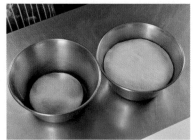

Before and after proving: the same amount of dough is twice the size after it has been left to prove

7 Bun wash

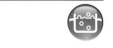

sugar	100 g
water or milk	125 ml

1 Boil ingredients together until the consistency of a thick syrup.

2 Use as required.

8 Chelsea buns

1 Take the basic bun dough (recipe 6) and roll out into a large square.

2 Brush with melted margarine or butter.

3 Sprinkle liberally with caster sugar.

4 Sprinkle with 25 g currants, 25 g sultanas and 25 g chopped peel.

5 Roll up like a Swiss roll, brush with melted margarine or butter.

6 Cut into slices across the roll 3 cm wide.

7 Place on a greased baking tray with deep sides.

8 Cover and allow to prove. Complete as for fruit buns.

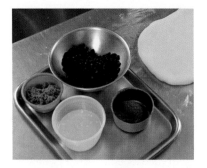

Ingredients for Chelsea buns

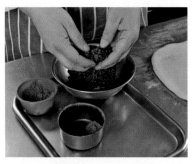

Combine the fruit and spices

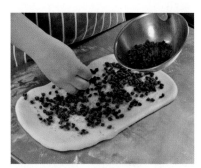

Sprinkle the fruit over the rolled dough

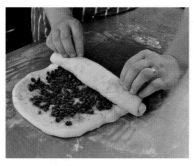

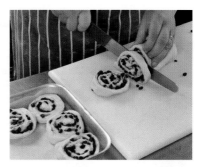

Roll up the dough as if you were making a Swiss roll

Cut the roll into slices to make the buns

9 Bath buns

1 Add to basic bun dough (recipe 6) 50 g washed and dried fruit (e.g. currants and sultanas), 25 g chopped mixed peel and 25 g sugar nibs.

2 Pull off into eight rough-shaped pieces.

3 Sprinkle with a little broken loaf sugar or nibs.

4 Place on a lightly greased baking sheet. Cover with a cloth and allow to prove.

5 Bake in a hot oven at 220°C for 15–20 minutes.

6 Brush liberally with bun wash (recipe 7) as soon as cooked.

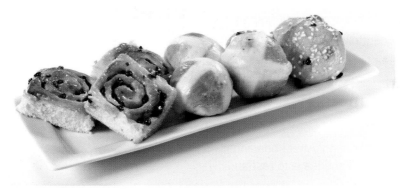

Recipes 8 to 10: Chelsea buns, hot cross buns and Bath buns

10 Hot cross buns

1 Add to basic bun dough (recipe 6), 50 g washed and dried fruit (e.g. currants and sultanas) and some mixed spice.

2 Mould into eight round balls. Make a cross on top of each bun with the back of a knife, or make a slack mixture of flour and water and pipe on crosses using a greaseproof paper cornet.

3 Place on a lightly greased baking sheet. Cover with a cloth and allow to prove.

4 Bake in a hot oven at 220°C for 15–20 minutes.

5 Brush liberally with bun wash (recipe 7) as soon as cooked.

11 Doughnuts

cal	kcal	fat	sat fat	carb	sugar	protein	fibre
918 KJ	218 kcal	13.3 g	4.0 g	22.6 g	4.0 g	3.6 g	1.2 g

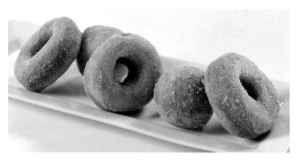

1 Take the basic bun dough (recipe 6) and divide into eight pieces.

2 Mould into balls. Press a floured thumb into each.

3 Add a little jam in each hole. Mould carefully to seal the hole. (For ring doughnuts, press your thumb right through each one and rotate to form a hole in the centre.)

4 Cover and allow to prove on a well-floured tray.

5 Deep-fry in moderately hot fat, 175°C, for 12–15 minutes.

6 Lift out of the fat, drain and roll in a tray containing caster sugar mixed with a little cinnamon.

Using hard margarine and peanut oil

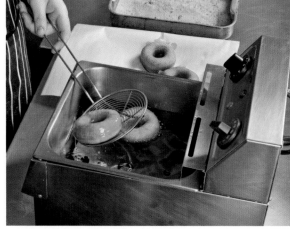

Carefully fry the doughnuts and lift them out with a spider

12 Parmesan rolls

1 Make a basic bread dough. After kneading it, cover with a tea towel and leave to rest and prove for 30 minutes.

2 Using a rolling pin, pin out the dough to a thickness of approximately 3 cm. Brush with a little water.

3 Pass finely grated Parmesan through a coarse sieve onto the dough.

4 Cut the dough into evenly sized pieces, each about 40 g.

5 Place each piece of dough onto a baking sheet with a silpat mat or non-stick parchment. Place in the prover and leave until they have doubled in size.

6 Bake in a pre-heated oven at 220°C for approximately 10 minutes. Cool on a wire rack.

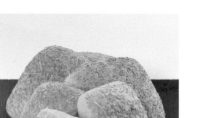

Try something different

Try adding white or black poppy seeds, sesame seeds or old bay seasoning to the dough.

13 Red onion and sage rolls

1 Finely dice the red onion. Sweat it, then leave to cool.
2 Chop the sage and add it to the onion.
3 Pin out bread dough in a rectangle. Spread the onion and sage mixture over 7/8 of the dough. Egg wash the exposed edge.
4 Roll the dough as you would for a Swiss roll, and seal the edge.
5 Cut into 50 g slices.
6 Place the slices on a prepared baking sheet and eggwash. Bake in a pre-heated oven at 220°C for approximately 10 minutes. Cool on a wire rack.

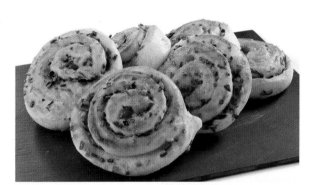

14 Seeded rolls

	8 rolls	16 rolls
strong flour	1 kg	2 kg
yeast	30 g	60 g
water at 37°C	600 ml	1175 ml
salt	20 g	40 g
caster sugar	10 g	20 g
sunflower oil	50 g	100 g

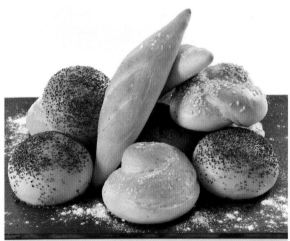

1 Sieve the flour onto paper.
2 Dissolve the yeast in half the water.
3 Dissolve the salt, sugar and oil in the rest of the water.
4 Add both liquids to the flour at once.
5 Mix on speed number 1 for 5 minutes, to a smooth dough.
6 Cover with cling film and leave for 1 hour.
7 Knock back the dough. Divide it into 8 or 16. Keep it covered at all times.
8 Shape the pieces of dough. Place on a silicon-covered baking sheet, in neatly spaced, staggered rows.
9 Prove until the rolls double in size.
10 Eggwash carefully. Bake at 243°C for 8–10 minutes with steam.

15 Chapatis

cal	kcal	fat	sat fat	carb	sugar	protein	fibre
1066 KJ	254 kcal	12.1 g	1.4 g	32.0 g	1.1 g	6.4 g	4.5 g

	4 portions	10 portions
wholewheat or chapati flour	200 g	500 g
pinch of salt		
water	125 ml	213 ml
vegetable oil		

1 Sieve the flour and salt, add the water and knead to a firm dough.

2 Knead on a floured table until smooth and elastic.

3 Cover with a damp cloth or polythene and allow to relax for 30–40 minutes.

4 Divide into 8 pieces (20 pieces for 10 portions), flatten each and roll into a circle 12–15 cm in diameter.

5 Lightly grease a frying pan with the oil, add the chapati and cook as for a pancake. Traditionally chapatis are allowed to puff by placing them over an open flame.

6 Just before serving reheat the chapatis under the salamander.

Chapatis are cooked on a tawa or frying pan. They are made fresh for each meal, and are dipped into sauces and used to scoop up food.

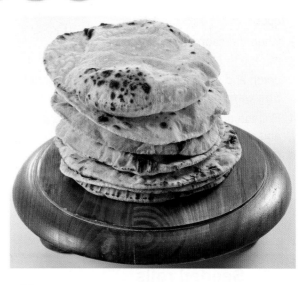

HEALTHY EATING TIP

- Use the minimum amount of salt.

- Lightly oil a well-seasoned pan to cook the chapati, or dry-fry.

- Chapatis are a useful accompaniment for fattier meat dishes.

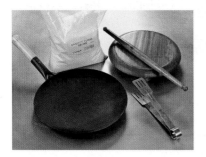

Equipment and ingredients for chapatis, including chapati flour from a specialist supplier, and a traditional rolling board

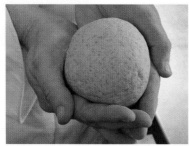

Knead the dough into a ball

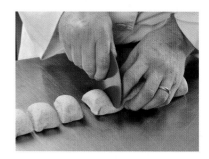

Divide the dough into evenly sized pieces

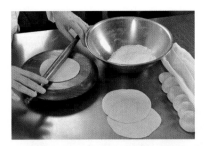
Roll out the dough

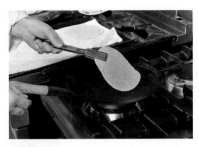
Fry the chapatis one at a time; this traditional pan is called a tawa

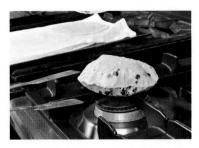
With care, place the chapati over the gas burner until it puffs up; use tongs to handle the chapati

16 Naan bread

cal	kcal	fat	sat fat	carb	sugar	protein	fibre	*
1619 KJ	386 kcal	20.5 g	12.0 g	48.3 g	5.0 g	10.1 g	1.8 g	

	6 portions
strong flour	350 g
caster sugar	1½ tsp
salt	1 tsp
baking powder	½ tsp
fresh yeast	15 g
warm milk (38°C)	150 ml
unsweetened plain yoghurt	150 ml
butter	100 g
poppy seeds	2 tbsp

1 Sift the flour into a suitable bowl and add the sugar, salt and baking powder.

2 Dissolve the yeast in the milk and stir in the yoghurt. Mix thoroughly with the flour to form a dough.

3 Knead the dough until it is smooth. Cover with a clean cloth and leave to rise in a warm place for about 4 hours.

4 Divide the risen dough into 12 equal portions and roll into balls, on a lightly floured surface.

5 Flatten the balls into oblong shapes, using both hands and slapping the naan from one hand to the other.

6 Cook the naan bread on the sides of the tandoori oven or on a lightly greased griddle or heavy-bottomed frying pan.

7 Cook the naan on one side only. Brush the raw side with clarified butter and poppy seeds, turn over, cook the other side or brown under a salamander.

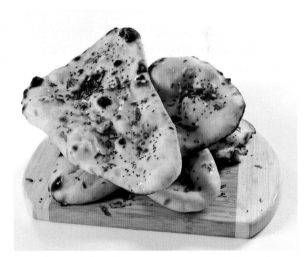

This recipe comes from Punjab and goes well with tandoori meat dishes as well as vindaloos. Traditionally, naans are baked in clay ovens. They must be eaten fresh and hot, and served immediately.

HEALTHY EATING TIP

- Cook the bread without added fat.
- Naan bread is a useful accompaniment for fattier meat dishes.

*With clarified butter – using ghee

17 Bagels

	12 bagels
water	125 ml
milk	250 ml
fresh yeast	12 g
or	
dried yeast	10 g
caster sugar	2 tbsp
bread flour	450 g
salt	15 g (3 tsp)
eggwash	
poppy seeds	1 tbsp
sea salt	10 g (2 tsp)

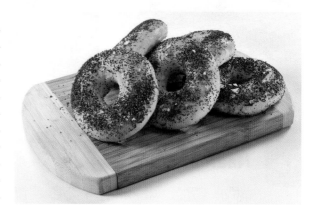

1 Warm the water and milk to 37°C, disperse the yeast in the water, add one tbsp of sugar, cover and leave to stand in a warm place for approximately 10 minutes.

2 Add the sifted flour and salt gradually, mixing into a firm dough. Add a little more flour, or some water, if necessary, to form a smooth and elastic dough.

3 Turn dough onto a floured surface. Knead well until dough is smooth and elastic. Place dough into a well-greased bowl, cover and leave to stand in a warm place in a prover for 1 hour or until the dough has doubled in size.

4 Turn dough out onto a floured surface, knead until smooth. Divide into 12, knead each into a ball. Make a hole in the centre of each.

5 Rotate each ball of dough with the finger until the hole is one-third of the size of the bagel.

6 Place bagels on a greased baking sheet approximately 3 cm apart. Cover and stand in a warm place or prover until double in size.

7 Drop bagels individually into a pan of boiling water. Do not allow them to touch. Turn bagels after 1 minute, simmer for a further 1 minute. Remove, drain well and place on greased baking sheet.

8 Brush each with eggwash, sprinkle with poppy seeds and sea salt. Bake in an oven 200°C for about 20 minutes. Remove, cool on a wire rack.

> Bagels are now very popular and are usually filled with a variety of fillings (e.g. smoked salmon and cream cheese) and served as a snack.
> The dough can be flavoured with herbs, cinnamon or sultanas.

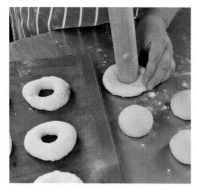

Use a rolling pin to make a hole in the centre of each bagel

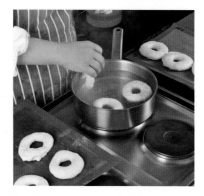

Poach the bagels in water

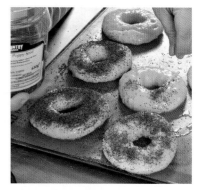

Eggwash the bagels and sprinkle with seeds before baking

18 Focaccia

	1 loaf
fresh yeast	30 g
sugar	1 tsp
lukewarm water (about blood temperature)	230 ml
extra virgin olive oil, plus extra to drizzle on the bread	70 g
salt	1½ tsp
unbleached all-purpose flour	725 g
coarse salt	
picked rosemary	

1 Dissolve the yeast and sugar in half of the lukewarm water in a bowl; let sit until foamy. In another bowl, add the remaining water, the olive oil, and the salt.

2 Pour in the yeast mixture.

3 Blend in the flour, a quarter at a time, until the dough comes together. Knead on a floured board for 10 minutes, adding flour as needed to make it smooth and elastic. Put the dough in an oiled bowl, turn to coat well, and cover with a towel.

4 Leave to rise in a warm draught-free place for 1 hour, until doubled in size.

5 Knock back the dough, knead it for a further 5 minutes, and gently roll it out in to a large disc or sheet to approx. 2 cm thick.

6 Let rise for 15 minutes, covered. Oil your fingers and make impressions with them in the dough, 3 cm apart. Let prove for 1 hour.

7 Preheat the oven to 210°C. Drizzle the dough with olive oil and sprinkle with coarse salt and picked rosemary.

8 Bake for 15–20 minutes in a very hot oven at 200°C, until golden brown. Sprinkle with additional oil if desired. Cut into squares and serve warm.

19 Pizza

cal	kcal	fat	sat fat	carb	sugar	protein	fibre	*
3956 KJ	941 kcal	46.3 g	13.0 g	114.4 g	20.1 g	23.6 g	8.4 g	

	2 × 18 cm		
flour, strong white	200 g	cornflour	10 g
pinch of salt		mozzarella cheese	100 g
margarine	12 g		
yeast	5 g		
water or milk at 24°C	125 ml		
caster sugar	5 g		
onions	100 g		
cloves garlic, crushed	2		
sunflower oil	60 ml		
canned plum tomatoes	200 g		
tomato purée	100 g		
oregano	3 g		
basil	3 g		
sugar	10 g		

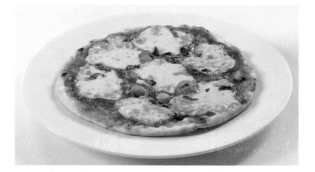

Pizza topped with cheese, tomato and basil

1 Sieve the flour and the salt. Rub in the margarine.

2 Disperse the yeast in the warm milk or water; add the caster sugar. Add this mixture to the flour.

3 Mix well, knead to a smooth dough, place in a basin covered with a damp cloth and allow to prove until doubled in size.

4 Knock back, divide into two and roll out into two 18 cm discs. Place on a lightly greased baking sheet.

5 Sweat the finely chopped onions and garlic in the oil until cooked.

6 Add the roughly chopped tomatoes, tomato purée, oregano, basil and sugar. Bring to the boil and simmer for 5 minutes.

7 Dilute the cornflour in a little water, stir into the tomato mixture and bring back to the boil.

8 Take the discs of pizza dough and spread 125 g of filling on each one.

9 Sprinkle with grated mozzarella cheese or lay the slices of cheese on top.

10 Bake in a moderately hot oven at 180°C, for about 10 minutes.

Try something different

Oregano is sprinkled on most pizzas before baking. This is a basic recipe and many variations exist, some have the addition of olives, artichoke bottoms, prawns, mortadella sausage, garlic sausage or anchovy fillets. Other combinations include:

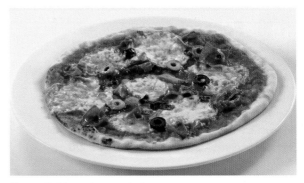

Pizza with Parma ham and olives

- mozzarella cheese, anchovies, capers and garlic
- mozzarella cheese, tomato and oregano
- ham, mushrooms, egg and parmesan cheese
- prawns, tuna, capers and garlic
- ham, mushrooms and olives.

* *Using 100 per cent strong white flour*

The pizza dough may also be made into rectangles so that it can be sliced into fingers for buffet work.

Pizza is a traditional dish originating from southern Italy. In simple terms it is a flat bread dough that can be topped with a wide variety of ingredients and baked quickly. The only rule is not to add wet ingredients, such as tomatoes, which are too juicy, otherwise the pizza will become soggy. Traditionally pizzas are baked in a wood-fired brick oven, but they can be baked in any type of hot oven for 8–15 minutes depending on the ingredients. The recipe given here is a typical one.

20 Savarin paste: basic recipe

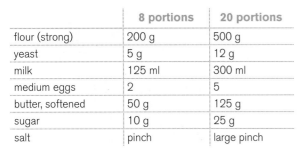

| cal 700 KJ | kcal 167 kcal | fat 7.4 g | sat fat 3.9 g | carb 21.5 g | sugar 2.5 g | protein 4.9 g | fibre 0.8 g | * |

	8 portions	20 portions
flour (strong)	200 g	500 g
yeast	5 g	12 g
milk	125 ml	300 ml
medium eggs	2	5
butter, softened	50 g	125 g
sugar	10 g	25 g
salt	pinch	large pinch

1 Sieve the flour in a bowl and warm.

2 Cream the yeast with a little of the warm milk in a basin.

3 Make a well in the centre of the flour and add the dissolved yeast.

4 Sprinkle with a little of the flour from the sides, cover with a cloth and leave in a warm place until it ferments.

5 Add the remainder of the warm milk and the beaten eggs, knead well to a smooth elastic dough.

6 Replace in the bowl, add the butter in small pieces, cover with a cloth and allow to prove in a warm place.

7 Add the sugar and salt, mix well until absorbed.

8 Half fill a greased savarin mould, and prove.

9 Bake in a hot oven at 220°C for about 30 minutes.

10 Turn out when cooked, cool slightly.

11 Soak carefully in hot syrup.

12 Brush over with apricot glaze.

Syrup for baba, savarin and marignans

	4 babas	10 babas
sugar	100 g	250 g
bay leaf	1	2–3
rind and juice of lemon	1	2–3
water	¼ litre	600 ml
coriander seeds	2–3	6–7
small cinnamon stick	½	1–1½

1 Boil all the ingredients together and strain.

2 Use as required.

* Using syrup, 1 portion of complete Savarin provides: 967 kJ/229 kcal Energy; 7.4 g Fat; 3.9 g Sat Fat; 38.2 g Carb; 19.1 g Sugar; 5.0 g Protein; 0.8 g Fibre

---

21 ## Savarin with fruit *(savarin aux fruits)*

cal	kcal	fat	sat fat	carb	sugar	protein	fibre
1224 KJ	292 kcal	13.5 g	7.7 g	39.1 g	20.6 g	5.9 g	1.0 g

1 Prepare the basic savarin mixture (recipe 20).

2 Prove and cook for about 30 minutes in a large greased savarin mould.

3 Turn out when cooked. Cool slightly.

4 Soak carefully in hot syrup (see recipe 20).

5 Sprinkle liberally with rum (optional). Brush all over with apricot glaze.

6 Fill the centre with fruit salad.

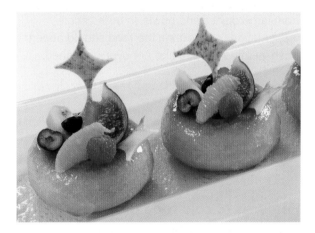

---

22 ## Marignans Chantilly

cal	kcal	fat	sat fat	carb	sugar	protein	fibre
1202 KJ	286 kcal	13.4 g	7.7 g	38.0 g	19.5 g	5.8 g	0.8 g

1 Marignans are prepared from a basic savarin mixture (recipe 20) and cooked in barquette moulds.

2 After the marignans have been soaked, carefully make a deep incision along one side.

3 Decorate generously with whipped, sweetened vanilla-flavoured cream.

4 Brush with apricot glaze.

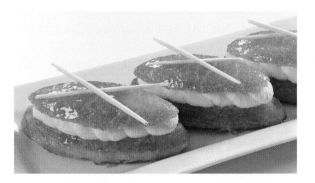

Appendix: Savouries, hors d'oeuvre and canapés

Cold food is popular in every kind of food service operation for at least three good reasons:

1 **Visual appeal:** when the food is attractively displayed, carefully arranged and neatly garnished, the sight of exactly what is being offered can stimulate the customers' appetites.
2 **Efficiency:** cold food can be prepared in advance, allowing a large number of people to be served in a short space of time. Self-service is also economic in terms of staffing.
3 **Adaptability:** if cold food is being served from a buffet, the range of foods can be simple or complex and wide-ranging, depending on the type of operation.

Cold foods can either be pre-plated or served from large dishes and bowls. In both cases presentation is important: the food should appear fresh, neatly arranged and not over-garnished.

Definition

Cold food preparation is the preparation of raw and/or cooked foods into a wide variety of cold items, such as hors d'oeuvre and salads.

Features of cold food preparation

Purpose

The purpose of cold dishes is to:

- add variety to the menu and diet by preparing food that looks good and tastes good
- produce a variety of flavours and textures, and provide food that is particularly suitable for hot weather
- prepare food that can be conveniently wrapped to take away.

Cold food characteristics

- Its appearance must be clean and fresh. It should be presented in a way that makes it look appealing (neither too colourful nor over-decorative) so that it stimulates the appetite.
- The mixture of raw and cooked foods provides good nutritional value.

Techniques associated with cold preparation

- **Peeling:** the removal of the outer skin of fruit or vegetables using a peeler or small knife, according to the thickness of the skin.
- **Chopping:** cutting into very small pieces (e.g. parsley, onions).
- **Cutting:** using a knife to divide food into the required shapes and sizes.
- **Carving:** cutting meat or poultry into slices.
- **Seasoning:** the light addition of salt, pepper and possibly other flavouring agents.
- **Dressing:** this can either mean an accompanying salad dressing, such as vinaigrette, or the arrangement of food for presentation on plates, dishes or buffets.
- **Garnishing:** the final addition to the dish, such as lettuce, quarters of tomato and sliced cucumber added to egg mayonnaise.
- **Marinade:** a richly spiced pickling liquid used to give flavour and to assist in tenderising meats such as venison. Simple marinades (e.g. olive oil with herbs or soy sauce with herbs and/or spices) can be used with cuts of fish, chicken or meat.

Equipment

You will need a variety of equipment when preparing cold foods, including bowls, tongs, whisks, spoons, and so on, as well as food processors, mixing machines and blenders.

Preparation for cold work

Good organisation is essential to ensure that enough pre-preparation (*mise-en-place*) has been done and that the workflow is efficient. This will mean that foods can be assembled quickly and will be ready on time. Before, during and after assembling, and before final garnishing, foods must be kept in a cool place, cold room or refrigerator to minimise the risk of contamination. Garnishing and final decoration should take place as close to the serving time as possible.

General rules

- Be aware of the texture and flavour of the many raw foods that can be mixed together or combined with cooked foods (e.g. coleslaw, meat salad).
- Understand what combination of foods (e.g. salads) is best suited to be served with other foods, such as cold meat or poultry.
- Develop simple artistic skills that require the minimum amount of time for preparation and assembly.
- Always ensure that the presentation of the food is attractive.
- Because of the requirements of food safety, cold foods are often served straight from the refrigerator. This is a mistake because, at refrigerator temperature, food flavours are not at their best. Individual portions should be removed from the fridge and allowed to stand at room temperature for 5–10 minutes before serving.

Types of hors d'oeuvre and salad

There is a wide variety of foods, combinations of foods and recipes available for preparation and service as hors d'oeuvre and salads. Hors d'oeuvre can be divided into three categories:

1 single cold food items (smoked salmon, pâté, melon, etc.)
2 a selection of well-seasoned cold dishes
3 well-seasoned hot dishes.

Hors d'oeuvre may be served for luncheon, dinner or supper, and the wide choice, colour appeal and versatility of the dishes make many items and combinations of items suitable for snacks and salads at any time of day.

Salads may be served as an accompaniment to hot and cold foods and as dishes in their own right. They can be served for lunch, tea, high tea, dinner, supper and snack meals. Salads may be divided into two types:

1 simple, using one ingredient
2 mixed, or composite, using more than one ingredient.

Some salads may form part of a composite hors d'oeuvre. Accompaniments include dressings and cold sauces.

1 Bruschetta

Bruschetta is a thick slice of toasted or grilled bread rubbed with a fresh clove of garlic and sprinkled with extra virgin olive oil. It can then be embellished with tomato, basil, anchovies, ricotta cheese or almost any type of topping. The recipe given here is a typical one.

Recipe 1

1 Toast or grill the slices of bread and rub them with garlic cloves while hot.

2 Cook the raw ingredients for the topping (see Try something different) in olive oil and pile on to the bread.

3 Add any final ingredients desired, such as cheese, anchovies and/or herbs.

Recipe 2

1 As mentioned above, one of the most popular ways of serving bruschetta is to toast or grill thick slices of ciabatta and rub with garlic cloves while hot.

2 Then add a generous topping of diced cheese (e.g. ricotta or mozzarella) and diced tomato flesh (skin and deseed the tomatoes).

3 Sprinkle with a good-quality olive oil and finely chopped onion or chives; serve.

🍎 HEALTHY EATING TIP

- Use a little olive oil to cook the topping ingredients.
- Ricotta cheese contains less fat than mozzarella.

Try something different

Toppings include mushrooms, aubergine, onions, spinach, tomatoes, ham, rocket, olives, Parmesan, mozzarella and anchovies. Traditionally an Italian-type bread (e.g. ciabatta) is used.

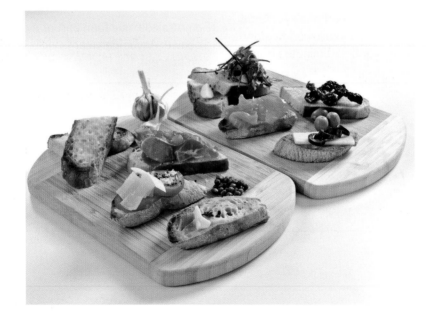

2   Canapés

A wide variety of cold canapés can be offered. Just a few examples are presented here.

- Cherry tomatoes, scooped out, filled with crab meat, seasoned and bound with mayonnaise.
- Avocado pear purée with lime juice, mixed with a fine dice of yellow peppers.
- Slices of rye bread with a slice of lobster, topped with asparagus, garnished with lobster eggs.
- Smoked duck on slices of rye bread, garnished with mango.
- Small new potatoes, cooked, scooped out, filled with sour cream and chives, garnished with caviar or lumpfish roe.
- Small choux pastry éclairs filled with liver pâté.
- Brioche croûtes with apricot chutney and Gorgonzola.
- Marinated and smoked salmon twisted onto the end of silver forms with a mustard dip. The marinade can be a combination of different flavours, e.g. beetroot and soya, lime juice and coriander.
- Various types of sushi.
- Profiteroles filled with prawns in cocktail sauce.

Some examples of hot canapés are as follows.

- Small Yorkshire puddings with a slice of beef topped with horseradish cream.
- Oyster beignets, garlic mayonnaise.
- Aubergine and goats' cheese tartlet.
- Monkfish spring rolls, remoulade sauce.
- Chicken and risotto croquettes.
- Small pizzas.
- Small pieces of chicken on skewers with bacon.
- Satay (peanut) sauce.
- Angels on horseback.

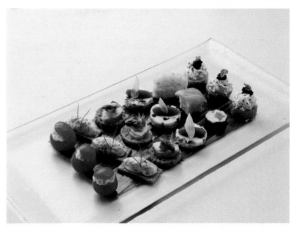

Selection of cold canapés

- Vegetable samosas (page 317).
- Latkes (recipe available on Dynamic Learning).

Dips for hot canapés:

- garlic mayonnaise
- yoghurt, cucumber and mint
- apricot chutney.

At some receptions, small finger pastries are requested. Some examples of what can be offered are:

- fruit tartlets, Bakewell tarts, lemon meringue tartlets
- éclairs
- palmiers with strawberries and cream
- scones filled with tropical fruit
- cornets made of brandy snaps filled with cream and stem ginger
- small scoops of ice cream dipped in white and dark chocolate
- lemon meringue tartlets
- various tuile shapes, caskets filled with lemon mousse.

3 Cheese soufflé (soufflé au fromage)

cal	kcal	fat	sat fat	carb	sugar	protein	fibre	*
3223 KJ	767 kcal	60.2 g	28.2 g	17.6 g	6.1 g	39.7 g	0.5 g	

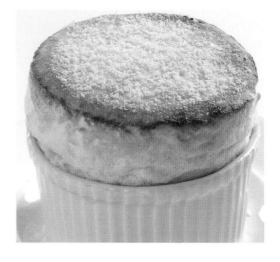

	4 portions	10 portions
butter or margarine	25 g	60 g
flour	15 g	50 g
milk	125 ml	300 ml
egg yolks	3	8
salt, cayenne		
cheese, grated	50 g	125 g
egg whites	4	10

1 Melt the butter in a thick-based pan.

2 Add the flour and mix with a kitchen spoon.

3 Cook out for a few seconds without colouring.

4 Gradually add the cold milk and mix to a smooth sauce.

5 Simmer for a few minutes.

6 Add one egg yolk, mix in quickly; immediately remove from the heat.

7 When cool, add the remaining yolks. Season with salt and cayenne.

8 Add the cheese.

9 Place the egg whites and a pinch of salt (a pinch of egg white powder will help strengthen the whites) in a scrupulously clean bowl, preferably copper, and whisk until stiff.

10 Add one-eighth of the whites to the mixture and mix well.

11 Gently fold in the remaining seven-eighths of the mixture, mix as lightly as possible. Place into a buttered soufflé case.

12 Cook in a hot oven at 220°C for 25–30 minutes.

13 Remove from the oven, place on a round flat dish and serve immediately.

🍎 HEALTHY EATING TIP

- Use sunflower margarine and semi-skimmed milk to make the sauce.

- No added salt is needed as the cheese has salt in it.

* Using hard margarine

4 Fried ham and cheese savoury (croque monsieur)

cal	kcal	fat	sat fat	carb	sugar	protein	fibre	*
1554 KJ	370 kcal	23.0 g	14.1 g	22.8 g	2.7 g	19.1 g	1.7 g	

	4 portions	10 portions
slices cooked ham	4	10
slices Gruyère cheese	8	20
slices thin toast	8	20
clarified butter, margarine or sunflower oil	50 g	125 g

1 Place each slice of ham between two slices of cheese, then between two slices of lightly toasted bread.

2 Cut out with a round cutter.

3 Gently fry on both sides in clarified butter or oil and serve.

* Using butter

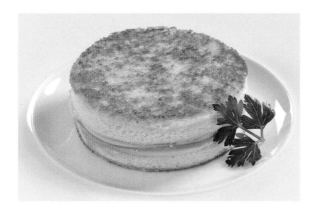

Cheese and ham savoury

5 Pumpernickel rounds with smoked salmon, sour cream and dill

1 Cut small rounds of pumpernickel and pipe on top a rosette of sour cream flavoured with chopped dill.

2 Arrange smoked salmon on top.

3 Garnish with lemon and dill.

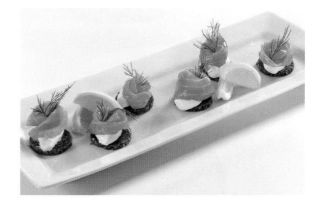

6 Sandwiches

For speed of production, sandwiches are made in bands by cutting the bread rectangularly. When filled, the crusts are removed and the sandwiches cut into fingers.

Today bakers will bake the bread to your specification and slice it ready for use. The specification may also include speciality breads like tomato, basil, walnut and olive bread.

Sandwiches may also be cut into small cubes and a variety placed on a cocktail stick like a mini kebab.

Sandwiches may be made from every kind of bread, fresh or toasted, in a variety of shapes, and with an almost endless assortment of fillings. They may be garnished with potato or vegetable crisps and a little salad.

Toasted sandwiches

These are made by inserting a variety of savoury fillings between two slices of hot, freshly buttered toast (e.g. scrambled egg, bacon, fried egg, scrambled egg with chopped ham) or by inserting two slices of buttered bread with the required filling into a sandwich toaster.

Club sandwich

This is made by placing between two slices of hot buttered toast a filling of lettuce, grilled bacon, slices of hard-boiled egg, mayonnaise and slices of chicken.

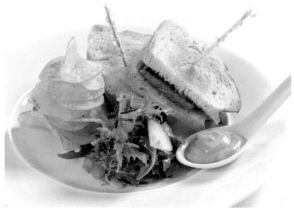

Bookmaker sandwich

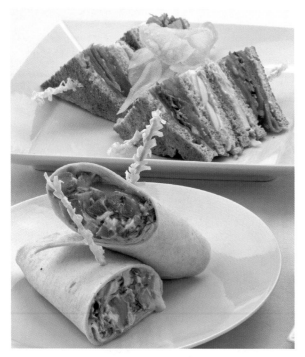

Club sandwiches and wraps

Bookmaker sandwich

This is an underdone minute steak between two slices of hot buttered toast.

Double-decker and treble-decker sandwiches

Toasted and untoasted bread can be made into double-decker sandwiches, using three slices of bread with two separate fillings. Treble- and quadro-decker sandwiches may also be prepared. They may be served hot or cold.

Open sandwich or Scandinavian smorgasbord

These are prepared from a buttered slice of any bread, garnished with any type of meat, fish, eggs, vegetables, salads, etc. The varieties of open sandwich include the following:

- smoked salmon, lettuce, potted shrimps, slice of lemon
- cold sliced beef, sliced tomato, fans of gherkins

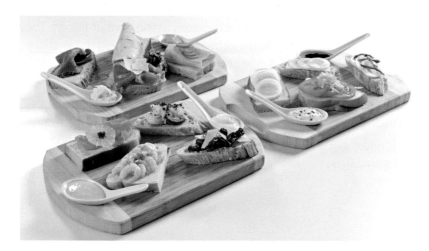

A selection of open sandwiches

- shredded lettuce, sliced hardboiled egg, mayonnaise, cucumber
- pickled herring, chopped gherkin, capers (sieved), hardboiled egg.

For further information contact the British Sandwich Association, 8 Home Farm, Ardington, Wantage, Oxfordshire OX12 8PN, www.sandwich.org.uk.

Wraps

These are made enclosing various fillings wrapped in tortillas (plain or flavoured – e.g. tomato, herbs). Any of a wide variety of fillings can be used – for example, chicken and roasted vegetables; beans and red pepper salad with guacamole (a well-flavoured avocado pulp). Flat breads (e.g. pitta, ciabatta) can be used with various fillings (e.g. chicken tikka).

7   Welsh rarebit

cal	kcal	fat	sat fat	carb	sugar	protein	fibre
1074 KJ	256 kcal	18.6 g	9.7 g	11.9 g	2.4 g	10.1 g	0.7 g

*

	1 portion
butter or margarine	25 g
flour	10 g
milk, whole or skimmed	125 ml
Cheddar cheese	100 g
egg yolk	1
beer	4 tbsp
salt, cayenne	
Worcester sauce	
English mustard	
butter or margarine	10 g
slices toast	2

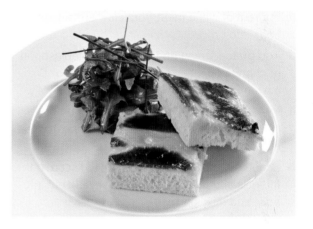

1 Melt the butter or margarine in a thick-based pan.
2 Add the flour and mix in with a kitchen spoon.
3 Cook on a gentle heat for a few minutes without colouring.
4 Gradually add the cold milk and mix to a smooth sauce.
5 Allow to simmer for a few minutes.
6 Add the grated or finely sliced cheese.
7 Allow to melt slowly over a gentle heat until a smooth mixture is obtained.
8 Add the yolk to the hot mixture, stir in and immediately remove from the heat.
9 Meanwhile, in a separate pan boil the beer and allow it to reduce to half a tablespoon.
10 Add to the mixture with the other seasonings.
11 Allow the mixture to cool.
12 Spread on the buttered toast.
13 Place on a baking sheet and brown gently under the salamander; serve.

Cheese contains a large amount of protein, which will become tough and strong if heated for too long or at too high a temperature.

HEALTHY EATING TIP

- A low-fat Cheddar may be used instead of the traditional full-fat variety.
- Use sunflower margarine and semi-skimmed milk to make the sauce.
- No added salt is needed as the cheese has salt in it.

* *Using hard margarine*

8 Dressed crab

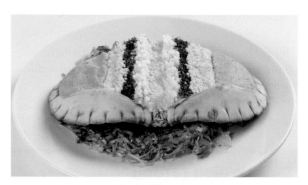

	Serves 2
crab, cooked and cooled	1 kg
lemon, grated rind and juice	1
fresh parsley, chopped	2 tbsp
mayonnaise	4 tbsp
soft brown breadcrumbs	4 tbsp
Dijon mustard	2 tsp
hard-boiled egg, finely chopped	1

1 Crack open the crab claws and remove the white meat, keeping it as intact as possible, and place into a bowl.

2 Put rest of white meat from claw arms, legs and body into bowl.

3 Add grated lemon rind, half juice, 1 tablespoon of chopped parsley and 3 tablespoons of mayonnaise to the white meat and mix lightly.

4 In a separate bowl, place the breadcrumbs, remaining mayonnaise and lemon juice and the mustard.

5 Scoop out brown meat from shell (discarding the gills and the sac behind the eyes), put into bowl and mix lightly.

6 Wash shell and dry.

7 Use brown meat mixture to fill the two sides of shell and pack the white meat into centre.

8 Sprinkle finely chopped hard-boiled egg and rest of parsley over top for decoration.

9 Serve with lots of brown bread and butter, and a green salad to follow.

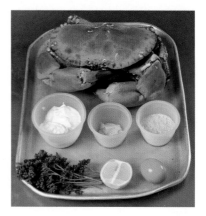

Ingredients for dressed crab

> To ensure freshness, purchase the crab live. When cleaning the cooked crab, ensure that the dead men's fingers (feathery gills) are removed.

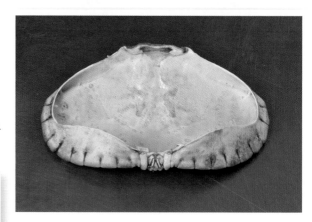

Empty, wash and dry the crab shell

9 Potted shrimps

	4 portions	10 portions
butter	100 g	250 g
chives, chopped	2 tbsp	5 tbsp
cayenne pepper to taste		
peeled brown shrimps	600 g	1½ kg
clarified butter	6 tbsp	15 tbsp

1 Put the butter, chives and cayenne pepper in a medium-sized pan and leave to melt over a gentle heat.

2 Add the peeled shrimps and stir over the heat for a couple of minutes until they have heated through, but don't let the mixture boil.

3 Divide the shrimps and butter between 4 small ramekins. Level the tops and then leave them to set in the refrigerator.

4 Spoon over a thin layer of clarified butter and leave to set once more. Serve with plenty of brown toast or crusty brown bread.

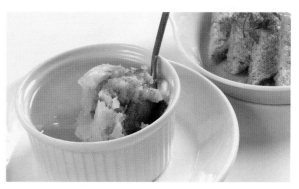

Chef's tip

Do not let the mixture boil (step 2) — if it does, the shrimps will become tough.

Remove from the fridge and allow to warm slightly before serving, to bring out the flavour.

A real seaside dish, full of flavour and eaten with plenty of brown bread and butter. Lobster or langoustine can be used — although timings will need to be adapted accordingly. The traditional seasoning for potted shrimps is ground mace.

10 Shellfish cocktails: crab, lobster, shrimp, prawn (cocktail de crabe, homard, crevettes, crevettes roses)

cal	kcal	fat	sat fat	carb	sugar	protein	fibre
966 KJ	230 kcal	21.0 g	3.2 g	0.6 g	0.6 g	9.6 g	0.3 g

	4 portions	10 portions
lettuce	½	1½
prepared shellfish	100–150 g	250–350 g
shellfish cocktail sauce (see page 191)	125 ml	300 ml

1 Wash, drain well and finely shred the lettuce, avoiding long strands. Place about 2 cm deep in cocktail glasses or dishes.

Chef's tip

Portion control is important so that this dish does not cost too much to produce. The cocktail needs to be presented well.

2 Add the prepared shellfish: crab (shredded white meat only); lobster (cut in 2 cm dice); shrimps (peeled and washed); prawns (peeled, washed and, if large, cut into two or three pieces).

3 Coat with sauce.

4 Decorate with an appropriate piece of the content, such as a prawn with the shell on the tail removed, on the edge of the dish or glass of a prawn cocktail.

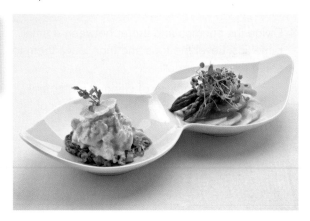

Glossary

à la In the style of

à la française In the French style

à la minute Cooked to order

à la carte Dishes prepared to order and priced individually

Abatis de volaille Poultry offal, giblets, etc.

Abats Offal, heads, hearts, liver, kidney, etc.

Accompaniments Items offered separately with a dish of food

Agar-agar A vegetable gelling agent obtained from seaweed, used as a substitute for gelatine

Aile Wing of poultry or game birds

Aloyau de boeuf Sirloin of beef

Ambient Room temperature, surrounding atmosphere

Amino acid Organic acids found in proteins

Antibiotic Drug used to destroy disease-producing germs within human or animal bodies

Antiseptic Substance that prevents the growth of bacteria and moulds, specifically on or in the human body

Aromats Fragrant herbs and spices

Arroser To baste, as in roasting

Ascorbic acid Known as vitamin C, found in citrus fruits and blackcurrants, necessary for growth and the maintenance of health

Aspic A savoury jelly mainly used for decorative larder work

Assorti An assortment

Au bleu When applied to meat it means very underdone

Au beurre With butter

Au four Baked in the oven

Au gratin Sprinkled with cheese or breadcrumbs and browned

Au vin blanc With white wine

Bactericide Substance that destroys bacteria

Bacterium (pl. bacteria) Single-celled micro-organisms; some are harmful and cause food poisoning; others are useful, such as those used in cheese making

Bain-marie
- A container of water to keep foods hot without fear of burning
- A container of water for cooking foods to prevent them burning
- A deep, narrow container for storing hot sauces, soups and gravies

Barder To bard = to cover breasts of birds with thin slices of bacon

Barquette A boat-shaped pastry case

Basting Spooning melted fat over food during cooking to keep it moist

Bat out To flatten slices of raw meat with a cutlet bat

Bean curd Also known as tofu (see below); a curdled, soft, cheese-like preparation made from soybean milk; a good source of protein

Beansprouts Young shoots of dried beans – e.g. mung beans, alfalfa and soybean

Beurre manié Equal quantities of flour and butter used for thickening sauces

Blanc A cooking liquor of water, lemon juice, flour and salt; also applied to the white of chicken (breast and wings)

Blanch
- To make white, as with bones and meat
- To retain colour, as with certain vegetables
- To skin, as for tomatoes
- To make limp, as for certain braised vegetables
- To cook without colour, as for the first frying of fried (chip) potatoes

Blanquette A white stew cooked in stock from which the sauce is made

Blitz to rapidly purée or foam a light sauce, generally using an electric hand blender at the last moment before service

Bombay duck Small, dried, salted fish; fried, it is used as an accompaniment to curry dishes

Bombe An ice cream speciality of different flavours in a bomb shape

Bone out To remove the bones

Botulism Rare form of food poisoning

Bouchée A small puff paste case, literally 'a mouthful'

Bouillon Unclarified stock

Bouquet garni A faggot of herbs (e.g. parsley stalks, thyme and bay leaf), tied in pieces of celery and leek

Brine A preserving solution of water, salt, saltpetre and aromats used for meats (e.g. silverside, brisket, tongue)

Brunoise Small dice

Butter
- Black butter (beurre noir)
- Brown butter/nut brown butter (beurre noisette)
- Melted butter (beurre fondu)
- Parsley butter (beurre maître d'hôtel)

Buttermilk Liquid remaining from the churning of butter

Calcium A mineral required for building bones and teeth, obtained from cheese and milk

Calorie A unit of heat or energy, known as a kilocalorie

Canapé A cushion of bread on which are served various foods, hot or cold

Carbohydrate A nutrient that has three groups – sugar, starch and cellulose; the first two provide the body with energy; cellulose provides roughage (dietary fibre)

Carbon dioxide A gas produced by all raising agents

Carrier A person who harbours and may transmit pathogenic organisms without showing signs of illness

Carte du jour Menu for the day

Casserole An earthenware fireproof dish with a lid

Cellulose The coarse structure of

fruit, vegetables and cereals that is not digested but is used as roughage (dietary fibre)

Châteaubriand The head of the fillet of beef

Chaud-froid A demi-glace or creamed velouté with gelatine or aspic added, used for masking cold dishes

Chiffonade Fine shreds, e.g. of spinach, lettuce

Chinois A conical strainer

Chlorophyll The green colour in vegetables

Ciseler To make slight incisions in the surface of a thick fillet of fish, on or off the bone, to allow even cooking

Civet A brown stew of game, usually hare

Clarification To make clear such as stock, jelly, butter

Clostridium perfringens Food-poisoning bacterium found in the soil, vegetables and meat

Coagulation The solidification of protein that is irreversible (e.g. fried egg, cooking of meat)

Cocotte Porcelain or earthenware fireproof dish

Collagen/elastin Proteins in connective tissue (e.g. gristle)

Compote Stewed (e.g. stewed fruit)

Concassée Coarsely chopped (e.g. parsley, tomatoes)

Confit A cooked meat, poultry or game preserved in good fat or oil

Consommé Basic clear soup

Contamination Occurrence of any objectionable matter in food

Contrefilet Boned-out sirloin of beef

Cook out The process of cooking flour in a roux, soup or sauce

Cordon A thread or thin line of sauce

Correcting Adjusting the seasoning, consistency and colour

Côte A rib or chop

Côtelette A cutlet

Coupe An individual serving bowl

Couper To cut

Court bouillon A well-flavoured cooking liquor for fish

Crème fraiche Whipping cream and buttermilk heated to 24–29°C

Crêpes Pancakes

Credit notes Issued when an invoice contains incorrect details; credit is therefore given

Croquettes Cooked foods moulded into a cylinder shape, coated in flour and egg, crumbed and deep-fried

Cross-contamination The transfer of micro-organisms from contaminated to uncontaminated hands, utensils or equipment

Croutons Cubes of fried or toasted bread served with soup; also triangular pieces served with spinach, and heart-shaped with certain vegetables and entrées

Crudités Small neat pieces of raw vegetables served with a dip as an appetiser

Cuisse de poulet Chicken leg

Cullis (coulis) Sauce made of fruit or vegetable purée (e.g. raspberry, tomato)

Danger zone of bacterial growth Temperature range within which the multiplication of pathogenic bacteria is possible; from 10–63°C

Dariole A small mould, as used for crème caramel

Darne A slice of round fish (e.g. salmon) on the bone

Déglacer To swill out a pan in which food has been roasted or fried, with wine, stock or water, in order to use the sediment for the accompanying sauce or gravy

Dégraisser To skim fat off liquid

Delivery note Form sent by supplier with delivery of goods

Demi-glace Brown stock reduced to a light consistency

Désosser To bone out meat

Detergent Substance that dissolves grease

Dilute To mix a powder (e.g. cornflour) with a liquid

Dish paper A plain dish paper

Disinfectant Substance that reduces the risk of infection

Doily A fancy dish paper

Drain Placing food in a colander, allowing liquid to seep out

Duxelle Finely chopped mushrooms cooked with chopped shallots

Eggwash Beaten egg with a little milk or water

Emulsion A mixture of oil and liquid (such as vinegar), which does not separate on standing (e.g. mayonnaise, hollandaise)

Entrecôte A steak cut from a boned sirloin

Enzymes Chemical substances produced from living cells

Escalope A thin slice such as escalope of veal

Farce Stuffing

Fecule Fine potato flour

Feuilletage Puff pastry

Fines herbes Chopped fresh herbs (e.g. parsley, tarragon, chervil)

First-aid materials Suitable and sufficient bandages and dressings, including waterproof dressings and antiseptic; all dressings to be individually wrapped

Flake To break into natural segments (e.g. fish)

Flan Open fruit tart

Fleurons Small crescent-shaped pieces of puff pastry

Flute A 20 cm diameter French bread used for soup garnishes

Food-borne Bacteria carried on food

Food handling Any operation in the storage, preparation, production, processing, packaging, transportation, distribution and sale of food

Frappé Chilled (e.g. melon frappé)

Freezer burn Affects frozen items, which are spoiled due to being left unprotected for too long

Friandises Sweetmeats, petits fours

Fricassée A white stew in which the meat, poultry or fish is cooked in the sauce

Friture A pan that contains deep fat

Fumé Smoked (e.g. saumon fumé = smoked salmon)

Garam masala A combination of spices

Garnish Served as part of the main item; trimmings

Gastroenteritis Inflammation of the stomach and intestinal tract that normally results in diarrhoea

Gâteau A cake of more than one portion

Ghee The Indian name for clarified butter; ghee is pure butter fat

Gibier Game

Glace Ice or ice cream from which all milk solids have been removed

Glaze To glaze
- To colour a dish under the salamander (e.g. fillets of sole bonne femme)
- To finish a flan or tartlet (e.g. with apricot jam)
- To finish certain vegetables (e.g. glazed carrots)

Gluten This is formed from protein in flour when mixed with water

Gratin A thin coating of grated cheese and/or breadcrumbs on certain dishes then browned under the grill or in an oven

Haché Finely chopped or minced

hors d'oeuvre Appetising first course dishes, hot or cold

Humidity Amount of moisture in the air

Incubation period Time between infection and first signs of illness

Infestations Insects breeding on the premises

Insecticide Chemical used to kill insects

Invoice Bill listing items delivered, with costs of items

Jardinière Vegetables cut into batons

Julienne Cut into fine strips

Jus-lié Thickened gravy

Larding Inserting strips of fat bacon into meat

Lardons Batons of thick streaky bacon

Liaison A thickening or binding

Macédoine
- A mixture of fruit or vegetables
- Cut into ½ cm dice

Magnetron Device that generates microwaves in a microwave oven

Marinade A richly spiced pickling liquid used to give flavour and assist in tenderising meats

Marmite Stock pot

Mascarpone An Italian cheese resembling clotted cream

Menu List of dishes available

Micro-organisms Very small living plants or animals (bacteria, yeasts, moulds)

Mignonette Coarsely ground pepper

Mildew Type of fungus, similar to mould

Mineral salts Mineral elements, small quantities of which are essential for health

Mirepoix Roughly cut onions and carrots, a sprig of thyme and a bay leaf

Mise-en-place Basic preparation prior to serving

Miso Seasoning made from fermented soybeans

Monosodium glutamate (MSG) A substance added to food products to increase flavour

Moulds Microscopic plants (fungi) that may appear as woolly patches on food

Mousse A dish of light consistency, hot or cold

Napper To coat or mask with sauce

Natives A menu term for English oysters

Navarin Brown stew of lamb

Niacin Part of vitamin B, found in liver, kidney, meat extract, bacon

Noisette (nut) A cut from a boned-out loin of lamb

Nutrients The components of food required for health (protein, fats, carbohydrates, vitamins, mineral salts, water)

Optimum Best, most favourable

Palatable Pleasant to taste

Pané Floured, egg and crumbed

Panettone A very light traditional Italian Christmas cake

Parsley butter Butter containing lemon juice and chopped parsley

Pass To cause to go through a sieve or strainer

Pathogen Disease-producing organism

Paupiette A stuffed and rolled strip of fish or meat

Paysanne Cut in even, thin triangular, round or square pieces

Persillé Finished with chopped parsley

Pesticide Chemical used to kill pests

Pests e.g. cockroaches, flies, silverfish

Petits fours Very small pastries, biscuits, sweets, sweetmeats

pH value A scale indicating acidity or alkalinity in food

Phosphorus A mineral element found in fish; required for building bones and teeth

Piquant Sharply flavoured

Piqué Studded clove in an onion

Plat du jour Special dish of the day

Poppadoms Dried, thin, large, round wafers made from lentil flour, used as an accompaniment to Indian dishes

Printanier Garnish of spring vegetables

Protein The nutrient needed for growth and repair

Prove To allow a yeast dough to rest in a warm place so that it can expand

Pulses Vegetables grown in pods (peas and beans) and dried; source of protein and roughage

Quark Salt-free soft cheese made from semi-skimmed milk

Ragout Stew (ragout de boeuf); brown beef stew

Rare When applied to meat, it means underdone

Réchauffer To reheat

Reduce To concentrate a liquid by boiling

Refresh To make cold under running cold water

Residual insecticide Insecticide that remains active for a considerable period of time

Riboflavin Part of vitamin B known as B2; sources in yeast, liver, eggs, cheese

Rissoler To fry to a golden brown

Rodents Rats and mice

Roux A thickening of cooked flour and fat

Sabayon Yolks of eggs and a little water or wine cooked until creamy

Saccharometer An instrument for measuring the density of sugar

Salamander Type of grill; heat from above

Salmonella Food-poisoning bacterium found in meat and poultry

Sanitiser Chemical agent used for cleaning and disinfecting surfaces and equipment

Sauté
- Toss in fat (e.g. pommes sautées)
- Cook quickly in a sauté pan or frying pan
- A brown stew of a specific type (e.g. veal sauté)

Seal To set the surface of meat in a hot oven or pan to colour and retain the juices

Seared Cooked quickly on both sides in a little hot fat or oil

Seasoned flour Flour seasoned with salt and pepper

Set
- To seal the outside surface
- To allow to become firm or firmer (e.g. jelly)

Shredded Cut in fine strips (e.g. lettuce, onion)

Silicone paper Non-stick paper (e.g. siliconised paper)

Singe To brown or colour

Smetana A low-fat product; a cross between soured cream and yoghurt

Sodium Mineral element in the form of salt (sodium chloride); found in cheese, bacon, fish, meat

Soufflé A very light dish, sweet or savoury, hot or cold

Soy sauce Made from soybeans and used extensively in Chinese cookery

Spores Resistant resting phase of bacteria, protecting them against adverse conditions such as high temperatures

Staphylococcus Food-poisoning bacterium found in the human nose and throat, and also in septic cuts

Starch A carbohydrate found in cereals, certain vegetables and farinaceous foods

Sterile Free from all living organisms

Sterilisation Process that destroys living organisms

Steriliser Chemical used to destroy all living organisms

Stock rotation Sequence of issuing goods: first into store 5 first to be issued

Strain To separate the liquid from the solids by passing through a strainer

Sweat To cook in fat under a lid without colour

Syneresis The squeezing out of liquid from an overcooked protein and liquid mixture (e.g. scrambled egg, egg custard)

Table d'hôte A meal at a fixed price; a set menu

Tahini A strong-flavoured sesame seed paste

Tartlet A small round pastry case

Terrine An earthenware dish used for cooking and serving pâté; also used as a name for certain products

Thiamine Part of vitamin B known as B1, it assists the nervous system; sources in yeast, bacon, wholemeal bread

Timbale A double serving dish

Tofu Low-fat bean curd made from soybeans (see also bean curd)

Tourné Turned, shaped in barrels or large olives

Tranche A slice

Trichinosis Disease caused by hair-like worms in the muscles of meat (e.g. pork)

Tronçon A slice of flat fish on the bone (e.g. turbot)

TVP Texturised vegetable protein, derived from soybeans

Vegan A person who does not eat fish, meat, poultry, game, dairy products, honey and eggs, and who does not use any animal products (e.g. leather)

Vegetarian A person who does not eat meat, poultry or game

Velouté
- Basic sauce
- A soup of velvet or smooth consistency

Viruses Microscopic pathogens that multiply in the living cells of their host

Vitamins Chemical substances that assist the regulation of body processes

Vol-au-vent A large puff pastry case

Wok A round-bottomed pan used extensively in Chinese cooking

Yeast extract A mixture of brewer's yeast and salt, high in flavour and protein

Yoghurt An easily digested fermented milk product

Index

Notes: recipes are indicated in **bold**

à la 99, 560
à la carte 100, 560
à la française 560
à la minute 560
à l'ancienne **319, 351**
abats *see* offal
accidents
    blue plasters 29, 32, 118
    causes 53, 56
    costs 61
    first aid 60
    prevention 53–7
    reporting 53–4, 60
    statistics 51
accommodation *see also* hotels
    establishments providing 8–9
    self-catering 4, 11
accompaniments 560
acids
    ascorbic acid (vitamin C) 76–7, 81–2,
        129, 560
    niacin (vitamin B) 76–7, 81–3, 130, 562
aerated, meaning 447
agar-agar 461, 560
airline/airport catering 15
al dente 131
alcohol 67
allergens 29
allergies 29, 84, 100
ambulance services 16
amino acids 73, 560
anaemia 82
antioxidants 80
ants 43–4
apples
    apple crumble tartlets **482**
    apple fritters (*beignets aux pommes*)
        474
    apple sorbet **495–6**
    baked apple (*pommes bonne femme*)
        472
    bramley apple spotted dick **469**
    French apple flan (*flan aux pommes*)
        505–6
    poached (*compote*) **487**
    tatin of apple **481**
apprenticeships 26, 91
apricots
    apricot and almond samosas **520**
    salsa **333**
aprons 61
aquatic, meaning 414
armed forces 1, 17
aromats 155, 560
arrowroot 137, 157
arson 66
artichokes
    à la grecque **253**

globe artichokes **245**
    risotto of Jerusalem artichoke and
        truffle **425–6**
ascorbic acid (vitamin C) 76–7, 81–2,
    130, 560
asparagus
    asparagus points/tips (*pointes
        d'asperges*) **244**
    soup (*crème d'asperges*) **165**
    wrapped in puff pastry with gruyère **245–6**
assault 66
assets, personal 2
Asylum and Immigration Act 1996 23, 25
attitude and behaviour 117–18
    towards customers 119–21
au beurre 560
au gratin 560, 561
aubergines
    ratatouille **238–9**
    spiced aubergine purée **243**
    stuffed aubergine (*aubergine farcie*)
        239–40
automation 205
avocado
    avocado and coriander salsa **195–6**
    preparation **219**

bacillus cereus 31, 414
bacon *see also* pork
    boiled bacon **332**
    griddled gammon with apricot salsa **333**
    joints and cuts 289–90
bacteria 29, 560
    aerobic bacteria 148
    anaerobic bacteria 148
    danger zone 36–7, 561
    food-borne 31, 148, 561
    heat, impact on 30–1, 36–7
    rate of multiplication 35
    and sous vide cooking 148
    types 30–2
bactericide 560
bain-marie 139, 560
baking 128, 137–9, 209 *see also*
    biscuits; cakes; dough products
    baking with increased humidity 139
    dry baking 139
    fish 368
baking powder 450–1, 522–3
ballotines 344
bananas
    banana bread **532–3**
    banana flan **511**
banqueting 98, 105
barbecuing 141–2
barley 217, 417
basil
    oil **201**
    pesto **197**
basting 140, 560

batter
    for cakes and biscuits 521–5
    for coating fish **386**
    Yorkshire pudding **292**
bavense (underdone) 443
bean curd *see* tofu
beans 207
    bean goulash **258**
    broad beans (*fèves*) **237**
    carrot and butterbean soup **162**
    dried beans 213
    haricot bean salad (*salade de haricots
        blancs*) **263**
    Mexican bean pot **259**
bed and breakfast accommodation 9
beef
    generally
        alayou de boeuf (whole on the bone)
            282, 560
        boned out 282, 560
        butchery 279–80
        cooking methods 282–3
        core temperatures 141, 271
        côte de boeuf (wing rib) 283
        forequarters 280
        hindquarters 279–80
        joints and cuts 279–82, 282–3
        offal 269–70, 281, 283
        roasting times 141
        selection and purchase 281
        storage 268
    recipes
        beef jus **176–7**
        beef olives (*paupiettes de boeuf*)
            296–7
        beef stroganoff (*sauté de boeuf
            stroganoff*) **297**
        boeuf bourguignonne **294–5**
        boiled silverside, carrots and
            dumplings **293–4**
        brown stock **158**
        carbonnade of beef (Belgian) **300**
        châteaubriand with Roquefort butter
            291
        Cornish pasties **300–1**
        cottage pie **316**
        Hamburg or Vienna steak (*bitok*) **302**
        Hungarian goulash **302–3**
        lasagne **426–7**
        roast beef (*boeuf rôti*) **291–2**
        sirloin steak with red wine sauce
            (*entrecôte bordelaise*) **293**
        spaghetti bolognaise **430**
        steak pie **299**
        steak pudding **298**
        white stock **158**
beetroot
    goats' cheese and beetroot tarts, with
        rocket salad **256**
    golden beetroot with parmesan **254**

behaviour 117–18
  towards customers 119–21
best before dates 39
beurre manié 136–7, 156, 560
birds 43–4
biscuits
  generally
    biscuit mixture methods 526–7
    biscuit pastes 528
    blending method 527
    convenience products 527
    filing 527
    finishing and decoration 527–8
    flour batter method 527
    foaming method 526
    piped sablé biscuits 528, **538–9**
    rubbing in method 526
    spreading and coating 527
    sugar batter method 527
  recipes
    brandy snaps **540**
    cats' tongues (*langues de chat*) **538**
    piped biscuits (*sablés à la poche*)
      538–9
    shortbread biscuits **537–8**
    sponge fingers (*biscuits à la cuillère*)
      536–7
    tuiles **539**
blanc **256,** 560
blanching 137, 143, 207, 560
blanquette 136, 560
blending, pastry work **499**
blinis 543
blond roux 156–7
blue plasters 29, 32, 118
blueberries
  baked blueberry cheesecake **488–9**
boiled buttercream **462–3**
boiling 128, 130–2, 207
  fish 373–4
  meat 131–2
  simmering 130–1
bones 270, 272
botulism 31, 560
bouchée 560
bouquet garni 560
brains 270, 286
braising 135–7
  meat 273, 275, 282, 285–6
brawn 270
breads *see* dough products
break-even point 6
breakfast 103
brioche 542–3
broccoli **236**
brown braising 136
brown roux 156–7
brunoise 207–8, 560
brusque, meaning 102
buckwheat 217, 417
budget hotels 5, 9
buffets 104
bulgar wheat 418
bulk fermentation time (BFT) 544
bullying 52–3

Burger King 20
burglary 66
business, catering for 18, 100
  corporate hospitality 19–20
  employees, catering for 18–20
  zero-subsidy establishments 99
butter 216, 448, 560
  butter sauce (*beurre blanc*) **183–4**
  clarified 144, 216
  compound butter sauces 202
  flavoured butters 202
  herb butters 202
buttermilk 215, 560
butternut squash, roast **247**
butterscotch, sauce **468**

cabbage
  braised red cabbage (*choux à la
    flamande*) **235**
  coleslaw **252–3**
  pickled red cabbage **257**
  stir-fried cabbage with mushrooms and
    beansprouts **234**
cafés 3
cakes
  generally 521
    baking powder 522–3
    batters 524–6
    blending method 522, 525
    boiling method 525
    convenience products 527
    creaming method 525
    faults in, reasons for 523–5
    filing 527
    finishing and decoration 527–8
    flour batter method 522–3
    foaming method 524
    Genoese sponges (*génoise*) 524–5,
      529–30
    high-ratio cake mixtures 522
    melting method 524
    methods 521–5
    separate yolk and white method 525
    sponge cakes 524–6, **533–4**
    spreading and coating 527
    stabilisers in 524
    steam or moisture in 525
    sugar batter method 521–3
  recipes
    banana bread **532–3**
    fresh cream and strawberry gateau
      530
    Genoese sponge (*génoise*) **529–30**
    lemon drizzle cake **533**
    madeleines **540**
    rich fruit cake **531–2**
    roulade sponge **531**
    scones **535**
    Swiss roll **534–5**
    Victoria sandwich **533–4**
calcium 78, 81, 560
calcium phosphate 451
calf *see* veal
calories 560
campylobacter 31

canapés 560, **563**
cancer 69, 80, 82, 84
canned products/canning 36, 38, 270,
  366
capital expenditure 93–4
caramel, sauce **468**
carbohydrates 71–3, 81, 560
  heat, impact on 129
  too much/too little in diet, impact of
    82–3
carbon dioxide 65, 420
  in fermentation 542–3
  as raising agent 450–1, 524, 560
care homes 18, 98
carob gum 461
carrageen 461
carrots
  carrot and butterbean soup **162**
  Vichy carrots **254**
carte du jour 560
carving 560
casinos 4, 9
casseroling 134–7, 560
  meat 273, 275, 282, 285–6
catering and hospitality industry *see also*
      hotels; restaurants; tourism; travel
  achieving balance 6
  chain catering 10
  characteristics 7
  in commercial sector 1
  contract catering 1, 3–4, 14, 16,
    19–20
  corporate hospitality 19–20
  cost sector catering 1, 3
  costs 6
  definitions 1, 7
  demand, fluctuations and patterns in
    6–7, 15
  employment in 21–6
  forecasting 6
  franchising 20
  globalisation of 5
  growth 3–4
  in-house catering development 9
  influences on 5–6
  leisure sector 3–4
  non-profit making sector 1
  outside catering 19–20
  outsourcing 9
  primary service sector 1
  profit sector catering 3
  in public sector 1, 16–18
  scale 1, 4–6
  secondary service sector 1, 16–18
  structure 1–5
  success, factors contributing to 10
  trends in 9
  types business 1–3
cauliflower
  à la grecque **253**
  au gratin (*chou-fleur mornay*) **246**
  polonaise **247**
ceilings 45
celeriac, buttered **255**
cellulose 560–1

Centre Parcs 12
cereals *see* grains and cereals
chain catering 10
chantilly cream **462**
chapati 543, **554–5**
châteaubriand 282, 561
chaud-froid 561
cheese
  generally
    for pasta dishes 416
    vegetarian cheese 216
  recipes
    cheese and ham savoury flan *(quiche lorraine)* **504**
    cheese soufflé *(soufflé au fromage)* **564**
    cheese straws *(paillettes au fromage)* **517**
    cheesecakes **488–9**
    fried ham and cheese savoury *(croque monsieur)* **564–5**
    goats' cheese and beetroot tarts, with rocket salad **256**
    macaroni cheese **432**
chef de partie 89–91
chefs
  attitude and behaviour 117–18
  celebrity chefs 8–9
  clothing and hats 32, 61, 67, 117–18
  hierarchy 89–91
  job description, for sous chef 24, 92
  nutrition, role in improving 85–6
  personal hygiene 32–4
  personal presentation 117–18
  sous chefs 24, 89–92
chemicals
  for cleaning 40, 42, 111
  food contamination by 29, 43
  in food premises 55
  hazardous substances, control 54–5
  storage 42
chicken
  generally
    ballotines 344
    core temperature 271
    health, safety and hygiene 346
    nutritional value 341
    preparation 341–4
    selection and purchase 341
    spatchcock 343
    storage 346
    trussing 341–2
    types 341
  recipes
    chicken à la king *(emincé de volaille à la king)* **347–8**
    chicken in red wine *(coq au vin)* **348–9**
    chicken jus **177**
    chicken Kiev **356**
    chicken sauté chasseur **346–7**
    chicken spatchcock *(poulet grillé à la crapaudine)* **349**
    chicken tikka **354–5**
    crumbed breast of chicken with

asparagus *(suprême de volaille aux pointes d'asperges)* **350**
    fricassée **350–1**
    fried chicken (deep-fried) **351**
    grilled chicken *(poulet grillé)* **352**
    roast, with dressing *(poulet rôti à l'anglaise)* **352–3**
    soup *(crème de volaille/crème reine)* **163**
    tandoori chicken **355**
    terrine of chicken and vegetables **353–4**
    white chicken stock **159**
chickpeas 213–14
  hummus (chickpea and sesame seed paste) **259–60**
chicory, shallow-fried *(endive meunière)* **244**
chiffonade 561
children
  catering for 17–18
  menus for 100
  nutritional requirements 84–5
  school meals 17
Children and Young Persons Act 1933 23
chlorophyll 207, 561
chocolate
  baked chocolate tart *(aero)* **510**
  éclairs **513–14**
  fondant **471–2**
  mousse **483–4**
  sauce **467**
  sorbet **496**
cholesterol 75, 80, 84
chopping 560
chopping boards 34–5
chutneys **196–7**
ciselé 372, 561
clams 367, 376
  New England clam chowder **170–1**
clarified butter 144, 561
cleaning
  fridges 35, 39
  importance 40, 98
  kitchen surfaces, methods for 40
  material costs 111
  products 40, 42, 111
  schedules 40
  spillages 56
  using heat for 40
closed-circuit televison (CCTV) 66
clostridium botulinum 31, 561
clostridium perfringens 31, 561
clothing 32, 61, 67, 117–18
clubs 1, 9
coagulation 129, 131–2, 561
  eggs 452, 455
  meat protein 135, 141, 272
cockles 376, 378–9
cockroaches 44
cocktail parties 104
cod, baked with a herb crust **393**
Coeliac disease 417–18
coffee shops 10

cold food preparation
  advantages of cold food 560
  health and safety 561
  methods 560
  presentation 560–1
  purpose 560
collagen 268, 272–3, 561
colour-coding 34, 271
commis chefs 89, 91
Compass Group 20
complaints 121
compotes **486–7**, 561
concassée 208, **257**, 561
condensed milk 215
conduction 128
confectioner's custard (pastry cream) *(crème pâtissière)* 455, **463–4**
consommé 561
consortia 9
conspicuous, meaning 65
constitutions, corporate 3
consumer protection 102
continental roux 157
contract catering 1, 3–4, 14, 16, 19–20
  corporate hospitality 19–20
  outside catering 19–20
contracting out 9
contrefilet 561
Control of Substances Hazardous to Health (COSHH) Regulations 54–5
convection 128
convenience products
  cakes and biscuits 527
  dough products 544
  and kitchen design 94
  in pastry work 453
  potato products 211
cooking methods 128
  baking 137–9, 209
  barbecuing 141–2
  boiling 130–2, 207
  braising 135–7
  casseroling/stewing 134–7
  cold food preparation 560–1
  deep frying 142–6
  grilling 141–2
  microwave cooking 148–51
  paper bag cooking 147–8
  poaching 130–3
  pot roasting 147
  roasting 137–8, 140, 209
  shallow frying 142–4
  simmering 130–1
  sous vide 148–9
  steaming 130–1, 133–4, 207
  tandoori cooking 147
'CookSafe' 48
cordon 562
corn on the cob (maize) *(maïs)* 217, **238**, 417
cornflour 137, 157
coronary heart disease 69, 75, 80
corporate hospitality 19–20
corrosive substances 62

COSHH (Control of Substances Hazardous to Health) Regulations 54–5
cosmetics 32
cost analysis 110
cost control
    advantages 110–11
    cleaning materials 111
    cost analysis 110
    food and material costs 111, 115
    influences on 115
    labour costs, direct/indirect 111
    operational control 115
    overheads 111
    profits, gross/net 112–15
    selling price 113–15
costs, fixed or variable 6
coulis 561
    fruit coulis **465**
country house hotels 8
courgettes
    courgette and potato cakes with mint and feta cheese **242**
    fettucini of courgette with chopped basil and balsamic vinegar **243**
    deep-fried (courgettes frites) **240**
    ratatouille **238–9**
    shallow-fried (courgettes sautées) **240**
court bouillon 132, 561
couscous 418
    couscous with chorizo sausage and chicken **436**
covering letters 123
crab 376, 378
    crab cakes with rocket salad and lemon dressing **405–6**
    crab stock **161**
    dressed crab **568**
crawfish 378
crayfish 376–7
cream
    alternate ingredients for 163
    chantilly cream **462**
    health, safety and hygiene 458
    heat, impact on 36
    pasteurisation 456–7
    soured 215
    sterilisation (UHT) 456–7
    types 215, 456
cream of tartar 451
credit notes 561
crème brûlée **490**
crème caramel **491**
crème fraîche 215, 561
crème renversée 455–6
crime prevention 66–7
croissants 542–3
croquettes 561
cross-contamination 33–5, 561
croutons 561
crudités 561
cruise liners 14–15
crustaceans 376–8 see also crab; lobster
curriculum vitae (CV) 122–3

custard
    confectioner's custard (pastry cream) (crème pâtissière) 455, **463–4**
    egg custard-based desserts 455–8, 459–60, **466, 507–8**
custard powder 458
customers
    behaviour towards 6–7, 119–21
    complaints 121
    customer care 119–21
    feedback from 121
    influence on kitchen layout and design 95
cutting 560
CVs 122–3

Dairy Product Regulations 1995 459
dairy products see also cream; milk
    delivery and storage 38
    types 215–16
danger zone, bacteria 36–7
Danish pastries 542–3
dariole 561
darne 561
Data Protection Act 1988 23
deep frying
    coatings for 143, **386**
    fats and temperatures for 145
    fish 366–7, 373–4
    flashpoint 145
    health and safety 146
    smoking point 145
deficiency 76
defrosting 38
deglazing 160, 561
dégraisser (skimming) 561
delicatessens 10
délice 372
deliveries
    delivery notes 561
    entrances for 91
    handling 37–8
    temperature 37–8
demand, fluctuations and patterns in 6
demi-glace 160, 561
deregulation 5
dermatitis 54
design and decor, trends in 94–5
desserts see also ice creams; pastry work
    apple, baked (pommes bonne femme) **472**
    apple, tatin of **481**
    apple crumble tartlets **482**
    apple fritters (beignets aux pommes) **474**
    baked Alaska (omelette soufflée surprise) **480**
    baked chocolate tart (aero) **510**
    Bakewell tart **508–9**
    banana flan **511**
    bavarois (basic) **483–4**
    Black Forest vacherin **493**
    blueberry cheesecake, baked **488–9**
    boiled buttercream **462–3**
    bramley apple spotted dick **469**

bread and butter pudding **474–5**
butterscotch sauce **468**
cabinet pudding **475**
caramel sauce **468**
chantilly cream **462**
chocolate fondant **471–2**
chocolate mousse **483–4**
chocolate sauce **467**
Christmas pudding **479**
crème brûlée (burned, caramelised or browned cream) **490**
crème caramel (cream caramel) **491**
crêpes Suzette **473**
custard sauce **467**
diplomat pudding **475**
egg custard-based desserts 455–8, 459–60, **466, 507–8**
egg custard tart **507–8**
Eve's pudding with gooseberries **471**
French apple flan (flan aux pommes) **505–6**
fresh egg custard sauce (sauce à l'anglaise) 455, **466**
fruit barquettes **512**
fruit slice (bande aux fruits) **512–13**
fruit tart **512**
ganache **463**
golden syrup pudding **470**
Italian meringue **464**
khoshaf (dried fruit with nuts, perfumed with rose and orange water) **494**
lemon tart (tarte au citron) **509**
lime and mascarpone cheesecake **488**
lime soufflé frappe **485**
mango soufflé **478**
meringues **491–2**
mince pies **510–11**
mousse, basic fruit **482–3**
pancakes with apple (crêpes normande) **473**
pear almond tart **506**
pear jalousie **516**
profiteroles and chocolate sauce **515**
raspberry bavarois (mousse) **484**
rice pudding **476**
soufflé pudding (basic) **478–9**
sticky toffee pudding **469–70**
stock syrup **468**
sweet samosas **520**
treacle tart **507**
trifle **489**
vacherin with strawberries (vacherin aux fraises) **492–3**
vanilla panna cotta served on a fruit compote **486**
vanilla soufflé (soufflé à la vanille) **476–7**
detergent 40, 561
dextrinisation 156
dextrose 459
dhal 214, **260**
diabetes 69, 75, 80, 85
diet see healthy eating; nutrition; special diets
digestible, meaning 541

digestive system 29
dinner 104
dirty areas 97
Disability Discrimination Act 1995 23
discrimination 23, 52
disease
  reporting 53–4
  risk assessment 53–4
dishwashing 42–3
disinfectant 40, 561
disposable income, real 3
dissemination, meaning 124
docking, pastry work **499**
doors 45
dough products
  generally 541–2
    breads 544
    bulk fermentation time (BFT) 544
    convenience products 544
    enriched dough 542–3
    faults in, reasons for 544
    fermentation 542–3
    laminated dough 543
    proving 543
    rules and tips for 542–3
    speciality dough 543
    storage 543
    types 543
    yeast 542–3
  recipes
    bagels **556**
    Bath buns **551**
    bun dough (basic) **549–50**
    bun wash **550**
    chapatis 543, **554–5**
    Chelsea buns **550–1**
    doughnuts **552**
    focaccia **557**
    hot cross buns **551**
    marignans chantilly **559**
    naan bread 543, **555**
    olive bread **548–9**
    parmesan rolls **552**
    pizza **557–8**
    red onion and sage rolls **553**
    rye bread **547**
    savarin paste (basic) **558–9**
    savarin with fruit **559**
    seeded rolls **553**
    soda bread **548**
    sun-dried tomato bread **545**
    syrup, for baba, savarin and marignans
      559
    wheatmeal bread **546**
Dover sole 371
drainage 45
dressings
  aioli dip **404**
  balsamic vinegar and olive oil dressing
    193–4
  cilantro vinaigrette **391**
  flavoured oils **200–1**
  lemon dressing **405–6**
  mayonnaise **188**
  mayonnaise variations **189–90**

shellfish cocktail sauce **191**
  thousand island dressing **190**
  tomato vinaigrette **191**
drive-in/drive-through restaurants 10
drugs 67
dry areas 96
dry goods, delivery and storage 38
Dublin Bay prawns 377
duck and duckling
  generally 345–6
    core temperature 271
  recipes
    confit duck leg with red cabbage and
      green beans **358–9**
    duckling with orange sauce (caneton
      bigerade) **359–60**
    roast duck or duckling (canard ou
      caneton rôti) **361**
due diligence 49
dumplings **293–4**
duxelle 179, 561

E coli 0157 31
eatwell plate 70
écrevisse 377
education sector 1, 3, 98
  school meals 17
EFK (electronic fly killer) 43
eggs
  generally 217
    coagulation 452, 455
    crème renversée 455–6
    egg custards 455–8
    egg whites 452–3, 491–2
    egg yolks 156, 188, 199, 460
    eggwash 561
    health, safety and hygiene 188, 199,
      420, 452, 458
    in ice cream 460
    nutritional value 420
    pasteurised 420, 452
    in pastry work 452
    poaching 132–3
    and salmonella 420, 452
    selection and purchase 419–20
    sizes 419
    in sponge cakes 524–5
    storage 38, 420, 452
    types 419
    versatility 420, 452
  recipes
    egg custard sauce, fresh (sauce à
      l'anglaise) 455, **466**
    egg custard tart **507–8**
    eggs in cocotte (oeufs en cocotte)
      444
    eggs sur le plat **445**
    French-fried eggs (deep-fried eggs)
      442
    fried eggs (oeufs frits) **441**
    hard-boiled eggs with cheese and
      tomato sauce (oeufs aurores)
      439–40
    Italian meringue **464**
    meringues **491–2**

omelettes (egg white) **443**
  omelettes (basic) (omelette nature)
    442–3
  poached eggs with cheese sauce
    (oeufs pochés mornay) **440–1**
  Scotch eggs **444**
  scrambled eggs (oeufs brouillés) **439**
  soft-boiled eggs (oeufs mollets) **440**
  Spanish omelette **443**
elastin 268, 272–3, 561
electricity 58, 63
electronic fly killer (EFK) 43
emergency procedures
  emergency exit signs (green) 63
  evacuation 60
  fire safety 63–5
empathy, meaning 121
employees
  absences 51
  attitude and behaviour 117–18
  catering for 18, 99–100
  clothing 32, 61, 67, 117–18
  costs, direct/indirect 111
  definition 23
  performance 120–1
  personal development plans 124–6
  personal hygiene 32–4
  personal presentation 117–18
  personal safety 62, 67
  references, checking 66
  right to search 66–97
  rights and responsibilities 23, 51–2
  staffing structures 21–2
  working with colleagues 122
  workplace skills 119–22
employers, rights and responsibilities 21,
  23
  accidents, reporting 53–4, 60
  bullying and harassment 52–3
  control of substances hazardous to
    health 54–5
  fire safety 63–5
  health and safety 23, 51–2
  risk management 57–9
  security risks 65–7
employment
  apprenticeships 26
  contracts of 21, 23
  discrimination 23
  job advertisements 23
  job applications 23, 122–3
  job descriptions 23–4
  job interviews 25, 123–4
  job offers 25
  and kitchen layout 93
  laws relevant to 23, 25
  qualifications 25–6
  recruitment and selection 23–6
  rights and responsibilities 21, 23
  scale of 4
  staffing structures 21–2, 89–91
  Statutory Sick Pay 25
emulsion 561
en papillotte (paper bag cooking) 147–8
entrecôte 282, 561

Environmental Health Officers 48–9
enzymes 129, 272, 365, 542, 561
equipment
    colour-coding 34
    dishwashing 42
    and kitchen layout 94
    for lifting 62, 67
    security marking 66
eradication 43
escalopes 284–6, 331, 561
Escoffier, Auguste 88
ethical, meaning 363
Eurostar 14, 16
evacuation procedures 60
evaporated milk 215
event management 13

farce 561
farms 13
fast-food outlets 3, 10, 98, 105
fats
    heat, impact on 129
    nutritional content 81–3
    saturated 75
    too much/too little in diet, impact of
        82–3
    types 448–9
fecule 561
feedback
    from colleagues 124
    from customers 121
fennel **392**
    poached **234**
feuilletage 561
fibre, dietary 72, 80, 82
finishing kitchens 87
fire safety 63–5
    fire detection and warning 65
    fire-fighting equipment 65
    fire precautions 64
    risk assessment 64–5
first aid 60, 561
    blue plasters 29, 32, 118
fish *see also* shellfish
    generally 363–4
    baking 368
    boiling 373–4
    canning 366
    cooking methods 366–8
    core temperature 374
    cuts 372–3
    deep frying 373–4
    freezing 365–6
    frying 366–7
    grilling 367, 373–4
    gutting and scaling 369
    health, safety and hygiene 368–9
    nutritional value 365
    oily fish 364, 373–4
    pickling 366
    poaching 367, 373–4
    preparation 369–72
    preservation 365–6
    roasting 367–8
    salting 366

seasonal availability 374–5
selection and purchase 364
shallow frying 366, 373–4
skinning and filleting 369–70
smoked fish 364, 366
steaming 368, 373–4, **389–90**
stir-frying 367, 373–4
storage 38, 365, 368–9
types 373–4
white fish 364, 373–4
recipes
    cod, baked with a herb crust **393**
    fillets of fish Véronique **383**
    fillets of fish with white wine sauce
        384
    fish, egg and breadcrumbed and fried
        381
    fish *belle meunière* **383**
    fish *bonne-femme* **384**
    fish Bretonne **383**
    fish *bréval* **384**
    fish Doria **383**
    fish Grenobloise **383**
    fish kebabs **397–8**
    fish kedgeree (*cadgery de poisson*)
        398
    fish *meunière* **382–3**
    fish pie **398–9**
    fish steamed with garlic, spring onions
        and ginger **389–90**
    fish stock **161**
    fish velouté **187**
    fried fish in batter **386**
    goujons of fish **381–2**
    grilled fish fillets (sole, plaice,
        haddock) **385–6**
    grilled round fish (herring, mackerel,
        bass, mullet) **390–1**
    haddock, smoked, poached **389**
    haddock and smoked salmon terrine
        400–1
    herring or mackerel, soused **400**
    mackerel, smoked, mousse **399**
    red mullet, nage with baby leeks **388**
    red mullet ceviche with organic leaves
        393–4
    salmon, grilled, with pea soup and
        quail's eggs **395**
    salmon, poached **394**
    sardines with tapenade **396**
    sea bass, pan-fried fillets, with
        rosemary mash and mushrooms
        387–8
    sea bass, roast fillet with vanilla and
        fennel **392**
    skate with black butter (*raie au beurre
        noir*) **385**
    sole, fried **381**
    swordfish, grilled with somen noodle
        salad and cilantro vinaigrette **391**
    trout, baked whole in salt **396–7**
    whitebait (*blanchailles*) **386–7**
flashpoint 145
fleurons 561
flies 43–4

floors
    materials/condition of 45
    slipping 53, 56
flour 447–8
    dextrinisation 156
    seasoned 563
folate 81, 83
folding **499**
folic acid 81, 83
fondant sugar 449
food and beverage (F&B) services 5
food and service management *see*
    contract catering
food contamination 561
    causes 29–32
    by chemicals 29, 43
    cross-contamination 33–5
    high risk foods 30–1, 96
    by pests 43–4
    time, impact on 30
food courts 98
food handling *see* food safety
Food Hygiene Regulations 2006 94
Food Hygiene (Amendments) Regulations
    1993 453
food intolerances 29, 84, 100, 417–18
food poisoning
    causes 28–32
    high-risk foods 30–1
    high-risk groups 28
    poisonous foods 29
    symptoms 28–9
food premises, design and layout *see*
    layout
food preparation *see* cold food preparation
food presentation 560–1
food purchasing
    buyer, role of 106, 109
    buying methods 106–7
    buying tips 107–8
    formal/informal buying 106
    influences on 107
    market awareness 105–6
    and portion control 106, 108–10
    principles 107
    product types 107
    standard purchasing specifications
        109–10
    suppliers, selection of 106
food safety
    cleaning and sanitising 35
    definition 28
    due diligence 49
    food safety management systems 45–9
    hygiene notices 48–9
    importance 28–9
    and kitchen design 94, 97
    legislation 48–9
    penalties for non-compliance 49
    training in 49
Food Safety Acts (1990, 1991, 1995) 94
food safety management systems
    'CookSafe' 48
    Hazard Analysis Critical Control Point
        (HACCP) 45–6

'Safer food, better business' 47–8
'Scores on the Doors' 49
Food Safety Temperature Control
    Regulations 1995 453
Food Standards Agency 47–9
food storage 37–9
    best before/use by dates 38
    cold food preparation 561
    food labelling codes 39
    stock rotation 39
food subsidies 115
forecasting 6, 118–19
formal buying methods 106
franchising 20
frangipane **465**
fraud 66
freezers
    putting hot food in 36
    temperature 38
freezing
    convenience foods 453
    defrosting 38
    fish 365–6
    freezer burn 561
    meat 270
    preparing cooked food for 37
    storage, of frozen food 38
friandises 561
fricassée 561
    chicken **350–1**
    veal **319–20**
fridges
    cleaning 35, 39
    putting hot food in 36
    temperature 38–9
frozen foods *see under* freezing
fructose 71, 449
fruit
    generally
        in healthy diet 80–1, 461
        selection and purchase 204
        storage 38, 205
    recipes
        apple, baked (*pommes bonne femme*)
            472
        apple, tatin of **481**
        apple fritters (*beignets aux pommes*)
            474
        apple sauce **192**
        apple sorbet **495–6**
        apple (bramley) spotted dick **469**
        apricot and almond samosas **520**
        apricot salsa **333**
        Black Forest vacherin **493**
        blueberries, baked cheesecake
            488–9
        Caribbean fruit curry **222**
        dried fruit compote **487**
        Eve's pudding with gooseberries
            471
        fresh fruit salad **220**
        fruit barquettes **512**
        fruit cocktail **220**
        fruit coulis **465**
        fruit slice (*bande aux fruits*) **512–13**

fruit tart **512**
grapefruit cocktail **218**
khoshaf (dried fruit with nuts,
    perfumed with rose and orange
    water) **494**
lemon curd ice cream **494**
lime and mascarpone cheesecake
    488
lime soufflé frappe **485**
mango soufflé **478**
mincemeat **511**
mousse, basic **482–3**
peach ice cream **495**
peach melba (*pêche melba*) **497**
pear almond tart **506**
pear and ginger samosas **520**
pear belle Hélène **497**
pear jalousie **516**
poached fruits/fruit compote **486–7**
raspberry bavarois (mousse) **484**
sweet samosas **520**
tropical fruit plate **221**
vacherin with strawberries (*vacherin
    aux fraises*) **492–3**
frying *see* deep frying; shallow frying;
    stir-frying

gambling establishments 4, 9
gammon 289–90
ganache **463**
garam masala 562
garlic
    garlic butter 202
    roast garlic **233**
garnishing 560, 562
gas 63
gastroenteritis 562
gelatine 131, 273, 460–1
gelling substances 460–1
ghee 216, 562
glazing 562
glazing, pastry work **499–500**
globalisation, of hospitality travel and
    tourism sectors 5
glucono-delta-lactose 451
glucose 71, 449–50, 459
    atomised glucose 459
gluten 447, 562
    gluten-free diets 84–5, 417–18
gnocchi
    gnocchi parisienne (choux paste) **437**
    gnocchi romaine (semolina) **438**
goats' milk 215
goose and gosling 345–6
grains and cereals
    couscous with chorizo sausage and
        chicken **436**
    gnocchi parisienne (choux paste) **437**
    gnocchi romaine (semolina) **438**
    polenta, crisp, with Mediterranean
        vegetables **435**
    types 217, 417–19
gravy
    health, safety and hygiene 154
    roast **327**

griddles 141, 142–3
grilling 141–2
    fish 367, 373–4
    health and safety 142
    meat 288, 290
gross profits 112–15
guar gum 461
guesthouses 9
guineafowl, suprêmes, with pepper and
    basil coulis **358**

HACCP (Hazard Analysis Critical Control
    Point) 45–6
haché 562
haddock
    haddock and smoked salmon terrine
        400–1
    smoked poached **389**
hair 32, 67, 118
halal 271
halitosis 75
hand washing 33
harassment 52–3
hats, chef's 61, 118
Hazard Analysis Critical Control Point
    (HACCP) 45–6
hazards, identifying 55–6
heads
    lamb or mutton 270
    pork 288
    veal 286
health and safety 23, 51–2 *see also* food
    safety
    accidents, prevention 53–7, 60
    deep frying 146
    fire safety 63–5
    grilling 142
    hot liquids 130, 132–3
    manual handling 62, 67
    microwave cooking 150
    oven cooking 137–40
    personal protective equipment 61–2
    safety signs 62–3, 67
    security risks 65–7
    shallow frying 144
    steam 134
    stovetop cooking 137
Health and Safety at Work Act 1974
    51–2
Health and Safety Executive (HSE) 55
Health and Safety (First Aid) Regulations
    1981 60
health clubs and spas 12
healthy eating
    chef's role in improving 85–6
    definition 69–71
    and desserts 454
    eatwell plate 70
    fruit and vegetables 80–1, 205, 461
    importance 69, 80
    nutritionally balanced diet, meaning 71
    school meals 17
hearts 269, 278
    braised lambs' hearts (*coeurs d'agneau
        braisés*) **335–6**

heat
  bacteria, impact on 30–1, 36–7
  carbohydrates, impact on 129
  in cleaning 40
  danger zone 36–7
  dry heat 128–9
  fat, impact on 129
  methods of applying to food 128–9
  moist heat 128–9
  protein, impact on 129
  uses 36–7, 40
  vitamins, impact on 129
herbs
  herb oils **200–1**
  mint sauce **192**
  parsley sauce **186**
  pesto **197**
herring, soused **400**
high blood pressure 69, 79, 83
Hindu diets 85
historical buildings 13
HM Revenue and Customs (HMRC) 2–3
hogget 274
holiday centres 4, 12
homogenisation 459
honey 450, 460
hors d'oeuvres 561, 562 see also salads;
      sandwiches
  bruschetta **562**
  canapés **563**
  cheese soufflé (soufflé au fromage)
      564
  dressed crab **568**
  fried ham and cheese savoury (croque
      monsieur) **564–5**
  potted shrimps **569**
  pumpernickel rounds with smoked
      salmon, sour cream and dill **565**
  shellfish cocktails **570**
  welsh rarebit **567**
hospitality industry see catering and
      hospitality industry
hospitals 1, 3, 17, 98, 100
hostels 4, 13, 18
hot dry areas 97
hot liquids/surfaces
  health and safety 130, 132–3
  risk assessment 58
hot wet areas 97
hotels 1, 4–5, 8, 98
Human Rights Act 1998 23, 25
humectant 522
hummus (chickpea and sesame seed
      paste) **259–60**
hydrolysis, meaning 449
Hygiene Emergency Prohibition Notices/
      Orders 49
Hygiene Improvement Notice 49
hygroscopic 273

Ice Cream Regulations (1959, 1963) 459
ice creams and sorbets
  generally
    health, safety and hygiene 459
    homogenisation 459
    ingredients for 459–61
    method 458
    pasteurisation 459
    ripening 459
    sorbets 460
    stabilisers 460–1
    storage 458–9
  recipes
    apple sorbet **495–6**
    caramel ice cream **495**
    chocolate sorbet **496**
    lemon curd ice cream **494**
    orange brandy granita **496**
    peach ice cream **495**
    peach melba (pêche Melba) **497**
    pear belle Hélène **497**
illness
  incubation period 562
  reporting 32
immobile, meaning 281
impeding, meaning 524
impermeable, meaning 447
in-house catering 9
industry, catering for 18, 98
infestations 43–4, 562
informal buying methods 106–7
information, dissemination 124
inhospitable, meaning 281
insecticide 29, 43, 55, 562–3
intimidation 52–3
intolerances see food intolerances
inverted sugar/sugar syrup/liquid inverted
      sugar 449, 459
invoices 108, 562
iodine 79
iron 78, 81
isomalt 450
Italian meringue **464**

jardinière (batons) 207–8, 562
jewellery 32, 67
Jewish diets 85
job advertisements 23
job applications 23, 122–3
job descriptions, for sous chef 24, 92
job interviews 25, 123–4
job offers 25
job titles 23
julienne (strips) 207–8, 562
jus lié **160,** 562

khoshaf (dried fruit with nuts, perfumed
      with rose and orange water) **494**
kidneys
  lambs' kidney bouchées **339**
  lambs' kidney grilled (rognons grillés)
      335
  lambs' kidney sauté (rognons sautés)
      337
  preparation 278, 283, 286, 288
kitchen areas
  eating in 32
  kitchen surfaces, cleaning methods 40
  layout and design 44, 87–8, 91–5
  need for organisation in 87–8

planning 91–5
  smoking in 32
  traffic flow in 56–7
kitchen brigades 89–91
kitchen cloths 35, 42–3
kitchen porters 89
kitchen waste see refuse
kneading **499**
knives
  health and safety 271
  risk management 58–9
kosher 271

lactose 71
lamb and mutton
  generally
    cooking methods 275–6
    core temperatures 141, 271
    joints and cuts 274–8
    offal 269–70, 278
    roasting times 141
    selection and purchase 274–5
    storage 268
  recipes
    best end or rack of lamb with
        breadcrumbs and parsley **303**
    braised lamb shanks with ratatouille
        312–13
    braised lambs' hearts (coeurs
        d'agneau braisés) **335–6**
    breadcrumbed cutlets (côtelettes
        d'agneau panées) **307**
    brown lamb or mutton stew (navarin
        d'agneau) **314**
    grilled cutlets (côtelettes d'agneau
        grillées) **306–7**
    grilled loin or chump chops or
        noisettes of lamb **307**
    hot pot of lamb or mutton **315**
    Irish stew **308–9**
    lamb fillets with beans and tomatoes
        311
    lamb jus **159–60**
    lamb kebabs (shish kebabs) **308**
    lamb samosas **317–18**
    lambs' kidney bouchées **339**
    lambs' kidney grilled (rognons grillés)
        335
    lambs' kidney sauté (rognons sautés)
        337
    liver and bacon, fried (foie d'agneau
        au lard) **336**
    mixed grill **313–14**
    roast leg of lamb with mint, lemon and
        cumin **304**
    roast loin of lamb, stuffed **305**
    roast saddle of lamb with rosemary
        mash **313**
    shepherd's pie **316**
    slow-cooked shoulder of lamb with
        vegetables **306**
    valentine of lamb **311–12**
    white lamb stew (blanquette
        d'agneau) **310–11**
langoustine 376

poached langoustines with aioli dip **404–5**
larding 283, 562
laws, relevant to catering and hospitality industry 23, 25
  on food safety 48–9, 459
layout, of food premises/kitchen 44, 87–8
  decor 94–5
  design, influences on 95–8
  equipment 94
  high risk/contaminated foods 96
  hygiene 91, 95–6
  multi-usage requirements 95
  planning, influences on 91–5
  product subdivisions 95–6
  refuse management 95
  work areas, separation of 95–8
  workflows, effective 91–6
leisure sector 3–4, 11–13
lemons
  lemon drizzle cake **533**
  lemon oil **200**
  lemon tart (*tarte au citron*) **509**
lentils 207, 214
  red lentil soup **174**
liaison 562
Licensing Act 1964 23
lifting equipment 62, 67
lighting 44–5, 56, 66
limes
  lime and mascarpone cheesecake **488**
  soufflé frappe **485**
limited liability companies 3
liquid inverted sugar 449, 459
listeria 31–2
liver 269
  lambs' liver and bacon, fried (*foie d'agneau au lard*) **336**
  liver pâté 202
  preparation 278, 283, 286, 288
lobster 376–8
  lobster thermidor (*homard thermidor*) **407–8**
local education
  school meals, responsibility for 17
lunches 104

McDonald's 105
macédoine 207–8, 562
mackerel
  smoked mackerel mousse **399**
  soused **400**
magnesium 83
Maillard reaction 273
maltose 71
management staff 21
mandatory signs (blue) 62–3
mangetout **238**
mangoes
  mango soufflé **478**
  preparation **221**
manual handling 62, 67
margarine 448–9
marinades/marinating 147, 272, 560, 562
marrow 270

mashing 209
mayonnaise **188**
  variations **189–90**
meat *see also* beef; lamb; offal; pork; veal
  generally
    boiling 131–2
    cooking methods 272–4
    core temperatures 141, 271
    frying 290
    grilling 288, 290
    hanging 268
    health, safety and hygiene 270–1
    Maillard reaction 273
    preservation 270
    roasting 282, 285–6, 287–8
    roasting times 141, 273–4
    searing 272––273
    selection and purchase 271–2
    slow cooking 273–4
    and special/religious diets 271
    stewing 273––276, 282, 285–6, 562
    storage 38, 268
    structure 268
    trimming 268
    vegetarian substitutes for 216–17
  recipes
    potted meats **333–4**
media, influence of 6, 115
mediocre, meaning 102
menus 562
  banquet menus 105
  breakfast menus 103
  buffet/party menus 104
  for children 100
  and consumer protection 102
  cyclical menus 101
  fast-food menus 105
  historical development 99
  for hospitals 100
  importance 99–100
  influences on 93–4, 99–100
  lunch and dinner menus 104
  planning 102
  pre-planned/pre-designed 101–2
  presentation 102
  speciality 100
  structure 102
  tea menus 104
  types 100
meringues **491–2**
  Italian meringue **464**
mice 43–4
microwave cooking 148–51
  health and safety 150
milk
  in desserts 455–6
  goats' milk 215
  impact of heat on 36
  pasteurisation 455
  poaching in 132
  sterilisation (UHT) 455
  uses for 215
millet 217, 417–18
mincemeat **511**
minerals 78–9, 81, 561, 562

mint
  oil **201**
  sauce **192**
mirepoix 155, 562
mise en place 87, 562
moderation, meaning 86
molluscs 376, 379–80 *see also* mussels; scallops; squid
money handling 66
monkfish, griddled with leeks and parmesan **390**
motorway service stations 15–16, 98
mould 562
mousses 562
  basic fruit mousse **482–3**
  bavarois (basic) **483–4**
  chocolate mousse **483–4**
  raspberry bavarois **484**
  smoked mackerel mousse **399**
museums 12
mushrooms
  Greek style (*champignons à la grecque*) **253**
  mushroom sauce **187**
  sauté of wild mushrooms **246**
  soup (*crème de champignons*) **164**
Muslim diets 85
mussels 376, 379
  mussels gratin with white wine **406–7**
'mutuality of obligation' 21, 23
myco-protein 216
myoglobin 271

naan bread 543, **555**
nage 155
National Health Service 17
National Insurance 2–3
National Minimum Wage Act 1998 23
nausea 29
navarin 562
nervous system 76
net profits 112
niacin (vitamin B) 76–7, 81–3, 129, 562
nicotinic acid (vitamin B) 76–7, 81–2, 129
noisettes 277, 307, 562
non-porous 45
noodles
  Chinese vegetables and noodles **248**
  noodles with butter **432–3**
norovirus 32
nursing homes 18
nutrition 562
  balanced diet, definition 70–1
  carbohydrates 71–3, 81–3, 560
  chef's role in 85–6
  cooking, impact on 131, 135, 138, 141, 149
  eatwell plate 70
  fats 81–3
  fibre, dietary 72, 80
  fruit and vegetables 80–1, 205
  health problems of poor diet 69
  minerals 78–9, 81–3, 560
  nutritional information, finding 72
  protein 73–4, 81–2, 129, 215–17, 562

school meals 17
too much/too little in diet, impact of 82–3
vitamins 76–7, 80–3, 365, 560–3
water 80
nuts 217
almond cream (frangipane) **465**
praline **514**
walnut oil **201**

oats/oatmeal 217, 418
obesity 69, 75
offal *see also* individual types
generally
preparation 278, 283, 286
storage 269
types 268–70
recipes
hearts, lamb's, braised (*coeurs d'agneau braisés*) **335–6**
kidney, lamb's, bouchées **339**
kidney, lamb's, grilled (*rognons grillés*) **335**
kidney, lamb's, sauté (*rognons sautés*) **337**
liver, lamb's, fried, and bacon (*foie d'agneau au lard*) **336**
liver pâté 202
oxtail with Guinness **334**
veal sweetbread escalope (*escalope de ris de veau*) **338**
veal sweetbreads, braised (white) (*ris de veau braisé – à blanc*) **337–8**
veal sweetbreads, grilled **339**
oils
herb oils **200–1**
lemon oil **200**
vanilla oil **201**
okra, in cream sauce (*okra à la crème*) **237**
olives
olive bread **548–9**
tapenade **197**
onions
bhajias **250**
braised (*oignons braisés*) **232**
caramelised button onions **233**
operating cycle 98
operational capacity 6–7
operational control 115
operational staff 21
osteoporosis 69
outside catering 19–20
outsourcing 9
oven cooking
health and safety 139, 140
preheating 139
recovery time 139
overheads 111
ox
offal 269–70
oxtail 270
oxtail with Guinness **334**
oysters 376, 380
natives 562

opening 402
tempura **403**

pans, choice of 131, 143–4
parmesan 216, 416
parsley, sauce **186**
parsnips, roast **255**
Part-time Workers (Prevention of Less Favourable Treatment) Regulations 2000 23
partie system 88
partnerships 2–3
pasta
generally
cheese, cooking with 416
cooking 415–16
dried 414–15
ingredients and sauces for 416
nutritional value 414
storage 414–15
tortellini, history of 415–16
types 415
recipes
cannelloni **429**
fresh egg pasta dough **433–4**
lasagne **426–7**
macaroni cheese **432**
pumpkin tortellini with brown butter balsamic vinaigrette **427–8**
ravioli **428–9**
spaghetti bolognaise **430**
spaghetti with tomato sauce (*spaghetti alla pomodoro*) **430**
stuffings for pasta **434**
tagliatelle carbonara **433**
pasteurisation 36
eggs 420, 452
ice cream 459
milk and cream 455–7
pastry cream (*crème pâtissière*) 455, **463–4**
pastry work
generally
convenience products for 453
eggs in 452
fats in 447–8
faults in, reasons for **501, 503**
finishing and presentation **500**
flour in 447–8
glazing **499–500**
health, safety and hygiene 453–4
milk and cream in 455–8
raising agents 450–1
storage 453
sugar in 449–50
techniques **499–500**
recipes
almond cream (frangipane) **465**
baked chocolate tart (aero) **510**
Bakewell tart **508–9**
baklavas (filo pastry with nuts and sugar) **520**
banana flan **511**
boiled buttercream **462–3**
cheese and ham savoury flan (*quiche lorraine*) **504**

cheese straws (*paillettes au fromage*) **517**
chocolate éclairs **513–14**
choux paste **502–3**
crème chiboust **464**
crème diplomat **464**
Eccles cakes **515**
egg custard sauce, fresh (*sauce à l'anglaise*) 455, **466**
flan **504–5**
French apple flan (*flan aux pommes*) **505–6**
fruit barquettes **512**
fruit slice (*bande aux fruits*) **512–13**
fruit tart **512**
ganache **463**
gâteaux pithiviers **519**
gnocchi parisienne (choux paste) **437**
hot water paste **330**
Italian meringue **464**
lemon tart (*tarte au citron*) **509**
mince pies **510–11**
palmiers **519**
Paris-Brest **514**
pastry cream (*crème pâtissière*) 455, **463–4**
pear almond tart **506**
profiteroles and chocolate sauce **515**
puff pastry slice (*mille-feuilles*) **517–18**
rough puff paste **502**
savarin paste 558–9, **558–9**
short paste (*pâte à foncer*) **501**
stock syrup **468**
suet paste **298**
sugar paste (*pâte à sucre*) **500**
sweet samosas **520**
treacle tart **507**
pathogenic bacteria 29–32, 562
paupiettes 372, 562
paysanne 207–8, 562
peaches
peach ice cream **495**
peach melba (*pêche Melba*) **497**
pears
pear almond tart **506**
pear and ginger samosas **520**
pear belle Hélène **497**
pear jalousie **516**
poached (compote) **487**
peas
dried 213–14
French-style (*petit pois à la française*) **236**
mangetout **238**
soup **395**
pectin 135, 461
peeling 560
penalties, for non-compliance with food safety law 49
peppers
roasted red pepper and tomato soup **174–5**
performance
measuring and monitoring 121
standards of 120

perishable goods/products 107
personal development plans 124–6
personal hygiene 32–4, 91, 96
personal protective equipment (PPE)
    61–2, 67
pesticides 29, 43, 562
pests 562
    control 44
    food contamination by 43–4
petits fours 562
pets 44
phosphorus 78–9, 82, 562
phytochemicals 80
pickling
    fish 366
    mixed pickle **198**
    pickled red cabbage **257**
    soused herring or mackerel **400**
piping, pastry work **500**
piquant 562
    sauce **180**
pitta bread 543
plat du jour 562
poaching 130–3
    deep poaching 132–3
    eggs 132–3, **440–1**
    fennel **234**
    fish and shellfish 367, 373–4, **389,
        394, 404–5**
    fruit (compote) **486–7**
    in milk 132
    shallow poaching 132
    in stock syrup 132
poêlé (pot roasting) 147
poisonous foods 29
polenta 417
    crisp polenta and Mediterranean
        vegetables **435**
police 16
pork
    generally
        bacon joints and cuts 289–90
        butchery 287, 289
        cooking methods 287–90
        core temperatures 141, 271
        HACCP stages for cooking and
            storage 46
        offal 269, 288
        pork joints and cuts 287–90
        roasting times 141, 327
        selection and purchase 290
        storage 268
    recipes
        bacon, boiled **332**
        gammon, griddled, with apricot salsa
            333
        pork escalopes **331**
        pork loin chops with pesto and
            mozzarella **329**
        pork pie, raised **330–1**
        roast leg of pork **327**
        sage and onion dressing for pork **327**
        slow roast pork belly **328**
        spare ribs in barbecue sauce **328–9**
        sweet and sour pork **331–2**

portion control
    portion size, influences on 108–9
    and product quality 108–9
    standard purchasing specifications
        109–10
    standard recipes 110
    weighing and measuring 110
pot roasting 147
potassium 81, 83
potatoes
    generally
        convenience products 211
        cooking methods 209–10
        nutritional value 211
        portion yields 211
        selection and purchase 209–11
        storage 211
        varieties 208–11
    recipes
        baked jacket potatoes (*pommes au
            four*) **225**
        château potatoes **230**
        courgette and potato cakes with mint
            and feta cheese **242**
        croquette potatoes **225–6**
        delmonico potatoes **229**
        duchess potatoes **223–4**
        fondant potatoes **227**
        fried/chipped potatoes (*pommes
            frites*) **227–8**
        hash brown potatoes **232**
        macaire potatoes (potato cakes) **231**
        mashed potatoes (*pomme purée*) **224**
        parmentier potatoes **229**
        parsley potatoes (*pomme persillées*)
            223
        potatoes cooked in milk with cheese
            (*gratin dauphinoise*) **231**
        potatoes with bacon and onions
            (*pommes au lard*) **226**
        roast potatoes (*pommes rôties*) **230**
        rosemary mash **313**
        samosas **317–18**
        sauté potatoes **226**
        sauté potatoes with onions (*pommes
            lyonnaise*) **228**
        soups **171, 173**
        Swiss potato cakes (rösti) **229–30**
poultry
    generally
        core temperatures 271
        health, safety and hygiene 346
        health and safety 346
        storage 346
        types 340–1
    recipes
        chicken, crumbed breast with
            asparagus (*suprême de volaille aux
            pointes d'asperges*) **350**
        chicken, fricassée **350–1**
        chicken, fried (deep-fried) **351**
        chicken, grilled (*poulet grillé*) **352**
        chicken, roast with dressing (*poulet
            rôti à l'anglaise*) **352–3**
        chicken, tandoori **355**

chicken, white stock **159**
chicken à la king (*emincé de volaille à
    la king*) **347–8**
chicken and vegetables, terrine
    353–4
chicken in red wine (*coq au vin*)
    348–9
chicken jus **177**
chicken Kiev **356**
chicken sauté chasseur **346–7**
chicken soup (*crème de volaille/
    crème reine*) **163**
chicken spatchcock (*poulet grillé à la
    crapaudine*) **349**
chicken tikka **354–5**
duck, confit duck leg with red cabbage
    and green beans **358–9**
duck or duckling, roast (*canard ou
    caneton rôti*) **361**
duckling with orange sauce (*caneton
    bigerade*) **359–60**
guineafowl, suprêmes with pepper
    and basil coulis **358**
turkey, roast (*dinde rôti*) **356–7**
turkey escalopes **357–8**
PPE (personal protective equipment)
    61–2
Pralus, George 148
prawns *see* shrimps and prawns
primary commodities/specifications 109
prisons 1, 16–17, 98
private companies 1–3
profits
    gross profits 112–15
    net profits 112
prohibition signs (red) 63
protein 562
    coagulation 129, 131–2, 272
    impact of heat on 129
    nutritional value 73–4, 81–2
    textured vegetable protein (TVP) 213,
        216, 563
    too much/too little in diet, impact of 82
    vegetarian proteins 215–17
proving, dough 543, 562
Public Interest Disclosure Act 1998 23
public limited companies 1–2
public sector catering 1, 16–18
    menu choices in 16
pubs and bars 1, 3–4
    categories of catering in 11
    influences on 11
pulses 562
    generally
        beans 213
        cooking methods 214
        health, safety and hygiene 212–13
        lentils 207, 214
        nutritional value 212
        peas 213–14
        pre-soaking 212–14
        storage 212
        uses 214
    recipes
        bean goulash **258**

dhal **260**
haricot bean salad (*salade de haricots blancs*) **263**
hummus (chickpea and sesame seed paste) **259–60**
Mexican bean pot **259**
red lentil soup **174**
pumpkin
pumpkin tortellini with brown butter balsamic vinaigrette **427–8**
pumpkin velouté **162**
punctuality 117

qualifications 25–6
quinoa 217, 419
Quorn 216–17
oriental Quorn stir-fry **261**

Race Relations Act 1976 23
radiation 129
raising agents 450–1
Ramsey, Gordon 9
raspberries
bavarois (mousse) **484**
poached (compote) **487**
Rastafarian diets 85
rats 43–4
réchauffer (reheating) 562
record keeping 2–3
recruitment and selection 23–6
red mullet
ceviche with organic leaves **393–4**
nage of, with baby leeks **388**
refreshing 137, 207, 563
refuse management 45, 95
Regulatory Fire Safety Order 2005 63–4
Rehabilitation of Offenders Act 1974 23, 25
relaxing, pastry work **499**
religion
influence on kitchen work 25
special diets for 85
Reporting Injuries, Diseases and Dangerous Occurrences (RIDDOR) Act 1996 53–4
residential establishments 18
resourcing 6–7
restaurants 1, 3–4, 98
speciality restaurants 10
Rhodes, Gary 9
rhubarb, poached (compote) **487**
Riboflavin (vitamin B2) 76–7, 129, 563
rice
generally
bacterial growth 31, 414
health and safety 31, 414
storage 414
varieties 217, 413
recipes
braised or pilaff rice (*riz pilaff*) (Indian pilau) **421**
paella (savoury rice with chicken, fish, vegetables and spices) **423–4**
plain boiled rice **422**
rice pudding **476**

risotto of Jerusalem artichoke and truffle **425–6**
risotto with parmesan **424–5**
steamed rice **422**
stir-fried rice **422–3**
rickets 83
RIDDOR (Reporting Injuries, Diseases and Dangerous Occurrences) Act 1996 53–4
ripening, ice creams and sorbets 459
risk assessment
crime prevention 66–7
disease 53–4
fire 64–5
harm, risk of 57–9
risk minimisation 57–9
security 66–7
risotto
Jerusalem artichoke and truffle **425–6**
with parmesan **424–5**
variations 425
roadside services *see* motorway
roasting 137–8, 140
fish 367–8, **392**
garlic **233**
low-temperature roasting 137–8
meat 273–6, 282, 285–6, 287–8
beef **291–2**
lamb **303–5**, **313**
pork **327–8**
poultry **352–3**, **356–7**, **361**
veal **321**
potatoes 209, **230**
roast gravy, for meat **327**
spit-roasting 137–8
vegetables **247**, **255**
robbery 66
rolling, pastry work **499**
roux 156–7, 563
rye 217, 418
rye bread **547**

sabayon **485**, 563
'Safer food, better business' 47–8
safety signs 62–3, 67
salad bars 10
salads 561
Caesar salad **266**
coleslaw **252–3**
haricot bean salad (*salade de haricots blancs*) **263**
Niçoise salad **263**
potato salad (*salade de pommes de terre*) **264**
Russian salad (*salade russe*) **265**
vegetable salad (*salade de légumes/salade russe*) **265**
Waldorf salad **265**
salamanders 141, 563
salmon
grilled, with pea soup and quail's eggs **395**
haddock and smoked salmon terrine **400–1**
poached **394**

salmonella 30, 188, 199, 420, 452, 563
salsify (*salsifi*) **256**
salt 79, 82
in pastry work 451
too much/too little in diet, impact of 83, 452
salting
fish 366
meat 270, 281
sandwich bars 10
sandwiches 565–7
bookmaker sandwich 566
club sandwich 566
double-decker/triple-decker sandwiches 566
open sandwiches/smorgasbord 566–7
toasted sandwiches 565–6
wraps 567
sanitisers 40, 563
sardines, with tapenade **396**
sauce flour 157
sauces
generally
basic principles 156–7
health, safety and hygiene 154
storage 154
recipes
Andalusian (*sauce andalouse*) **190**
anglaise (*sauce à l'anglaise*) (fresh egg custard) 455, **466**
apple **192**
avocado and coriander salsa **195–6**
balsamic vinegar and olive oil dressing **193–4**
barbecue **328**
Béarnaise **199–200**
béchamel (white) 156, **184**
beef jus **176–7**
beurre blanc (butter sauce) **183–4**
brown onion (*sauce lyonnaise*) **180**
brown sauce (*espagnole*) 157
butter sauce (*beurre blanc*) **183–4**
butterscotch **468**
caramel **468**
chasseur **179**
chicken jus **177**
chocolate **467**
Choron sauce **199**
compound butters 202
cranberry and orange, for duck **192–3**
custard **467**
espagnole 157
fish velouté **187**
flavoured butters 202
Foyot **199**
fresh egg custard sauce (*sauce à l'anglaise*) 455, **466**
fruit coulis **465**
green (*sauce verte*) **190**
hollondaise **198–9**
horseradish (*sauce raifort*) **194**
Italian **179**
lyonnaise (brown onion) **180**
Madeira sauce **178**

mayonnaise **188**
mint **192**
mornay **185**
mushroom **187**
paloise **200**
parsley **186**
pepper and basil coulis **358**
pesto **197**
piquant **180**
red wine jus **177–8**
reduction of wine, stock and cream **182**
remoulade **189**
Robert **180–1**
salsa verde **195**
sauce suprême **186**
shellfish cocktail sauce **191**
soubise **185**
stock reduction (glaze) **182**
sweet and sour **183**
syrup for baba, savarin and marignans **559**
tapenade **197**
tartare **189**
thousand island dressing **190**
tomato and cucumber salsa **194–5**
tomato sauce **181**
tomato vinaigrette **191**
valois **199**
white sauce *(béchamel)* 156, **184**
yoghurt and cucumber raita **193**
sautéing 143, 563
savarin paste 558–9
basic recipe **558–9**
savarin with fruit **559**
scallops 376, 379
with caramelised cauliflower **401–2**
ceviche with organic leaves **408–9**
scampi 377
scheduling, of resources 6–7
schools and colleges 1, 3, 98
school meals 17
'Scores on the Doors' 49
scurvy 82
sea bass
pan-fried fillets, with rosemary mash and mushrooms **387–8**
roast fillet, with vanilla and fennel **392**
sea ferries 14
sea kale *(chou de mer)* **247**
searing, meat 272–3, 563
seasoning 560
secondary commodities/specifications 109
secondary service sector catering 1, 16–18
security risks 65–6
personal safety 67
risk assessment 66–7
seeds 217
self-catering accommodation 4, 11
self-employed catering 2
self-service/self-assisted service 98
selling price 113–15
semolina 418

gnocchi romaine **438**
septicaemia 31
Sex Discrimination Act 1975 23
shallow frying 142–4
fish 366, 373–4
health and safety 144
shares 2
shellfish
generally
cooking 376–80
seasonal availability 376
selection and purchase 376–80
storage 377, 379–80
types 376–80
recipes
crab, dressed **568**
crab cakes with rocket salad and lemon dressing **405–6**
kalamarakia yemesta (stuffed squid) **409**
langoustines, poached with aioli dip **404–5**
lobster thermidor *(homard thermidor)* **407–8**
mussels gratin with white wine **406–7**
New England clam chowder **170–1**
oysters tempura **403**
prawn bisque **169–70**
scallops, ceviche with organic leaves **408–9**
scallops with caramelised cauliflower **401–2**
seafood in puff pastry *(bouchées de fruits de mer)* **411**
seafood stir-fry **410**
shellfish cocktail sauce **191**
shellfish cocktails **570**
shrimp butter 202
shrimps, potted **569**
shortening 449
shrimps and prawns 376–7
prawn bisque **169–70**
shrimp butter 202
shrimps, potted **569**
sickness
absence from work due to 51
reporting 32, 53–4
Statutory Sick Pay 25
silicone paper 563
simmering 130–1
skate, with black butter *(raie au beurre noir)* **386**
skimming *(dégraisser)* 131, 561
small to medium-sized business enterprises (SMEs) 1–2
smetana 563
smoking
cigarettes 11, 32
fish 366
smoking point 145
sodium 79, 82–3, 563
sodium aluminium sulphate 451
sodium bicarbonate 450
sole, fried **381**

sole traders 2
solvents 54
sorbets *see* ice creams and sorbets
soufflés 563
cheese soufflé *(soufflé au fromage)* **564**
lime soufflé frappe **485**
mango soufflé **478**
soufflé pudding (basic) **478–9**
vanilla soufflé *(soufflé à la vanille)* **476–7**
soups
generally
basic principles 155–6
health, safety and hygiene 154
recipes
asparagus *(crème d'asperges)* **165**
carrot and butterbean **162**
chicken *(crème de volaille/crème reine)* **163**
chive and potato *(vichyssoise)* **171**
gazpacho **172**
minestrone **167–8**
mushroom *(crème de champignons)* **164**
New England clam chowder **170–1**
Paysanne *(potage)* **169**
pea soup **395**
potato and watercress *(purée cressonnière)* **173**
prawn bisque **169–70**
pumpkin velouté **162**
red lentil **174**
roasted red pepper and tomato **174–5**
Scotch broth **176**
spinach and celery, cream of **167**
tomato *(crème de tomates fraiche)* **166**
vegetable *(purée de légumes)* **172–3**
vegetable and barley **175**
sous chef 89–91
job description for 24, 92
sous vide 148–9, 366
soya beans/soybeans 212–13
soya protein 216
special diets
children and teenagers 83–4
diabetes 85
elderly 84
food allergies or intolerances 84
gluten-free diets 84–5
on health grounds 84–5
ill persons 84, 100
on moral/religious grounds 85, 271
pregnant and breastfeeding women 83
vegetarian 84, 215–17
spelt 418
spillages 56
spinach
purée *(epinards en purée)* **235–6**
spinach and celery, soup, cream of **167**
spit-roasting 137–8
spores 30, 36, 563
squid, kalamariaka yemesta (stuffed) **409**

stabilisers
  in ice creams and sorbets 460–1
  in sponge cakes 524
staffing hierarchies/structures 21–2, 89–91
standard operational procedures (SOP) 7
standard purchasing specifications
  109–10
standard recipes 110
staphylococcus aureus 31, 563
staple goods/products 107
star ratings 8
starches 72, 563
  for thickening 156–7
Statutory Sick Pay 25
steaming 130–1, 133–4, 207
  atmospheric steaming 133
  cleaning steamers 134
  combination steaming 133
  fish 368, 373–4, **389–90**
  high-pressure steaming 133
  vegetables 207
sterilisation 36, 455, 456–7, 563
stewing 134–7, 563
  meat 273–6, 282, 285–6
stir-frying 143, 207
  fish 367, 373–4
  oriental Quorn stir-fry **261**
  seafood stir-fry **410**
  stir-fried cabbage with mushrooms and
    beansprouts **234**
  stir-fried rice **422–3**
stock
  generally
    basic principles 155
    boiling in 131
    braising in 137
    demi-glace 160
    health, safety and hygiene 154
    poaching in 132
  recipes
    brown stock **158**
    crab stock **161**
    fish stock **161**
    lamb jus **159–60**
    stock reduction (glaze) **182**
    veal stock, reduced for sauce **160**
    white chicken stock **159**
    white stock **158**
    white vegetable stock **158**
stock control 115
stock rotation 39, 563
stock syrup **468**
  poaching in 132
strawberries
  poached (compote) **487**
  vacherin with strawberries (*vacherin aux
    fraises*) **492–3**
stress 51
stroke 80, 84
stuffings
  for lamb **305**
  for pasta **434**
  for pork **327**
  sage and onion **327**
  for veal **321–2**

sucrose 71, 449, 459
suet 270, 272
  suet paste **298**
sugar *see also* carbohydrates
  types 449–50
supervisory staff 21
suppliers, selection of 106
sushi 563
swede, buttered **255**
sweetbreads 269, 278, 283
  veal sweetbread escalope (*escalope de
    ris de veau*) **338**
  veal sweetbreads, grilled **339**
  veal sweetbreads (white), braised (*ris de
    veau braisé – à blanc*) **337–8**
swordfish, grilled with somen noodle salad
  with cilantro vinaigrette **391**
syneresis 455, 563

table d'hôte/set price menus 100, 563
tahini 563
takeaways 3
tandoori cooking 147
  tandoori chicken **355**
targets
  operational 121–2
  personal 121–2, 124–6
taxation 2–3
tea, menus for 104
tea-towels 35, 42
teamwork 89–90, 122
temperature
  bacteria, impact on 30–1, 36–7
  core temperatures 36–7
    fish 374
    meat 141, 271
  danger zone 36–7
  dishwashing water 42
  for holding cooked food 37
temperature probes 36
terrorism 66
tertiary commodities/specifications 109
testing panels 108
textured vegetable protein (TVP) 213,
  216, 563
theft 65–6
theme parks 12
Thiamin (vitamin B1) 76–7, 129, 563
thickening
  beurre manié 137, 156, 560
  egg yolks 156
  roux 156–7
  sauce flour 157
  sauces 156
  stews/casseroles 136
  thickening agents 136, 137, 156–7
timbale 563
time and motion (workflows) 91–5
timeshare villas 11
tofu (bean curd) 560, 563
  barbecued **262**
  crispy deep-fried **261–2**
tomatoes
  generally
    concassée (basic preparation) **257**

standard purchasing specification,
  example 109
  recipes
    chutney **196–7**
    sauce **181**
    soup (*crème de tomates fraiche*) **16**
    stuffed (*tomates farcies*) **241**
    tomato and cucumber salsa **194–5**
    vinaigrette **191**
tongue 270
  preparation 278, 283
tooth decay 69
tortellini 415–16
  pumpkin tortellini with brown butter
    balsamic vinaigrette **427–8**
tourism 3–4
tournedos 283
toxins 29–31, 36
Trade Descriptions Act 1968 102
training
  in customer interaction 7
  in food safety 49
  in money handling 66
  in safety and risk management 59
travel catering outlets 3, 9
  airport and airline services 15
  rail services 16
  roadside services 15–16
  at sea 14–15
tripe 270, 283
trout, whole baked in salt **396–7**
turbot 371–2
turkey
  generally 344–5
  health, safety and hygiene 271, 346
  roast turkey (*dinde rôti*) **356–7**
  storage 346
  turkey escalopes **357–8**
turnips, buttered **255**
TVP (textured vegetable protein) 213,
  216, 563

UHT 36, 455–7
Ultra Heat Treatment (UHT) 36, 455–7
use by dates 39

vacuum packaging 148
value added tax (VAT) 2–3
vandalism 66
vanilla
  oil **201**
  panna cotta served on a fruit compote **486**
  soufflé (*soufflé à la vanille*) **476–7**
variables 6–7
veal
  generally 283
    butchery 283–5
    cooking methods 285–6
    core temperatures 141, 271
    joints and cuts 284–5
    offal 269–70, 286
    roasting times 141
    selection and purchase 286
  recipes
    escalopes **325**

escalopes, with Parma ham and mozzarella cheese (involtini di vitello) **326**
fricassée **319–20**
grilled cutlet (côte de veau grille) **322**
roast veal four-bone rib **321**
shin of veal, braised (osso buco) **323–4**
sweetbread escalope (escalope de ris de veau) **338**
sweetbreads, grilled **339**
sweetbreads (white), braised (ris de veau braisé – à blanc) **337–8**
veal and ham pie **324**
veal stock, reduced for sauce **160**
veal stuffing **321–2**
white stew of veal (blanquette de veau) **320**
vegan 563
vegetables
generally
blanching 207
boiling 131, 207
classification 205
cuts/preparation 207–8
EU grading 206
green vegetables 206
health, safety and hygiene 206
in healthy diet 80–1
nutritional value 205
preparation areas for 97
root vegetables 206
selection and purchase 205–6
steaming 207
storage 38, 206
washing 33, 97, 206
recipes
artichokes à la grecque **253**
asparagus points/tips (pointes d'asperges) **244**
asparagus wrapped in puff pastry with gruyère **245–6**
aubergine, stuffed (aubergine farcie) **239–40**
aubergine purée, spiced **243**
beetroot, golden with parmesan **254**
broad beans (fèves) **237**
broccoli **236**
butternut squash, roasted **247**
cabbage, stir-fried with mushrooms and beansprouts **234**
carrots, Vichy **254**
cauliflower à la grecque **253**
cauliflower au gratin (chou-fleur mornay) **246**

cauliflower polonaise (chou-fleur polonaise) **247**
celeriac, turnips or swedes, buttered **255**
chicory, shallow-fried (endive meunière) **244**
Chinese vegetables and noodles **248**
coleslaw **252–3**
corn on the cob **238**
courgette, deep-fried (courgettes frites) **240**
courgette, fettuccine of, with chopped basil and balsamic vinegar **243**
courgette, shallow-fried (courgettes sautées) **240**
courgette and potato cakes with mint and feta cheese **242**
crisp polenta and Mediterranean vegetables **435**
fennel, poached **234**
globe artichokes (artichauts en branche) **245**
goats' cheese and beetroot tarts, with rocket salad **256**
ladies' fingers (okra) in cream sauce (okra à la crème) **237**
mushrooms, Greek-style (champignons à la grecque) **253**
mushrooms, wild, sauté of **246**
onions, braised (oignons braisés) **232**
onions, caramelised button **233**
onions bhajias **250**
parsnips, roasted **255**
peas French-style (petit pois à la française) **236**
ratatouille **238–9**
red cabbage, braised (choux à la flamande) **235**
red cabbage, pickled **257**
salsify (salsifi) **256**
sea kale (chou de mer) **247**
seaweed, deep-fried **248**
spinach purée (epinards en purée) **235–6**
tomato concassée (basic preparation) **257**
tomatoes, stuffed (tomates farcies) **241**
vegetable salad (salade de légumes/ salade russe) **265**
white vegetable stock **158**
vegetable tempura **250–1**
vegetarian curry (alu-chole) **249**
vegetarian strudel **251–2**
vegetarians 563 see also vegetables generally

diets 84, 215–17
proteins for 215–17
vegans 563
recipes
oriental Quorn stir-fry **261**
tofu, barbecued **262**
tofu, crispy deep-fried **261–2**
vegetarian curry (alu-chole) **249**
vegetarian strudel **251–2**
velouté 563
vending machines 18
venison 141
ventilation 44–5, 56
viruses 32, 563
visitor attractions 4, 13
vitamins 76–7, 80, 562–3
heat, impact on 129
too much/too little in diet, impact of 82–3
voiding 271
vol-au-vent 563

walls 45
warning signs (yellow) 62, 67
wasps 43–4
waste management see portion control; refuse management
water
nutritional importance 80
water vapour, as raising agent 451
weevils 44
weighing and measuring ingredients 110
wet areas 96
wheat 418–19
intolerance of 417–18
wheat flour 447–8
whelks 380
white braising 136
white roux 156
whitebait (blanchailles) **386–7**
windows 45
winkles 380
workers, definition 23
workflows, effective 91–6
Working Time Regulations 1998 23, 25
workplace skills 118–22

yeast
dried 542
fermentation 542–3, 544
yeast extract 81, 215, 563
yield 108
yoghurt 215, 563
Youth Hostels Association 13

zero-subsidy establishments 99